OXFORD MEDICAL PUBLICATIONS

Oxford Desk Reference:

Respiratory Medicine

Oxford Desk Reference
Respiratory Medicine

Nick Maskell

Senior Lecturer and
Consultant Physician in Respiratory Medicine
North Bristol Lung Centre
University of Bristol

and

Ann Millar

Professor of Respiratory Medicine
North Bristol Lung Centre
University of Bristol

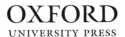

OXFORD
UNIVERSITY PRESS

Great Clarendon Street, Oxford OX2 6DP

Oxford University Press is a department of the University of Oxford.
It furthers the University's objective of excellence in research, scholarship,
and education by publishing worldwide in

Oxford New York

Auckland Cape Town Dar es Salaam Hong Kong Karachi
Kuala Lumpur Madrid Melbourne Mexico City Nairobi
New Delhi Shanghai Taipei Toronto

With offices in

Argentina Austria Brazil Chile Czech Republic France Greece
Guatemala Hungary Italy Japan Poland Portugal Singapore
South Korea Switzerland Thailand Turkey Ukraine Vietnam

Oxford is a registered trade mark of Oxford University Press
in the UK and in certain other countries

Published in the United States
by Oxford University Press Inc., New York

British Library Cataloguing in Publication Data
Data available

Library of Congress Cataloguing in Publication Data
Data available

Typeset by Cepha Imaging Private Ltd., Bangalore, India
Printed in Great Britain
on acid free paper by
CPI Antony Rowe,
Chippenham, Wiltshire

ISBN 978–0–19–923912–2

10 9 8 7 6 5 4 3 2 1

Preface

This book aims to act as a rapid reference for busy health professionals and covers the main respiratory disorders that would be encountered both in the inpatient and outpatient setting. Each section has been written by an expert in a particular field and is focused on providing a clear, concise clinical message on how best to investigate the relevant condition. In order to make the book as user-friendly as possible we have included a lot of images and illustrations to make the information more accessible. We believe it is one of the only books in the field where chest radiology lies alongside clinical information. Each chapter also includes authors' tips and key messages and is laid out in a format which makes the information easy to find and digest.

The book includes many common-sense approaches and has a guide for further reading in each area. It should be possible to use as a 'first-line' reference book either to jog your memory or to read about a condition with which you are not familiar. It is likely that you will also need to consult other texts and data sources. However, this is a very portable book which can be carried around with you in your bag or left on the ward for quick and easy reference. We hope that you will enjoy this new approach.

Acknowledgements

In editing this book we are indebted to colleagues and friends who have kindly given up their time and expertise to write each of the separate sections of the book. We acknowledge that many of them are national and international experts in their field and we know that this has helped to enhance the quality and clarity of the book, Our special thanks to our families for tolerating our endeavour with this book.

Brief contents

Detailed contents

Abbreviations

∴	therefore
∝	proportional
~	approx
≻	greater than
≺	less than
α	alpha
β	beta
κ	kappa
γ	gamma
ARDS	acute respiratory distress syndrome
ASA	American Society of Anaesthesiologists
AT	antitrypsin
BAL	bronchoalveolar lavage
BALF	bronchoalveolar lavage fluid
BAPE	benign asbestos pleural effusion
BOOP	bronchiolitis obliterans organising pneumonia
BOS	bronchiolitis obliterans syndrome
BR	breathing reserve
BTS	British Thoracic Society
CABG	coronary artery bypass graft
CAP	community-acquired pneumonia
CBAVD	congenital bilateral absence of the vas deferens
CF	cystic fibrosis
CFA	cryprogenic fibrosing alveolitis
CFLD	cystic fibrosis liver disease
CFRD	cystic fibrosis-related diabetes mellitus
CFTR	cystic fibrosis transmembrane conductance regulator
CHF	chronic heart failure
CKD	chronic kidney disease
cm	centimetre
CMV	cytomegalovirus or controlled mechanical ventilation
CNS	central nervous system
CO	carbon monoxide
CO_2	carbon dioxide
COAD	chronic obstructive airways disease
COP	cryptogenic organising pneumonia
COPD	chronic obstructive pulmonary disease
CPAP	continuous positive airway pressure
CPET	cardiopulmonary exercise testing
CPG	central pattern generator
CRQ	Chronic Respiratory Questionnaire
CRT	cardiac resynchronisation therapy
CSF	cerebrospinal fluid
CSS	Churg–Strauss syndrome
CTD	connective tissue disorder
CTEPH	chronic thromboembolic pulmonary hypertension
CVID	common variable immunodeficiency
CVS	chorionic villus sampling
CWR	constant work rate
CXR	chest X-ray
DAD	diffuse alveolar damage
DH	dynamic hyperinflation
DIP	desquamative interstitial pneumonia
$D_{L}co$	diffusing capacity for carbon monoxide
DRG	dorsal respiratory group
EAA	extrinsic allergic alveolitis
EB	eosinophilic bronchitis
EBUS	endobronchial ultrasound
ECG	electrocardiogram
EELV	end-expiratory lung volume
EMG	electromyography
EPAP	expiratory positive airway pressure
EPP	equal pressure point or extrapleural pneumonectomy
ERV	expiratory reserve volume
ESR	erythrocyte sedimentation rate
ESWT	endurance shuttle walk test
ETT	endotracheal tube
FBC	full blood count
FEF_{25-75}	forced mid-expiratory flow rate
FEV_1	forced expiratory volume in 1 second
FNA	fine needle aspiration
FOB	fibre-optic bronchoscopy
FRC	functional residual capacity
FVC	forced vital capacity
g	gram
GCS	Glasgow coma scale
GI	gastrointestinal
GMCSF	granulocyte monocyte colony stimulating factor
GOR	gastro-oesophageal reflux
GORD	gastro-oesophageal reflux disease
GR	glucocorticoid receptor
GVHD	graft versus host disease
HAART	highly active antiretroviral therapy
HAP	hospital-acquired pneumonia
HCAP	health-care-associated pneumonia
HDM	house dust mite
HDU	High Dependency Unit
HIV	human immunodeficiency virus
HLA	human leucocyte antigen

HME	heat and moisture exchanger	NRT	nicotine replacement therapy
HPV	hypoxic pulmonary vasoconstriction	NSAID	non-steroidal anti-inflammatory drug
HRCT	High-resolution computed tomography	NSIP	non-specific interstitial pneumonia
HSCT	haematopoietic stem cell transplantation	NYHA	New York Heart Association
IC	inspiratory capacity	O_2	oxygen
ICU	Intensive Care Unit	OGTT	oral glucose tolerance test
Ig	immunoglobulin	OI	opportunistic infections
IIP	idiopathic interstitial pneumonia	OSA	obstructive sleep apnoea
ILD	interstitial lung disease	OSAH	obstructive sleep apnoea/hypopnoea
IPAP	inspiratory positive airway pressure	OSAS	obstructive sleep apnoea syndrome
IPF	idiopathic pulmonary fibrosis	PA	postero-anterior
IRIS	immune reconstitution inflammatory syndrome	$PaCO_2$	partial pressure of carbon dioxide in arterial blood
IRT	immunosuppressive trypsin	PaO_2	partial pressure of oxygen in arterial blood
IRV	inspiratory reserve volume	PAH	pulmonary arterial hypertension
ISWT	incremental shuttle walk test	PAP	pulmonary alveolar proteinosis
ITU	Intensive Therapy Unit	PAVM	pulmonary arteriovenous malformation
IV	intravenous	PCD	primary ciliary dyskinesia
kPa	Kilopascal	PCP	*Pneumocystis* pneumonia
KS	Kaposi sarcoma	PCR	polymerase chain reaction
LABA	long-acting beta agonist	Pcrit	critical collapsing pressure
LAM	lymphangioleiomyomatosis	PDT	photodynamic therapy
LC	Langerhans' cells	PE	pulmonary embolism
LCH	Langerhans' cell histiocytosis	PEA	pulmonary endartectomy
LDH	lactate dehydrogenase	PEEP	positive end-expiratory pressure
LIP	lymphoid interstitial pneumonia	PEF	peak expiratory flow
LMWH	low-molecular-weight heparin	PET	positron emisson tomography
LTBI	latent tuberculosis infection	PFT	pulmonary function test
LTOT	long-term oxygen therapy	PI	phosphoinositide
LTRA	leukotriene receptor antagonist	PIV	parainfluenza
LVF	left ventricular failure	PKA	protein kinase A
LVRS	lung volume reduction surgery	PLCH	pulmonary Langerhans' cell histiocytosis
m	metre	PLMS	periodic leg movement in sleep
MALT	mucosa-associate lymphoid tissue	PPH	primary pulmonary hypertension
MAU	Medical Admission Unit	PRG	pontine respiratory group
MDI	metered dose inhaler	PSV	pressure support ventilation
MDR	multi-drug resistant	PTLD	post-transplantation lymphoproliferative disorder
MEF	maximal expiratory flow	RA	rheumatoid arthritis
MIF	maximal inspiratory flow	RAR	rapidly adapting receptor
ml	millilitre	RAST	radio-allergo-sorbent test
MND	motor neuron disease	RBILD	respiratory bronchiolitis-associated interstitial lung disease
MPA	microscopic polyangiitis	RCT	randomised controlled trial
MPE	malignant pleural effusion	REM	rapid eye movement
MPO	myeloperoxidase	RSI	rapid sequence intubation
MRC	Medical Research Council	RSV	respiratory syncitial virus
MRI	magnetic resonance imaging	RV	residual volume
MSLT	multiple sleep latency testing	s	second/s
MVC	maximum voluntary contraction	SaO_2	arterial oxygen saturation
NETT	National Emphysema Treatment Trial	SAR	slowly adapting receptor
NG	nasogastric	SARS	severe acute respiratory syndrome
NHL	non-Hodgkin lymphoma	SBOT	short-burst oxygen therapy
NIV	non-invasive ventilation		
NO	nitric oxide		

SCC	squamous cell carcinoma
SEPCR	European Society of Clinical Respiratory Physiology
SGRQ	St George's respiratory questionnaire
SIADH	syndrome of Inappropriate antidiuretic hormone
SLE	systemic lupus erythematosus
SNIP	sniff nasal inspiratory pressure
SNP	single nucleotide polymorphism
SOT	solid organ transplant
SPECT	single-photon emission computed tomography
SPN	solitary pulmonary nodule
SSc	systemic sclerosis
SVC	superior vena cava
SVCO	superior vena cava obstruction
TB	tuberculosis
TBB	transbronchial biopsy
TBNA	transbronchial needle aspiration
TLC	total lung capacity
TMN	tumour–nodal–metastasis
TNF	tumour necrosis factor
TOSCA	transcutaneous oxygen and carbon dioxide monitoring
TTAB	transthoracic aspiration biopsy
TV	tidal volume
U&E	urea and electrolytes
UARS	upper airway resistance syndrome
UIP	usual interstitial pneumonia
V/P	ventilation/perfusion
VAP	ventilator-associated pneumonia
VATS	video-assisted thoracoscopic surgery
VC	vital capacity
VCD	vocal cord dysfunction
VEGF	vascular endothelial growth factor
VILI	ventilator-induced lung injury
VRG	ventral respiratory group
WG	Wegener's granulomatosis
WLL	whole-lung lavage

Contributors

Dr Anthony Arnold
Department of Respiratory Medicine
Castle Hill Hospital
Hull

Dr Janice Ash-Miles
Department of Radiology
University Hospitals Bristol
Bristol

Dr Angela Atalla
Department of Respiratory Medicine
Derriford Hospital
Plymouth

Dr David Baldwin
Department of Respiratory Medicine
Nottingham University Hospitals
Nottingham

Dr Phillip Barber
North West Lung Centre
University Hospital of South Manchester
Manchester

Professor Peter Barnes
Airway Diseases Section
National Heart & Lung Centre
Imperial College
London

Dr Nick Bell
Dept of Respiratory Medicine
University Hospitals Bristol
Bristol

Dr Diane Bilton
Adult CF Unit
Papworth Hospital
Cambridge

Dr Stephen Bourke
Department of Respiratory Medicine
Royal Victoria Infirmary
Newcastle-upon-Tyne

Professor Sherwood Burge
Department of Respiratory Medicine
Birmingham Heartlands Hospital
Birmingham

Professor Peter Calverley
School of Clinical Sciences
University of Liverpool
Liverpool

Dr James Calvert
North Bristol Lung Centre
Southmead Hospital
Bristol

Dr G Cardillo
Department of Surgery
Glenfield Hospital
Leicester

Dr Jim Catterall
Respiratory Department
Bristol Royal Infirmary
Bristol

Dr Colin Church
Scottish Pulmonary Vascular Unit
Western Infirmary
Glasgow

Dr Ian Coutts
Department of Respiratory Medicine
Royal Cornwall Hospitals
Cornwall

Dr Michael Darby
Department of Radiology
Southmead Hospital
Bristol

Dr Chris Davies
Department of Respiratory Medicine
Royal Berkshire Hospital
Reading

Dr Helen Davies
Oxford Centre for Respiratory Medicine
Churchill Hospital
Oxford

Professor Robert Davies
Oxford Centre for Respiratory Medicine
Churchill Hospital
Oxford

Professor David Denison
Emeritus Professor in Clinical Physiology
Hospital Royal Brompton
London

Dr Paddy Dennison
Department of Respiratory Medicine
Dorset County Hospital
Dorset

Dr A Degryse
Vanderbilt University Medical Center
Nashville
Tennessee, USA

Dr Amber Degryse
Fellow in Pulmonary Disease
Vanderbilt Medical Center
Nashville

Dr David Derry
Department of Respiratory Medicine
Derriford Hospital
Plymouth

Dr Lee Dobson
Respiratory Department
Torbay Hospital
Torquay

Dr James Dodd
Department of Respiratory Medicine
Royal Devon & Exeter NHS Foundation Trust
Exeter

Dr Anne Dunleavy
Department of Respiratory Medicine
Royal Free Hospital
London

Professor Jim Egan
Department of Respiratory Medicine
Master Misericordiae Hospital
Dublin

Dr Ugo Eleowa
Cambridge Institute for Medical Research
University of Cambridge
Cambridge

Dr Rachel Evans
Department of Respiratory Medicine
University Hospitals of Leicester
Leicester

Professor Tim Evans
Department of Intensive Care Medicine
Royal Brompton Hospital
London

Dr Hosnieh Fathi
Division of Cardiovascular and
Respiratory Studies
Castle Hill Hospital
Cottingham

Dr Tony Fennerty
Department of Respiratory Medicine
Harrogate District Foundation Trust
Harrogate

Dr Rhian Finn
North Bristol Lung Centre
Southmead Hospital
Bristol

Dr Andrew Fisher
Department of Respiratory Medicine
Freeman Hospital
Newcastle-upon-Tyne

Dr Helen Firth
Consultant Clinical Geneticist
Addenbrookes Hospital
Cambridge

Jane French
Nurse Consultant
Papworth Hospital
Cambridge

Dr Peter Froeschle
Department of Thoracic and Upper GI Surgery
Royal Devon and Exeter Hospital
Exeter

Professor Duncan Geddes
Royal Brompton Hospital
London

Dr Fergus Gleeson
Department of Radiology
The Churchill Hospital
Oxford

Dr Mark Glover
Hyperbaric Medicine Unit
St Richard's Hospital
Chichester

Dr Anna Goodman
Wellcome Trust Centre for Human Genetics
University of Oxford
Oxford

Dr Mark Grover
Hyberbanic Medicine Unit
St Richard's Hospital
Chichester

Dr Melissa Hack
Chest Clinic
Newport Hospital
Wales

Dr P. Halder
Institute of Lung Heath
Glenfield Hospital
Leicester

Dr Praneb Haldar
Institute for Lung Health
Glenfield Hospital
Leicester

Dr David Halpin
Department of Respiratory Medicine
Royal Devon & Exeter NHS Foundation Trust
Exeter

Dr Kim Harrison
Respiratory Unit
Morriston Hospital
Swansea

Dr John Harvey
North Bristol Lung Centre
Southmead Hospital
Bristol

Dr Melissa Heightman
Department of Thoracic Medicine
University College Hospital
London

Dr Martin Hetzel
Department of Respiratory Medicine
University Hospitals Bristol
Bristol

Dr Bernard Higgins
Respiratory Medicine Department
Freeman Hospital
Newcastle-upon-Tyne

Dr Mathew Hind
Royal Brompton Hospital
London

Dr Nik Hirani
MRC Centre for Inflammation Research
Queen's Medical Research Institute
Edinburgh

Professor Margaret Hodson
Department of Cystic Fibrosis
Royal Brompton Hospital
London

Dr Clare Hooper
North Bristol Lung Centre
Southmead Hospital
Bristol

Dr John Hurst
Academic Unit of Respiratory Medicine
Royal Free Hospital Medical School
London

Professor Richard Hubbard
Division of Epidemiology and Public Health
University of Nottingham
Nottingham

Dr Phil Hughes
Chest Clinic
Derriford Hospital
Plymouth

Dr Jane Hurst
Consultant in Clinical Genetics
Oxford Radcliffe Hospitals NHS Trust
Oxford

Dr Nabil Jarad
Department of Respiratory Medicine
University Hospitals Bristol
Bristol

Dr Simon Johnson
Division of Therapeutics and Molecular Medicine
University of Nottingham
Nottingham

Dr Andrew Jones
Adult Cyctic Fibrosis Centre
University Hospitals
NHS Foundation Trust
Wythenshawe
Manchester

Dr Adrian Kendrick
Consultant Clinical Scientist
University Hospitals Bristol
Bristol

Professor Keith Kerr
Department of Pathology
University of Aberdeen
Aberdeen

Dr Ayaz Khan
North Bristol Lung Centre
Southmead Hospital
Bristol

Dr Will Kinnear
Department of Respiratory Medicine
University Hospital
Nottingham

Dr Malcolm Kohler
Oxford Centre for Respiratory Medicine
Churchill Hospital
Oxford

Dr Sophie Kravinskas
Division of Therapeutics and Molecular Medicine
University of Nottingham
Nottingham

Dr Gabriel Laszlo
Department of Respiratory Medicine
Bristol Royal Infirmary
Bristol

Professor Y C Gary Lee
University of Western Australia
Sir Charles Gairduer Hospital
Perth

Professor Richard Light
Vanderbilt University Medical Center
Nashville

Dr Lim Wei Shen
Department of Respiratory Medicine
Nottingham University Hospitals
Nottingham

Dr Marc Lipman
Consultant in Respiratory and HIV Medicine
Royal Free Hospital
London

Professor David Lomas
Cambridge Institute of Medical Research
Cambridge University
Cambridge

Dr Toby Maher
Royal Brompton Hospital
London

Dr Adam Malin
Respiratory Unit
Royal United Hospital
Bath

Dr William Man
Royal Brompton Hospital
London

Dr Nick Maskell
North Bristol Lung Centre
University of Bristol
Bristol

Dr Matthew Masoli
North Bristol Lung Centre
University of Bristol
Bristol

Dr Andrew R L Medford
Department of Respiratory Medicine
Derriford Hospital
Plymouth

Professor Ann Millar
North Bristol Lung Centre
University of Bristol
Bristol

Professor Rob Miller
Centre for Sexual Health & HIV Research
University College Hospital
London

Dr Robert Milroy
Department of Respiratory Medicine
Stobhill Hospital
Glasgow

Dr John Moore-Gillon
Department of Respiratory Medicine
Barts and the London NHS Trust
London

Professor Alyn Morice
Division of Cardiovascular and
Respiratory Studies
Castle Hill Hospital
Cottingham

Dr Cliff Morgan
Department of Critical Care & Anaesthesia
Royal Brompton Hospital
London

Professor Mike Morgan
Department of Respiratory Medicine
University Hospitals of Leicester
Leicester

Professor Nick Morrell
Division of Respiratory Medicine
Department of Medicine
University of Cambridge

Dr Suranjan Mukhersee
Directorate of Respiratory Medicine
University Hospitals of North Staffordshire
Stoke-on-Trent

Dr John T Murchison
Department of Radiology
Royal Infirmary of Edinburgh
Edinburgh

Dr Mitzi Nisbet
Host Defence Unit
Royal Brompton Hospital
London

Professor Marc Noppen
International Endoscopy Clinic
University Hospital
Brussels

Professor Peter Ormerod
Department of Respiratory Medicine
Royal Blackburn Hospital
Blackburn

Professor Paulo Palange
Department of Clinical Medicine
University of Rome
Rome

Dr Timothy Palfreman
Adult Intensive Care Unit
Royal Brompton Hospital
London

Dr Timothy Palfreyman
Department of Intensive Care Medicine
Royal Brompton Hospital
London

Dr Manish Pareek
Infectious Disease Unit
Leicester Royal Infirmary
Leicester

Dr S Parker
Department of Respiratory Medicine
Freeman Hospital
Newcastle-upon-Tyne

Dr Bipen Patel
Department of Respiratory Medicine
Royal Devon & Exeter NHS Foundation Trust
Exeter

Dr Sam Patel
Dept of Respiratory Medicine
University Hospitals Bristol
Bristol

Professor Ian Pavord
Institute of Lung Heath
Glenfield Hospital
Leicester

Professor Andrew Peacock
Scottish Pulmonary Vascular Unit
Western Infirmary
Glasgow

Dr Mike Peake
Dept of Respiratory Medicine
University Hospitals of Leicester
Leicester

Dr Justin Pepperell
Department of Respiratory Medicine
Taunton and Somerset Hospital
Taunton

Dr Gerrard Phillips
Department of Respiratory Medicine
Dorset County Hospital
Dorset

Dr Martin Plummeridge
North Bristol Lung Centre
Southmead Hospital
Bristol

Professor Jose Porcel
Department of Internal Medicine
Lleida, Spain

Dr Susan Poutanen
University Health Network & Mount
Sinai Hospital
Department of Microbiology
Toronto, Canada

Dr R Ragendram
Department of General Medicine
John Redcliffe Hospital
Oxford

Dr Kasper F Remund
Department of Respiratory Medicine
Mater Misericordiae Hospital
Dublin

Dr Gerrit Van Rensburg
Respiratory Unit
Royal United Hospital
Bath

Professor Douglas Robinson
Laboratories Leti, Madrid
and Imperial College, London

Dr Grace Robinson
Department of Respiratory Medicine
Royal Berkshire Hospital
Reading

Dr Francisco Rodriguez-Panadero
MD El Mirador
Tomares (Sevilla)

Dr Robin Rudd
Consultant Physician
London

Dr Pallav Shah
Royal Brompton Hospital
London

Dr Clare Shovlin
National Heart & Lung Institute
Imperial College
London

Dr Anita Simonds
Sleep and Ventilation Unit
Royal Brompton & Harefield
NHS Trust
London

Dr Nicholas Simmonds
Department of Cystic Fibrosis
Royal Brompton Hospital
London

Dr Pasupathy Sivasothy
Department of Respiratory Medicine
Addenbrooke's Hospital
Cambridge

Dr David Smith
North Bristol Lung Centre
Southmead Hospital
Bristol

Professor Monica Spiteri
Department of Respiratory Medicine
University Hospital of North Staffordshire
Stoke-on-Trent

Professor Stephen Spiro
Department of Thoracic Medicine
University College Hospital
London

Dr Iain Stephenson
Infectious Diseases Unit
Leicester Royal Infirmary
Leicester

Dr John Strading
Oxford Centre for Respiratory Medicine
Churchill Hospital
Oxford

Dr Jay Suntharalingam
Respiratory Unit
Royal United Hospital
Bath

Dr Richard Teoh
Department of Respiratory Medicine
Castle Hill Hospital
Hull

Dr Matthew Thornber
Department of Acute Medicine
North Bristol NHS Trust
Bristol

Dr Joseph Unsworth
Department of Immunology
Southmead Hospital
Bristol

Mr David Waller
Department of Surgery
Glenfield Hospital
Leicester

Dr Neil Ward
Department of Respiratory Medicine
Royal Devon and Exeter Hospital
Exeter

Professor Kevin Webb
Adult Cystic Fibrosis Centre
University Hospitals NHS Foundation Unit
Manchester

Professor Jadwiga Wedzicha
Academic Unit of Respiratory Medicine
Royal Free Hospital Medical School
London

Professor Athol Wells
Royal Brompton & Harefield NHS
London

Dr Adam Whittle
Department of Respiratory Medicine
University Hospitals Bristol
Bristol

Dr R Wilson
Host Defence Unit
Royal Brompton Hospital
London

Dr Robert Winter
Addenbrooke's Hospital
Cambridge University Hospitals
NHS Foundation
Cambridge

Dr Nick Withers
Department of Respiratory Medicine
Royal Devon and Exeter Hospital
Exeter

The healthy lung

Chapter contents

1.1 Pulmonary anatomy

Lobes and fissures

Each lung is divided into lobes by the presence of fissures; the left lung by the oblique fissure into an upper and lower lobe, whilst the right is split into an upper, middle, and lower lobe by the oblique and transverse fissures (Fig. 1.1.1). Accessory fissures can occur, of which the one formed if the azygos vein arches laterally to the mediastinum instead of medially, giving rise to the 'azygos lobe' is the most common (up to 1%).

AUTHOR'S TIPS
- The visceral pleura is continued on to the major fissures, its visibility as a horizontal hairline is a normal finding in almost half of all chest X-rays.
- The horizontal fissure is often incomplete medially, allowing collateral ventilation between lobes.

Airways

The trachea bifurcates into the right and left main bronchi at the level of the manubrio-sternal joint. The right is typically wider, shorter (3cm) and less steeply angled than the longer (5cm) left. The main bronchi divide into lobar and segmental branches which continue until they reach 1mm in diameter, when they lose their cartilage and become bronchioles.

Both lungs have 10 wedge-shaped bronchopulmonary segments, each with its own air and blood supply.

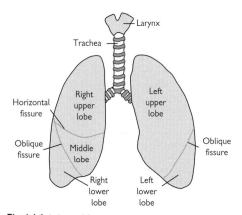

Fig. 1.1.1 Lobes and fissures.

Parenchyma

Terminal bronchioles (0.5mm diameter) are the last airway before the alveolar lined respiratory bronchioles start. There are 20,000–30,000 terminal bronchioles, each ending in an acinus (primary bronchiole). Respiratory bronchioles within an acinus will branch several times until they reach the further divided alveolar ducts which lead to the alveolar sacs and their alveoli.

The secondary lobule is the smallest section of lung which can be seen on high resolution computed tomography (HRCT); it contains 5 or 6 acini, whose interlobular septum consists of pulmonary lymphatics, veins and a discrete layer of connective tissue (Fig. 1.1.2).

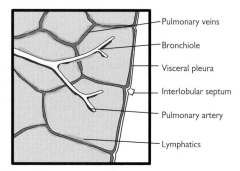

Fig. 1.1.2 Secondary lobule.

Nerve supply to the lung

Sympathetic supply is from thoracic segments 3 to 5 via the sympathetic chain which supplies the bronchial airway and pulmonary artery muscle.

Parasympathetic supply is from the vagus nerve which constricts bronchial muscle and has secretomotor action to the mucous glands.

Sensory supply is stretch sensation to the lung and visceral pleura and pain to the parietal pleura. The diaphragmatic portion is via the phrenic nerve whilst the costal portion is from intercostals nerves.

Blood supply

The lung receives both a pulmonary and a bronchial artery supply. The pulmonary arterial circulation follows the branching of the bronchi, the bronchial arterial circulation supplies the airways, visceral pleura and lymphoid tissue.

Lymphatic drainage

There are no lymphatic vessels in the alveoli. The lymphatic vessels from the alveolar duct and bronchioles follow the bronchial tree back to the hilum and then the mediastinum. Lymph nodes may occur along their intrapulmonary course.

Beneath the visceral pleura a plexus of lymphatics are present, they drain into the peribronchial lymphatics, through vessels that run in septae through the acini and segments. It is distension of these horizontally placed septae which causes Kerley B lines.

AUTHOR'S TIP
Since there is communication between the pulmonary and bronchial circulation in the parenchyma, the bronchial arteries may contribute to gas exchange in pulmonary vascular disorders.

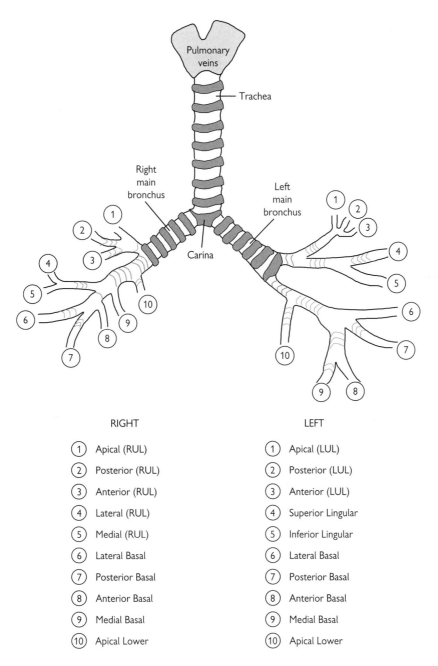

	RIGHT		LEFT
①	Apical (RUL)	①	Apical (LUL)
②	Posterior (RUL)	②	Posterior (LUL)
③	Anterior (RUL)	③	Anterior (LUL)
④	Lateral (RUL)	④	Superior Lingular
⑤	Medial (RUL)	⑤	Inferior Lingular
⑥	Lateral Basal	⑥	Lateral Basal
⑦	Posterior Basal	⑦	Posterior Basal
⑧	Anterior Basal	⑧	Anterior Basal
⑨	Medial Basal	⑨	Medial Basal
⑩	Apical Lower	⑩	Apical Lower

Fig. 1.1.3 Diagram of the bronchial tree with typical segmental bronchi. Nomenclature is that used most commonly in the UK.

1.2 Radiology of the healthy chest

The plain chest X-ray (CXR)

Technical factors

PA (postero-anterior)

Full inspiration (mid-diaphragm crossed by 5th–7th anterior ribs) necessary to assess heart size and mediastinal contours.

Less = reduced lung volume, obesity or poor patient cooperation.

More = asthma, emphysema/chronic obstructive airways disease (COAD) or fit healthy young adult.

Heart size <50% of max. internal chest diameter.

- Emphysema/COAD, 'normal' heart size may be significantly less, due to over expansion of rib cage – changes from previous may be more useful.
- In elderly/osteoporosis, chest diameter may be relatively less, and so 'normal' heart size could be up to 2/3rds chest diameter.
- Rotation – spinous processes over mid trachea; clavicles and ribs symmetrical. If not, can cause apparent lucency/increased density of one lung.

Beware the 'hidden' zones – nearly 50% of lung area may be partially obscured on PA view by mediastinum and diaphragm (anterior and posterior costophrenic recesses). These areas are even less well seen on portable films.

AP (antero-posterior) supine

Magnification of mediastinum makes sizes inaccurate, but gives useful information on gross lung pathologies and position of lines, drains and tubes.

Lateral

Allows visualisation of 'hidden' areas and localises to a lobe a lesion seen on PA view.

Normal appearances (Fig 1.2.1)

Mediastinum

Left heart border made up of 4 'moguls' = aortic knuckle (indents trachea), pulmonary artery, left atrial appendage and left ventricle.

Right heart border made up from ascending aorta and right atrium.

Hilar points formed by the crossing of upper and lower zone broncho-vascular bundles. Left lies 1–1.5cm higher than right.

Lung parenchyma

Branching pattern of bronchovascular bundles which taper towards periphery. Arteries accompany airways, but latter not discernable except above each hilum when seen end-on as rings.

Absence of discernable structures in outer 1/3 of lungs.

Interstitium only visible when pathological.

Fissures may undulate and frequently incomplete (NB cause of collateral air drift between lobes). Horizontal fissure joins right hilum. Obliques pass from few centimetres behind anterior chest wall to 6th thoracic vertebra.

Diaphragms

Right up to 2cm higher than left. If not 'dome' shape, suggests hyperinflation. Localised bulge – 'eventration' due to muscle deficiency, usually antero-medial portion.

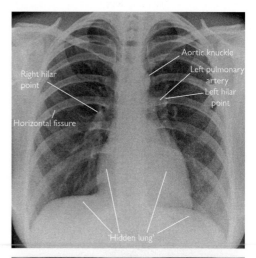

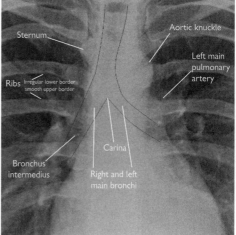

Fig. 1.2.1 Normal PA CXR.

Assessing the CXR

Systematic approach

Mediastinum, lungs, bones and soft tissues.

Mediastinum

Aorto-pulmonary window is concave (if not, is there nodal disease?).

Additional, 'double' contours to heart border signify abnormal pathology.

Shift of Hilar points indicates either traction due to collapse/fibrosis or pressure from space-occupying lesions.

Left heart border obscuration indicates lingular disease.

Right heart border obscuration indicates middle lobe disease.

Superior mediastinal borders may widen in elderly due to ectasia of vessels, or by obesity.

Lungs

Overall picture – lung volumes, symmetry of density and size. Variations within a lung. Refer to 'zones', not lobes unless obvious or have a lateral film.

Lateral CXR (Fig. 1.2.2)

Retrosternal and retrocardiac areas should be more 'black'. Gradual transition from whiter to blacker lung over spine as pass cranio-caudally.

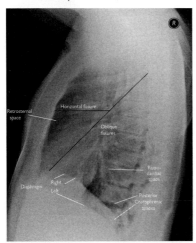

Fig. 1.2.2 Normal lateral CXR.

Common normal variants

Pectus excavatum. Steeply angled anterior ribs, horizontal posterior ribs. Compression of mediastinum cause straight left heart border and poor definition right heart border – mimicking middle lobe disease – confirmed by lateral.

Azygos fissure (Figs. 1.2.13 and 1.2.14). <1% of population. Azygos vein at medial end, as joins with SVC. Other accessory fissures occasionally visible.

Right-sided aortic arch (Fig. 1.2.11). <1%. May be associated with congenital heart disease. Indents right side of trachea.

Rib anomalies. Cervical ribs <8%. Congenital fused ribs or forked anterior ends (Fig 1.2.3).

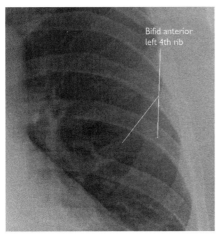

Fig. 1.2.3 Normal variant – bifid rib.

Beware

• 'Hidden' areas – behind heart, lung apices (partially obscured by overlying bones), through diaphragm in anterior and posterior costophrenic recesses.
• Bones – lower borders of posterior ribs often indistinct, upper borders smooth and clear margins. Fractures, metastases.
• Soft tissues – beware extra thoracic soft tissue lines mimicking pathology (e.g. pneumothorax). Mastectomy causes unilateral lucency of a lung.

Computed tomography (CT)

Techniques

Helical = spiral = multidetector CT

Constant acquisition of images as patient passes through scanner. Modern scanners can acquire 64 (or more) images per rotation of X-ray tube. A volume of information is acquired which can be manipulated to give reformations in sagittal, coronal or oblique planes.

IV contrast allows improved visualisation of vascular structures.

Protocol varies depending on clinical question:
• PE scans need high volume at high flow rates, to preferentially visualise pulmonary arteries.
• Staging scans may be in 2 phases; first to show mediastinum and second delayed to show liver in portal venous phase.
• Pleural disease is better shown at delayed phase to improve soft tissue enhancement.

> **AUTHOR'S TIP**
> Clinical information vital to ensure correct protocol followed.

HRCT

Conventionally, HRCT is performed as single axial sections at intervals throughout chest. Therefore there are gaps, making it inadequate for excluding nodules or masses. There is better resolution of fine detail. With latest generation scanners detail of a 'volume' scan can be good enough to show fine detail adequately and the advantages of not 'missing' some portions of lung outweigh marginal quality differences.

Uses:
• Assessment of interstitial lung disease.
• Expiratory scans improve visualisation of air-trapping in suspected small airway disease.
• Prone scans show if apparent posterior abnormalities disappear when patient is turned, So-called 'dependent' changes (normal).

Normal appearances (Figs. 1.2.4, 1.2.8–10)

Mediastinum

Trachea – posterior wall deficient in cartilage and bows inwards in expiration. Diameter 12–18mm in females; 16–20mm in males.

Aorta – ascending <35mm; descending <25mm.

Main pulmonary artery <3cm diameter.

Lymph nodes – in high superior mediastinum 'normal' <5mm; in hila <3mm; pre-tracheal and aorto-pulmonary <10mm but subcarinal and upper right hilum can be 10–15mm and still be 'normal'.

Thymus – up to early 20s can still be present as band of soft tissue in anterior mediastinum, moulding around adjacent structures. Later in life small nodular remnants can still be seen.

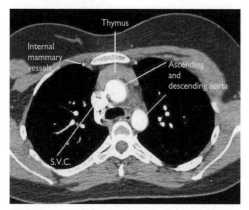

Fig. 1.2.4 Normal superior mediastinum.

Pericardial recesses (Fig. 1.2.5) contain small amounts of pericardial fluid which may measure up to 15mm and can mimic adenopathy. Seen in pretracheal and aortopulmonary areas, but usually identifiable due to their moulding to adjacent structures rather than being round or oval.

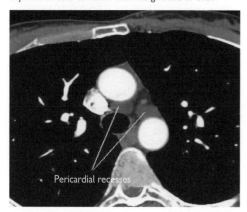

Fig. 1.2.5 Pericardial recesses (mimic adenopathy).

Normal variants – left SVC in 0.5%; aberrant right subclavian artery in 0.5% (originates from distal aortic arch, passing from left to right, behind oesophagus).

Lung parenchyma (Figs. 1.2.6 and 1.2.7)
Can see
- Broncho-vascular bundles seen to 8th generation (diameter of bronchus up to that of accompanying artery when seen end-on).
- Pulmonary veins.
- Interlobular septae only occasionally seen peripherally.
- Visceral pleura only seen when double layer in fissures.

Occasional intrapulmonary lymph nodes.

Cannot see
- Lymphatic vessels.
- Alveoli and acini.
- Capillary vessels.

NB Relatively 'bare' or featureless zone in peripheral 1cm of subpleural lung is normal.

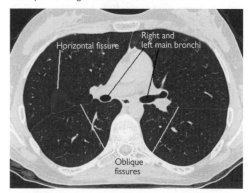

Fig. 1.2.6 HRCT of normal lungs (a).

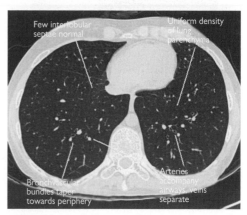

Fig. 1.2.7 HRCT of normal lungs (b).

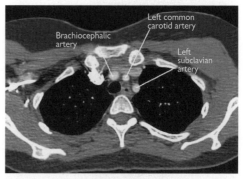

Fig. 1.2.8 Arteries arising from aortic arch.

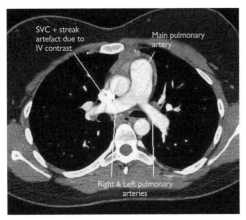

Fig. 1.2.9   Mediastinal structures just below carina.

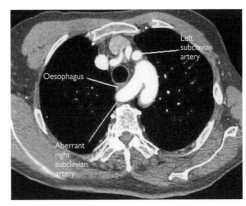

Fig. 1.2.12   Normal variant – aberrant right subclavian artery.

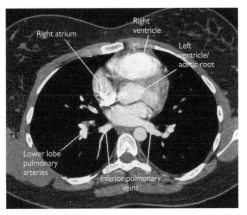

Fig. 1.2.10   Mediastinal structures at level of aortic root.

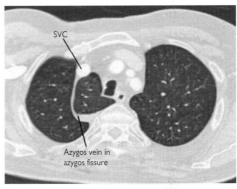

Fig. 1.2.13   Normal variant – azygos lobe (CT).

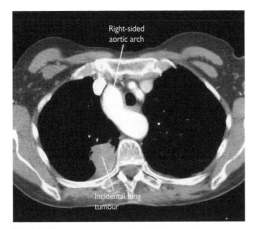

Fig. 1.2.11   Normal variant – right-sided aortic arch.

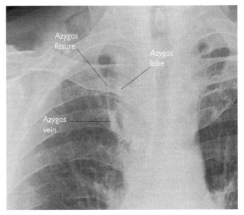

Fig. 1.2.14   Normal variant – azygos lobe (PA CXR).

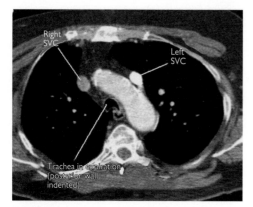

Fig. 1.2.15 Normal variant – left-sided SVC.

CT artefacts

Cardiac motion – blurring and double contours in middle lobe and lingular.

Respiratory motion – blurring and double contours throughout scan.

'Streaking' – next to SVC/brachiocephalic veins when contain high density IV contrast.

Mixing defects – contrast in SVC may have apparent filling defect due to unopacified blood entering from below, e.g. azygos flow, or from opposite arm.

Assessing CT of the chest

Systematic approach

Have a system and use it every time e.g. heart, pericardium and mediastinal vessels, lymph nodes, airways, lungs, pleura, bones and soft tissues, outside the thorax.

Mediastinum

Know the normal anatomy (see p.4) and what should be where.

Follow structures up and down the scan to see if they are vessels or masses.

Check for lymphadenopathy; pre/para-tracheal and sub carinal region, anterior mediastinum, aortopulmonary window; axillary and supra-clavicular regions.

Lungs

If you find an abnormality, assess it for position, size, shape and outline, density and presence of calcification or fat.

Look at lung, mediastinum and bones on appropriate 'window' settings.

Multi-planar reformats in coronal and saggital planes help localisation.

Other imaging modalities

Ventilation/perfusion scans (Fig. 1.2.16)

Perfusion performed by IV injection of radioactively labelled micro-particles which lodge in pulmonary capillaries. A more proximal obstruction (i.e. embolus) will cause a 'defect' in the perfusion image.

Ventilation images performed by inhalation of a radioactive gas (usually krypton) or radioactively labelled particles.

A normal V/Q scan has 95–98% accuracy in excluding a recent pulmonary embolus.

Best performed in patient with no pre-existing lung complaints and normal CXR.

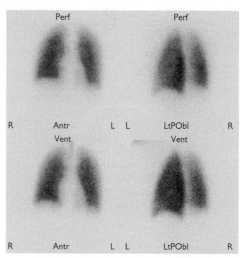

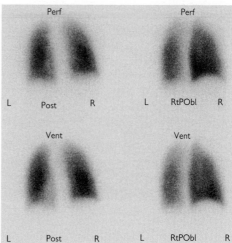

Fig. 1.2.16 Normal ventilation/perfusion lung scan.

Ultrasound

Useful in assessing pleural collections and pleurally based masses.

Good at differentiating fluid from solid.

Can show septations within fluid.

Guidance for drainage and biopsy procedures.

In normals, unreliable at showing all layers of the chest wall/pleura but 'real-time' ultrasound demonstrates the normal movement of lung against pleura.

Magnetic resonance imaging (MRI)

Of most use as a complementary test to CT in assessing chest wall invasion by masses, especially for diaphragmatic and apical lesions.

Good non-invasive tool for assessment of congenital cardiac disease and myocardial ischaemia.

Further reading

Hansell DM, Armstrong P, David A, *et al. Imaging of Diseases of the Chest.* Elsevier Health Services: UK 2004.

Respiratory physiology

Chapter contents

2.1 Basic physiology

The primary function of the lungs is gas exchange. This requires the movement of O_2 into the blood to support aerobic respiration in the mitochondria and the removal of the metabolic by-product CO_2 from the blood. To achieve this, an integrated system of external respiration (lungs), circulatory system linking the pulmonary and peripheral circulations and cellular respiration (internal respiration) must function harmoniously. This integration allows the system to (1) maintain the acid–base balance and (2) respond to applied stresses, such as exercise. Any part of the system that becomes compromised may affect gas exchange, the degree of which can be assessed at rest or during exercise.

The external respiratory system consists of:
- the ventilatory pump;
- the gas exchanger;
- the respiratory controller.

The ventilatory pump consists of the structures that form the bellows of the respiratory system, and enables gas exchange between the alveoli and the pulmonary capillaries. The respiratory controller receives information from inputs throughout the body and alters the rate and depth of breathing appropriately.

The ventilatory pump

This moves, by bulk flow, air from the atmosphere to the alveoli and back out. The pump must:
- generate sufficient pressure within the thorax to move gas down the airways to the alveoli;
- distribute the inhaled air throughout the lungs;
- overcome obstacles to gas movement, i.e. narrowed airways, as observed in COPD;
- achieve this with minimal energy expenditure;
- respond to increased demands, e.g. exercise.

Statics: the main static lung volumes (Fig. 2.1.1) are:

Total lung capacity (TLC) – the maximal volume of the lungs after a full inhalation.

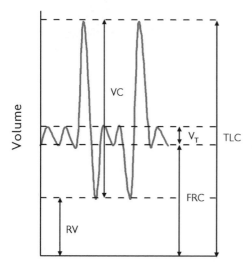

Fig. 2.1.1 Static lung volumes: V_T – tidal volume, TLC – total lung capacity, VC – vital capacity, FRC - functional residual capacity, RV – residual volume.

Functional residual capacity (FRC) – volume of air at the start of a tidal breath. Also known as end-expiratory lung volume (EELV).

Residual volume (RV) – volume of air left after a full exhalation.

Vital capacity (VC) – volume of air that can be exhaled from TLC to RV, or vice versa, either forcibly (FVC) or relaxed (VC).

What determines FRC?

- The chest wall and lungs are elastic structures coupled together by the pleural fluid.
- If air enters the pleural space, the lungs and chest separate with the chest wall expanding outwards and the lungs collapse inwards.
- At FRC, the chest wall and lungs are not at their ideal equilibrium volumes. The chest wall is being held at a lower volume and the lungs are being stretched open at a higher volume.
- At some point, the outward pull of the chest wall and the inward collapse of the lungs are of equal magnitude, but of opposite direction, and hence a balance point occurs (Fig. 2.1.2). This is the FRC.

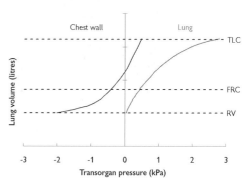

Fig. 2.1.2 Pressure–volume (P–V) relationships of the lungs and chest wall.

What determines TLC and RV?

- At TLC the P–V relationship of the lungs shows a plateau, whereas the chest wall does not. Hence it is the elasticity of the lungs that determines TLC. At TLC, the inspiratory muscles are shortened and are less effective at generating tension.
- At RV, the P–V relationship of the chest wall shows a plateau, whereas the lungs do not. Hence it is the chest wall that determines the RV. At this volume, the diaphragm and the external intercostal muscles are long and are more effective at generating tension.

For gas exchange to occur, air is bought to the alveoli (inhalation) and returned to atmosphere (exhalation).
- Inhalation is an active process requiring inspiratory muscles, the diaphragm being the primary muscle.
- As the diaphragm contracts, it shortens, moves downwards and moves the rib cage outwards. This change in chest wall shape results in the pleural pressure (P_{pl}) and alveolar pressure (P_{alv}) becoming more negative so air flows into the lungs.

Exhalation at rest is a passive process.
- When the inspiratory muscles stop contracting at the end of inhalation, the normal elastic properties of the lungs lead to a flow of air out of the lungs.

During exercise, exhalation is a combination of the passive recoil of the lungs and active contraction of the expiratory muscles of the abdominal wall and internal intercostals.

Normal breathing
Changes in the volume of the lungs requires pressure to be generated:
- To breathe in, a pressure must be generated within the thorax to move air into the alveoli.

- The magnitude of the pressure required is dependent on the compliance of the chest wall and the lungs:
$$\rightarrow \text{Compliance (C)} = \Delta\text{Volume} \div \Delta\text{Pressure} \quad (Eq.1)$$
- In emphysema, the lungs are compliant (floppy) so a small ΔP results in a large ΔV. In fibrosis the lungs are stiff, so a small ΔP results in a small ΔV.
- The compliance of the lungs (C_L) changes with lung volume (Fig 2.1.2). At FRC, the P–V curve is steep and the lungs are compliant (measured – 2.0 l.kPa^{-1}). At TLC, the curve is flatter, the lungs are stiffer and less compliant (measured – 0.56 l.kPa^{-1}).

The process of ventilation is summarised in Fig 2.1.3.
- At FRC the system is balanced, there is no airflow, P_{alv} is zero and P_{pl} is negative.

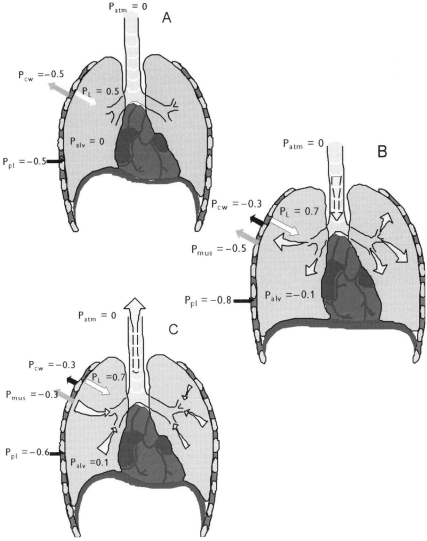

Fig. 2.1.3 Changes in various pressures during normal inhalation and exhalation.

- On inhalation, respiratory muscles contract, and P_{pl} becomes more negative. These changes in P_{pl} are transmitted to the alveoli, resulting in P_{alv} becoming negative with respect to atmospheric pressure (P_{Atm}), so air moves down the airways into the alveoli.
- When the system 'switches off' inhalation, the system relaxes resulting in a $P_{alv} > P_{Atm}$, so air moves out of the lungs.

In terms of force vectors, when inhaling from FRC:
- The respiratory muscle vector increases in magnitude as force is exerted to move the chest wall.
- The chest wall vector becomes smaller in magnitude as the chest wall approaches its equilibrium position.
- The lung force vector increases in magnitude as the lung moves further from its equilibrium position.
- On reaching the maximum VT for that breath, the system relaxes back to FRC.

Surfactant
As the alveolus is the site of gas exchange function, it is essential that the alveoli remain open. If we assume an alveolus is a sphere, we can apply:

$$\rightarrow \text{Laplace's law} - P = 2T \div r \qquad (Eq.2)$$

where P is pressure inside a sphere, T is the tension in the sphere wall and r is the radius of a sphere:
- As r decreases, P must increase inside the alveolus to prevent it from collapsing.
- Alveoli increase and decrease in radius during the breathing cycle, but do not do this uniformly.
- In an unstable state, small alveoli will have a greater P_{Alv} than large alveoli, and as pressure moves from high to low pressure small alveoli will empty into large alveoli. This does not happen in reality!

To ensure stable alveoli, Type II pneumocytes in the alveoli produce a detergent like substance called surfactant, which lines the alveolar surface.
- On inhalation, surfactant ↓T, so the lungs expand more easily.
- On exhalation surfactant ↓T, preventing alveolar collapse and minimising any effects on gas exchange.
- Surfactant minimises fluid transudation from the pulmonary capillaries, i.e. it helps keeps the alveoli dry.

Dynamics
The respiratory system is a dynamic organ. The movement of air into and out of the airways and lungs are affected by:

Airflow
This is either laminar or turbulent.
- Laminar flow, occurs in the peripheral airways, where flow (V) is proportional to driving pressure (ΔP):

$$\rightarrow \Delta P \propto V \qquad (Eq.3)$$

- Turbulent flow conditions occurs in the larger airways:

$$\rightarrow \Delta P \propto V^2 \qquad (Eq.4)$$

Where laminar and turbulent airflow occurs depends on the structural–functional relationship at that location, and may be determined by the Reynolds number (Re):

$$\rightarrow Re = (2ru\rho) \div \eta \qquad (Eq.5)$$

r – radius, ρ – gas density, u – gas velocitys η – gas viscosity. A value <2000 indicates laminar airflow.
- In the trachea (r = 15mm) breathing air, Re is >2000, hence turbulent airflow. Gas velocity is high.

- In peripheral airways (r = 0.5mm) Re is <1000 indicating laminar airflow. Gas velocity is low.
- Changing the radius of an airway or the gas composition affects Re. Breathing 20% O_2, 80% helium reduces Re to <1000 in the trachea, indicating laminar airflow and resulting in a higher peak expiratory flow (PEF).

Airway radius
The radius of the airways is important.
- Poiseuille's law states that:

$$\rightarrow V = \Delta P \pi r^4 \div 8\eta l \qquad (Eq.6)$$

where l is the tube length.

$$\rightarrow \text{Airways resistance } (R_{aw}) = \Delta P \div V \qquad (Eq.7)$$

- Combining Eq.6 and Eq.7:

$$\rightarrow R_{aw} \propto 1/r^4 \qquad (Eq.8)$$

Hence if r decreases by 50%, R_{aw} increases 16-fold.
- Most of the resistance to airflow occurs in the 5th–7th airway generations (large airways).
- As air moves from the periphery of the lungs to the central airways, velocity increases.
- Small airways in the periphery are tethered open by the elastic recoil of the lung tissue.
- Smooth muscle of medium-sized airways is controlled by the autonomic system. Bronchial smooth muscle tone is a major determinant of the cross-sectional area and hence the R_{aw} of the medium sized airways.

Flow–volume relationships
The system can generate flows of $>10l.s^{-1}$. At TLC high flows occur because:
- the elastic recoil of the lung tissue is maximal;
- the density of surfactant is least at TLC, so the surface forces are greatest;
- expiratory muscles are at their greatest length, and the chest wall at its farthest above relaxation volume;
- pleural pressure is at its most positive;
- airway radius is at its greatest so R_{aw} is low.

As lung volume decreases from TLC to RV, airflow decreases because:
- driving pressure decreases as lung volume decreases;
- elastic recoil of the lung and chest wall decreases;
- expiratory muscles are shorter, producing less tension
- airway radius decreases, so R_{aw} increases (Eq.6);
- the pressure across the airways is normally positive. In forced exhalation, this pressure becomes negative and small airways collapse;
- when pressure in the airways equals P_{pl}, the pressure across the airways = 0 and the equal pressure point (EPP) is attained so airway compression may follow;
- when the EPP is reached, flow limitation exists;
- the EPP is determined principally by the elastic recoil of the lungs. Low elastic recoil (emphysema) shifts the EPP towards the periphery of the lungs;
- after PEF, most of the expiratory portion of the flow-volume curve is effort independent and flow limitation has been attained;
- flow rates after 75% VC has been exhaled ($MEF_{25\%FVC}$) may be used as a guide to small airways function;
- inspiratory F–V curves are effort dependent.

Work of breathing (W)

To move the lungs and chest wall requires energy.

- Total W is the sum of elastic and resistive work.
- Resistive work decreases with increasing lung volume and widening of the airways ($\uparrow$r, $\downarrow$R – $Eq.8$).
- Elastic work increases at low and high lung volumes.
- W is normally at a minima close to FRC.
- Changes in W occur when the balance of elastic and resistive work are altered as in emphysema ($\uparrow$FRC to $\downarrow$R to $\downarrow$W) or fibrosis ($\downarrow$FRC to $\downarrow$Elastic to $\downarrow$W, BUT a $\downarrow$FRC leads to $\uparrow$R).
- At rest, W requires 1–2% of O_2 uptake (VO_2), which increases during exercise.
- Breathing frequency (f_b) at rest is 10–15/min, which is efficient. With increased elastic resistance f_b increases, whilst in increased airflow resistance, f_b decreases.

The gas exchanger

For gas exchange to occur 3 simple rules must be met:

- The alveoli are ventilated.
- The alveoli are perfused.
- Ventilation and perfusion are matched.

Ventilation

May be described in terms of total ventilation and alveolar ventilation.

Total ventilation (V_E, l.min^{-1}) is

- measured at the mouth;
- the sum of alveolar (V_A) and dead space ventilation (V_D), hence:

$$\rightarrow V_E = V_A + V_D \qquad (Eq.9)$$

The product of f_b and tidal volume (V_T), hence:

$$\rightarrow V_E = f_b \times V_T \qquad (Eq.10)$$

Note V_T must be $>V_D$ for gas exchange to occur.

Dead space ventilation is composed of the:

- anatomical dead space (2.2ml = 1kg body weight);
- alveolar dead space – 20 to 50ml.

A 70kg person therefore has a $V_D \approx$ 180ml/breath and a V_D/V_T ratio = 180/500 = 0.36.

If f_b = 15/min and V_T = 500ml, then V_E = 7500ml.

If V_D = 180ml/breath, total V_D = 2700ml.min^{-1}, and V_A = 4800ml.min^{-1}. If V_D = 300ml/breath, V_A = 3000ml.min^{-1}

Questions

1 Is a V_A = 4800ml.min^{-1} able to maintain arterial PO_2 and PCO_2 at the required levels?

2 What effect does increasing V_D have on arterial PO_2 and PCO_2?

CO$_2$ elimination

CO_2 is eliminated by the ventilatory pump, so any compromise to this, will affect the P_aCO_2.

$$\rightarrow V_A = k.VCO_2 \div P_aCO_2 \qquad (Eq.11)$$

where k is a constant and VCO_2 is the CO_2 produced by cellular respiration.

- $V_A \propto VCO_2$, $\therefore \uparrow$ or $\downarrow$ in VCO_2 must be matched by appropriate changes in V_A to maintain P_aCO_2.
- If V_A does not increase with increases in VCO_2, the P_aCO_2 will increase – **hypoventilation**.
- If V_A is greater than that required to match for VCO_2, then P_aCO_2 will be reduced – **hyperventilation**.

- If VCO_2 $\uparrow$ and V_A $\uparrow$ in sync, i.e. exercise – **hyperpnoea**.
- If f_b is >20/min, without $\uparrow$ V_E, then V_T $\downarrow$ (Eq.10) – BUT V_D/V_T $\uparrow$, so P_aCO_2 $\uparrow$ (Eq11) – **tachypnoea**.

Distribution of ventilation

At FRC in the upright position the lung apex, compared to the lung base:

- have larger alveoli which are less compliant;
- have a more negative P_{pl} (-0.8 kPa vs -3 kPa);
- requires greater ΔP to expand each alveolus;
- has less volume distributed i.e. ΔV of the basal alveoli is greater.

Distribution of perfusion

The pulmonary circulation is a high-compliance, low-resistance system, enabling it to adjust to changes in flow with little change in resistance.

- Gravity distributes blood flow (Q) to the lung bases.
- Some capillaries receive little or no blood flow, particularly at the lung apex – hence $V_{D,alv}$.
- With $\uparrow$Q or $\uparrow$pulmonary vascular resistance, capillaries may be recruited and participate in gas exchange.
- Pulmonary capillaries have very compliant walls, so if P_{Alv} > pulmonary capillary pressure (Pc), the capillary will narrow or collapse.
- What determines flow is the relationship of P_a, P_{Alv} and pulmonary venous pressure (P_v).

The lung may be divided into three zones (Table 2.1.1)

Table 2.1.1 The three zones of the lung.

Zone	Pressures	Flow
Apical	$P_{Alv} > P_a > P_v$	Little flow
Central	$P_a > P_{Alv} > P_v$	$\uparrow$Flow from upper to lower part of zone
Basal	$P_a > P_v > P_{Alv}$	Unimpeded flow

Pulmonary artery walls contain smooth muscle, and the tone of this muscle plays an important role on determining the radius of the vessel, and hence its resistance (Eq.8).

Pulmonary vessels constrict:

- when exposed to low levels of O_2 – **hypoxic vasoconstriction** – which reflects reduced alveolar ventilation due to airflow obstruction or alveoli filled with fluid, thereby affecting gas exchange;
- $\uparrow$R and resulting in redistribution of blood to areas that are well ventilated.

Pulmonary vessels dilate:

- when exposed to nitric oxide (NO) produced by nitric oxide synthase. NO acts locally. Its production is increased by mechanical or by biochemical stimulation. As flow increases, NO production increases to dilate the vessel and hence diminish resistance;
- when prostacyclins are produced in the lungs as they act as vasodilators.

For gas exchange to occur, ventilation must match perfusion. At the lung apices, ventilation exceeds perfusion (V/Q <1), whilst at the lung base, perfusion exceeds ventilation (V/Q >1). Hence V/Q matching is not perfect.

CO$_2$ transport

CO_2 is carried by blood:

- Bound to haemoglobin.
- Dissolved in the plasma.
- Dissolved CO_2 in equilibrium with carbonic acid:

$$\rightarrow CO_2 + H_2O \Leftrightarrow H_2CO_3 \Leftrightarrow H^+ + HCO_3^- \qquad (Eq.12)$$

- The P_aCO_2 of normal blood is 4.8–5.9 kPa.
- CO_2 is in high concentration in the tissues relative to the blood, so diffuses from the tissues into the blood.
- The relationship of CO_2 content and P_aCO_2 is linear over the normal physiological range. This relationship allows hyperventilation of normal alveoli to compensate for hypoventilation of diseased lung units.
- The *Haldane Effect* describes the shift to the right of the CO_2–Hb curve in the presence of O_2. CO_2 is displaced from Hb and enters the blood as dissolved gas.

An elevated P_aCO_2 may occur because of:
1. $\downarrow V_E$ – refer to *Eq.9* and *Eq.10* for changes in f_b and V_T;
2. $\downarrow V_A$ (*Eq.11*);
3. $\uparrow VCO_2$ with no change in V_E or V_A;
4. V/Q mismatch.

A decreased P_aCO_2 indicates an $\uparrow V_A$ (*Eq.11*) and the cause of this may be acute (whilst taking the blood sample) or due to other causes, i.e. hyperventilation syndrome

O_2 transport
The binding of O_2 to haemoglobin is different to that of CO_2.
- The P_aO_2 of normal blood is 11.3–13.3 kPa.
- The O_2–Hb curve is sigmoid shaped and relates O_2 saturation (SO_2) to P_aO_2 (Fig. 2.1.4).

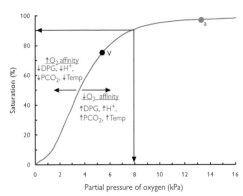

Fig. 2.1.4 Oxyhaemoglobin dissociation curve. V – mixed venous blood, a – arterial blood. The effects of changes in temperature, PCO$_2$, [H$^+$] and 2-3 diphosphoglycerate (DPG) on the affinity of Hb for O_2 are shown.

- The upper flat portion of the curve (PO$_2$ > 8 kPa) allows for quite large changes in PO$_2$ with little change in SO_2 – $SO_2 \geq 90\%$.
- Within the steeper middle portion of the curve, small changes in PO$_2$ result in large changes in SO_2. It is essential to record the on-air SO_2 if studying changes overnight in SO_2 using pulse oximetry.
- Consciousness is lost when PO$_2 \approx 3.5$ kPa ($SO_2 \approx 50\%$).
- The amount of O_2 carried is the O_2 content and is the sum of the O_2 bound to Hb and of that dissolved in the plasma.

$$\rightarrow O_2 \text{ content} = (1.39[Hb] \times SO_2) + (0.023P_aO_2) \quad (Eq.13)$$

- For an [Hb] = 14.6 g.dl^{-1}, SO_2 = 98% and P_aO_2 = 13.33 kPa, the O_2 content = 20.18 ml.dl^{-1}.

- A $\downarrow$[Hb] i.e. anaemia $\downarrow O_2$ content, so the amount of O_2 delivered to the tissues is lower. It does not change the P_aO_2 and hence there is no change in S_aO_2.
- The alveolar gas equation estimates P_AO_2 in an ideal alveolus and is a guide to alveolar gas exchange:

$$\rightarrow P_AO_2 = P_IO_2 - (P_aCO_2 \div R) \quad (Eq.14)$$

P_IO_2 – PO$_2$ in inspired air; R is $VO_2 \div VCO_2$ and is assumed to be 0.8.

From *Eq.14* a number of inferences can be made:
- For a given P_IO_2 and R, there is only one P_aCO_2 for each value of P_AO_2.
- A mild reduction in P_AO_2 can be normalised by $\uparrow V_A$, so $\downarrow P_aCO_2$.
- Hypoventilation results in an $\uparrow P_aCO_2$ and $\therefore \downarrow P_AO_2$.
- Maximum P_aO_2 breathing room air is determined by how low the P_aCO_2 and hence P_ACO_2 can be reduced to. Normally P_aO_2 does not exceed 16 kPa.
- In respiratory failure, P_aCO_2 may increase to 12 kPa, if the P_aO_2 decreases to 4 kPa. Chronically hypoxic patients may manage on a P_aO_2 of 2.5 kPa.

> For - P_IO_2 = 19.7kPa, P_aCO_2 = 5.33kPa and R = 0.8, the P_AO_2 = 13.0 kPa. If P_aO_2 is 13.2kPa, the alveolar–arterial O_2 difference (AaDO$_2$) is 0.2kPa. This is within 2kPa and reflects the V/Q mismatch that occurs in normal lungs.

Gas diffusion
Having ventilated and perfused the alveoli, gas exchange of O_2 and CO_2 across the alveolar capillary membrane must take place.
- Gas moves from a high pressure to a lower pressure, i.e. O_2 moves from the alveoli to the capillary blood.
- Gas uptake (V) depends on - pressure difference ($P_1 - P_2$), the properties of the gas (D), membrane surface area (A) and membrane thickness (t). Fick's law of diffusion states:

$$\rightarrow V = [D \times A \times (P_1 - P_2)] \div t \quad (Eq.15)$$

- D, A and t cannot be measured and are lumped together as T_L – transfer factor or D_L – diffusing capacity (D_L), so *Eq.15* becomes.

$$\rightarrow T_L = V \div (P_1 - P_2) \quad (Eq.16)$$

- T_L is a number of resistances in parallel; Dm – diffusing membrane capacity, Θ - the reaction rate of CO with haemoglobin and Vc - pulmonary capillary blood volume. These are combined as:

$$\rightarrow 1/T_L = 1/Dm + 1/\Theta Vc \quad (Eq.17)$$

- Disease states may reduce gas uptake and T_L due to:
1. loss of surface area ($\downarrow A$ or $\downarrow Dm$ - emphysema);
2. $\uparrow$membrane thickness ($\uparrow t$ or $\downarrow Dm$ - fibrosis);
3. $\downarrow \Theta$ (anaemia);
4. $\downarrow Vc$ (reduced cardiac output).
- Blood flow through the capillary at rest takes $\approx 0.75s$ and equilibrium between pulmonary venous and alveolar gas takes $\approx 0.25s$ for PO$_2$ and $\approx 0.30s$ for PCO$_2$.
- At maximal exercise, blood flow through the capillary takes $\approx 0.25s$, but generally there is little affect on the equilibration of PO$_2$ and PCO$_2$.
- O_2 and CO_2 diffusion are *perfusion-limited* in normal lungs, but may be *diffusion-limited* in diseased lungs.

The respiratory controller

The control of breathing is complex and not fully understood. Respiratory control involves both autonomic and volitional elements.

Autonomic control

The neural structures responsible for the autonomic control are:

- located in the medulla oblongata;
- the dorsal (DRG) and ventrolateral (VRG) respiratory groups, each with inspiratory and expiratory neurons.

The DRG:

- processes information from the receptors in the lungs, chest wall and chemoreceptors;
- has a key role in the activation of the diaphragm and the VRG;
- shows increased neuron activity during inhalation;
- has an important role in (a) determining the rhythm of breathing and (b) regulating the changes in upper airway radius, by stimulating muscles to expand the upper airway during inhalation.

In the pons, the pontine respiratory group (PRG):

- contributes to switching from inhalation to exhalation;
- if damaged, there is ↑inhalation time (T_i), ↓f_b and ↑V_T.

In the medulla there are:

- inspiratory neurons with a pacemaker function, firing at a given rate, but may be modified by other factors;
- neurons that fire during (a) inspiration, (b) exhalation or (c) transition from inhalation to exhalation.

Hence, the neurons responsible for the autonomic rhythmic breathing form the **central pattern generator** (CPG), which controls the minute-to-minute breathing in the normal person.

Volitional breathing

The system permits:

- breath-holding for periods of time;
- hyperventilation by ↑f_b and ↑V_T;
- alteration of the T_i and time of exhalation, by ↓f_b and ↑V_T under conscious controlled breathing conditions;
- changes in the breathing pattern in the presence of discomfort and anxiety. When experiencing pain or shortness of breath, ↑f_b and ↑V_E are observed.

Inputs to autonomic controller

The brain receives information from a variety of sources (Fig. 2.1.5):

Mechanoreceptors: Activated by distortion of their local environment. Includes receptors in:

- **Upper Airways**: sense and monitor flow, probably by temperature change. Inhibit central controller.

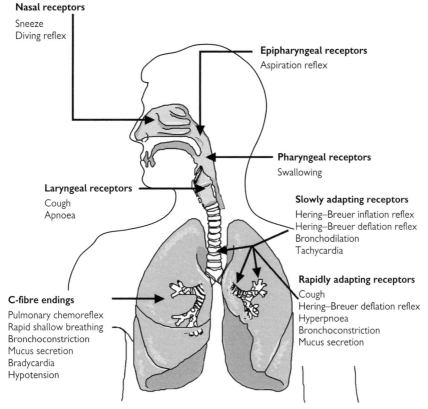

Nasal receptors
Sneeze
Diving reflex

Epipharyngeal receptors
Aspiration reflex

Pharyngeal receptors
Swallowing

Laryngeal receptors
Cough
Apnoea

Slowly adapting receptors
Hering–Breuer inflation reflex
Hering–Breuer deflation reflex
Bronchodilation
Tachycardia

Rapidly adapting receptors
Cough
Hering–Breuer deflation reflex
Hyperpnoea
Bronchoconstriction
Mucus secretion

C-fibre endings
Pulmonary chemoreflex
Rapid shallow breathing
Bronchoconstriction
Mucus secretion
Bradycardia
Hypotension

Fig. 2.1.5 The location of the major upper and lower airway and lung sensory receptors and the primary reflexes activated by these receptors.

- **Pulmonary system**, which include stretch receptors in the lungs:
  - **Slowly adapting receptors (SARs):** located in smooth muscle in the intra- and extrathoracic airways. When stimulated by lung inflation, the expiratory phase of respiration is prolonged. May also be involved in the early termination of inhalation when $\uparrow V_T$.
  - **Rapidly adapting receptors (RARs):** located in airway epithelial cells around the carina and in the large bronchi. Stimulated by chemical (tobacco smoke, histamine etc.) and mechanical stimuli. Activation may lead to cough, bronchospasm or increased mucus production. Lung deflation activates RARs and can contribute to an $\uparrow f_b$ and prolonged breaths, i.e. sighs.
  - **Hering–Breuer reflex:** a reflex that prevents over-inflation of the lungs. Pulmonary stretch receptors respond to excessive stretching of the lung during large inhalations. When activated, the receptors send action potentials to the pons, inhibiting the inspiratory neurons, so exhalation occurs. This reflex may only apply in newborn humans.
  - **C-fibres:** believed to be stimulated by chemical (histamine, prostaglandins etc.) and mechanical stimuli ($\uparrow$pulmonary capillary pressure). May contribute to changes in f_b and V_T.
- **Chest wall:** monitor respiration and alert the controller that the physiology of the ventilatory pump has changed i.e. $\uparrow R_{aw}$ or $\downarrow C_{RS}$.
- **Chemoreceptors:** located centrally and peripherally, and monitor chemical changes in the blood:
  - **Peripheral chemoreceptors:** located in the carotid body and the aortic arch, they monitor changes in P_aO_2, P_aCO_2 and pH A $\downarrow P_aO_2$ or a $\uparrow P_aCO_2$ or a $\downarrow$pH results in a $\uparrow V_E$ and vice versa.
  - **Central chemoreceptors:** located in the medulla and monitor changes in P_aCO_2 and pH. A $\uparrow P_aCO_2$ or a $\downarrow$pH results in a $\uparrow V_E$ and vice versa.
  - The ventilatory response to hypoxia is relatively flat until 8 kPa, after which V_E rapidly increases
  - The ventilatory response to hypercapnia is linear, and compared to an awake normal subject the slope of relationship of V_E to P_aCO_2 becomes increasingly flatter with the effects of sleep, narcotics and anaesthesia.

Ageing and the lungs

Ageing causes important changes in the structure and function of the respiratory system. From birth, the lungs develop and reach their maximum around the age of 18–25 years. From aged 25 years there is:

- Progressive loss of alveolar elastic recoil.
- Calcification of the costal cartilages.
- Decreased spaces between the spinal vertebrae and a greater degree of spinal curvature.

This results in the following gradual changes, which vary from person to person:

- $\uparrow C_L$ and $\downarrow C_{Chest\,Wall}$.
- $\uparrow$FRC, $\uparrow$RV and $\downarrow$VC as TLC remains fairly constant.
- $\downarrow$PEF and other flow rates.
- $\uparrow V_D$ and $\downarrow V_A - V_E$ and V_T unchanged.
- $\downarrow VO_2$ at rest, but $\uparrow VO_2$ for a given exercise level.
- $\downarrow$Cardiac output and Cardiac frequency (220 – age).
- $\downarrow P_aO_2$ and $\downarrow S_aO_2$, but $\uparrow$AaDO$_2$ as P_AO_2 unchanged.
- $\downarrow$Dm and $\downarrow$A (*Eq.15 & Eq.17*) and $\downarrow V_C$ resulting in $\downarrow T_L$.
- Poorer distribution of ventilation.
- $\downarrow$maximum inspiratory (MIP) and expiratory (MEP) mouth pressures.
- $\downarrow$exercise capacity – however assessed.

When assessing the normal physiology of an individual, it is essential to take into account the age of the subject.

Further reading

Cloutier MM. *Respiratory physiology*. Mosby Physiology Monograph Series, 2006.

Lung Model 4.2: http://oac.med.jhmi.edu/LungMode 14.2/

Lumb AB. *Nunn's Applied Respiratory Physiology*, 6th edn. Oxford: Butterworth-Heinemann, 2005.

Schwartzstein RM, Parker MJ. *Respiratory Physiology – A Clinical Approach*. Philadelphia: Lippincott Williams & Wilkins, 2006.

West JB. *Respiratory Physiology: The Essentials*, 7th rev. edn. Philadelphia: Lippincott Williams & Wilkins, 2004.

Answers

If V_A = 4800ml.min^{-1} then P_aCO_2 = 5.8 kPa and P_aO_2 = 12.97 kPa. By doubling V_D, P_aCO_2 = 9.3 kPa and P_aO_2= 8.7 kPa. V_T or f_b would need to increase to 620ml or 24/min respectively to achieve the original V_A

2.2 Lung function tests: a guide to interpretation

Introduction

Breathing tests are used:

- To look for evidence of respiratory impairment.
- If present, to measure lung function using tests which are sensitive to changes in the severity of the patient's condition.

Clinicians may look for diagnostic patterns of impairment as part of the investigation of symptoms, especially breathlessness; these are most informative when the CXR shows no localising disorder. Epidemiologists use them to study the effects of disease and the environment on the lung.

This section describes the investigation of conscious, cooperative adults who can perform the required voluntary breathing manoeuvres. Reference values are available for most populations; numerical results may be interpreted using population means and upper and lower 90% confidence intervals. Good technique is essential.

The three main types of lung function disturbance are:

- Ventilatory impairment: mechanical damage to the lungs or chest wall that make the breathing more difficult).
- Damage to the gas exchanging surface: a reduction of the number of pulmonary capillaries in contact with healthy alveoli.
- Abnormalities of blood gases: these are caused by
  1. Lung failure (damage to the gas exchanging mechanism).
  2. Pump failure (weakness, fatigue or paralysis of the respiratory muscles).

3. Abnormal control of the rate and depth of breathing leading to inadequate or excessive ventilation.

These disturbances can cause breathlessness on exertion or at rest. Breathlessness on exertion usually occurs in a predictable way; at rest the symptom may be chronic or occur episodically. In disease states, some correlation is found between the severity of the abnormalities of lung function and the amount of breathlessness suffered. In individuals, the impact of impaired lung function is modified by co-morbidity, general health and current psychological state as well as personality, level of habitual exercise and expectations.

Spirometric tests of expiratory and inspiratory flow and volume

Spirometry is simple and inexpensive. Its interpretation depends on an understanding of static lung volumes.

VC: *vital capacity* is the volume of air that can be delivered by a full expiration from total lung capacity to residual volume or inspiration by the reverse procedure. This may be reduced because of

1. **Airflow obstruction** which can cause airway closure at the end of expiration. RV is increased.
2. **Restriction to inspiration** caused by reduced volume of the alveolar gas, by abnormalities of the chest wall or by weakness of the respiratory muscles. Total lung capacity TLC is reduced.

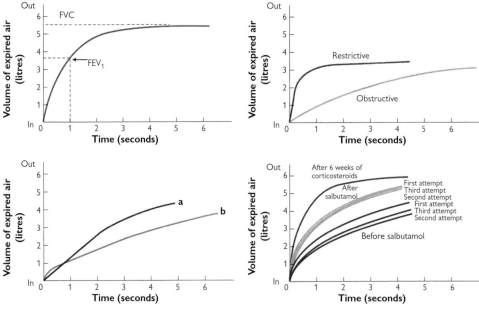

Fig. 2.2.1. Volume–time curves obtained during forced expiration using a wedge-bellows spirometer. **(a)** The subject has taken a full breath in and exhaled forcibly and fully. Maximal flow decelerates as forced expiration proceeds, because the airways decrease in size as the lung volume diminishes. Exhalation is terminated when the expired flow rate falls to <0.25 litres/sec (as here) or at 14 sec, whichever is sooner. **(b)** Obstructive and restrictive patterns. In obstruction, FEV_1/FVC is low; in restrictive disorders it is normal or high. **(c)** Straight line traces (a) in central airways obstruction, flow is constant through the first half of expiration; (b) Tracheo-bronchial collapse occurs in severe emphysema and tracheomalacia the first 200 ml is exhaled rapidly after which the compressed airway behaves like a fixed central obstruction. **(d)** Response of FEV_1 to treatment. A patient with moderate asthma tested before and after salbutamol and after a course of prednisolone. FEV_1 improves more than FVC.

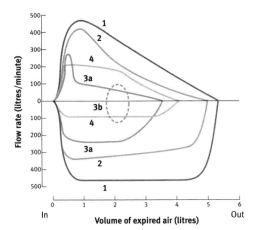

Fig. 2.2.2 Maximal expiratory and inspiratory flow–volume loops **(1)** Normal. The subject has taken a full breath in and exhaled forcibly and fully. Maximal flow decelerates as forced expiration proceeds, because the airways decrease in size as the lung volume diminishes. Maximal flow rates are much greater than flow rates during quiet breathing (3b). MIF is approximately the same as MEF but is sustained throughout mid-inspiration because there is no impediment to the opening of the airways when negative pressure is applied to the outside of the lung. **(2)** Mild airflow obstruction showing reduction of flow rate at mid-expiration and near RV. MIF = MEF. **(3a)** Severe airflow obstruction demonstrating airways collapse shortly after the beginning of forced expiration. MIF = MEF. **(3b)** Tidal breathing without forcing may achieve higher flow rates than forced expiration, which may cause the airways to collapse. **(4)** Obstruction of a central airway (glottis, larynx or trachea). In this example, MIF < MEF, indicating that the obstruction is in a collapsible airway outside the thorax. If the obstruction is fixed, MIF = MEF.

- FVC: *forced vital capacity* is the volume of air that can be delivered by a forced expiration from total lung capacity to residual volume (RV).
- FEV_1 (*the volume expired from full inspiration in the initial sec of a forced expiration from full inspiration*) should be greater than about 75% of FVC (according to age). Reduction of the ratio of FEV_1/FVC points towards airflow

obstruction, i.e. narrowing of the calibre of the airways. This is exaggerated by the effort of forced expiration; exhalation is impeded and therefore flow rate during expiration is reduced. COPD (chronic obstructive pulmonary disease) is defined as an irreversible reduction of FEV_1/FVC to below 70%.

- PEF: *peak expiratory flow rate* is the maximum flow at the start of a short forced exhalation. (Peak flow meters measure the first 10 milliseconds. The results from these are similar to the first part of an expiratory flow-volume loop.) PEF is reduced if there is narrowing of either proximal or distal airways or both, so it is very useful for identifying variability when spirometry indicates the presence of airflow obstruction. When a diagnosis of asthma has been made, PEF is used to assess daily and hourly variation. PEF is deceptively simple and has to be interpreted cautiously because:

1. Weakness or sub-maximal effort will produce low results.
2. Very low readings are obtained when there is obstruction of the larynx or trachea.
3. PEF does not reflect accurately the severity of COPD.

Flow volume loops

Graphic displays of maximal expiratory and inspiratory flow during forced expiration and inspiration between TLC and RV plotted against lung volume (see Fig. 2.2.2). During forced expiration flow is characteristically greatest at TLC, because the lung is at its most elastic, the airways are wide open and the respiratory muscles are at their greatest length and efficiency ('peak flow'). In normal subjects flow decelerates steadily towards RV when the lung is empty and no further flow occurs. This is because the airways progressively narrow and may collapse one by one because of the pressure around them. In COPD, particularly emphysema, airway collapse occurs at relatively high lung volumes. Tracheal or laryngeal obstruction is characterised by a very low peak flow and a constant flow rate throughout expiration. Forced inspiration opens the airways maximally so the inspiratory loop shows a more or less constant flow. Maximum inspiratory flow is usually the same as PEF in normal subjects, greater in COPD and less in some cases of central or upper airway obstruction.

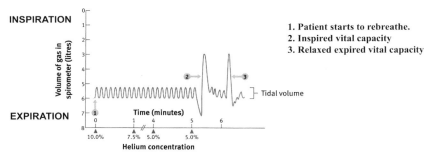

Fig. 2.2.3a Subdivisions of total lung capacity – measurement of static lung volumes by closed-circuit helium dilution. The patient rebreathes quietly from a spirometer of known volume initially containing about 10% helium, 21% oxygen and nitrogen. Oxygen is added as it is consumed and carbon dioxide removed to maintain a constant volume of gas. The test ends when the helium concentration ceases to fall. FRC is calculated using an equation which depends on the fact that the amount of helium is constant though its concentration falls as it diffuses into the lungs. [ ] denote concentrations. [Initial helium] × initial spirometer volume = (Initial spirometer volume + FRC) × [final helium]. In this example (emphysema) FRC = 6(10 5)/5 = 6 litres. Residual volume (RV) is derived by measuring a full expiration from FRC. After this a full inspiration yields the inspired vital capacity (IVC) and thence total lung capacity (TLC). In patients with airflow obstruction IVC is usually greater than FVC and relaxed expired VC. In this example IVC = 4.25, EVC 3.5, TLC = 9, the best estimate of RV = 4.75 litres. For abbreviations see text and Fig. 2.2.3a.

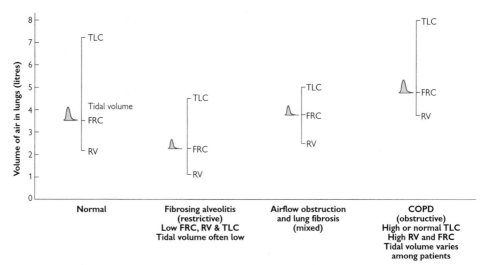

Fig. 2.2.3b Static lung volumes in obstructive and restrictive disorders.

Static lung volumes

The volume of air in the lungs can be measured by:
- Insoluble gas analysis, e.g. helium dilution. The subject is connected to a closed circuit of known volume containing helium. Oxygen is supplied and carbon dioxide absorbed. The helium concentration falls by an amount which reflects the volume of the lung. A similar test involves plotting the change of expired nitrogen concentration when an oxygen-rich mixture is inhaled.
- Body plethysmography. The subject sits in a closed booth ('body box', plethysmograph) of known volume and breathes in and out against a closed tube for a few seconds. According to Boyle's Law the ratio of the pressures in the mouth and around the subject is determined by the ratio of the volumes of the lungs and the box.

Both these methods measure *functional residual capacity (FRC)*: the volume of air at the end of a quiet expiration.
- FRC is reduced when the elasticity of the lungs is increased, e.g. in lung fibrosis; it is increased when the elastic recoil is reduced, as in emphysema. In health, the respiratory muscles are inactive at FRC. In airflow obstruction the need to take another breath may be felt while the patient is still exhaling. This phenomenon is known as dynamic hyperinflation and occurs mainly in exercise and during exacerbations of asthma and in COPD. Dynamic hyperinflation is important because the work of breathing and the sensation of respiratory effort increase markedly at high lung volumes
- RV: *residual volume* is the volume of air in the lungs after a full expiration. As stated before, it is increased when the lungs fail to empty because of airway obstruction. It is reduced when the lung volumes are small; a fall of RV without any other abnormality may occur early in the course of interstitial pulmonary fibrosis or granulomatous disease.
- TLC: *total lung capacity* is the volume of air in the lungs at full inspiration. Inspiration is maximal when the lungs are at full stretch. It follows that TLC is increased when lung elasticity is lost, as in emphysema, and reduced when

there is lung fibrosis. Removal of lung tissue leaving normal lung in place causes only a slight fall of TLC because the healthy lung can expand to compensate.
- ERV: *expiratory reserve volume* is the difference between FRC and RV. It is reduced in obesity; obese subjects breathe at low lung volumes and this accounts for the ease with which they develop low arterial oxygen levels if the breath is held
- IC: *inspiratory capacity* is the volume that can be inhaled from FRC to TLC. It can be measured using a portable spirometer and is used to identify dynamic hyperinflation. The test is helpful because TLC usually does not vary very much in individual cases of asthma and COPD, while any situation which increases the rate of breathing tends to cause the resting lung volume to increase.

Ways of assessing changes in airflow obstruction without maximal effort
- *Total airways resistance* can be determined by measuring the flow at the lips during quiet breathing and estimating the pressure difference between the pleura and the mouth. Resistance is normally low and it requires little physical effort to achieve the relatively low flow rates required during tidal breathing; greater pressure differences are required if all or some of the airways are narrowed. Resistance can be measured directly with the subject breathing normally while seated in a closed body plethysmograph. The higher the resistance to the flow of air in the airways, the greater is the pressure swing in the box because the flow of air in and out of the lungs is impeded. Flow at the mouth is measured at the same time; resistance can be calculated as pressure swing/flow rate.
- *Resistance and impedance of the lung* can be estimated during quiet breathing by a commercial device which generates pressure waves at the mouth using a loudspeaker. The flow waves that result depend on the resistance to flow and the elasticity of the lungs and airways. The test is easy to apply and repeatable and the concept

is quite simple but the assumptions and calculations are complex and the results are not directly comparable to other measurements.

Response to bronchodilators and bronchoconstrictors

The response of FEV_1 and other measures of airflow obstruction to bronchodilators is measured routinely, without any consensus as to how this should be performed or interpreted. It is mainly used to identify untreated asthma, when dramatic improvements of 0.5 litres or more may be seen after only 200 mcg of inhaled salbutamol. Disappointingly there is no test which identifies asthma in the presence of COPD. An improvement of 15% or 0.4 litres (the greater) after 2.5 mg nebulised salbutamol points towards some potential for reversibility, but current guidelines emphasise the need for several days of therapy rather than a single laboratory test to assess this potential. In COPD, post-bronchodilator FEV_1 and VC vary less than pre-bronchodilator readings and should ideally be used to measure changes of lung function over time in longitudinal studies of obstructive disorders.

Bronchial challenges with histamine, methacholine, cold air or intensive exercise are used to confirm asthma in individuals with normal resting spirometric tests. Asthmatic subjects react to pharmacological bronchoconstrictors with a 20% fall of FEV_1 at a much lower dose than non-reactive individuals.

Diffusing capacity (synonym transfer factor) of the lung for carbon monoxide (D_Lco)

Carbon monoxide (CO) combines avidly with haemoglobin. The uptake of a trace of CO can therefore be used to measure the capacity of the whole lung to transfer CO from inspired air to haemoglobin and thus assess the integrity of the gas-exchanging function of the whole lung. In practice the single breath breath-holding test is commonly used and normal values are available for many populations (see Fig. 2.2.4).

The patient inhales from full expiration from a reservoir containing a trace of CO (0.03%), about 10% helium (or other non-absorbed gas) and 16–20% oxygen. Helium dilution is used to measure the accessible volume of alveolar gas (V_A). Carbon monoxide is both diluted and absorbed, thus:

inspired[CO]/expired[CO] is greater than inspired[He]/expired[He]; i.e. the ratio of CO uptake to helium dilution (CO ratio) >1. It is assumed that CO is absorbed exponentially during the period of breath-holding; because Pco is zero in the pulmonary blood the pressure gradient is the alveolar pressure of the gas. Therefore:

$D_Lco = V_A$ × loge(CO ratio) × (1/breath-holding time) × (1/dry barometric pressure). The units are CO uptake per unit time per pressure unit difference from alveolar gas to blood, corrected to 0 deg C and dry.

D_Lco/V_A is calculated by dividing D_Lco by V_A measured at body temperature and pressure, saturated with water vapour.

The amount of CO extracted depends on:

The *diffusing capacity of the alveolar membrane*, comprising:
- The area of the gas exchanging surface of the lung.
- The thickness of the alveolar capillary barrier.

The *pulmonary capillary blood volume* (the volume of haemoglobin in contact with the inhaled gas).

D_Lco depends mainly on alveolar function except:
- When the airways are abnormal and a deep breath is not evenly distributed to all parts of the lung.
- When the concentration of haemoglobin in the red cells is not normal.

There are two ways of reporting diffusing capacity. D_Lco is the rate of uptake of CO per unit of alveolar Pco in the whole lung. In some situations it can be helpful to divide this by the lung volume; this yields an index known as diffusion

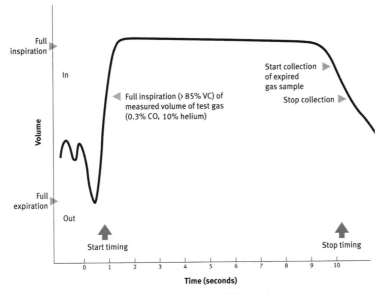

Fig. 2.2.4 Measurement of CO diffusing capacity by the single breath breath-holding method.

or transfer coefficient D_L/V_A. In practice both are useful in separate situations.

The calculation of $D_{L}co$ assumes that regional variations of ventilation, perfusion and diffusion are averaged out. In patients with respiratory failure severe ventilation–perfusion mismatching can result in marked abnormalities of CO_2 and O_2 exchange when $D_{L}co$ is normal. Conversely, a low $D_{L}co$ is compatible with a normal resting arterial Po_2. Oxygen exchange in exercise is invariably abnormal when $D_{L}co$ is low.

Interpretation of $D_{L}co$

$D_{L}co$ and D_L/V_A are useful clinically in a number of situations.
- When VC, FEV_1, FVC and [Hb] are all normal, **a low DLco strongly suggests disease involving the alveoli**.
- In airflow obstruction a low $D_{L}co$ and $D_{L}co/V_A$ suggest alveolar destruction (emphysema). In contrast, they are sometimes abnormally high in asthma.
- In restrictive pleural and chest wall disease, a high $D_{L}co/V_A$ suggests that there is no underlying lung disease.
- When there are widespread radiological lung shadows, such as in sarcoidosis or some occupational lung diseases, $D_{L}co$ reflects lung impairment and disability but is not correlated directly with the extent of the abnormality on the plain CXR.
- Polycythaemia, pulmonary plethora such as in heat failure or left-to-right shunting and pulmonary haemorrhage cause an increase in $D_{L}co$ because of increases in the volume of haemoglobin in contact with the inspired air.

Practice points: frequently asked questions

What are reference (normal) values?

Lung volumes and diffusing capacity are dependent on height, age, sex, and sometimes influenced by body mass. There are substantial published racial differences. The most striking of these is the relatively lower lung volumes seen in those of black African descent; their higher diffusing capacity and coefficient result in an overall advantage in athletics. A reading of 1.64 standardised residual deviations from the predicted population mean can be interpreted as abnormal in that only 5% of a healthy population will be below this reading; greater deviations obviously can be interpreted with greater confidence. The use of '% predicted' is helpful in giving a feel for the size and shape of the lungs and in tables describing the abnormalities found among groups of patients with specific disorders. The common assumption that 80% usually defines the lower limit of normal is highly misleading and often leads to over-reporting of abnormalities.

COPD guidelines use FEV_1/FVC rather than FEV_1/VC; does this matter?

Physiologists prefer FEV_1/VC because it is a better diagnostic tool. In obstructive diseases, FVC almost always underestimates VC even if care is taken to continue the breath for the full 14 sec. Forcing expiration causes more airway closure and true residual volume is easier to each with a relaxed expiration. In normal subjects FVC is the same as VC or better according to the equipment used. When both are measured, FEV_1/vital capacity is the taken to be the lower of the estimates. However, most COPD guidelines have employed FEV_1/FVC for simplicity. In most healthy subjects this ratio is greater than 70%. 14 sec forced expirations are uncomfortable. 6-sec readings of FVC, yielding FEV_1/FEV_6, are receiving increasing attention; the lower limit of normal being 73%.

Why are D_L/VA (diffusion or transfer coefficient) and $D_{L}co$ both used?

As shown in the calculation, diffusing capacity is the product of the diffusion coefficient (uptake per litre of lung volume) and the lung volume at which the measurement was made. In normal subjects the pulmonary capillary blood is distributed to the alveoli which are ventilated; as a result the diffusion coefficient is much higher than in full inspiration. As the lung volume is increased the coefficient falls but proportionally less than the rise of lung volume. Therefore, overall, diffusing capacity is higher near TLC. When TLC is high, as in pulmonary emphysema, D_L/V_A is found to be more sensitive to changes in pulmonary vascularity than $D_{L}co$. In restrictive alveolar diseases such as advanced pulmonary fibrosis, diffusing capacity is low but the coefficient D_L/V_A is usually within or near normal limits. If it were not, the gas exchanging capacity might be insufficient to sustain life. When restriction to inspiration is caused by pleural or chest wall disease, without lung disease, transfer coefficient is high as it is in normal subjects who have taken an incomplete inspiration; this can be used to help determine whether there is underlying lung disease.

Further reading

Hughes JMB, Pride NB. (eds). *Lung Function Tests: Physiological Principles and Clinical Applications.* London: Saunders, 1999.

MacIntyre N, Crapo RO, Viegi G, et al. Standardisation of the single-breath determination of carbon monoxide uptake in the lung. *Eur Resp J* 2005; **26**: 720–735.

Miller MR, Crapo RO, Hankinson J, et al. General considerations for lung function testing. *Eur Resp J* 2005; **26**: 153–161.

Miller MR, Hankinson J, Brusaco V, et al. Standardisation of spirometry. *Eur Resp J* 2005; **26**: 319–338.

Pellegrino R, Viegi G, Brusaco V, et al. Interpretative strategies for lung function tests. *Eur Resp J* 2005; **26**: 948–968.

Wanger J, Clausen JL, Coates A, et al. Standardisation of the measurement of lung volumes. *Eur Resp J* 2005; **26**: 511–522.

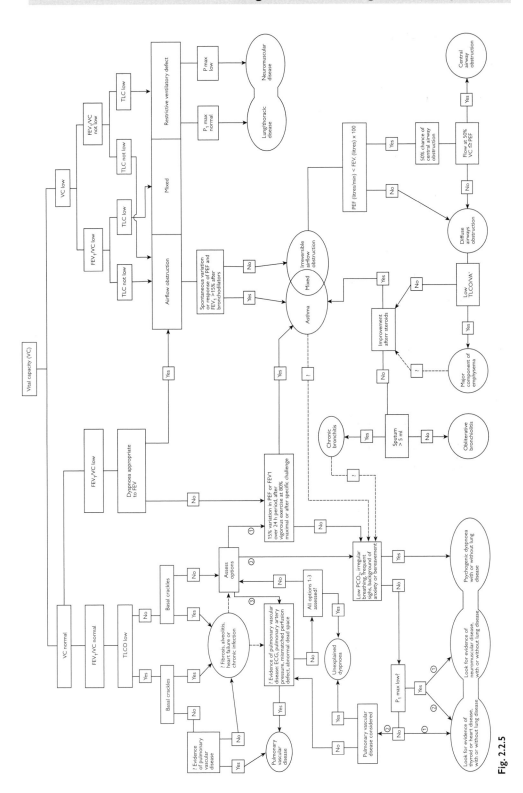

Fig. 2.2.5

2.3 Exercise testing

The ability to exercise largely depends on the efficiency of the integrated physiologic responses of the cardiovascular and respiratory systems to couple the metabolic needs of contracting skeletal muscles. In healthy subjects, exercise tolerance is largely influenced by age, gender, level of day life activity and fitness. In patients with heart or lung diseases, exercise tolerance is limited by symptoms (e.g. dyspnoea, leg fatigue) caused by abnormal cardiovascular, ventilatory and metabolic responses to exercise load.

The causes of exercise intolerance can classified as 'central' (e.g. ventilatory limitation, circulatory limitation) and 'peripheral' (e.g. muscle dysfunction). In patients with chronic pulmonary or heart diseases, central and peripheral abnormalities often co-exist.

> The principal causes of reduced exercise tolerance that can be ruled out at cardiopulmonary exercise testing (CPET) are the following:
> - Reduced oxygen (O_2) delivery to exercising muscles.
> - Ventilatory limitation to exercise.
> - Pulmonary gas exchange abnormalities.
> - Muscle dysfunction including deconditioning.
> - Excessive perception of symptoms.

Protocols and variables

CPET is considered the gold standard for evaluating the causes of exercise intolerance in lung and heart diseases.

CPET comprises the imposition of symptom-limited incremental exercise in combination with comprehensive breath-by-breath monitoring of cardiopulmonary variables (e.g. ventilation (V'_E), heart rate (HR), oxygen uptake ($V'O_2$), CO_2 output ($V'CO_2$)), perceptual responses (e.g. dyspnoea, leg discomfort) and, as needed, measurements such as exercise-related arterial O_2 desaturation, dynamic hyperinflation and limb-muscle strength.

> **AUTHOR'S TIP**
> There are some CPET response patterns (e.g. ventilatory limitation, circulatory limitation) that are not disease-specific but point to particular sites of system dysfunction, narrowing the differential diagnosis. The absence of these response patterns can be taken as evidence against a significant involvement of these systems in the exercise limitation.

The classical criterion for defining exercise intolerance and classifying degrees of impairment is $V'O_2$ peak standardised by body mass ($mlV'O_2$/min/kg). Values below 80% predicted should be considered abnormal while values below 40% of the predicted indicate severe impairment.

Walking tests, such as the 6-minute walking test (6MWT) and the 'shuttle' walking test, are increasingly utilised for the assessment of exercise tolerance in chronic diseases; measurement of arterial O_2 saturation by pulse oxymetry (SpO_2), HR and exertional symptoms are recommended during these tests.

Protocols: key points

- *CPET*. It is a symptom-limited incremental protocol, performed on a cycle ergometer or on a treadmill. Work rate is increased every minute or in a ramp fashion.

Suggested exercise duration: 10–12 minutes. Pulmonary gas exchange should be measured breath-by-breath. EKG and blood pressure are monitored. Symptoms (e.g. dyspnoea and leg fatigue) are recorded at the end of exercise by the use of dedicated scales (e.g. Borg scale).

- *Constant work rate (CWR)*. CWR protocols, on a cycle ergometer or on a treadmill, are utilised for the measurement of exercise 'endurance' tolerance, pulmonary gas exchange kinetics, arterial blood gases and flow-volumes curves during exercise. CWR exercise results in steady-state responses when work rate is of moderate intensity (i.e. below the lactate threshold, θ_L); conversely, high intensity CWR exercise (i.e. above the θ_L) results in continually changing in most physiologic variables.

- *6MWT*. The object of this test is to walk as far as possible for 6 minutes. The test should be performed indoors along a 30 m long, flat, straight corridor; encouragement significantly increase the distance walked.

- *Safety*. Careful selection of patients prevents serious complications during maximal incremental exercise. Myocardial infarction (within 3–5 days), unstable angina, severe arrhythmias, pulmonary embolism, dissecting aneurism, respiratory failure, and severe aortic stenosis represent absolute contraindication to CPET.

Variables: key points

- *$V'O_2$-work rate relationship ($\Delta V'O_2/\Delta WR$)*. In normal subjects, the slope of the linear phase from 'unloaded pedaling' to peak cycle ergometer exercise is ~9–12 ml/min/watt. This index is used as an approximate index of work efficiency. $\Delta V'O_2/\Delta WR$ is relatively independent of age, gender, fitness and body mass.

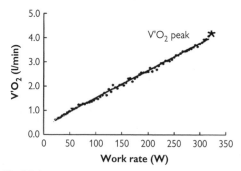

Fig. 2.3.1

- *$V'O2$ peak*. Is the highest $V'O_2$ value (ml/min or corrected for body mass, ml/min/kg) measured at peak exercise. With good subject effort, $V'O_2$ peak reflects subject's maximal aerobic capacity ('maximum' $V'O_2$). This index is taken to reflect the attainment of a limitation in the O_2 conductance pathway from the lungs to the mitochondria.

- *Lactic threshold (θL)*. The lactate threshold is the highest WR or $V'O_2$ at which arterial lactate is not systematically increased; it is considered an important functional demarcator of exercise intensity. Sub-θ_L work rates can normally be sustained for prolonged periods. θ_L is dependent on age, gender, body mass and fitness.

Non-invasive estimation of θ_L requires the demonstration of an augmented $V'CO_2$ in excess of that produced by aerobic metabolism.

- *Ventilatory equivalents for CO_2.* Measured as the slope of the increase of V'_E over $V'CO_2$ ($\Delta V'_E/\Delta V'CO_2$) from 'unloaded pedalling' to the respiratory compensation point (RCP) or as the value at θ_L ($\Delta V'_E/\Delta V'CO_2$ @ θ_L). It is considered a non invasive index of 'ventilatory efficiency'. In normal individuals $\Delta V'_E/\Delta V'CO_2$ values of ~25–28 have been reported. Several factors may increase ventilatory response to exercise, namely hypoxemia, acidosis, increased levels of wasted ventilation and pulmonary hypertension.
- *Breathing reserve (BR).* BR provides an index of the proximity of the ventilation at the limit of tolerance (V'_E max) to the maximal achievable ventilation (MVV, estimated from the subject's resting FEV_1 x 40). BR can be defined as V'_E max as a percentage of MVV (i.e. $1-V'_E$ max/MVV). In chronic lung diseases BR is reduced or absent at peak CPET exercise.
- *Dynamic hyperinflation (DH).* In normal subjects end-expiratory lung volume (EELV) decreases with increasing WR by as much as 0.5–1.0 litres below functional residual capacity (FRC). Changes in EELV during exercise can be estimated by asking the subject to perform an inspiratory capacity (IC) manoeuvre at a selected point in the exercise test. In obstructive lung diseases, such as chronic obstructive pulmonary disease (COPD), EELV increases during exercise in spite of expiratory muscle activity.
- *Arterial O_2 desaturation.* During exercise arterial O_2 saturation (SpO_2) is maintained in the region of 97–98%. However, it is not uncommon for highly-fit endurance athletes and women to exhibit arterial desaturation at peak exercise. Arterial oxygen desaturation can be observed in patients with moderate–severe interstitial lung disease (ILD) and in patients with primary pulmonary hypertension (PPH). A more pronounced arterial O_2 desaturation as been reported during walking compared to cycling in patients with COPD.
- *T_{LIM} and 'isotime' measurements.* T_{LIM} is the tolerable limit of exercise, expressed as function of time (e.g. minutes) measured during CWR protocols. In clinical practice high intensity (~80% watt max) CWR protocols are utilised for the evaluation of interventions. In addition to T_{LIM}, measurement of pertinent physiologic variables (e.g. V'_E, IC, dyspnoea) at standardised time ('isotime') are obtained.

Exercise testing in clinical practice

Evaluation of heart and lung functional reserves measured at rest (e.g. spirometry, lung diffusion for CO, echocardiography) do not allow accurate prediction of the level of exercise tolerance in health and disease states such as COPD and chronic heart failure (CHF). Importantly, exercise intolerance predicts poor prognosis in chronic diseases. Well established indications for exercise testing are the diagnosis of myocardial ischaemia and exercise-induced bronchoconstriction. In the last decade, however, exercise testing has been increasingly utilised for the functional and prognostic evaluation of patients with chronic lung and heart diseases and for the evaluation of the effects of interventions. CPET variables as well as distance covered during walking tests have proven to be useful in the functional and prognostic evaluation of patients with COPD, CHF, ILD, PPH and cystic fibrosis (CF).

The principal indications to exercise testing in clinical practice are the following:
1 Provide an objective measure of exercise capacity.
2 Identify the mechanisms limiting exercise tolerance.
3 Establish indices of the patient's prognosis.
4 Monitor disease progression and/or the response to interventions.

AUTHOR'S TIPS

- $V'O_2$ peak, θ_L, oxygen pulse ($V'O_2/HR$), BR, $\Delta V'_E/\Delta V'CO_2$, DH, SpO_2 are the exercise variables/indexes that have been shown to be particularly useful in the functional and prognostic evaluation of patients with chronic heart and lung diseases.
- $V'O_2$ peak values of <14 ml/min/kg, $V'O_2$ values at θ_L of <11 ml/min/kg and $\Delta V'E/\Delta V'CO_2$ slopes of >34 all suggest poor prognosis in patients with CHF $V'O_2$ peak has also been utilised as a prognostic variable in patients with COPD, ILD, CF and PPH.
- High intensity CWR tests, performed on a cycle ergometer or on a treadmill, to the T_{LIM} seems to provide the best information on the effects of therapeutic interventions.

Further reading

ATS/ACCP Statement on cardiopulmonary exercise testing. *Am J Respir Crit Care Med* 2003; **167**: 211–277.

ATS statement: guidelines for the six-minute walking test. *Am J Respir Crit Care Med* 2002; **166**: 111–117.

Beaver WL, Wasserman K, Whipp BJ. A new method for detecting the anaerobic threshold by gas exchange. *J Appl Physiol* 1986; **60**: 2020–2027.

Casaburi R, Kukafka D, Cooper CB, et al. Improvement in exercise tolerance with the combination of tiotropium and pulmonary rehabilitation in patients with COPD. *Chest* 2005; **127**: 809–817.

ERS task force on standardisation of clinical exercise testing. Clinical exercise testing with reference to lung diseases: indications, standardisation and interpretation strategies. *Eur Resp J* 1997; **10**: 2662–2689.

Gitt AK, Wasserman K, Kilkowski C, et al. Exercise anaerobic threshold and ventilatory efficiency identify heart failure patients for high risk of early death. *Circulation* 2002; **106**: 3079–3084.

Myers J, Prakash M, Froelicher V, et al. Exercise capacity and mortality among men referred for exercise testing. *N Engl J Med* 2002; **347**: 288–90.

O'Donnell DE, Revill SM, Webb KA. Dynamic hyperinflation and exercise intolerance in chronic obstructive pulmonary disease. *Am J Respir Crit Care Med* 2001; **164**: 770–777.

O'Donnell DE, Fluge T, Gerken F, et al. Effects of tiotropium on lung hyperinflation, dyspnoea and exercise tolerance in COPD. *Eur Respir J* 2004; **23**: 832–840.

Oga T, Nishimura K, Tsukino M, et al. The effects of oxitropium bromide on exercise performance in patients with stable chronic obstructive pulmonary disease. A comparison of three different exercise tests. *Am J Respir Crit Care Med* 2000; **161**: 1897–1901.

Palange P, Crimi E, Pellegrino R, et al. Supplemental oxygen and heliox: 'new' tools for exercise training in chronic pulmonary diseases. *Curr Opin Pulm Med* 2005; **11**: 145–148.

Palange P, Valli G, Onorati P, et al. Effect of heliox on lung dynamic hyperinflation, dyspnoea, and exercise endurance capacity in COPD patients. *J Appl Physiol* 2004; **97**: 1637–1642.

Palange P, Forte S, Onorati P, et al. Ventilatory and metabolic adaptation to walking and cycling in patients with COPD. *J Appl Physiol* 2000; **88**: 1715–1720.

Palange P, Ward SA, Carlsen K-H, et al. Recommendations on the use of exercise testing in clinical practice. *Eur Respir J* 2007; **27**: 529–41.

Singh SJ, Morgan MDL, Scott S, et al. Development of a shuttle walking test of disability in chronic airways obstruction. *Thorax* 1992; **47**: 1019–1024.

Wasserman K, Hansen JE, Sue DY, et al. *Principles of Exercise Testing and Interpretation*, 4th edn. Philadelphia: Lea & Febiger, 2004.

2.4 Interpretation of arterial blood gases and acid/base balance

This chapter describes a simple approach to interpreting PaO_2, $PaCO_2$, pH, and Hb, as obtained from standard blood gas machines. The information is divided into what can be learnt about gas exchange, and what can be learnt about acid/base balance. Considering that only four numbers are actually measured by blood gas machines (the rest are calculated), a considerable amount of information can be derived.

Interpretation of arterial blood gases–gas exchange

Normal ranges
Breathing air:
$PaO_2 > 12$ kPa (>10 kPa in normal elderly), $PaCO_2$ 4.6–5.9 kPa.

How to take an arterial sample
Arterial blood gases are best taken from the radial, rather than the brachial, artery due to the dual radial/ulnar supply to the hand. Occasionally the radial and ulnar arteries do not anastomise in the hand and damage to the radial artery can lead to infarction of the thumb and first finger. In reality this is not a problem if fine needles (22 or 23G) are used to sample the arterial blood, but is an issue when an indwelling radial artery cannula is to be inserted. The presence of an adequate anastamosis can be proven by pressure occlusion of the radial and ulnar arteries, while asking the patient to make a tight fist (to squeeze out blood from the superficial capillaries), then release the pressure on the ulnar artery and show that the whole palm becomes pink again within a few seconds, despite continuing radial artery pressure (Allen test). Cock the wrist back, use quick vertical penetration of the skin (to lessen pain), followed by slower penetration down to the artery at a slight angle along the line of the artery towards the elbow. Use a specific heparinised syringe designed for arterial use which should only self fill if in the artery. Analyse immediately, or within 30 minutes if kept cool on ice. Always record date, time, and the % inspired O_2 (FiO_2) during sampling.

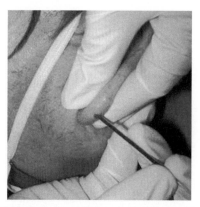

Fig. 2.4.1 Taking an arterialised sample of capillary blood from an earlobe.

An alternative is an arterialised capillary sample, an underused technique. This technique utilises a small glass preheparinised tube to draw up blood milked from a lancet puncture on the end of the ear lobe (Fig. 2.4.1). Some units

use a small magnetic 'flea' in the tube to mix the blood with the heparin, by sliding an external magnet up and down the tube immediately after obtaining the sample. The blood gas machine must be able to take microsamples (most do). Although the sample is only an 'arterialised' capillary sample, and not pure arterial, $PaCO_2$ levels are accurate enough for clinical practice. However, with good arterialisation, with rubefacients (Algipan™/Deep Heat™) or heat and vigorous rubbing, a reasonably accurate PaO_2 is obtainable: the accuracy of the latter is less important as arterial oxygenation can also be assessed by oximetry. This ear lobe technique is easily performed by nursing staff, for example, to monitor $PaCO_2$ response to non-invasive ventilation (NIV) and O_2 therapy.

The three main things blood gases tell you about gas exchange.

1 How much is the patient ventilating their alveoli? This is derived from the $PaCO_2$. $PaCO_2 \geq 6$ kPa is due to underventilating the alveoli, $PaCO_2 \leq 4.5$ kPa is due to overventilating the alveoli. This is not the same as total ventilation, which includes dead-space of course.

2 Is the PaO_2 high enough to adequately oxygenate tissues and thus prevent anaerobic metabolism? $PaO_2 > 6$ kPa ($SaO_2 \approx 80\%$) is probably adequate; $PaO_2 > 7$ kPa ($SaO_2 \approx 87\%$) is definitely adequate.

3 Is there any evidence of V/Q mismatch? Evidence of low V/Q units is derived from the calculated alveolar to arterial (A–a) gradient for oxygen.

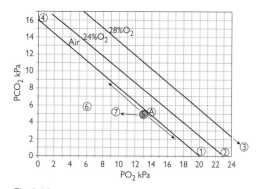

Fig. 2.4.2 Alveolar air line graph showing the graphical derivation of the A–a gradient for O_2.

The A–a gradient calculator graph (Fig. 2.4.2) sets out the graphical representation of gas exchange.
• Point ❶ = the pO_2 and pCO_2 of alveolar air. (Atmospheric pressure $\approx$ 100 kPa, water vapour pressure in warm/humified air $\approx$ 7 kPa, and 21% of (100 − 7) $\approx$ 20.)
• Point ❷ = the pO_2 and pCO_2 when breathing 24% O_2 via a Ventimask. (24% of (100 − 7) $\approx$ 23.)
• Point ❸ = the pO_2 and pCO_2 when breathing 28% O_2 via a Ventimask. (28% of (100 − 7) $\approx$ 26.)
• Point ❹ = the theoretical pO_2/pCO_2 of alveolar gas when breathing air, if all the O_2 were removed and replaced by CO_2 (equivalent to extreme hypoventilation and of course impossible!), when the respiratory quotient (RQ = CO_2 produced/O_2 consumed) is 0.8 (usual value).

- The line between ❶ and ❹ with a gradient of 0.8 describes all possible combinations of alveolar gas: moving towards ❶ if ventilating more, and towards ❹ is ventilating less - called the alveolar air line.
- Point ❺ = is the area in which PaO_2 and $PaCO_2$ of arterial blood normally sit. If the lungs are perfect gas exchangers, then blood leaving the lungs and entering the systemic arterial circulation (❺) should be perfectly equilibrated with the alveolar gas (A).
- Point ❻ = However, the mixed venous point (the pulmonary arterial blood) is well to the left of the alveolar air line, because capillary PO_2 falls more kPa (≈7) than the PCO_2 kPa rises (≈1 to 2) during gas exchange in the tissues (because the CO_2 solubility curve is steeper than the PaO_2/SaO_2 dissociation curve).
- If the lungs fail to oxygenate mixed venous blood properly (e.g. pneumonia, or low V/Q from asthma/COPD) then it is as if mixed venous blood has bypassed the lung and spilled into the systemic arterial blood, which therefore moves the eventual arterial $PaO_2/PaCO_2$ point to the left of the alveolar air line, point ❼.
- The horizontal distance that the actual arterial point is to the left of the 'ideal' alveolar air line is called the alveolar to arterial (A–a) gradient and is a measure of how efficiently mixed venous blood is being equilibrated with alveolar gas, i.e. it is a measure of V/Q mismatch and right-to-left shunts.

As well as being read from the graph, the A-a gradient can be calculated. The following formula essentially adds the RQ-corrected $PaCO_2$ to the PaO_2, and finds out how far away from the inspired PO_2 (PIO_2) this number is.

$$\underset{\text{*Inspired } PO_2}{\underset{\nearrow}{\text{Aa gradient}}} = PIO_2 - \underset{\text{Arterial } PO_2}{(\overset{\searrow}{PaO_2}} + \frac{\overset{\swarrow}{PaCO_2}}{\underset{\nwarrow}{0.8}})}$$

Arterial PO_2 Arterial PCO_2

Aa gradient = $PIO_2 - (PaO_2 + \dfrac{PaCO_2}{0.8})$

*Inspired PO_2 Respiratory quotient

*Calculation of inspired PO_2 breathing either air, 24% or 28% O_2:
Air: 21% of (100 − 7) ≈ 20 kPa, (where 100 kPa = atmospheric pressure, 7 kPa = H_2O vapour pressure)
24%: 24% of (100 − 7) ≈ 23 kPa
28%: 28% of (100 − 7) ≈ 26 kPa

On the graph, the position of the 'alveolar air' line depends on the inspired %O_2, and the two extra lines, for 24% and 28% O_2, are shown approximately. In the calculation the PIO_2 has to be adjusted accordingly, see above*.

In normal lungs, matching of V/Q is not totally perfect, and this is due to relative under-perfusion of the apices and over-perfusion of the bases (gravity effects on pulmonary arterial blood flow, not fully compensated for by hypoxic vasoconstriction of pulmonary arterioles). These imperfections in V/Q, and direct drainage of some of the cardiac muscle's venous blood into the left ventricular cavity (and thus systemic arterial circulation), lead to a small A–a gradient of 1 to 2 kPa in the young and middle aged, and 2 to 3 in the elderly. Figures in excess of these values are abnormal and indicate areas of low V/Q or increased right-to-left shunt.

Use of A–a gradient diagram: examples (Fig. 2.4.3)
Case 1. Consider point (W) in the pO_2/pCO_2 graph, the blood gases on air of a young non-smoker complaining of chest pain 7 days postop. The PaO_2 of 13 is normal; does this reassure you, or does it provide supporting evidence for a pulmonary embolus? $PaCO_2 = 2$. Ask the following questions:

- How much is the patient ventilating? $PaCO_2 ≤4.5$ kPa; therefore there is hyperventilation.
- Is the patient adequately oxygenated? $PaO_2 > 7$ kPa; therefore OK.
- Is there an abnormal A–a gradient? Measure the horizontal line between W and the alveolar line off the graph, or calculate:
$$20 - (13 + \frac{2}{0.8}) = 4.5 \text{ kPa}$$

>2 kPa, hence yes; the V/Q matching is not normal. This provides supporting evidence for a pulmonary embolus, but could also be due to consolidation from a pneumonia, for example. This makes the point that PaO_2 cannot be used to assess V/Q matching in the lung without an associated $PaCO_2$ to tell you 'what the PaO_2 ought to be'.

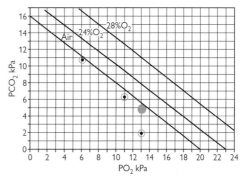

Fig. 2.4.3 Examples of the use of the A–a gradient for O_2 when interpreting blood gases.

Case 2. Consider point (X) on the pO_2/pCO_2 graph. These gases are on air from a young man following an overdose of methadone tablets, $PaO_2 = 6$, $PaCO_2 = 11$.

- How much is the patient ventilating? $PaCO_2 > 6$ kPa; therefore he is hypoventilating
- Is the patient adequately oxygenated? PaO_2 only 6 kPa, therefore no, he needs added O_2.
- Has the patient got an increased A–a gradient? Measure the horizontal line between X and the alveolar line off the graph, or calculate:
$$20 - (6 + \frac{11}{0.8}) = 0.8 \text{ kPa}$$

<2 kPa, hence no; therefore there is nothing wrong with the lungs, despite the abnormal gases, this therefore represents pure hypoventilation.

After a messy stomach wash-out he is sent to the ward and 24 h later is febrile. Blood gases on 24% O_2 are point (Y) on the graph, thus both $PaCO_2$ and PaO_2 are better.

- How much is the patient ventilating? $PaCO_2$ just >6 kPa; therefore is still hypoventilating a bit.

- Is the patient adequately oxygenated? $PaO_2 > 7$ kPa; therefore adequately oxygenated.
- Has the patient got an A–a gradient?

$$23 - (11 + \underline{6.5)} = 4.2 \text{ kPa}$$
$$\,\underline{Z}0.8$$

(23, not 20, because on 24% O_2, not air)

>2 kPa so yes; may now have an aspiration pneumonia.

Relationship between SaO_2 and PaO_2 – 'discrepancies' between oximetry and blood gases

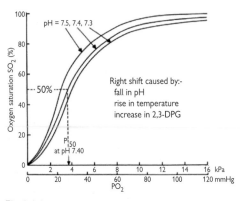

Fig. 2.4.4 Haemoglobin dissociation curve.

A fall in pH (more acidotic), or a rise in body temperature, will move the dissociation curve to the right. This has the effect of making the PaO_2 higher for any given SaO_2, e.g. at pH 7.20, a measured saturation (e.g. by oximetry) of 90% is equivalent to a higher PaO_2 of 9.7 kPa than the usual 7.7 kPa: a rise in body temperature to 41°C will do the same, and the effects of pH and temperature are additive.

Conversely, for a given PaO_2, pyrexia and acidosis will lower the SaO_2 and thus oxygen carriage to the tissues, e.g. a PaO_2 of 7.7 kPa will normally give an SaO_2 of 90%, but if the temperature rises to 41°C, and pH falls to 7.20, then the SaO_2 falls to 70%. Increasing 2,3-DPG levels shift the curve to the right, but levels fluctuate unpredictably and any changes are small.

Changes in body temperature are often the reason why measured pulse oximetry saturations apparently 'do not agree' with the measured blood gases (pH is taken into account in the theoretical calculation of SaO_2 by blood gas analysers, but the patient's correct body temperature is rarely entered and thus not taken into account). This is particularly important in hypothermia when the curve is left shifted leading to impaired oxygen unloading anyway. Furthermore, an apparently adequate oximetry reading can mask a low PaO_2, which will further lessen oxygen availability to the tissues (although somewhat mitigated by the reduced metabolic rate of hypothermic tissues).

Interpretation of arterial blood gases – acid/base balance

Normal ranges
pH 7.37–7.43 (H^+ 37–43 nmol/l), $PaCO_2$ 4.6–5.9 kPa, base excess ±3 mmol/l.

The two main things blood gases tell you about acid/base balance.

- What is the respiratory (or ventilatory) component to an abnormal pH? This is derived from the $PaCO_2$.
- What is the metabolic component to an abnormal pH? This is derived from the calculated standard base excess/deficit.

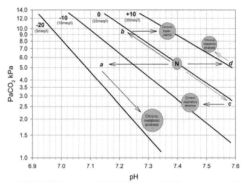

Fig. 2.4.5 Relationship between pH and $PaCO_2$ (log scale) with calculated iso $[HCO_3^-]$ lines added.

Interpretation of acid/base relationships are best plotted as a log $PaCO_2$ versus pH graph (Fig. 2.4.5), because these are the two primary measurements made by blood gas machines (everything else to do with acid/base balance, except the Hb, is calculated). Normality lies in the area labelled (N), the pH between 7.37 and 7.43, and the $PaCO_2$ around 5 kPa. As ventilation is decreased or increased ($PaCO_2$ going up or down respectively), the pH will change; the amount depends on the buffering capacity of the blood (CO_2 is an acid gas, combining with water to give $[H^+]$ and $[HCO_3^-]$ ions).

$$CO_2 + H_2O \leftrightarrow HCO_3^- + H^+$$

Removed by combination with Hb and other proteins

Following small rises in $PaCO_2$, the pH would fall disastrously without buffering of H^+ ions. This buffering capacity depends mainly on Hb (hence an estimate is made of Hb by the blood gas machine) and other proteins, producing the normal buffer line running through (N) on the graph (Fig. 2.4.5). This line would be much flatter without buffering.

Therefore acute hypoventilation and hyperventilation will move the patient up and down this line, in directions b or c, respectively. If hypoventilation at point b becomes chronic (e.g. as it may in COPD), then the kidney retains HCO_3^- (by excreting H^+) to try and correct the pH towards normal, and the patient moves onto a new iso HCO_3^- buffer line displaced to the right, e.g. the one labelled +10 meq/l (35 meq/l). The degree of displacement represents the metabolic component to the acid/base status and, in this case, because the $[HCO_3^-]$ has risen, will be higher than the normal figure of about 25 meq/l. When the raised figure is quoted relative to the normal 25 meq/l (by subtracting 25), this is called the 'base excess'. Thus buffer lines to the right of the normal buffer line represent a metabolic alkalosis or base excess.

These figures are calculated assuming a normal or 'standard' $PaCO_2$ (i.e. not using the patient's real value), called the 'standard bicarbonate' (SBC on the blood gas machine printout), or 'standard base excess' (usually SBE). Two other similar figures on some printouts (usually HCO_3^- and TCO_2) are calculated at the patient's actual $PaCO_2$ and are not much use. They will be higher when the real $PaCO_2$ is above normal (thus more HCO_3^- made), and lower when below normal, as HCO_3^- will fall having combined with H^+ to replace the CO_2.

Chronic hyperventilation (e.g. at altitude due to the hypoxia) produces the opposite, a resorption of $[H^+]$ by the kidney, and thus the buffer line shifts to the left giving a negative value for the 'base excess', a 'base deficit'. Thus a metabolic acidosis compensates for a respiratory alkalosis. Note that these homeostatic corrections do not bring the pH back to normal as there needs to be an error signal to keep the correction process going.

A metabolic acidosis (such as in ketoacidosis) will also move the line to the left (a), producing a base deficit (or negative base excess – a curious invention!), followed by hyperventilation to try and correct the pH (i.e. a respiratory alkalosis to correct a metabolic acidosis). This pure ventilatory stimulation in the absence of abnormal lungs often produces deep breathing with little increase in rate and is called Kussmaul's breathing. Thus lines to the left of the normal buffer line represent a metabolic acidosis or base deficit.

A metabolic acidosis due to anaerobic metabolism (and hence lactic acid production) can reverse the compensatory metabolic alkalosis secondary to chronic hypercapnia during a severely hypoxic COPD exacerbation, removing the evidence for chronic CO_2 retention. Thus a fall in pH during a COPD exacerbation reflects not only impaired alveolar ventilation (increased airways obstruction) but also reduced PaO_2 (anaerobic metabolism) – hence a low pH is the best guide to how sick such a patient is.

Finally, metabolic alkalosis e.g. during hypokalaemia (when the kidney is forced to use H^+ ions, instead of potassium ions, to swap for the sodium that needs resorbing from the tubular fluid, $[H^+]$ is lost in the urine and HCO_3^- returned to the blood). This will move the buffer line to the right (d), but only limited hypoventilation is available to compensate, due to the inevitable ventilatory stimulation that the attendant hypoxaemia produces.

Thus the mixture of respiratory and metabolic contributions to a patient's acid/base disturbance can be established by plotting the $PaCO_2$ and pH on the graph (Fig. 2.4.5).

Anion gap

The anion gap $[(Na^+ + K^+) - (Cl^- + HCO_3^-)]$ shows you the amount of other anions, apart from $Cl^- + HCO_3^-$, that

exist, and helps differentiate the cause of any metabolic acidosis. Depending on methods of measurement, the normal value is between 8 and 16mmol/l (or meq/l) and mainly due to albumin. A high anion gap indicates that there is loss of HCO_3^- without a subsequent increase in Cl^-. Electroneutrality is maintained by the increase in anions such as ketones, lactate, PO_4^-, and SO_4^-. Because these anions are not part of the anion-gap calculation a high anion gap results.

An acidosis with a normal anion gap will be a simple HCO_3^-/Cl^- exchange such as might occur, for example, in:
- renal tubular acidosis;
- acetazolamide therapy;
- HCO_3^- loss from profuse diarrhoea.

An anion gap is likely to be present, for example, when the metabolic acidosis is due to:
- diabetic ketoacidosis (ketones are acids);
- renal failure (although can be in the normal range too);
- lactic acidosis;
- salicylate poisoning;
- methanol poisoning;
- ethylene glycol (antifreeze) poisoning.

AUTHOR'S TIPS

There are only **three** main things to think about when assessing **gas exchange**:
- How much is the patient ventilating their alveoli?
- Is the PaO_2 high enough to adequately oxygenate tissues and thus prevent anaerobic metabolism?
- Is there any evidence of a V/Q mismatch, assessed from the A–a gradient for oxygen?

There are only **three** main things to think about when assessing **acid/base**:
- Is there a ventilatory/respiratory contribution from an abnormally high or low $PaCO_2$?
- Is there a metabolic component evidenced by a shift of the buffer line to the left or right, numerically the base excess (or deficit)?
- If there is an acidosis, is there an increased anion gap?

Further reading

Williams AJ. http://www.bmj.com/cgi/content/full/317/7167/1213

2.5 Respiratory muscle function

Overview of function

- The respiratory muscles ventilate the lungs with a pumping action that is as significant as that of the heart. The most important inspiratory muscle is the diaphragm. Contraction of diaphragm muscle fibres leads to downward movement of the dome of the diaphragm with outward movement of the lower chest wall. This generates negative intrathoracic pressure, drawing air down a pressure gradient from mouth to alveoli.
- Exhalation is predominantly a passive phenomenon: as the inspiratory muscles relax, lung elastic recoil causes air to move out of the lungs.
- As ventilatory requirements rise during exercise, the accessory inspiratory muscles are recruited. The external intercostals muscles assist inspiration by raising the lower ribs up and out, increasing the anterior-posterior diameter of the thoracic cavity. The scalene and sternomastoid muscles raise the upper ribs and the sternum.
- During active expiration and coughing, the most important muscles are those of the abdominal wall. By increasing intra-abdominal pressure when they contract, they push up the diaphragm raising intrathoracic pressure above atmospheric pressure, expelling air from the lungs.
- The internal intercostals assist active expiration by pulling the ribs down and in, thus decreasing thoracic volume.

> **AUTHOR'S TIPS**
>
> - Consider respiratory muscle weakness in unexplained breathlessness.
> - In generalised neuromuscular disease the respiratory muscles are usually affected and ventilatory failure may develop insidiously.

Why are the respiratory muscles important?

Any disease affecting the motor nerves or striated muscles can affect the respiratory muscle pump as can any condition requiring increased effort to ventilate the lungs. There is increasing awareness that respiratory muscle weakness compounds malnutrition, steroid therapy, heart failure, COPD and delayed weaning from mechanical ventilation in intensive care. Respiratory muscle weakness is often overlooked as a cause of breathlessness or poor cough, despite wide availability of techniques that can detect respiratory muscle weakness and quantify its severity.

Ventilatory assistance can support respiration during acute episodes of respiratory muscle weakness (e.g. polio, Guillain–Barré syndrome). Patients with chronic respiratory muscle impairment can be supported with a variety of techniques to assist ventilation (e.g. non-invasive positive pressure ventilation, negative pressure 'iron-lung' ventilation)

It is therefore important for respiratory physicians to initiate and interpret simple tests of respiratory muscle function when appropriate.

Causes of respiratory muscle weakness

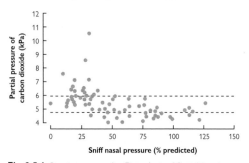

Fig. 2.5.1 Respiratory muscles. Data obtained from 81 patients with motor neuron disease Source: Lyall R *et al.*, Brain 2001; **124**: 2000–13. Respiratory failure. Medicine 2004. The Medicine Publishing Company.

Approach to the patient

History and examination

Dyspnoea that is unexplained by other cardio-respiratory factors, particularly if combined with orthopnoea or dyspnoea when partly submerged in water, should induce suspicion of respiratory muscle weakness. However, patients with generalised weakness may have limited mobility, so exertional dyspnoea may only manifest at a late stage. If respiratory muscle weakness is severe or there is increased work of breathing due to obesity or other thoracic pathology, symptoms of ventilatory failure may develop: daytime somnolence, poor concentration, morning headaches, peripheral oedema.

Evidence of generalised neuromuscular disease, e.g. wasting and fasciculation, or features characteristic of specific conditions, e.g. myxoedema, dystrophia myotonica may be present. Inspiratory muscle weakness leads to reduced tidal volume and tachypnoea. Accessory muscle action may be required to maintain ventilation and may be apparent.

Patients with bilateral diaphragm weakness will develop orthopnoea and paradoxical inward movement of the abdominal wall during inspiration as diaphragm strength falls to about 25% of normal. Weakness of bulbar and expiratory muscles may impair speech, swallowing and cough, predisposing to aspiration and pneumonia.

Lung function

The usual lung function abnormality is a restrictive defect with a low VC and reduced TLC. In patients with diaphragm weakness the VC falls when supine. A fall of >25% when moving from standing to supine is considered unequivocally abnormal. The demonstration of a normal supine VC indicates that a patient does not have clinically significant inspiratory muscle weakness.

If there is no pre-existing pulmonary condition the diffusion coefficient (KCO) will be normal or slightly increased. Because alveolar volume is decreased, carbon monoxide diffusing capacity (TLCO) is also decreased.

Overnight oximetry with transcutaneous CO_2 may be useful as demonstration of nocturnal hypoventilation signifies that respiratory muscle weakness is severe enough to lead to ventilatory failure.

Imaging

A chest radiograph showing small lungs may indicate inspiratory muscle weakness, a raised hemi-diaphragm may be due to a phrenic nerve lesion causing hemi-diaphragm paralysis. Ultrasound or fluoroscopic screening may be able to detect paradoxical diaphragm movement where there is severe unilateral or bilateral diaphragm weakness.

Direct measurement of respiratory muscle strength

Mouth pressures

Measurement of maximum inspiratory and expiratory pressures (MIP and MEP) generated at the mouth are the most widely used tests of global inspiratory and expiratory muscle strength. The manoeuvres required can be difficult for some patients and rely on maximum volitional effort. Normal ranges are available, but there is considerable variability even in healthy subjects. A value at the lower end of the normal range can be due to mild weakness or a

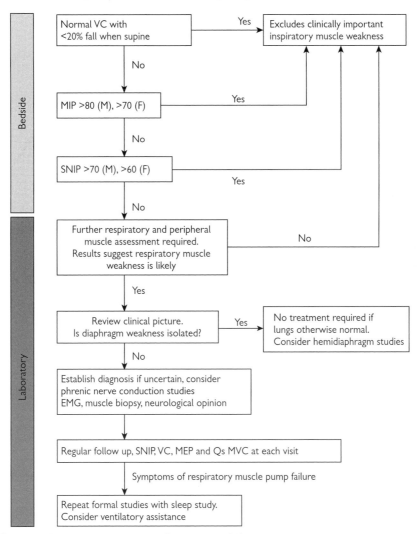

Fig. 2.5.2 Algorithm for the approach to assessment of respiratory muscle function.

sub-maximal effort in a normal subject. Unequivocally normal pressures are useful in excluding respiratory muscle weakness.

Nasal pressure

Sniff nasal inspiratory pressure (SNIP) relies on a manoeuvre that is easier to perform than MIP and provides an accurate, easy and non-invasive assessment of global inspiratory muscle strength. It can be particular helpful when deciding whether to pursue the finding of a low MIP, but may under-estimate inspiratory strength in COPD where pressure transmission from within the thorax may be delayed. The equipment required for this test is becoming more widely available.

Cough pressures

Pressure or peak flow generated during a cough can help determine expiratory muscle strength.

Specific or invasive tests

The non-invasive tests rely on rapid pressure transmission from thorax to mouth as well as good patient comprehension, cooperation and motivation to estimate global inspiratory or expiratory strength. By swallowing pressure catheters into the oesophagus and stomach, specific measurements of inspiratory, expiratory and trans-diaphragmatic pressures can be obtained during sniffing and coughing. By combining invasive pressure measurement with electrical or magnetic phrenic nerve stimulation, a non-volitional measure of diaphragm strength is available. These tests may detect unilateral diaphragm weakness or a phrenic nerve lesion, but are rarely available outside specialist laboratories.

Conclusion

An appreciation of respiratory muscle activity is important in understanding how the lungs are ventilated. A graded approach to testing the respiratory muscles can provide insight into the progress of various disease states and into unexplained respiratory symptoms.

Further reading

Polkey M, Green M, Moxham J. Measurement of respiratory muscle strength. *Thorax* 1995; **50**: 1131–1135.

Troosters T, Gosselink R, Decramer M. Respiratory muscle assessment. *Eur Respir Mon* 2005; **31**: 57–71.

Clinical presentations

Chapter contents

3.1 Chronic cough

Definition
Cough is an expulsive expiration with a characteristic sound. It is a protective reflex designed to combat aspiration and the stimulus to cough may arise anywhere within the territory of the vagus nerve. When cough persists for over 8 weeks it is arbitrarily defined as chronic.

Epidemiology
Cough is the commonest complaint for which medical attention is sought. Chronic cough is reported by 12% of the population and is considered to have a significant impact by 7%. Women cough more than men. Smoking has a dose-related effect on cough. Other significant associations are obesity, regurgitation, and irritable bowel syndrome.

Causes
In the absence of obvious other chest disease (normal CXR) three common causes of chronic cough are said to exist; gastric reflux, asthma syndrome (cough-variant asthma and eosinophilic bronchitis), and rhinitis (upper airways cough syndrome in the USA). However a common typical clinical history, histological and inflammatory profile point to reflux as the major cause of undiagnosed chronic cough. Atypical causes of chronic cough are as follows:
- Medication (e.g. angiotensin-converting enzyme (ACE) inhibitors) – relief may be delayed by 18 months following cessation of treatment.
- Inhaled foreign body – particularly in toddlers.
- Tonsillar enlargement – may be lingular.
- Auricular pathology – stimulation of Arnolds' nerve which is the auricular branch of the vagus nerve.
- Tic disorders (Tourette's) – mainly adolescent boys.

Impact of chronic cough
The impact of cough on quality of life has been shown to be comparable to that of severe COPD.

A patient with chronic cough suffers numerous physical and psychological consequences from their condition:
- Physical: cough syncope, urinary incontinence.
- Psychological: social exclusion, marital disharmony, depression.

Pathophysiology
Cough reflex sensitivity
In almost all forms, upregulation of the various cough receptors (such as the capsaicin receptor (TRPV1)) heightens cough sensitivity and leads to paroxysms of cough. Changes in atmospheric conditions (i.e. either going from a hot to a cold room or vice versa), perfumes, gastro-oesophageal reflux (GOR), and ACE inhibitors are its known triggers.

Reflux pathophysiology
Non-acid reflux as well as acid reflux causes chronic cough, hence the greatest association of regurgitation rather than heart burn with chronic cough. The reasons for reflux are:

Lower oesophageal sphincter incompetence: this results in irritation of the larynx or perhaps aspiration of gastric contents, and is caused by:
- Physiological transient opening:
  - To combat aerophagy and occurs 10 min post-prandial or on rising in the morning.

- Pharyngeal lower oesophageal sphincter reflex during swallowing.
- Pathological:
  - Loss of its natural tone e.g. hiatus hernia.

Movements:
- Gastrointestinal dysmotility: there is a strong correlation between oesophageal dysmotility, irritable bowel syndrome, and chronic cough. Reverse oesophageal peristalsis also occurs.
- Diaphragmatic movements: specifically during phonation, typically on the telephone.

Clinical approach
History: key questions and hints in answers pointing to reflux as the cause
- Is the cough worse at night or during the day? During the day.
- When is the first cough of the morning ? On rising.
- What makes you cough? Talking specifically on the phone or laughing.
- How many minutes after a meal does the cough come? Roughly 10 min, sometimes the swallowing can trigger cough.
- Does your voice go after a coughing bout? Yes, sometimes.
- Does any one else in the family have the cough? 10% yes.
- Is it related to your posture? Change in position makes it worse; like bending, lying.
- Do you have any funny taste in your mouth? Metallic taste.
- Do you produce sputum? Not much, white colour sputum sometimes.
- Do you wheeze at all? If yes, wheezing bouts immediately following cough indicates aspiration.

Physical exam
General exam (e.g. weight, clubbing) added to the examination of the upper airways as well as listening to the lungs may provide clues to diagnosis.

Risk factors
Smoking, sex, obesity, and family history.

Investigations
Baseline evaluation should look for pulmonary and extra-pulmonary conditions which cause cough. A chest radiograph and lung function tests are mandatory in an early stage. Next steps are recommended as follows:

Respiratory investigations
- Laryngoscopy.
- Bronchoscopy (when foreign body suspected).

AUTHOR'S TIP
Ventricular obliteration is highly characteristic for GOR. (Fig. 3.1.1).

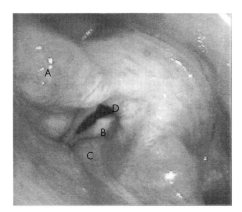

Fig. 3.1.1 Typical reflux variations in laryngoscopy: A. Arythenoid erythema, B. Vocal cord oedema, C. Ventricular obliteration, D. Posterior commisure hypertrophy.

Reflux investigations

Most tests for the diagnosis of GOR are only partially helpful, as pH studies are designed to detect acid component in GOR. Non-acid reflux can precipitate severe coughing with no trace with regard to pH monitoring; pH studies and manometry can be useful in deciding whether fundoplication should be offered.

Other useful investigations are:

- Oesophageal impedance: it detects both acid and non-acid reflux.
- High resolution oesophageal manometry.
- Salivary pepsin (a new pepsin analyser which will commercially be available soon).

Treatment

We aim to either tackle the specific cause of cough or, if this fails, to suppress it. The European Respiratory Society (ERS) and British thoracic Society (BTS) guidelines endorse therapeutic trials. The following ladder for reflux cough is recommended (Fig. 3.1.2).

Further reading

Dicpinigaitis P, Tso R, Banuch G. Prevalence of depressive symptoms among patients with chronic cough. *Chest* 2006; **130:** 1839–1843.

Ford AC, Forman D, Moayyedi P, Morice AH. Cough in the community: a cross sectional survey and the relationship to gastrointestinal symptoms. *Thorax* 2006; **61** (11): 975–979.

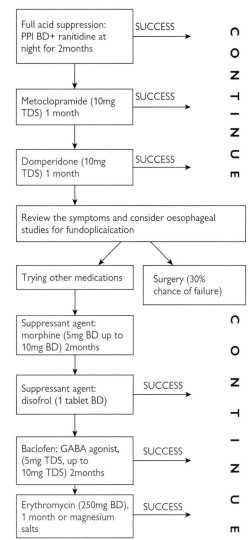

Fig. 3.1.2 Treatment ladder for reflux cough. Note: disofrol is an anti-histaminic medication recommended in American College of Chest Physicians (ACCP) guidelines which is an inhibitor of TRPV1 cough receptor and this explains its efficacy in cough.

3.2 Breathlessness

What is breathlessness?

We all know what breathlessness feels like, but defining it is difficult. Breathing is something that we are not normally aware of; when it encroaches into our consciousness we call this sensation breathlessness. This term probably covers several different sensory experiences, meaning different things to different people in various situations. For example, the air hunger you experience after running as fast as you can is not likely to be the same as the feeling some patients report of not being able to take a deep enough breath in, or indeed the distress experienced by a patient with an exacerbation of COPD who is struggling to breathe out through obstructed airways.

The physiology of breathlessness is complex and incompletely understood. It seems to arise when there is a mismatch between what the brain expects and what it receives in terms of afferent information from the lungs, airways and receptors in the tendons and muscles of the chest wall. Heart–lung transplant patients – in whom the vagus nerves are cut–experience breathlessness, as do those with complete transection of the cervical spinal cord. Breathlessness can be related to changes in blood gas tensions, but often it is not. Psychological, emotional and social factors also play a part.

Causes of breathlessness

The list of diseases that can cause breathlessness is very long. It may be helpful to think of the route an oxygen molecule takes from the inspired air to reach an end organ – such as the quadriceps muscle. This ensures considering diseases affecting the following:

- ventilatory pump (central drive and muscles);
- upper airway;
- lower airways ;
- alveoli;
- pulmonary vasculature;
- red blood cells;
- cardiac output;
- peripheral circulation;
- skeletal muscle.

It is important to remember that breathlessness can just be the result of increased oxygen requirement. This might just be obesity, but someone with bad arthritis may complain of breathlessness because of the energy they expend in struggling up stairs, rather than because of any respiratory or circulatory problem.

> **AUTHOR'S TIP**
> Think about the possibility of pulmonary embolism every time you see a patient who is breathless.

History

Speed of onset

Although it is important to ask the patient what they mean by 'breathlessness', you are more likely to find out the cause by asking how long they have had it and in what situations it occurs. Sudden onset is seen in pulmonary emboli, pneumothorax, left ventricular failure, inhalation of a foreign body and asthma; more gradual onset suggests fibrotic lung disease, pleural effusion, anaemia or lung cancer.

Precipitating factors

Breathlessness is usually made worse by exercise, which can be used to quantify the degree of breathlessness.

Medical Research Council dyspnoea scale

0 Breathlessness only on strenuous exercise
1 Short of breath when hurrying or walking up a slight hill
2 Walks slower than contemporaries on the level because of breathlessness, or has to stop for breath when walking at own pace
3 Stops for breath after about 100 m or after a few minutes on the level
4 Too breathless to leave the house, or breathless when dressing or undressing

Most patients with breathlessness – not just those with heart failure – feel worse when they lie down (orthopnoea). Occasionally you will see someone who feels better when they lie down; this is called platypnoea.

Causes of platypnoea

(shortness of breath worse in the upright posture)
- Intra-cardiac shunt:
  - Atrial septal defect*
- Intra-pulmonary shunt:
  - Arterio-venous malformations.
  - Cirrhosis, with pulmonary spider naevi.
  - Lung disease, predominantly affecting the lower lobes.
- Other rarities:
  - Supraglottic tumour.
  - Autonomic failure.

* Platypnoea may only occur when there is a right-to-left shunt rise in right-sided pressure (for example with a pulmonary embolism), after thoracic surgery, or if the patient develops a pericardial effusion.

Although unusual, breathlessness on wading into water is a characteristic symptom of bilateral diaphragm paralysis, because the diaphragm is pushed up in to the chest by the pressure of the water.

Associated symptoms

Wheeze is the most useful associated symptom in terms of a diagnosis, whereas the presence of cough doesn't usually help. Sudden onset or offset palpitations can be a useful clue to breathlessness caused by a cardiac dysrhythmia. Tingling in the tips of the fingers or around the mouth suggests hyperventilation, usually of dysfunctional breathing; there are other features which will lead you to make an active diagnosis of this syndrome, rather than just excluding any other pathology.

Other things to ask about are smoking, drug therapy, recreational drug use, pets, hobbies and occupational exposure.

Feature suggestive of dysfunctional breathing

- Sensation of inability to inflate lungs fully.
- Feeling of the need to take deep breaths or sigh.
- Breathlessness varies with social situation.
- Breathless when talking but not on exercise.
- Very variable exercise tolerance.
- Dizziness.
- Tingling in the fingers or around the mouth.
- Symptoms reproduced by taking 20 deep breaths in the clinic.
- Previous 'somatisation' disorders.

Clinical examination

Particular things to look out for when examining a breathless patient:

- An elevated jugular venous pressure alerts indicates the possibility of pulmonary emboli or primary pulmonary hypertension (as well as heart failure, obviously).
- In-drawing of the lower ribcage towards the end of inspiration (Hoover's sign) indicates that the patient is chronically hyper-inflated from COPD.
- Paradoxical inspiratory inward motion of the abdomen is seen in bilateral diaphragm paralysis. It is easier to see when the patient is lying down, and when they sniff. If the accessory muscles in the neck are contracting when the patient is at rest, think of a more generalised muscle or nerve problem which has affected the diaphragm and the intercostal muscles.
- Inspiratory squeaks usually mean extrinsic allergic alveolitis (which is really a bronchiolitis), although sometimes they are heard in bronchiectasis.

Investigation

- Full blood count, D-dimer (negative result will help exclude pulmonary emboli), renal, liver and thyroid function.
- CXR, HRCT (to look for early diffuse parenchymal lung disease if the transfer factor is low (see below).
- An ECG and an echocardiogram are useful as exclusion criteria as well as diagnostic tools.

AUTHOR'S TIP

In hyperventilation, the ECG can be abnormal with widespread T-wave inversion and ST segment depression.

- Spirometry, lung volumes , carbon monoxide transfer factor.

If these are also normal it is useful to proceed to a 'respiratory' exercise test, where gas exchange is measured whilst the patient exercises on a treadmill or cycle ergometer. A simpler exercise test such as a shuttle or six minute walk may be undertaken first, just to confirm that exercise capacity is impaired. Check the oxygen saturation on air, and proceed to arterial blood gas analysis if it is less than 94%.

AUTHOR'S TIP

Patients often hyperventilate transiently when they are having an arterial blood gas sample taken. You can only confidently diagnose dysfunctional breathing if there is a chronic respiratory alkalosis, with a bicarbonate concentration of <20 mmol/litre.

Management

Obviously the best treatment for breathlessness is to cure the underlying disease. In some instances this is not possible, and the symptom are treated rather than the cause.

Drugs

Opiates are the most effective drugs, but benzodiazepines are also helpful. It is better to use short-acting preparations, so that the patient can get more rapid relief when they get breathless. They should be taken orally – nebulised therapy for breathlessness has proved disappointing, whether it be opiates, local anaesthetic or (more recently) furosemide.

Oxygen

Oxygen is an expensive and potentially dangerous therapy. It should only be used when the patient has been documented to be hypoxic. It is considered in detail in Chapter 6 There are three ways of giving oxygen:

- Long-term oxygen therapy (LTOT) is used from an oxygen concentrator for at least 12 hours per day in patients with chronic lung disease (usually COPD).
- Ambulatory oxygen therapy (AOT) is used to improve exercise capacity. Ideally patients should have completed a pulmonary rehabilitation program first. During a walk test, oxygen saturation should fall by at least 4% and to below 90% to qualify for AOT assessment.
- Short burst oxygen therapy (SBOT) is used for a few minutes to relieve breathlessness. There is very little evidence to support its use, and it is probably greatly overused. An argument can be made for using cylinders of air as comparison when assessing patients for SBOT, because of the relief obtained simply by blowing gas onto the face.

Other therapies

- Physiotherapists can teach patients with dysfunctional breathing to slow and regularise their breathing rhythm.
- Pulmonary rehabilitation is effective in reducing the breathlessness of COPD and other chronic lung diseases.
- Non-invasive ventilation will help patients with neuromuscular problems who are struggling to maintain adequate ventilation.
- Many other non-drug therapies have been tried in patients who are breathless, but here is little evidence to support their use.

Further reading

Jennings AL, Davies AN, Higgins JPT, *et al.* Opioids for the palliation of breathlessness in terminal illness. *Cochrane Database of Systematic Reviews* 2001; **4**.

The adult clinical component for the home oxygen service in England and Wales.http://www.brit-thoracic.org.uk/page294.html

3.3 Haemoptysis

This is a common presentation of respiratory disease defined as the expectoration of blood from haemorrhage into the respiratory tract. It can vary from streaks of blood within sputum to massive, life-threatening haemorrhage. All patients with unexplained haemoptysis require further investigation to identify one of the many causes. The urgency of investigation and treatment will depend on the rate of bleeding and source, and the severity of underlying lung disease. Most patients do not require admission for investigation or management.

Causes of haemoptysis

Most common causes	Bronchiectasis
	Tuberculosis *
	Pneumonia especially *Streptococcal pneumoniae* *
	Bronchial carcinoma *
	Pulmonary embolism *
Other rarer causes	**Pulmonary infections**
	Acute bronchitis
	Lung abscess
	Aspergilloma or invasive fungal disease
	Tumours
	Carcinoid tumour
	Endobronchial metastasis, e.g. breast, melanoma, colon
	Pulmonary parenchymal diseases
	Pulmonary vasculitis/alveolar haemorrhage syndromes
	Pulmonary fibrosis
	Pulmonary vascular disease
	Severe pulmonary hypertension
	AV malformation
	Mitral stenosis (rare nowadays)
	Congenital malformation
	Aortic aneurysm
	Miscellaneous causes
	Endometriosis
	Anticoagulant therapy or coagulopathy, e.g. DIC
	Iatrogenic, e.g. Swan–Ganz catheter, bronchial biopsy
	Drugs, e.g. cocaine, thrombolytics

Evaluation of a patient with haemoptysis

History: key points
- Identify time course and likely volume of blood.
- Identify symptoms suggestive of malignancy, infection, bronchiectasis or embolism.
- Smoking history.
- Ask about risk factors for aspiration.
- Medications including illicit drugs.

Examination: key points
- The examination may be normal.
- Look for signs of bronchiectasis or malignancy.
- In patients with massive haemoptysis, assessment of airway and circulation are essential (see Investigations).

AUTHOR'S TIP
Always examine the mouth and nasal cavities for possible causes of bleeding and consider the possibility of GI haemorrhage. NB In up to 20% patients a source will not be identified – cryptogenic haemoptysis.

Investigations

Chest radiograph
The chest radiograph may be normal or show signs of the likely origin of the bleeding, e.g. a mass, consolidation, bronchiectactic changes.

Laboratory investigations
- FBC and clotting.
- Group and save/cross match if massive bleeding.
- ANCA, autoantibodies and anti-GBM antibodies if vasculitis is suspected.

CT scan
- A CT scan should be performed in most subjects unless the cause is already known (e.g. a patient with recurrent bleeding from bronchiectasis or a tumour).
- CT scanning may show the cause of bleeding or may direct the clinician to the likely site of bleeding at subsequent investigations such as bronchoscopy.
- Patients suspected of bronchiectasis will also require high resolution CT imaging or image reconstruction to identify parenchymal disease.
- When pulmonary embolic disease is considered within the differential diagnosis, CT pulmonary angiography should be performed.
- For some diagnoses further diagnostic investigations may be unnecessary after the CT scan, e.g. bronchiectasis, pulmonary embolism, AV malformation, pulmonary fibrosis.

Bronchoscopy
Bronchoscopy and CT scanning should be considered complementary investigations in patients with haemoptysis. The timing of bronchoscopy has not been shown to affect the outcome of investigating the cause of haemoptysis and it is usual for CT scanning to be performed prior to bronchoscopy.

AUTHOR'S TIP
Bronchoscopy should be considered in patients with massive haemoptysis, to identify possible source of bleeding when CT is normal, and when CT scan has identified a likely abnormality responsible for the bleeding. Bronchoscopy may help obtain tissue or microbiological samples to confirm the diagnosis, e.g. bronchial tumour, TB, parenchymal lung disease (by transbronchial biopsy) and can help locate anatomical origin of bleeding when considering bronchial arterial embolisation

---

Other investigations
Where the clinical picture indicates an alternative cause for bleeding further investigations may include:
- Echocardiography, e.g. to identify pulmonary hypertension or mitral valve disease.
- Bronchial arterial angiography and embolisation (see below).

Massive haemoptysis

Massive haemoptysis is fortunately rare (about 5% of episodes of haemoptysis) and is often defined as expectoration of blood exceeding between 100–600 ml in 24 hours. This definition is rather arbitrary as the outcome will depend on the volume, rate and cause of the bleeding, and the underlying respiratory reserve and ability of the patient and medical staff to maintain a clear airway.

Commonest causes

- Bronchiectasis – due to dilated, ectatic and tortuous vessels around the abnormal airways. Bleeding may be triggered by inter-current infection.
- TB – either due to active infection or damaged airways from previous infection.
- Aspergilloma.
- Bronchial tumours – usually large, centrally located.
- More common with squamous cell carcinoma.
- Lung abscess.

Early involvement of a respiratory specialist is recommended. In some cases, e.g. patients with cancer, the main approach to management may be entirely palliative.

Management of massive haemoptysis

Initial resuscitation and investigations

- Airway protection.
- Administer oxygen.
- Assess cardiovascular status and resuscitate with IV fluids as necessary.
- Move patient to a higher monitoring area or intensive care setting. Early anaesthetic input may be required.
- Check FBC and coagulation and take measures to correct any coagulopathy. Discussion with a haematologist may be needed.
- Cross match blood.
- Assess arterial blood gases.
- Chest radiograph – may reveal likely cause.
- Chest CT (and/or CT angiography).

Protection of the non-bleeding lung

AUTHOR'S TIP

- Protection of the non-bleeding lung is a major priority as spillage of blood into the other lung can cause airway obstruction and lead to respiratory failure or asphyxia. To achieve this requires identification of the likely site of bleeding. If known:
- Position the patient onto their side, either flat or at about 30°, so that the bleeding lung is in the dependent position.

Introduce a single lumen endotracheal tube into either main stem bronchus so that the tube protects the non-bleeding lung. This is easier to achieve when bleeding is from the left side as the tube is more likely to enter the right main bronchus. Intubation of the left main bronchus is more difficult. An alternative is to use a double lumen endotracheal tube, although experience of insertion and subsequent care may be lacking in some centres. They tend to have a smaller lumen too, which may block with blood.

Drugs

- Tranexamic acid is a drug that inhibits fibrinolysis, is useful to reduce bleeding. Usual dose is 15–25 mg/kg 2–3 times daily oral or 0.5–1g 3 times daily IV.
- Antibiotics – when infection is a likely trigger (e.g. in bronchiectasis).
- Nebulised adrenaline – 5–10 ml of 1 in 10,000.

Bronchoscopy

Bronchoscopy is useful in massive haemoptysis. Rigid bronchoscopy may allow a clearer view of the airway but requires expertise and anaesthesia. In practice most clinicians will have access to fibreoptic bronchoscopy in the first instance. General anaesthesia and intubation may still be required. Bronchoscopy may allow:

- Identification of the likely origin of the bleeding.
- Introduction of topical adrenaline (5–10 ml of 1:10000 or 1:20000) directly to the source of bleeding or blindly into the main bronchi.
- Lavage with iced 0.9% saline to induce vasoconstriction and reduce bleeding.
- Introduction of a balloon catheter (e.g. 14Fr Foley 100 cm long) to tamponade the main bronchus leading to the bleeding site or introduction of a smaller catheter (e.g. 4–7 Fr Foley 200 cm long) can be passed through the scope into a segmental bronchus.
- Laser or electrocautery to the visualised bleeding lesion.

Pulmonary angiography and embolisation

Once the patient has been resuscitated and stabilised a definitive procedure to prevent further bleeding may be necessary depending on clinical circumstances. As bleeding is usually from a bronchial artery, abnormal vessels may be identified at angiography and then occluded using either non-absorbable glue or steel coils. This technique is usually only available in a few specialist centres but has success rates of up to 85%. Bronchial wall necrosis may occur after embolisation and there is a risk of spinal cord paralysis due to inadvertent embolisation of a spinal artery. Rebleeding may occur in 10–20% of patients, and definitive treatment of the cause should be initiated afterwards to reduce risk.

Surgery

In selected cases surgical resection of the affected bleeding site, e.g. by lobectomy, can be successful, but surgery in setting of acute massive haemoptysis has reported mortality between 20–30%. Surgery may still be indicated after successful embolisation of a bleeding site or for selected patients with bleeding from resectable lesions such as AV malformations, bronchial adenoma, aspergilloma.

Further reading

Lordan JK, Gascoigne A, Corris PA. The pulmonary physician in critical care. Illustrative case 7: assessment and management of massive haemoptysis. *Thorax* 2003; **58**: 814–819.

3.4 Chest pain

Chest pain is a frequently encountered symptom in all areas of medical practice, being the most common site of pain that prompts the sufferer to seek medical attention. It may signal the onset of a severe or life-threatening condition but more commonly will have a less serious cause. A focused history with a careful clinical examination may be sufficient to decide the cause of the chest pain but further investigation is often required. Knowledge of disease prevalence and awareness of risk factors can help formulate an appropriate differential diagnosis and guide further investigation.

Initial assessment of chest pain may include questions about character of the pain, onset, location, radiation, severity, duration, exacerbating or relieving factors and its relationship to breathing, coughing and movement. Readers should be aware that cardiac chest pain can present with atypical symptoms such as pleuritic pain and chest wall tenderness in a small proportion of patients. The presence of associated symptoms such as breathlessness, cough, sputum or haemoptysis may help point to a respiratory cause of the chest pain.

An algorithm for the initial approach to a patient with chest pain is suggested in Fig. 3.4.1.

When considering respiratory causes of chest pain, knowledge of the thoracic neuro-anatomy will help understanding of how certain pathologies present. The lung parenchyma and visceral pleura have no pain innervation. Parietal pleura is supplied by the intercostal nerves giving rise to pleuritic chest pain. Central diaphragmatic pleurisy can present with referred shoulder tip pain as it is supplied by pain fibres which run in the phrenic nerve. The outer diaphragm is innervated by the lower 6 intercostal nerves and can give rise to referred upper abdominal pain. Chest wall pain can be of differing character depending on the cause and tissue affected. It may be pleuritic type pain (e.g. with rib pathology), it may be localised or diffuse dull pain and can be associated with chest wall tenderness. Pain in a dermatomal distribution, particularly with hyperaesthesia can occur with herpes zoster infection and with lesions affecting the intercostal nerve or nerve root. The trachea and large bronchi have pain fibres running in the vagus nerve and can give rise to retrosternal or anterior chest pain which is often raw or burning in character and worse on inspiration. Rarely, massive mediastinal adenopathy can give rise to anterior chest pain although more commonly invasive adenopathy will present with ipsilateral chest pain.

A limited list of differential diagnoses for respiratory causes of chest pain is shown in the box.

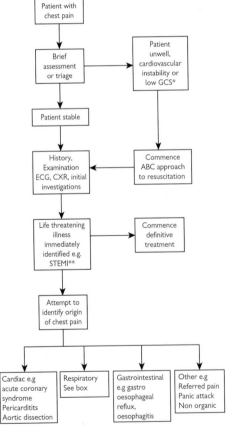

Differential diagnosis of respiratory causes of chest pain
Pleuritic pain
Sudden onset
Pulmonary embolus
Spontaneous pneumothorax
Onset over hours
Pneumonia
Pleurisy
Pericarditis
Onset over days
Connective tissue associated pleurisy
Empyema
Onset over weeks
Malignancy
Tuberculosis
Chest wall pain
Sudden onset
Trauma e.g. assault, violent coughing
Developed over days
Costochondritis
Vertebral body collapse
Developed over weeks
Malignancy e.g. mesothelioma
Nerve root irritation
Tracheobronchial pain
Infection
Irritant inhalation
Mediastinal pain
Invasive adenopathy

Fig. 3.4.1 Algorithm for initial approach to a patient with chest pain.
*GCS = Glasgow coma score
**STEMI = ST elevation myocardial infarction

An approach to investigation of the patient with chest pain due to a suspected respiratory cause is suggested in Fig. 3.4.2.

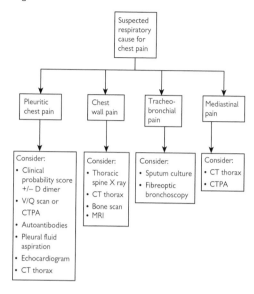

Fig. 3.4.2
V/Q scan = ventilation perfusion scan; CTPA = Computed tomography pulmonary angiogram

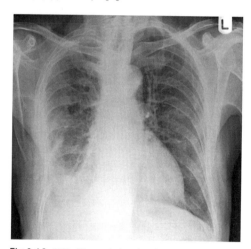

Fig. 3.4.3 CXR of former dockyard worker presenting with chest wall pain and weight loss, showing volume loss in the right hemithorax with diffuse right pleural thickening and right pleural effusion typical of mesothelioma.

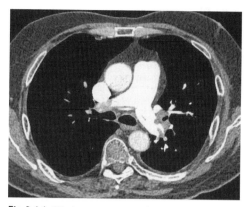

Fig. 3.4.4 CT pulmonary angiogram showing bilateral proximal pulmonary artery thromboembolic disease with a saddle embolus.

In recent years several biomarkers such as D-dimer and cardiac troponins have become readily available to aid the diagnosis of chest pain. It is important, however, to be aware that these tests have low specificity and should not be used in isolation of other clinical findings.

In a proportion of people the cause of the chest pain can not be conclusively identified. The authors feel that it is important to avoid the temptation to attach a diagnostic label that is not proven. It is generally best to explain diagnostic uncertainty to the patient and the referring physician.

AUTHOR'S TIPS
- Biomarkers such as D-dimer and cardiac troponin have a large number of false positive causes.
- When considering the diagnosis of pulmonary embolism the clinical probability score must be calculated first to assess if a D-dimer assay will be helpful. Only a normal result (which excludes PE) is of any clinical value; an abnormal result (however high) does not imply a significantly increased probability of PE.
- Patients with airways diseases such as asthma and COPD can complain of chest wall pain particularly worsened by breathlessness.
- Pleuritic pain may ease or become duller in character as a pleural effusion develops.

Further reading

BTS Guidelines for the Management of Suspected Acute Pulmonary Embolism. The British Thoracic Society Standards of Care Committee, Pulmonary Embolism Guideline Development Group. *Thorax* 2003; **48**: 470–484.

D-Dimer in Suspected Pulmonary Embolism. A statement from the British Thoracic Society Standards of Care Committee, Dec 2006. www.brit-thoracic.org.uk/c2/uploads/ddimerstatement.pdf

Mahajan N, Mehta Y, Rose M, et al. Elevated troponin level is not synonymous with myocardial infarction. *Int J Cardiol* 2006; **111**: 442–449.

Swap C J, Nagurney J T. Value and limitations of chest pain history in the evaluation of patients with suspected acute coronary syndromes. *JAMA* 2005; **294**: 2623–2629.

Von Korff M, Dworkin SF, Le Resche L, et al. An epidemiologic comparison of pain complaints. *Pain* 1988; **32**(2): 173–183.

3.5 Pre-operative assessment

Respiratory physicians are not infrequently asked by surgical colleagues to assess fitness for surgery, either in a patient with known respiratory disease or where respiratory disease has been suggested by pre-operative tests. This chapter will deal with the pre-operative assessment of the respiratory patient and ways of assessing specific risks posed to such patients by particular operations, together with strategies for 'optimising' a patient preoperatively.

Pre-operative assessment

- Should be undertaken before the operation in a time-frame that allows any essential preoperative investigations to be performed and optimisation strategies to be implemented.
- Should include full history and examination to clarify the respiratory diagnosis.
- Should include targeted investigations and a plan for optimisation of the patient's pre- and post-operative well-being.
- Should consider that surgery may exacerbate the underlying respiratory disease and/or that the respiratory disease itself may lead to peri-operative and/or post-operative complications which may be pulmonary and/or non-pulmonary.

History and examination: key points

- Clarify the respiratory diagnosis.
- Assess disease severity.
- Determine whether or not there are any reversible factors.
- Establish what treatment has already been tried, whether or not this can be escalated, and what treatment has not yet been tried.

Preoperative investigations

Preoperative tests can be useful in several ways:
- Assessing risks and potential complications of a particular operation in a particular patient.
- Changing the clinical management of the patient to reduce morbidity/mortality:
  - (a) **Preoperatively**
    Optimising the patient's condition.
    Avoiding last-minute cancellations or delays.
  - (b) **Intra-operatively**
    Anaesthetic technique e.g. general versus local anaesthetic/sedation.
    Operative type e.g. staged operations.
  - (c) **Post-operatively**
    Timing of operation.
    Level of care post-operatively e.g. HDU/ICU/ward.
- Incidental findings, e.g. lung mass noted on shoulder X-ray, interstitial markings on a CXR. Care must be taken, however, not to unnecessarily delay surgery by carrying out further investigations based on false positive or insignificant results.

Recent guidelines have been published by NICE on preoperative testing in all patients. They take into account physical status as judged using the ASA (American Society of Anaesthesiologists) classification (Table 3.5.1) and the extent of the operation.

Table 3.5.1 ASA Physical Status classification system

I.	A normal healthy patient
II.	A patient with mild systemic disease
III.	A patient with severe systemic disease
IV.	A patient with severe systemic disease that is a threat to life
V.	A moribund patient who is not suspected to live without the operation
VI.	A declared brain-dead patient whose organs are being removed for donation purposes

The investigations that are commonly considered pre-operatively include:

Blood tests (FBC, renal function, coagulation)
There is no evidence from randomised controlled trials that testing will alter the health outcomes in patients. However there is an increasing prevalence of abnormality with age.

Pre-operative CXR
- The proportion of pre-operative abnormal CXR results increases with age and severity of respiratory disease. Many of these changes will be chronic, however, and may not lead to changes in clinical management.
- The CXR may be useful for clarification of the respiratory diagnosis and for comparison if peri-operative pulmonary complications arise.
- When no CXR is available, consider performing one if ASA status is ≥3, in major operations or operations for malignant neoplasm.
- If symptoms have changed since the previous CXR consider repeating it.

Electrocardiogram (ECG)
- Consideration should be given to obtaining a preoperative ECG unless pulmonary disease is mild and the operation is minor.
- There is an increasing prevalence of ECG abnormalities with age and severity of disease. Abnormalities on the preoperative ECG have been associated with increased risk of in-hospital cardiovascular death in major operations.

Arterial blood gas analysis (ABG)/oxygen saturations
- There is a lack of data suggesting that measuring preoperative ABGs can independently predict post-operative complications or affect clinical management in extra-thoracic or non-resective lung surgery, and they should therefore not be considered to be a routine test.
- In resective lung surgery, earlier studies suggested increased complications with hypercapnoea ($PaCO_2$ > 6 KPa) and it was initially considered a strong relative contraindication to such surgery (ATS/ERS guidelines). However, later studies did not show a predictive effect on complications. Whilst such patients may be excluded surgery on other grounds e.g. FEV_1, preoperative assessment of ABGs is not routinely recommended in current BTS guidelines for lung resection.
- Low arterial oxygen saturations (<90% at rest) are associated with increased complications and are incorporated in lung resection assessment (see Chapter 13.4: pp. 292–297).

Pulmonary function tests.
- Post-operative pulmonary complications in extrathoracic/non-resective lung surgery seem to be associated with lower FEV_1 and TLCO values. Particular risk is associated with FEV_1 <1L or <60% predicted.
- Spirometry is helpful in clarifying the respiratory diagnosis and objectively assessing response to optimisation strategies.
- In resective lung surgery, spirometry is mandatory to assess fitness for operation. If the post-bronchodilator FEV_1 >1.5L (for lobectomy) or >2L (for pneumonectomy), no further tests are required. If FEV_1 is below these values, predictive postoperative FEV_1 ± cardiopulmonary exercise testing should be undertaken (see Chapter 13.4, pp. 292–297).

Cardiopulmonary exercise testing
- This is not widely available in the UK, but can be useful in high risk patients undergoing extra-thoracic/non-resective lung surgery.
- Patients with anaerobic thresholds <11 ml/kg/min are at high risk for major surgery, particularly if this occurs in combination with evidence of myocardial ischaemia. They should be considered for either aggressive pre- and post-operative optimisation in a critical care setting or reconsideration of the need, if the procedure is not life saving.
- In resective lung surgery, cardiopulmonary exercise testing is helpful in predicting risk. VO_2 max <15ml/kg/min predicts that the patient is at increased risk (see Chapter 13.4, pp. 292–297).

Risk assessment

Risk from a particular operation can be assessed by looking at patient factors, operative factors and anaesthetic factors.

Patient factors
Risk factors for postoperative pulmonary complications include cigarette smoking (2–5 fold increase in risk), and COPD (2–3 fold increase in risk). To a lesser extent age, functional dependence, alcohol use, impaired sensorium and weight loss are also risk factors. Severity of asthma does not predict complications in elective procedures.

Other patient risk factors are useful in assessing preoperative risk. The most important of these are the cardiac risk factors, as postoperative cardiac complications are common. Several indices are available for predicting cardiac risk, one of which is the Lee risk index (Table 3.5.2).

Operative characteristics
Thoracoscopic and upper abdominal procedures in particular have a deleterious affect on respiratory function through pain, reduction of diaphragmatic function and sometimes pleural effusion. Decreased ability to breathe deeply or cough due to pain leads to atelectasis, mucus retention, increased incidence of pulmonary infection and reduced gas exchange. Video assisted thoracoscopic surgical (VATS) procedures with smaller thoracotomy ports result in fewer such complications. Duration of operation may also contribute to the risk of pulmonary complications, especially in operations lasting >3–4 hours.

Anaesthetic characteristics
Intubation can cause intra-operative bronchospasm, although most induction agents are bronchodilators. In general, regional anaesthesia is safer than general anaesthesia.

Optimising the respiratory patient

Optimisation of the patient may involve escalation/addition of therapy, or modification of current therapy, e.g. inhaler

Table 3.5.2 Lee index for estimating perioperative cardiac risk in noncardiac surgery

No. of risk factors	Risk of major postoperative cardiac event (death or non-fatal myorcardial infarction or cardiac arrest) % (95% CI)
0	0.4 (0.1–0.8)
1	1.0 (0.5–1.4)
2	2.4 (1.3–3.5)
≥3	5.4 (2.8–7.9)

Score 1 for each of the following:
(a) High-risk surgery (intrathoracic, intraperitoneal, suprainguinal vascular surgery)
(b) History of ischaemic heart disease (history of myocardial infarction, positive exercise test result, current ischaemic chest pain or nitrate use, Q waves on ECG, or any of the above after CABG/angioplasty procedure)
(c) History of congestive heart failure (history of heart failure, pulmonary oedema, or paroxysmal nocturnal dyspnoea, S3 gallop rhythm or bilateral rales on examination, or CXR showing increased pulm vasc resistance)
(d) History of cerebrovascular disease (stroke/TIA)
(e) Insulin dependent diabetes
(f) Preoperative serum creatinine >175µmol/L

technique. Close liaison with surgical and anaesthetic colleagues is essential, and sometimes the operative risks cannot be altered. Some general points apply, however:

Smoking cessation
Cigarette smokers are at increased risk of cardiovascular and pulmonary complications. Smoking increases carboxyhaemoglobin levels, decreasing oxygen delivery, whilst nicotine increases blood pressure, heart rate and causes systemic vasoconstriction. Smokers have increased mucus production, decreased ciliary activity and impaired pulmonary immune function, together with impaired wound healing and increased incidence of wound infections.

Clear benefit is seen from periods of abstinence of >6–8 weeks before surgery and, even if this is not possible, abstinence of 24–48 hours pre-surgery also has important beneficial physiological effects.

Postoperative care
Recognising patients at increased risk for postoperative complications allows appropriate decisions to be made ahead of time to try to minimise those risks. These include determining the site of post-operative or even pre-operative care e.g. HDU/ITU, together with (if appropriate) postoperative aggressive physiotherapy with lung expansion exercises, or selective nasal decompression after abdominal surgery. Patients may benefit from 'shared care' postoperatively from both respiratory physicians and surgeons.

Further reading

Guidelines on the selection of patients with lung cancer for surgery. British Thoracic Society. *Thorax* 2001; **56**; 89–108.

Joo HS, Wong J, Naik VN, *et al*. The value of screening preoperative chest X-rays: a systematic review. *Can J Anesth* 2005; **52**: 568–574.

Noordzij PG, Boersma E, Bax JJ, *et al*. Prognostic value of routine preoperative electrocardiography. *Am J Cardiol* 2006; **97**(7): 1103–1106.

Pre-operative tests, National Institute of Clinical Evidence.

Pretreatment evaluation of non small cell lung cancer, ATS/ERS guidelines. *AJRCCM* 1997; **156**: 320–332.

Smetana GW, Lawrence VA, Cornell JE, *et al*. Preoperative pulmonary risk stratification for non-cardiothoracic surgery: systematic review for the American College of Physicians. *Ann Int Med* 2006; **144**(8): 581–595.

3.6 Solitary pulmonary nodule

Definition

A solitary pulmonary nodule (SPN) is a single lesion ≤3cm in diameter surrounded by normal lung without lymphade-nopathy or atelectasis. Lesions >3cm are almost always malignant and are called masses.

Epidemiology

A nodule is seen on 0.1-0.2% of CXRs. It is usually > 8mm in diameter before it is clearly visible. CT is more sensitive and finding nodules as small as 2mm is common.

The reported prevalence of malignancy varies widely between studies but the risk of malignancy in nodules detected on CXR is probably 30–40%. Small nodules (<8mm) are difficult to investigate but fortunately are much more likely to be benign.

Aetiology

There are several possible causes for a SPN (Table 3.6.1), but > 95% are neoplasms (usually primary), granulomas (usually infection) or hamartoma (Table 3.6.2).

Table 3.6.1 Causes of solitary pulmonary nodules

Neoplastic (malignant or benign)
Bronchogenic carcinoma
Single metastasis
Lymphoma
Carcinoid
Connective tissue & neural tumours – fibroma, neurofibroma, blastoma, sarcoma
Hamartoma
Lipoma

Inflammatory (infectious)
Granuloma – TB, histoplasma, coccidioidomycosis, blastomycosis, *Cryptococcus, Nocardia*
Lung abscess
Round pneumonia
Hydatid cyst

Inflammatory (non-infectious)
Rheumatoid arthritis
Wegener's granulomatosis
Sarcoidosis
Lipoid pneumonia

Congenital
Arteriovenous malformation
Sequestration
Lung cyst

Others
Pulmonary infarct
Round atelectasis
Mucoid impaction

Initial detection of a SPN: CXR and CT

Chest radiography: provides information on size, shape, cavitation, growth rate, and calcification. These features can help suggest whether the lesion is benign or malignant. However, none are specific (see below).
CT has many advantages over CXR e.g. better resolution and detection of small nodules. Regions that are difficult to

assess with CXR (e.g. lung apices, perihilar, costophrenic angles) are seen well on CT. CT can also stage malignancy and help guide needle biopsy.

Table 3.6.2 Common causes of benign and malignant nodules

Malignant nodules	Percentage	Benig nodules	Percentage
Adenocarcinoma	47%	Healed/ non-specific granulomas	25%
Squamous cell carcinoma	22%		
Solitary metastasis Undifferentiated	8%	Granulomatous infections	15%
NSCLC	7%	Hamartomas	5%
SCLC	4%		
Bronchioloalveolar cell	4%		

CT densitometry measures the attenuation of a lesion and aids detection of calcification. Enhancement with IV contrast also suggests malignancy. However, the sensitivity and specificity of these measurements are low and combination with other clinical and radiological features increases their usefulness.

Low-dose techniques should be used to reduce the dose of radiation if multiple follow-up CT scans are required.

Nodule characteristics

Size: Table 3.6.3 shows the relationship between size and risk of malignancy. Lesions >3cm in diameter are very likely to be malignant, but other possible causes include lung abscess, Wegener's granulomatosis, round pneumonia, rounded atelectasis, and hydatid cyst.

Nodules <8mm are too small to biopsy or assess with positron emission tomography (PET) so the most sensible option is follow-up CT.

Shape: generally unhelpful but, a very irregular edge, corona radiata (spiculation), lobulation, or notching suggest bronchogenic carcinoma. A well-defined, smooth edge suggests a benign lesion or metastasis.

Table 3.6.3 Method of detection, size of nodule and risk of malignancy

Method of detection	Size (mm)	Approximate risk of malignancy
CT only	≤4	<1%
CT, Rarely CXR	>4–8	6%
CXR or CT	>8–30	50%

Attenuation: nodules may be solid, non-solid (ground glass; underlying lung parenchyma preserved and visible through nodule) part solid (mixed solid and ground glass). Table 3.6.4 shows how the risk and growth rate of malignancies vary between these types of nodule.

Rate of growth: serial CXR or CT can assess growth (doubling time; Td i.e. doubling of nodule volume). A 26% increase in diameter (e.g. 11mm to 14mm) on CXR reflects a doubling of volume as nodules are seen in 2-D rather than 3-D and the volume of a sphere is $4/3\uparrow$ r3. However, a 3mm change is difficult to detect using CXR.

The Td of bronchogenic carcinoma is generally 1–18 months (mean 4–8). Outside this range bronchogenic carcinoma is unlikely but not impossible; <1 month suggests infections; >18 suggests benign processes (e.g. granuloma, hamartoma, carcinoid, rounded atelectasis). If there is no change over 2 years, the SPN is probably benign. Further follow-up (up to 5 years), may be indicated particularly for non-solid nodules as indolent malignancies with Td >730 days may be missed (see Table 3.6.4).

Table 3.6.4 Nodule characteristics, doubling time and risk of malignancy

HRCT characteristics	Risk	Mean Td of malignancy (days)
Non-solid (ground glass)	34%	813
Partly solid (<15mm)	40–50%	457
Solid (<10mm)	15%	149

Calcification: often indicates that the SPN is benign. CT is the most sensitive technique for detecting calcification. Patterns of calcification usually seen in benign lesions are diffuse, central, laminar, concentric and popcorn. Stippled or eccentric patterns are associated with malignancy.

Fat: within a SPN can be seen with CT and suggests hamartoma or lipoma but metastases from a liposarcoma or renal cell cancer may rarely contain fat.

Other features: invasion of adjacent bone = bronchogenic carcinoma. Cavitation with thin (<1mm), smooth walls suggests lung abscess or a benign lesion, but thick walls may be present in benign or malignant lesions.

False positives/negatives: up to half of the nodules seen on CXR are false-positive findings; the presence of the nodule not seen on subsequent CT. SPN mimics include nipple shadows, summation shadows, soft tissue tumours, bone shadows, pleural plaques, pseudotumours and round atelectases.

Differential diagnosis

Whether to biopsy, resect, or observe a nodule should be decided within 1 month of presentation. Patients with a SPN are usually asymptomatic but symptoms, signs and baseline imaging studies (CXR and CT) can be used to determine differential diagnoses and perform a risk assessment for malignancy.

The SPN should be classified as likely to be benign, malignant, or indeterminate. Bayesian analysis which uses likelihood ratios of malignancy for various clinical and imaging factors may guide risk assessment. The ratios are combined to produce a probability of malignancy (PCa).

Management of clearly benign or malignant nodules is straightforward. The management of the indeterminate nodule, however, is more difficult. The aim is to resect (cure) early-stage malignancy whilst avoiding the morbidity and mortality of surgery for benign nodules.

Most studies have focused on investigation and very few outcome studies have been performed. The suggestions in this review are therefore based on evidence that is graded 1B-2C at best.

The mortality associated with lung cancer is generally high (5-year survival rate 14%), but early lung cancer, (stage 1A; T1N0M0; primary tumour <3cm), may have a 5-year survival rate of 70-80%. Metastastectomy also offers the potential of cure to some patients with treated extra-pulmonary malignancy. Thus, the patient with cancer who presents with a SPN could be cured.

It is impossible to ignore the emotional and medicolegal implications of missing a potentially curable cancer. Most recommendations (and current practice) at least partly reflect this anxiety. This must be balanced against the substantial radiation exposure this group of patients may receive and which may itself induce malignancy.

Further investigations

Lab studies: the role of lab studies is limited. Anaemia or elevated inflammatory markers may suggest malignancy or infection. Deranged liver function tests or bone profile may suggest metastases. Histoplasma or coccidioidomycosis serology may identify infections with these fungi. A gamma interferon blood test (e.g. Elispot) can be used to detect tuberculosis.

Sputum cytology: is generally only indicated for investigation of patients with central nodules who are unable to tolerate or unwilling to undergo other invasive tests.

PET: the metabolic rate and glucose uptake of malignant nodules is greater than normal lung. Thus enhancement on 18-F-2 fluorodeoxyglucose (FDG) PET makes it likely to be malignant. The sensitivity and specificity are >90% and mediastinal metastases can be detected, improving the staging of non-invasive lung cancer. Furthermore, the yield from biopsy may be increased if the metabolically active regions of nodules are sampled.

However, false-positives occur in infectious or inflammatory nodules which are metabolically active. Tumours with low metabolic rates (e.g. carcinoid and bronchoalveolar carcinoma) may be difficult to distinguish from background activity. Furthermore, FDG-PET is less sensitive for nodules <20mm in diameter and may miss lesions <10mm.

Single-photon emission computed tomography (SPECT): cheaper than PET but the sensitivity, specificity and diagnostic accuracy (89%, 67%, and 81%, respectively) are similar. It is performed using a radiolabeled somatostatin-type receptor binder, technetium Tc P829. SPECT has not been assessed in large studies; in a smaller series, the sensitivity fell significantly for nodules <20mm.

Bronchoscopy and transbronchial needle aspiration (TBNA): may be helpful if the SPN is endobronchial, near a large airway or mediastinal nodes need to be sampled. Because the diagnostic yield from bronchoscopy is generally <20% if the SPN is <2cm, bronchoscopy has a limited role in the investigation of SPN.

Transthoracic aspiration biopsy (TTAB): the accuracy is high (90–95%) when the SPN is ≥2cm, but is less (60–80%) in lesions <2cm. Sensitivity for specific benign diagnosis is lower (11–68%); so most specimens are non-diagnostic. Complications include pneumothorax which occurs in up to 30% (of these 5% require a chest drain) and haemoptysis which occurs in 5–10% (usually minor and resolves spontaneously).

As samples may be taken from normal tissue adjacent to a SPN the negative predictive value is low. Further management depends on PCa and patient-related factors such as operative risk. Thoracotomy should be considered if PCa is high.

Thoracoscopy or thoracotomy: thoracotomy should be considered in patients with an indeterminate nodule and a high PCa, if lung function is adequate. Peripheral nodules can also be removed using VATS. If frozen sections confirm malignancy complete resection can be performed by open thoracotomy. If benign, thoracotomy and lobectomy can be avoided.

Summary

The incidental finding of a SPN on CXR or CT is common. The possibility of malignancy must be considered. The aim of management is curative surgery for early cancers whilst preventing the morbidity associated with resection of benign lesions. It is vital to involve the patient in the complicated decisions involved in the investigation and treatment of pulmonary nodules.

AUTHOR'S TIPS

- Cancers (primary and secondary) that present as a SPN may be curable.
- Always compare current imaging with previous imaging if available.
- Pulmonary nodules with diagnostic imaging features and solid nodules that are stable for over 2 years are benign. Part-solid and non-solid nodules require longer follow-up.
- Estimate the probability that the SPN is malignant (PCa). A risk calculator is available online at www.chestx-ray.com.
- If PCa is high (>60%) consider VATS and resection. If PCa is low (<5%), observation is appropriate. Lesions with intermediate Pca (5-60%) require further investigation.
- Lesions <8mm are too small to biopsy or use PET; follow-up with CT.
- New nodules detected during follow-up should be investigated independently.
- Patient preferences and operative risk must be considered, particularly if recommending invasive tests such as VATS. Discuss the risks and benefits of either invasive intervention or observation.

Further reading

Diagnosis and treatment of lung cancer. National Collaborating Centre for Acute Care. London 2005. Available from www.rcseng.ac.uk.

Gould MK, Fletcher J, Iannettoni MD, *et al.* Evaluation of patients with pulmonary nodules: when is it lung cancer?: ACCP evidence based clinical practice guidelines. *Chest* 2007; **132**: 108–130.

Miller JC, Shepard JA, Lanuti M, *et al.* Evaluating pulmonary nodules. *J Am Coll Radiol* 2007; **4**: 422–426.

Winer-Muram HT. The solitary pulmonary nodule. *Radiology* 2006; **239**: 34–48.

3.7 Wheeze

Wheeze is one of the commonest medical presentations and always implies airway obstruction. Asthma or COPD are the most likely diagnoses in first world adults but such generalisation is not possible in developing world populations where viral, bacterial and parasitic infection may be important or in children where congenital causes for wheeze must also be considered.

Definition

Wheezing is a high-pitched, continuous sound produced as the result of obstruction at any level within the airways. It is generated as the airway walls oscillate in response to the acceleration of air through a narrowed lumen. Flow may be impeded by intraluminal obstruction or extrinsic compression.

Approach

Correct diagnosis depends on complete assessment of the patients history and physical examination.

History

For refinement of the differential diagnosis the following factors must be taken into consideration:

- Age of the patient (Tables 3.7.1 and 3.7.2).
- Speed of onset of symptoms.
- Potential triggers (occupational, infectious, atopic).
- Past medical history.
- Family history.

Physical examination

The level and nature of the obstruction in part determines the nature of the wheeze. During physical examination it is important to distinguish the following features:

- Wheeze vs stridor.
- Monophonic vs polyphonic wheeze.
- Unilateral vs symmetrical wheeze.
- The presence of symptoms in inspiration or expiration.

Stridor is a harsh, inspiratory, monophonic sound loudest centrally on examination of the thorax which implies central airway obstruction. Wheeze is higher pitched and audible on more general examination of the chest. Monophonic wheeze implies fixed obstruction of medium-sized airways whilst polyphonic wheeze, which is usually bilateral, implies obstruction in medium to small airways.

Unilateral wheeze suggests a fixed obstruction such as an endobronchial tumour or extrinsic compression causing partial airway obstruction, e.g. as the result of vascular enlargement or lymphadenopathy, a foreign body or airway stenosis (congenital or acquired).

Table 3.7.1 Causes of adult wheeze by speed of onset/chronicity

Adults	
Acute onset	• Asthma (exacerbations)
	• Congestive heart failure
	• Pneumonia
	• Pulmonary embolism
	• Anaphylaxis
	• Aspiration syndromes
	• Foreign body aspiration
	• Vocal cord dysfunction

Table 3.7.1 Causes of adult wheeze by speed of onset/chronicity (continued)

Adults	
Slow onset	• COPD
	• Primary endobronchial tumours
	• Endobronchial metastasis (colon, breast, melanoma, kidney, pancreas)
	• Tracheal stenosis
	• Vocal cord paralysis
	• Asthma
	• Churg–Strauss/pulmonary eosinophilia syndrome

Table 3.7.2 Causes of wheeze in infants and young children by speed of onset/chronicity

Children	
Acute onset	• Infections e.g. bronchiolitis, pertussis
	• Reflux/aspiration
	• Asthma/wheezing syndromes
	• Pneumonia
	• Anaphylaxis
	• Foreign body aspiration
Slow onset	• Congenital anomalies
	• Bronchopulmonary dysplasia
	• Bronchomalacia
	• Vascular rings
	• Cystic fibrosis
	• Tracheal stenosis
	• Vocal cord paralysis
	• Asthma

Investigations

Laboratory

Few laboratory investigations assist in diagnosis of wheeze - particularly at the time of presentation. The following tests may assist in investigation:

Specific IgE (RAST testing): the presence of IgE specific for inhaled or food allergens may indicate an atopic precipitant for wheeze. A significant association between atopic sensitisation and wheeze is generally not observed until after the age of 4 years. In adults a general screen for sensitisation to inhaled aeroallergens may include testing for cat dander, house dust mite, and a mix of tree or grass pollens – selected on the basis of seasonality of symptoms reported by the patient. If allergic bronchopulmonary aspergillus is suspected then testing for total IgE, specific IgE to aspergillus, aspergillus precipitins (IgG) and sputum examination for fungal hyphae is required. Where available skin prick testing can be substituted for RAST testing.

Serology: routine testing for immunoglobulin sub-classes may identify subjects at increased risk of respiratory infections. In children in whom an infectious cause for symptoms is suspected blood for viral serology can be taken and stored for comparison with results of a paired sample taken 4–6 weeks later, at which point antibodies raised during the acute infection should have returned to normal.

Appropriate culture of nasopharyngeal aspirates may also be of assistance in identifying infectious causes of wheeze in children. Finally if tuberculosis is suspected then Mantoux testing or testing for T cells reactive to *M. tuberculosis* proteins (Elispot, Quantiferon Gold) can be considered.

Autoantibody testing: definitive diagnosis of pulmonary vasculitis is likely to require tissue biopsy obtained via VATS or fibreoptic bronchoscopy but autoantibody testing may be of assistance in suggesting a possible diagnosis. Two-thirds of subjects with Churg–Strauss syndrome will have a positive p-ANCA (anti-nuclear cytoplasmic antibody) and anti-MPO detected. Subjects are also likely to have a peripheral eosinophilia (>10%). 90% of subjects with extensive Wegener's granulomatosis and 75% with limited Wegener's will have a positive c-ANCA and staining for anti PR-3.

Cystic fibrosis: in children with recurrent respiratory tract infections, fat malabsorption or a number of other suggestive symptoms (see Chapter 11) testing for cystic fibrosis should be considered. In specialist centres this may involve sodium sweat testing. Alternatively genetic testing for common CF-genotypes is widely available.

Radiological investigation

A postero-anterior (PA) or lateral CXR may be normal in wheezing patients however the presence of lobar collapse/volume loss may indicate proximal airways obstruction and areas of atelectasis may suggest pulmonary embolus. If parenchymal infiltrates are present they may suggest infection or a vasculitic cause for symptoms. Examination of congenital abnormalities will be facilitated by contrast CT. Where detailed examination of the lung parenchyma is necesary high resolution CT scanning is required. Newer modalities such as spiral CT with multi-planar and 3D reconstructions allows assessment of airways in their long axis which may assist in diagnosis of obstruction.

Bronchoscopy

Where obstruction in the central or segmental airways or a dynamic abnormality such as tracheomalacia is suspected fibreoptic bronchoscopy is required. Rigid bronchoscopy is the method of choice for removal of foreign bodies. It should be noted that normal radiographic examination does not preclude foreign body aspiration and in such cases direct bronchoscopic visualisation of the airways is mandatory.

Lung function testing

In adult patients a reduced FEV_1 (forced expiratory volume in 1 second) indicates airway obstruction. Reversibility of the degree of obstruction by $\geq$ 15% (if this is >150ml) is diagnostic of reversible airflow obstruction. Where spirometry is normal peak flow variability of >20% on a peak flow diary or a positive response to an inhalational challenge such as methacholine may assist in diagnosis. Flow volume loops have a characteristic appearance in asthma with scalloping in the mid portion of the expiratory flow loop. In subjects with a compatible exposure history an FEV_1 of less than 80% predicted with an FEV_1/FVC ratio of <70% is considered diagnostic of COPD.

Flow-volume loops are most frequently used for differentiating between intra and extra-thoracic airflow obstruction. Three patterns are recognised. Variable intrathoracic, variable extrathoracic and fixed airflow obstruction. Where the obstruction is fixed, limitation in the inspiratory and expiratory flow volume loops will be seen (Fig. 3.7.1). Variable extrathoracic airway obstruction (e.g. bilateral vocal cord paralysis) is associated with a truncated inspiratory limb due to the area of obstruction being drawn inwards during the inspiratory manoeuvre, so limiting flow, and blown apart during expiration. Conversely variable intrathoracic flow obstruction is associated with a truncated expiratory loop but normal inspiratory limb.

Specific conditions

Bronchiolitis

Bronchiolitis is the commonest cause of wheeze in infants. Respiratory syncytial virus (RSV) should be considered in children aged less than 24 months during the epidemic season between November and April. Typical associated symptoms include low grade fever and rhinorrhoea. Coronaviruses are also commonly associated with wheezing in younger children, influenza A and adenovirus are found in older children and rhinovirus is found in children of all ages. Wheeze in the context of infection in infants occurs as the result of mucosal oedema leading to narrowing of the airway lumen.

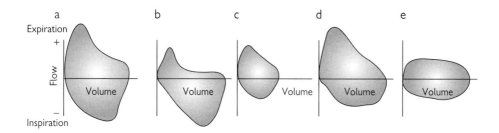

a: Normal

b: Intrathoracic obstruction

c: Restriction

d: Variable extrathoracic obstruction

e: Fixed airway obstruction

Fig. 3.7.1 Flow volume loop demonstrating fixed airway obstruction.

Vocal cord dysfunction (VCD)

VCD is inappropriate adduction of the vocal cords during inspiration, resulting in marked inspiratory stridor. This is often misdiagnosed as asthmatic wheeze resulting in treatment with escalating doses of glucocorticoids. This is generally ineffective at relieving symptoms leading to increased psychological and physical morbidity in the patient. Prevalence is highest in women aged 20–40 years. Subjects have normal lung function during testing or a flow volume loop consistent with variable extrathoracic flow obstruction. On arterial blood gas analysis the A–a gradient will be normal. The gold standard for diagnosis is direct visualisation of the vocal cords during a wheezing episode with observation of adduction of the anterior 2/3 during inspiration. Asthma may co-exist with VCD – bronchoprovocation testing may be safely carried out to distinguish VCD from variable airflow obstruction as the result of asthma. Treatment is challenging and often includes breathing re-training with a specialist physiotherapist and psychological support.

Asthma and COPD are the commonest clinical conditions associated with wheeze in adults. They are covered in detail in Chapters 4 and 5.

3.8 The acute admission with a new unilateral pleural effusion

Background

Undiagnosed pleural effusions are a common reason for admission to the Medical Admission Unit (MAU). Their clinical presentation ranges from an asymptomatic patient with an incidental finding on a CXR to a patient in extremis with severe dyspnoea and cyanosis.

The management focus of these patients should be aimed at quick relief of troubling symptoms with prompt targeted investigations to obtain an early diagnosis whilst undertaking as few invasive procedures as possible.

A plain CXR, focused history, thorough examination and diagnostic tap are often all that is necessary to make a diagnosis. This should be easily achievable by the team on take.

Key questions to ask yourself when seeing a patient with an undiagnosed pleural effusion on the MAU

1   Is this patient septic? If so it is likely that they will need to stay in for further investigation and management of their likely pleural infection.

2   Is the patient symptomatic? If not, and pleural infection is unlikely, could they be investigated as an urgent outpatient? Before discharge 30ml of pleural fluid under ultrasound guidance, needs to be removed and sent for analysis (also see Chapter 14.2). An urgent outpatient CT thorax with pleural contrast also needs to be arranged with rapid clinic follow up (Fig. 3.8.1).

3   If their main symptom is breathlessness (and pleural infection is unlikely) together with a moderately large pleural effusion on chest radiograph, then removing 1–1.5L with a venflon and three-way tap will give relief of symptoms, whilst leaving some of the fluid in situ for the CT scan and possible thoracoscopy if appropriate. After this fluid has been removed you need to ask could this patient now go home and have an urgent out-patient appointment after a CT thorax?

4   Do they require an urgent chest drain (e.g. empyema and haemothorax)? If so are you adequately trained to insert one? If not, you need to find an appropriately trained colleague. In addition, wherever possible, a chest drain should always be inserted with ultrasound guidance.

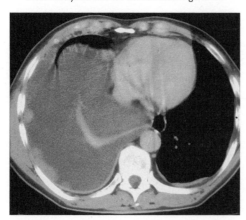

Fig. 3.8.1 CT with pleural contrast showing a pleural effusion with enhancement of the nodular pleural thickening.

Clinical presentation

The main presenting features of effusions are cough, dyspnoea and chest pain. Despite this, many patients are asymptomatic with an effusion first being found on examination or their admission CXR. Identifying the degree of respiratory compromise caused by the effusion is essential, as this is a deciding factor in where the patient may be best managed. It also helps to point towards an underlying cause; particularly in cases of pulmonary embolism where the degree of dyspnoea may be out of proportion to the size of the effusion.

History

On a busy MAU it is essential to be able to take a focused history ensuring all the most salient points are addressed. For any patient with an effusion this should include:

- Any evidence of associated infection – pyrexia, fevers, sweats, presence, or absence of a productive cough.
- Associated constitutional symptoms – particularly pointing towards an infective or malignant cause.
- Skin, joint or eye symptoms raising the possibility of underlying connective tissue disease.
- A full occupational history including any previous asbestos exposure – > 90% of patients with mesothelioma develop a pleural effusion and its incidence is continuing to rise (see Chapter 14.7).
- A thorough past medical history especially including any previous malignancies – breast cancer in particular can recur 10–20 years later, presenting with a unilateral pleural effusion.
- Risk factors for TB including foreign travel and place of birth.
- A full drug history – over 40 drugs can cause pleural effusions (further details in Chapter 14.2 or at www. pneumotox.com).

Examination

Chest examination can provide clues to the underlying cause of an effusion but examination of associated systems often produces the crucial diagnostic signs. Lymphadenopathy, intra-abdominal masses, cachexia and focal neurology can all indicate a malignant cause. Examination of joints, eyes and skin must be performed if there is any suspicion of underlying connective tissue disease. Looking for supporting signs of cardiac failure is also important.

The cardinal signs of an effusion are
- Reduced chest expansion.
- Reduced tactile vocal fremitus.
- Stony dull percussion note.
- Quiet breath sounds.
- Patch of bronchial breathing above effusion.

Initial investigations

CXR

Despite the multiple imaging modalities available a plain CXR is still the best initial investigation for a pleural effusion. A lateral X-ray is able to pick up 50ml of fluid, whilst 200ml is needed to be visible on a PA film.

However some pleural effusions can be easily missed. These include:

- Subpulmonary effusions – due to fluid accumulating between diaphragm and inferior part of the lung, they often mimic a raised hemidiaphragm.

- A patient on ITU will often have a supine chest radiograph. In this situation a pleural effusion will be distributed eveningly (if not loculated) over the posterior hemithorax, seen as diffuse opacification on the supine film.

Ultrasound

With an almost 100% sensitivity for fluid ultrasound can detect an effusion as small as 50ml (Fig. 3.8.2). It is particularly useful in detecting loculation and identifies a safe site for aspiration and/or chest tube insertion.

Ideally, all patients should undergo this type of imaging. Respiratory SpR's should be aiming to obtain a certificate of level 1 competency in pleural ultrasound during their training. This would then allow them to undertake this task on the MAU. Otherwise departmental imaging is recommended.

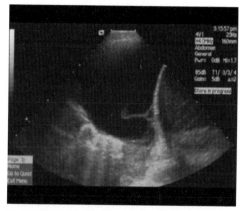

Fig. 3.8.2 Ultrasound image of a pleural effusion. D= diaphragm, P= pleural fluid, L= liver, and B = lung

CT

Most patients with an undiagnosed pleural effusion will require a CT thorax at some stage.

CT is especially useful to:
- Differentiate between empyema and lung abscess.
- Identify any underlying lung disease which may affect further management.
- Allow visualisation of an underlying mass lesion obscured by fluid on the plain film.
- Stage any underlying malignancy by assessing its spread throughout the body.
- Where malignancy is likely it will determine if there is any nodular pleural thickening. amenable to CT guided biopsy in patients unsuitable for thoracoscopy (see Fig. 3.8.1).

Blood tests

Essential initial blood tests that should be performed in all new patients presenting with a pleural effusion are:
- FBC & CRP – to identify possible underlying infection and allow monitoring of response to treatment.
- Clotting screen – to allow correction of any abnormalities prior to any invasive procedures.
- Liver function tests and calcium – often abnormal in malignancy.

Diagnostic pleural aspiration

All patients with an unilateral pleural effusion should have a diagnostic aspiration. This is easily done with a 21F bore needle on the MAU.

It should be sent for:
Biochemistry:
- Protein, LDH – to help differentiate the transudates from exudates.
- Glucose – low levels seen in pleural infection and rheumatoid effusions.
- pH – A pH <7.2 is an indication for chest tube drainage in cases of pleural infection. However, it is important to remember that in cases of advanced malignancy the pH may also be low.

Cytology:
- At least 15 mls must be sent, ideally in a container containing citrate as this reduces the risk of clots. It also allows the sample to be stored at four degrees Celsius for 4 days – useful over a weekend!
- The sensitivity of cytology is around 60% but this can be increased by sending a second sample.
- If there is any suspicion of Lymphoma. Flow cytometry is recommended.

Microbiology:
- Sending samples in blood culture bottles and a universal container increases the yield. A gram stain should be performed on all samples as well as AAFB and TB culture.

Please find further details in Chapter 14.2.

Key points

- Many patients with pleural effusions can be managed and investigated safely as outpatients.
- Early CT with contrast prior to fluid drainage provides more accurate diagnosis in underlying pleural disease.
- Always use ultrasound when undertaking pleural procedures.
- Always ask yourself – does this patient really need a chest tube now. If so, am I properly trained to insert it safely?

Further reading

Light RW, Gary Lee YC (eds.). *Textbook of Pleural Diseases,* 2nd edn. London: Edward Arnold Publisher Ltd, 2008.

Maskell NA, Butland RJA. BTS guidelines for the investigation of a unilateral pleural effusion in adults. *Thorax* 2003; **58**(2): 8–17.

3.9 Unexplained respiratory failure

The introduction of bedside ABG measurement and non-invasive ventilation has revolutionised the management of respiratory failure in the acute setting. The history, examination and initial investigations of these patients usually points to a straightforward diagnosis and subsequent management plan. In this section we will highlight a clinical approach to patients where the cause of respiratory failure is not obvious on initial assessment.

Respiratory failure is commonly classified into 2 types dependent on the arterial partial pressure of carbon dioxide; type 1 – hypoxaemia (PaO_2 < 8kPa) with a normal or low carbon dioxide, and type II – hypoxaemia and hypercapnoea (PaO_2 < 8kPa, $PaCO_2$ >6kPa). The underlying pathophysiology of these disorders is quite different. Type 1 respiratory failure is due to an increased alveolar–arterial (A–a) gradient with a normal or increased ventilatory response. This is a final common path for many diseases not just those with lung pathology, e.g. left ventricular failure. Patients presenting with type 2 respiratory failure or ventilatory failure can have a normal A–a gradient and it is these patients that we will consider below. A logical approach is to firstly to examine the causes of unexpected respiratory failure

Causes of unexplained respiratory failure

Failure of ventilatory drive

Neural suppression	Opiates
	Overdoses
	Metabolic alkalosis
Brainstem disease	Polio/postpolio
	Brainstem stroke
	Arnold–Chiari malformation
	Syringobulbia
	CNS infection (encephalitis, toxoplasmosis, tuberculoma)
	Brainstem tumour

Failure of the ventilatory pump

Myopathies	Acid maltase deficiency
	Duchene muscular dystrophy
	Ulrich's muscular dystrophy
	Myotonic dystrophy
	Limb-girdle dystrophy
	Inflammatory myopathies
Neuropathy	Motor neuron disease
	Neuralgic amyotrophy
	Guillain–Barré syndrome
	Spinal muscular atrophy (II-IV)
	Cord injury
Neuromuscular junction	Myasthenia gravis
	Lambert–Eaton syndrome
	Post-muscle relaxants e.g. suxamthonium
	Anti-cholinesterase poisoning (organophosphate poisoning)
Mixed	Critical care neuropathy/myopathy
Chest wall abnormalities	Obesity
	Scoliosis
	Thoracoplasty
	Flail chest
	Pneumothorax or large effusion
	Ankylosing spodylitis
Airways obstruction/ mixed	Unrecognised COPD/ severe asthma
	Obstructive sleep apnoea/obesity/ muscle weakness

History

A careful and thorough history with clear timelines, particularly for neuromuscular weakness, often points to a particular disorder. Sleep disturbance is often an early feature of many neuromuscular disorders and may predate breathlessness. Shoulder pain might suggest neuralgic amyotrophy. Orthopnoea, breathlessness when bathing or swimming is suggestive of diaphragm weakness. Swallowing and speech difficulties are important clues. Collateral history from partners and/or family is important particularly if the patient presents with a reduced level of consciousness.

Examination

A full examination can reveal subtle diagnostic clues; the rate, depth and pattern of breathing should be noted e.g. abnormal slowing of breathing seen in opiate use or Cheyne–Stokes periodic respiration seen in cerebral and cardiac disease; scars and evidence of previous surgery might point to phrenic nerve injury; neurological signs such as fatigability, fasciculation, myotonia, and weakness should be looked for; abdominal paradox (inward drawing of the abdomen during inspiration) points to diaphragm weakness.

Initial investigations

ABGs

- Assessment of blood gasses off supplementary oxygen.
- The level of $PaCO_2$.
- The base excess/base deficit.
- A–a gradient (normal <2.5 changes with age).

Chest radiograph/HRCT

This may reveal evidence of unsuspected lung disease

Lung function

- Unexpected airway obstruction.
- Reduction in vital capacity (chest wall or neurological).
- Fall in supine VC (diaphragm weakness).
- If supine VC <1 litre then this likely to be cause of failure.
- Mouth pressure, sniff pressures and trans-diaphragm pressures can be useful in specific situations.

Other tests

- Sleep study – to exclude REM related hypoxaemia, obstructive sleep apnoea.
- CK – elevated in some myopathies.
- ANA, ANCA – repeated measurements are helpful in vasculitis.
- Acetyl cholinesterase receptor antibodies – myasthenia gravis.
- ECG – assessment of right and left heart function, estimation of pulmonary artery pressure and exclusion of structural lesions is often helpful.
- Electromyography/nerve conduction studies – diagnostic for MND, myotonia, myasthenia.
- Muscle biopsy – acid maltase deficiency.

Brainstem imaging – gadlinium-enhanced MRI to exclude structural lesions

CSF sampling – lumbar puncture to exclude CNS inflammation/infection

Clinical cases

Case 1

A 65-year-old man, following an elective left total hip replacement, was noted to have frequent oxygen desaturations in recovery. Daytime ABGs on room air demonstrated a P_aO_2 8.5kPa and a P_aCO_2 6.8kPa. Chest radiograph was normal. Further questioning of his wife revealed a several year history of heavy snoring, witnessed apnoeas, and unrefreshing sleep. The patient also suffered from significant daytime hypersomnolence and had been involved in a car accident 4 months previously where he dozed off during driving and crossed the central reservation. Examination revealed a BMI of 36 and a bull neck. Overnight oximetry is shown in Fig. 3.9.1. The patient was commenced on CPAP therapy with good symptomatic effect, and at 3 months, ABGs on air revealed a P_aO_2 10.5kPa and a P_aCO_2 5.8kPa.

Diagnosis – severe obstructive sleep apnoea.

Case 2

A 33-year-old lady admitted from Accident & Emergency with a 2-week history of generalised lethargy, culminating in being bed-bound for 24 hours. 4 weeks prior to admission, she had a viral upper respiratory tract infection that was self-resolving. On examination she had a symmetrical distal weakness of her lower limbs associated with lower limb areflexia. She developed progressive muscle weakness and a steady deterioration in limb function on the general ward. She began complaining of breathlessness and difficulty in coughing, and vial capacity was measured at 900ml. ABGs demonstrated a pH 7.28, P_aO_2 9.4kPa and a P_aCO_2 8.0kPa. The patient was intubated and admitted to intensive care. Brain and lung imaging revealed no abnormalities. CSF examination demonstrated normal cell count but elevated protein level, and neurophysiology showed evidence of demyelination with significant slowing of nerve conduction. The patient was treated with IV immunoglobulin, and made a progressive recovery and was eventually extubated. At 2 months, however, she still required nocturnal non-invasive ventilation due to moderate respiratory muscle weakness and nocturnal hypoventilation.

Diagnosis – Guillain–Barré syndrome.

Case 3

A 68-year-old woman was admitted to the ICU following an elective mediastinoscopy and biopsy of a mediastinal mass imaged incidentally on chest radiograph and subsequent CT. Following general anaesthesia, she was unable to ventilate adequately unaided or clear bronchial secretions. Reversal of muscle relaxant initially showed a good response but then ventilation deteriorated again. She remained intubated and ventilated, and eventually required a tracheostomy. There was a history from the daughter that the patient had been complaining of intermittent tiredness and muscle weakness for several months before the operation. Electrophysiological studies showed a decrement in compound muscle action potential amplitude on repetitive nerve stimulation (Fig. 3.9.2), whilst single fibre EMG demonstrated abnormal jitter. Histology from the mediastinal mass confirmed a thymoma. Tensilon test demonstrated an immediate improvement in maximum inspiratory pressure measured via the tracheostomy from 18cmH$_2$O to 65cmH$_2$O. Serologic testing confirmed autoantibodies to the acetylcholine receptor. The patient was started on pyridostigmine and underwent plasmapheresis, followed by prednisolone. The patient was eventually decannulated, and managed without the need for non-invasive ventilation.

Diagnosis – myasthenia gravis.

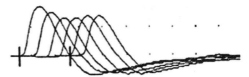

Fig. 3.9.2

Case 4

A 44-year-old man presented with a 4-month history of progressive shortness of breath and reducing exercise tolerance. Symptoms were particularly worse on lying flat at night. He was a keen swimmer, but in the last 2 months, he had stopped going to the pool as he was getting breathless even standing in the deep end. In the previous month, he was feeling muzzy-headed and getting frequent headaches in the morning. Examination revealed evidence of abdominal paradox and tongue fasiculations. Vital capacity dropped from 2.0 to 1.1 litres from sitting to supine positions. Sniff nasal pressure was markedly reduced at 22cm H$_2$O (normal >70cm H$_2$O). Chest radiograph demonstrated small lung volumes. ABGs on room air were P_aO_2 11.1kPa and a P_aCO_2 6.7kPa. Overnight sleep study showed REM related oxygen desaturations (Fig. 3.9.3) and a rise in transcutaneous CO_2 to above 9kPa. The patient was started on domiciliary non-invasive ventilation with good palliation of symptoms. EMG demonstrated fibrillations, positive sharp waves and fasciculation potentials. The patient subsequently developed significant

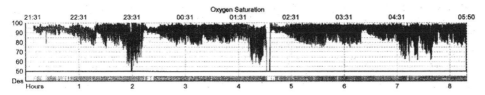

Fig. 3.9.1

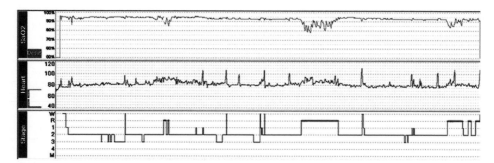

Fig. 3.9.3
SaO2 Plot – oximetry data recorded over the entire night.
Heart Plot – heart rate data recorded over the entire night
Stage Plot – sleep stages recorded the entire night.

bulbar symptoms, rapidly progressing to dysphonia, dysphagia and pooled secretions.

Diagnosis – motor neurone disease.

Clinical pointers

- Does the patient require immediate ventilatory support?
- Is the clinical setting appropriate for the patient e.g. general ward, level 2 (HDU) or level 3 (ICU) care?
- Is there an appropriate ceiling of treatment?
- Does the patient require intubation and ventilation?

Asthma

Chapter contents

4.1 Pathophysiology

Definition and epidemiology

- Asthma is usually defined clinically as reversible airflow limitation, but current definitions also recognise the presence of airway hyper-responsiveness to bronchoconstricting stimuli such as histamine, and eosinophilic airway inflammation.
- It affects 2.5 million children and 3 million adults in the UK. Around 70% of asthmatics are atopic (that is they make IgE responses to common allergens such as pollen, dust or animal danders), and 30% non-atopic.
- Asthma may be triggered by occupational exposure, drugs (including aspirin: around 1%). Asthma attacks or exacerbations may be triggered by viral infections, allergen exposure or non-specific irritants (see Acute asthma, p. 78).
- Genetic analysis of asthma has defined genes linked to atopy, airway hyper-responsiveness or asthma symptoms: including genes of the IgE receptor and genes associated with defective epithelial repair.

Diagnosis

- Asthma is diagnosed on the basis of variable symptoms of cough, wheeze, chest tightness and breathlessness and confirmed by demonstration of reversible airway narrowing either spontaneously over time or in response to inhaled β2 agonists.
- This can be documented as 15% or more improvement in peak expiratory flow rate or FEV_1. Radiology may show hyper-inflation but is not useful in diagnosis except to rule out other conditions.

AHR

A characteristic feature of asthma is exaggerated narrowing of the airways in response to specific or non-specific stimuli, termed AHR. This can be measured in the lung function laboratory by controlled inhalation of agents such as histamine to determine the dose of histamine causing a 20% fall in FEV_1 from baseline (PD20). Such measurement is not usually required for diagnosis but can be helpful if there is doubt.

Allergy and asthma

- A majority of asthmatics are atopic and allergic and most have co-existent nasal airway disease.
- Treatment of rhinitis is important for symptom control and may in itself help with asthma control although direct evidence is scant.
- Assessment of allergy in asthma by skin prick testing and history is important if anti-IgE therapy is considered. Allergen avoidance measures were ineffective in trials where they were applied broadly in house dust mite sensitised asthmatics. Further studies will be needed to determine whether focused interventions could be effective in severe asthmatics with predominant mono-sensitisation to house dust mites together with exposure in the home.
- Acute severe asthma associated with anaphylaxis may form type 1 'brittle asthma', and should be investigated for allergic sensitisation. These rare patients may require injectable epinephrine (EpiPen®) to self-inject to treat attacks.

> **AUTHOR'S TIP**
>
> On a practical clinical level patients may find it useful to confirm sensitisation to pets or pollen allergens. *Aspergillus* sensitisation and screening for allergic bronchopulmonary aspergilosis should form part of the work-up of all symptomatic asthmatics (skin test or RAST for specific IgE, blood (and/or sputum) eosinophil count, *Aspergillus* precipitins and CT if indicated by symptoms of chronic sputum production).

Airway inflammation in asthma

- Patients who die of asthma show massive inflammatory infiltration of the airway at post-mortem, often with marked eosinophilia and mucus plugging.
- The use of bronchial biopsies and induced sputum to sample the airways showed that epithelial shedding and airway eosinophilia together with mast cell and lymphocytic infiltration are present even in mild or asymptomatic asthma.
- Exactly how inflammation contributes to airway narrowing and AHR in asthma remains controversial although many of these features have been correlated to disease severity measured by symptoms, airflow obstruction or AHR.
- Bronchial biopsy is not helpful in diagnosis of asthma at present as generally changes are not specific. However, a 'normal' biopsy (no remodelling or inflammation) may be helpful in apparent refractory asthma to focus on other causes for symptoms.

IgE and mast cells and basophils

- A proportion of asthmatics are atopic and make IgE to common allergens.
- In these patients, allergen exposure may trigger attacks through cross linking high-affinity IgE receptors on mast cells and basophils leading to release of histamine, cytokines and growth factors from pre-stored sources in granules as well as *de novo* synthesis of leukotrienes and cytokines.
- Histamine and lipid mediators may cause acute airway narrowing (within minutes) due to oedema, vascular engorgement and muscle contraction and may be important in acute severe asthma linked to anaphylaxis or some cases of 'brittle asthma'.
- Cytokines and growth factors are thought to contribute to further airway inflammation and airway remodelling (see below). These factors laid the basis for development of anti-IgE treatment for asthma (Xolair®: see Key Issues: antibody therapy in asthma box): this antibody blocks the association of IgE with its receptor on mast cells and basophils. Of note IgE is also involved in 'antigen trapping' since dendritic cells have high affinity IgE receptors which can act to 'catch' allergens for processing into peptides within the cell for subsequent presentation to and activation of T lymphocytes: anti-IgE also blocks this process.
- It is of note that non-atopic asthmatics also have increased IgE receptor-bearing cells in the airway, together with evidence of local airway synthesis of IgE and marginally raised serum IgE. Whether this is mechanistically important or a target for treatment remains unclear.

Eosinophils in asthma

- Blood and sputum eosinophilia are characteristic but not diagnostic of asthma (atopic and non-atopic).
- Eosinophils contain specific basic granule proteins which probably function in host defence against parasites and helminths, but which can also damage airway epithelium in vitro and cause AHR if instilled into the airway of experimental animals.
- Eosinophils can produce mediators such as leukotriene C4 which act to contract airway smooth muscle, recruit inflammatory cells and increase mucus production.

Given these findings, together with studies that related airway eosinophilia and granule proteins to asthma severity and results of animal models, the eosinophil hypothesis of asthma suggested that eosinophils were an important cause of much of the airway pathology of asthma. Certainly inhaled or oral steroid treatment dramatically reduces eosinophilic inflammation in asthma.

- However, more recent data has cast some doubt on the importance of eosinophils in asthma.
- Anti-IL-5 antibody treatment which dramatically reduced blood and sputum eosinophils failed to have clinical impact on asthma.
- Studies of a condition termed eosinophilic bronchitis (EB: associated with cough but normal lung function and no AHR), showed similar eosinophilic airway inflammation in asthma and EB. The only difference detected between the two conditions was infiltration of airway smooth muscle with mast cells in asthma but not EB.
- It is important to note that these studies do **not** definitively rule out an important role for eosinophil in asthma. Eosinophils were not completely removed from the airway by anti-IL-5 treatment (a 50% reduction was seen) and further studies are required to show whether eosinophil activation differs between EB and asthma.

Eosinophils may play a role in asthma exacerbations.

- In a study comparing use of sputum eosinophil measurement to usual guideline management of asthma, the control of sputum eosinophilia more than halved exacerbation rates.
- In the clinical anti-IL-5 studies, exacerbations rates were reduced (also 50% but not statistically significant) at the highest anti-IL-5 dose.
- Some studies suggest persistent eosinophilia in a proportion (around 50%) of asthmatics who remain symptomatic despite inhaled steroid and other treatment but that others have persistent symptoms with non-eosinophilic inflammation. Whether there is a subgroup of asthmatics in whom analysis of airway eosinophilia will be incorporated into management guidelines remains to be seen.

KEY ISSUES: EOSINOPHILS IN ASTHMA

- Eosinophilia is characteristic of asthma in blood, sputum and bronchial biopsies but is not diagnostic (also seen in some COPD and in eosinophilic bronchitis)
- Eosinophilia has been correlated with disease severity and these cells have the potential to contribute to epithelial damage, AHR and inflammation
- Animal models can reproduce features of asthma pathology by activating eosinophils in the airway and block AHR and remodelling by removing or reducing eosinophils
- Intervention studies with anti-IL-5 in humans were not effective clinically but did not fully deplete airway eosinophils or target eosinophilic patients

T cells, cytokines, and asthma

- T lymphocytes are thought to be important drivers of airway inflammation in asthma.
- These cells are pivotal to specific immune responses and are activated by antigens processed and presented by cells such as dendritic cells.
- In asthmatic airways, CD4+ T cells or helper T cells appear to be activated by allergens presented by dendritic cells leading to production of a particular pattern of messenger chemicals termed cytokines.
- These T-helper-2 (Th2) cytokines include interleukin (IL)-4 and IL-13 which turn on IgE antibody production and activate airway epithelium, and IL-5 which acts to recruit and retain eosinophils to the airway.
- T cells producing these cytokines are the predominant cell type in asthmatic airways and strategies to block these cytokines with monoclonal antibodies or other therapies have been developed, based on expression studies of human asthma and intervention studies in animal models.
- Other cell types including mast cells and eosinophils and airway structural cells can also produce these cytokines so may amplify and perpetuate Th2 type inflammation in asthma.
- More recently, cytokines that favour development of a Th2 type of response have been described: these include IL-25 and IL-33 which act on the T cells and TSLP (thymic stimulating lymphopoietin) which acts on dendritic cells.
- Clinical testing of anti-IL-4 and anti-IL-5 strategies was disappointing to date, whilst anti-IL-13 agents are currently being evaluated.
- In addition other inflammatory cytokines such as TNF and IL-6 are over-expressed in asthmatic airways: although anti-TNF therapies are useful in other inflammatory pathologies such as rheumatoid arthritis and Crohn's disease, data in asthma is less compelling. Agents to target IL-25, IL-33 or TSLP may be of interest in the future.

KEY ISSUES: ANTIBODY THERAPY IN ASTHMA

- Anti-IgE (Xolair®) is the only currently licensed antibody therapy: data suggest it can reduce exacerbation rates by 50% and may reduce steroid requirement. No effect on lung function in trials. It can only be used if total IgE is between 30 and 700IU/l. No clear guidance on how to assess response.
- Anti-IL-5: clinical studies negative although trend to reduce exacerbation rates. Did not fully deplete airway eosinophils. Not licensed.
- Anti-TNF: one positive but at least 2 other negative trials in severe/moderate asthma. Not licensed.
- Others: anti-IL-4, anti-IL-13 receptor, anti-IL-5 receptor, antichemokines (eotaxin) either discouraging or no current data, but investigating may guide use to subgroups.

Corticosteroids

Corticosteroids are the main anti-inflammatory agent in asthma and act in part through suppressing T-cell cytokine production. Other specific immunosuppressive agents have been successful in trials including cyclosporin A and methotrexate, but have not found wide application in severe asthma and their use should be restricted to specialist units in refractory asthma.

Allergen immunotherapy

Allergen immunotherapy has been used for many years to desensitise patients with severe hay fever or anaphylaxis to bee or wasp venom. This treatment involves subcutaneous injection of escalating doses of allergen extracts which appears to induce immune suppression or tolerance. This treatment has been shown to be effective for house dust mite-related asthma and is widely used in countries other than the UK. The limitation is the risk of anaphylaxis: modification of the allergen for injection may allow more widespread use of this therapy although at present it remains **contraindicated** for asthma in the UK.

Regulatory T cells

This arm of the immune system naturally suppresses immune responses and seems to prevent autoimmunity and immune-mediated organ damage due to over-exuberant immune responses to infection. There is increasing evidence that allergic diseases including asthma are associated with a relative failure of this arm of immunoregulation and strategies to redress regulatory T cell function may be of interest.

Anti-viral interferons

Recent data also suggest that there may be reduced production of anti-viral interferons in asthmatic airways: whether this predisposes to viral exacerbations of asthma or is amenable to therapy remains to be seen.

Chemokines

Recruitment of inflammatory cells such as eosinophils and T cells depends in part on production of chemoattractant cytokines (chemokines) by airway epithelial and other cells. Chemokine receptors are also co-factors for HIV infection, thus there is a huge push for development of agents to block these pathways. As yet such treatment has not been studied in human asthma.

Airway remodelling in asthma

- One of the characteristic histopathological findings in the asthmatic airways is epithelial change with increased goblet cells, increased airway collagen and extracellular matrix deposition and airway smooth muscle hypertrophy. These changes are referred to as 'airway remodelling'.
- Such changes are present even in children with asthma, and their relation to airway inflammation and pathophysiology remains uncertain. Mathematical modelling suggests that airway smooth-muscle changes may be important in airway hyper-responsiveness. It is also suggested that remodelling may predispose to fixed airway narrowing and the accelerated loss of lung volumes that occurs in asthma. Current therapies (including inhaled steroids) have little impact on airway remodelling and until reversal is achieved in animal or human studies the real impact of these changes will remain a subject of speculation.

Severe or 'refractory' asthma: the future challenge

For most asthmatic patients, excellent disease control can be achieved with inhaled steroids, long acting bronchodilators and or other agents as suggested by international guidelines. However, around 2% remain symptomatic despite treatment and these patients represent a major management challenge as they account for 50% of resource use in asthma and are at increased risk of dying of asthma and of morbidity from their disease or oral steroid treatment. Thorough investigation is vital, as a substantial proportion have other chest disease, non-adherence or other

factors to explain their persistent symptoms. Of note, asthmatics who smoke are less responsive to inhaled steroids than non-smokers. However around 1% of severe asthmatics have asthma largely refractory to current treatment and there is a pressing need to evaluate the airway pathophysiology of these patients to define whether indeed there are different immunopathological patterns (eosinophilic and non-eosinophilic disease or neutrophilic airway inflammation). Such studies should define which patients will benefit from expensive biological therapies of the present and future.

KEY ISSUES: DIFFICULT OR REFRACTORY ASTHMA

- Systematic assessment protocols have identified up to 15% non-asthma diagnosis and 30% non-adherence with treatment.
- Some evidence of fixed airway narrowing in a sub group.
- May be subtypes (eosinophilic and non-eosinophilic).
- Regional specialist 'difficult asthma' units may help in assessment.

AUTHOR'S TIPS

- Prednisolone and cortisol levels (sent to regional reference laboratory for HPLC) and trial of injected triamcinalone can be very helpful in assessing adherence and treatment response.
- Full lung function tests are essential.
- Think of and exclude other diagnoses: just because the notes have said 'asthma' for 20 years does not necessarily mean this is correct!
- Nurse specialist and psychologist input is invaluable.

Further reading

Bousquet J, Rabe K, Humbert M, et al. Predicting and evaluating response to omalizumab in patients with severe allergic asthma. Respir Med 2007; **101**: 1483–1492.

British Thoracic Society. Scottish Intercollegiate Guidelines Network. British guideline on the management of asthma. Thorax 2003; **58** (Suppl 1): 1–94.

Busse WW, Lemanske RF Jr. Asthma. N Engl J Med 2001; **344**: 350–362.

Heaney LG, Robinson DS. Severe asthma treatment: need for characterising patients. Lancet 2005; **365**: 974–976.

Holgate ST, Davies DE, Powell RM, et al. Local genetic and environmental factors in asthma disease pathogenesis: chronicity and persistence mechanisms. Eur Respir J 2007; **29**: 793–803.

O'Byrne PM, Inman MD, Parameswaran K. The trials and tribulations of IL-5, eosinophils, and allergic asthma. J Allergy Clin Immunol 2001; **108**: 503–508.

Papadopoulos NG, Xepapadaki P, Mallia P, et al. Mechanisms of virus-induced asthma exacerbations: state-of-the-art. A GA2LEN and InterAirways document. Allergy 2007; **62**: 457–470.

Robinson DS. Regulation: the art of control? Regulatory T cells and asthma and allergy. Thorax 2004; **59**: 640–643.

Robinson DS, Hamid Q, Ying S, et al. Predominant TH2-like bronchoalveolar T-lymphocyte population in atopic asthma. N Engl J Med 1992; **326**: 298–304.

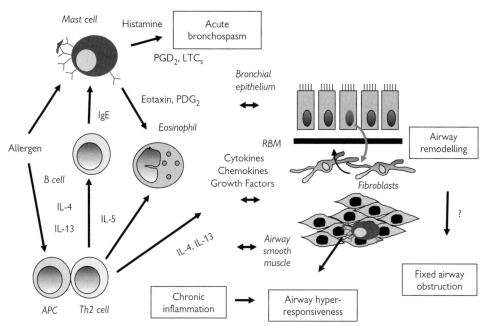

Fig. 4.1.1 Mechanisms in asthma. Allergen activates inflammation through direct interaction with IgE on mast cells and basophils but also via dendritic cell processing and antigen presentation (APC) including activity of IL-25, IL-33 and TSLP, leading to activation of a Th2 response. Th2 cytokines IL-4 and IL-13 switch on IgE production andf activate the asthmatic epithelium. Il-5 acts on eosinophil. These inflammatory cells interact with structural cells including epithelium, smooth muscle and fibroblasts to induce inflammatory cytokines and chemokines but also tissue remodelling though production and activation of growth factors such as TGFβ (transforming growth factors) which activate fibrosis. Together with goblet cell hyperplasia and smooth muscle cells hypertrophy and interaction with mast cells these changes may contribute both to AHR and development of fixed airway narrowing.

4.2 Allergic rhinitis

Infection (especially viral) is the commonest cause of rhinitis overall, but this section focuses on allergic rhinitis.

Background

Pathogenesis

Type 1 (IgE mediated) immediate hypersensitivity accounts for most allergic rhinitis. Typically, the allergic immune response is directed against airborne protein-based allergens. Local nasal inflammation arises in the context of TH2 type immune responses. Clinically, symptoms (sneezing, dripping, blockage) occur within minutes of exposure to trigger substances (allergens).

Epidemiology

The problem is seen worldwide. Prevalence has increased in the industrialised 'West'. Around 20% of the UK population have allergic rhinitis. A familial pattern of predisposition is recognised, but the specific genetic factors have not been fully defined.

Rhinitis and asthma

It is increasingly clear, that allergic rhinitis is a risk factor for asthma. The supporting evidence includes:
- Perennial rhinitis is an independent risk factor for asthma. Asthma is commoner in patients with perennial rhinitis, irrespective of whether they are atopic individuals.
- Children, who develop seasonal rhinitis, are more likely to develop asthma, but the risk is reduced if the seasonal allergic rhinitis is adequately treated.
- In patients with both asthma and rhinitis, there are fewer seasonal admissions for asthma, if the rhinitis is adequately treated.
- Bronchial hyper-reactivity increases in the hay fever season.

Aspirin sensitivity/nasal polyps and asthma

'Samter's' triad. Rhinitis is often the first symptom.

All non-steroidal anti-inflammatories should be avoided. Nasal polyposis can be reduced medically (nasal corticosteroid) or surgically. Accidental exposure to aspirin (or similar drugs) can provoke life-threatening adverse effects. Clinical features can include urticaria, and angioedema, as well as asthma.

Differential diagnosis

Pointers against allergy include:
- Asymmetric/unilateral symptoms/signs.
- Symptoms which fail to respond to adequate doses of corticosteroid (see Treatment p.65).
- Mid-life onset with no previous allergic problems and no family history of atopy.

Non-allergic diagnoses

- Congenital defects (e.g. ciliary dysmotility) – rare.
- Infection – common but typically acute/short lived, and with associated systemic features (malaise, fever, 'flu-like symptoms').
- Iatrogenic – medical (e.g. excessive decongestant medication).
- Iatrogenic – surgical.
- Autoimmune (Wegener's – rare).

Non-allergic irritation/inflammation

Cigarette smoke, pungent inhaled chemicals (e.g. perfumes), dusty environments (building sites), and chemical contact sensitivity (e.g. chlorine in swimming pools), are all common examples of non-allergic rhinitis. It is common for healthy individuals to find these factors irritant. Note however, in any circumstance where the nasal mucosa is damaged (e.g. viral infection), these irritants will be more problematic.

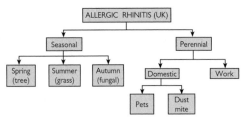

Fig. 4.2.1 Diagnostic algorithm.

KEY POINT

Non-specific irritants do exacerbate true allergic rhinitis.

One key clue is whether symptoms are all year round (perennial), seasonal, or perennial with seasonal exacerbation (e.g. house dust mite (HDM) with grass pollen sensitivity).

Another consideration is whether symptoms suggest a domestic- or work-related trigger. Work-related symptoms (which may be due to true allergy or non-allergic irritation) would reduce at weekends and evenings typically, and be maximal towards the end of the working day. Examples might include vets, bakers (flour dust), latex (hospital staff), and chemicals / paints.

In the UK, seasonal allergic rhinitis may be due to
- Tree pollen: February–May.
- Grass pollen: May–August.
- Fungal spores: July–September.
- Weed pollen: April–September.

Most seasonal rhinitis in the UK will be tree and or grass (weed and fungal spores are less of a problem)

Diagnostic tests

Skin prick tests

These tests detect functional IgE specific antibody, in vivo. They are sensitive and at least for the common inhaled allergens (including HDM, pollens, pets) are reliable with sensitivity and specificity both approaching 80–90%. Purified allergen is applied externally to the patients skin, and the allergen is scratched into the epidermis by gentle use of a sharp sterile blade. Positive results (itchy wheal and flare reactions) develop within 15 minutes, and the patient can leave the clinic knowing their results. This test has an extremely good safety record.

Specific IgE blood tests

Originally 'RAST' tests were performed. Nowadays simpler non-radioactive assays are performed. Purified allergen in vitro is used to detect small amounts of allergen specific IgE. A sample of clotted blood (serum) is required by the laboratory, and results are routinely available the same day.

Total serum IgE
This test is of little value. Elevated levels point to an allergic (atopic) tendency but elevated IgE per se does not prove allergic rhinitis.

Results from skin prick tests and from allergen specific IgE blood tests largely agree with one another, and costs are comparable.

Provocation tests
Allergen challenge, to determine if symptoms are reliably provoked is rarely necessary, and in some circumstances (e.g. asthmatics) carries some risk.

Treatment
Allergen avoidance
This can be difficult or near impossible. Some situations are easier to manage than others – e.g. removing feather pillows from the home.

> **KEY POINT**
> Some pet epithelial allergens, (notoriously cat), can persist for many years after a cat has died or been removed, despite house cleaning.

HDM – a very common culprit

Typical features include:
- Symptoms worst first thing in the morning.
- Tendency to wake with nasal obstruction.
- Symptoms with vacuum cleaning / dusting.

> **KEY POINT**
> HDM can be strangly limked to eczema and reduced exporure can lead to improvement of eczema in many cases.

HDM reduction measures include:
- Purchase of barrier bedding (pillow cases and sheets). HDM feeds on shed human epithelium, and large reservoirs of HDM are found in bedding.
- Use of chemicals (acaricides), which kill HDM.
- Maintaining a domestic environment which is unfavourable to HDM (increased ventilation, low humidity, use of air filters).

Clinical trials of these methods have suffered from design limitations. Isolated use of barrier bedding is unlikely to be successful. In the UK, in the winter especially, low humidity is hard to achieve. Acaricides offer most promise. Combining interventions may prove to be most effective, but again the evidence base is poor.

Irritant avoidance
Non-specific irritants (cigarette smoke, dust, swimming pools (chlorine, perfumes)) can exacerbate allergic rhinitis and should be avoided.

> **KEY POINT**
> The commonest reason for treatment failure is non-compliance or inappropriate drug administration. Drugs will **not** work if the nasal passages are blocked in the first place (here use of topical decongestant drops helps open up the airways before switching to topical corticosteroid and or other medications).

Table 4.2.1 Topical medications

	Sneez	Drip	Blockage
Saline douches			++
Decongestant			+++
Anti-histamine	++	+	
Ipatropium bromide		+++	
Topical corticosteroid	+++	+++	+++
Chromoglycate	++	+	+

In the same way that many asthma suffers may not have been taught how to optimally use their inhalers, the majority of patients with allergic rhinitis do not employ the correct delivery technique. A 'head down' position (with the head bent forward, akin to kneeling on a prayer mat) helps ensure that medication does not simply drip into the oro-pharynx. Administration should be passive (no violent sniffing).

Systemic decongestants are often less effective than topical equivalents and are best avoided. Both preparations risk rebound congestion if overused (more than 1 week). Ephedrine is the safest topical sympathomimetic, and can be effective within hours.

Mild rhinitis
Often, the first step should be to try saline washouts and or topical decongestants (e.g. ephedrine). These simple treatments with or without anti histamine (anti-H1 receptor) topically or orally may be sufficient on an as required basis. Oral anti-histamines have few side effects and are easier to administer than their topical counterparts.

Moderately severe rhinitis
For more severe symptoms, (see Table 4.2.1), topically administered corticosteroid is the gold standard. Aim to use the lowest effective doses topically. Concurrent anti-histamine will usually also be required.

Severe rhinitis
Treatment options include addition of:
- Topical chromoglycate.
- Topical ipatropium bromide – very useful for vasomotor drip.
- Oral leukotriene antagonists (reduce obstruction/dripping).

Oral corticosteroid
Under certain circumstances, it is generally agreed that oral prednisolone or similar, can be justified to cover short periods of either severe symptoms, or where avoidance of symptoms needs to be guaranteed (e.g. weddings, examinations). Doses would be similar to those used to control asthma exacerbations.

Prophylaxis/prevention
Where problems can be predicted (e.g. hay fever) it is good practice to start treatment a week or two before onset of symptoms, and maintain it daily throughout the season.

Benefit/harmful effects
The estimated minimum number of treated patients required to demonstrate benefit (5 patients for topical anti-H1 or for injection immunotherapy, and 15 for oral monteleukast), can be contrasted with the number of

patients on the same medication before significant side effects are noted (approximately 15, 25, 150 respectively). Thus monteleukast is 'safer' but less effective than topical steroid.

Desensitisation

This involves planned, controlled, cautious, repeated exposure to purified allergen (e.g. grass pollen prior to the hay fever season) administered in such a way that the resulting immunological response favours 'tolerance' with reduced symptoms, and reduced need for rescue medication. The efficacy is dose dependant.

Subcutaneous injection

This has been most used over the last 25 years. Recently, better defined allergen preparations, exclusion of brittle asthmatics, and limitation to experienced secondary care centres, has led to fewer severe side effects.

Consent for desensitisation by injection must highlight the following considerations:
- Only successful in approximately 75% patients (varies according to the allergen).
- minor/local injection site irritation (25% or more).
- Severe systemic immediate hypersensitivity reactions in fewer than 5% (risks reduced if asthmatic patients are excluded).
- Patients must be detained for observation for 1 hour post treatment.

Note percentages quoted here vary, with some allergens (e.g. cat epithelium) being more likely to provoke adverse reactions than other allergens.

Oral desensitisation

Immunological tolerance can be generated by mucosal (e.g. oral) antigen / allergen exposure, rather than by subcutaneous injection. This logistically easier approach shows promise, and early observations suggest that adverse hypersensitivity reactions are less than with subcutaneous immunotherapies. This approach offers the prospect of potentially safe home therapy. However, direct comparisons of subcutaneous and oral delivery employing the same allergen preparations are awaited.

Results to date suggest improved outcomes when compared to placebo, but further studies are required.

Pollen sensitivity and 'oral allergy' (pollen/food allergy) syndrome

A sub-group of pollen-sensitive individuals develop additional food-related problems typically several years after onset of their hay fever. Immunological hypersensitivity to particular pollen proteins (namely profilins) leads to specific and predictable cross – reactions and immediate 'oral' or throat symptoms when certain foods (which contain the shared allergen) are handled or eaten.

The problem relates to
- Fruits (apples, cherries, peaches and several others).
- Vegetables (potatoes, celery, carrots and others).
- Some tree nuts (hazelnut, walnut and almond).

KEY POINT

With the exception of nuts (which may resist cooking) profilin proteins are heat sensitive and easily destroyed by cooking/tinning/microwaving.

Further reading

Durham SR. Allergen immunotherapy (desensitisation) for allergic diseases. *Clin Med* 2006; **6**: 348–351.

Leynaert B, Bousquet J, Neukirch C, et al. Perennial rhinitis: an independent risk factor for asthma in non-atopic subjects. *J Allergy Clin Immunol* 1999; **104**: 301–304.

Madonini E, Briatico-Vangosa G, Pappacoda A, et al. Seasonal increase of bronchial reactivity in allergic rhinitis. *J Allergy Clin Immunol* 1987; **79**: 358–363.

Portnoy J M, Van Osdol T, Brock Williams P. Evidence based strategies for the treatment of allergic rhinitis. *Curr Allergy Asthma* Rep 2004; **6**: 439–446.

4.3 Pharmacology

The pharmacology of asthma largely involves the use of drugs to treat airway obstruction. Two types of drug are used in its treatment:

- Relievers (bronchodilators) give immediate reversal of airway obstruction, largely by relaxing airway smooth muscle.
- Controllers (preventers) suppress the underlying disease process and provide long-term control of symptoms. These drugs include anti-inflammatory treatments.

Asthma is characterised by airway narrowing secondary to a chronic inflammatory process. Eosinophilic and sometimes neutrophilic) inflammation occurs throughout the respiratory tract. Bronchodilators cause immediate reversal of airway obstruction as a result of an effect on airway smooth muscle; other pharmacological effects on other airway cells (reduced micro-vascular leakage, reduced release of bronchoconstrictor mediators from inflammatory cells) may contribute to the reduction in airway narrowing.

β_2-adrenoceptor agonists

Inhaled β_2-agonists are the bronchodilator treatment of choice in asthma because they are the most effective bronchodilators, reverse all known bronchoconstrictor mechanisms and have minimal side-effects when used correctly. Short-acting and non-selective β-agonists (e.g. isoprenaline, orciprenaline) have no role.

Mode of action

β_2-agonists produce bronchodilatation by:

- Directly by stimulating β_2-receptors in airway smooth muscle, leading to relaxation of central and peripheral airways. β_2-agonists act as 'functional antagonists' and reverse bronchoconstriction irrespective of the contractile agent; this is important in asthma, because many bronchoconstrictor mechanisms (neural and mediators) are likely to constrict airways. Occupation of β_2-receptors by agonists results in the activation of adenylyl cyclase via the stimulatory G-protein (Gs), which increases intra-cellular cAMP, leading to relaxation.
- Indirectly by inhibiting mast cell mediator release, cholinergic neurotransmission and microvascular leakage.

By binding to β_2-adrenoceptors β_2-agonists activate adenylate cyclase resulting in an increase in intracellular cyclic AMP (cAMP) (Fig. 4.3.1).

β_2-agonists relax airway smooth muscle via several mechanisms:

- Lowering of intracellular calcium ion (Ca^{2+}) concentration by active removal of Ca^{2+} from the cell and into intracellular stores.
- Inhibitory effect on phosphoinositide hydrolysis.
- Inhibition of myosin light chain kinase.
- Activation of myosin light chain phosphatase.

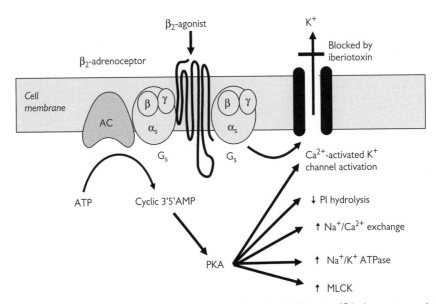

Fig. 4.3.1 Molecular mechanism of action of β 2-agonists on airway smooth muscle cells. Activation of β 2-adrenoceptors results in activation of adenylyl cyclase (AC) via a stimulatory G-protein (Gs) and increase in cyclic 3'5' adenosine monophosphate (AMP). This activates protein kinase A (PKA) which then phosphorylates several target proteins which result in opening of calcium-activated potassium channels (KCa) or maxi-K channels, decreased phosphoinositide (PI) hydrolysis, increase sodium/calcium ion (Na⁺/Ca²⁺) exchange, increase Na⁺/K⁺ ATPase and decrease myosin light chain kinase (MLCK) activity. In addition, β2-receptors may be coupled directly via Gs to KCa. (ATP = adenosine trithosphate).

- Opening of a large conductance calcium-activated potassium channels (KCa) which repolarise the smooth muscle cell

β2-agonists have no significant inhibitory effects on the chronic inflammation of asthmatic airways, and do not reduce airway hyperresponsiveness in asthma.

Clinical use

Short-acting inhaled β_2-agonists (e.g. salbutamol, terbutaline) have a duration of action is 3–4 hours (less in severe asthma). They are convenient, easy to use, rapid in onset and without significant side effects. They also protect against bronchoconstrictor stimuli such as exercise, cold air and allergen. They are the bronchodilators of choice in acute severe asthma, in which the nebulised route of administration is as effective as IV use. The inhaled route of administration is preferable to the oral route because side effects are less common, and because it may be more effective (better access to surface cells such as mast cells). Short-acting inhaled β_2-agonists should be used as required by symptoms, and not on a regular basis. Increased usage indicates a need for more anti-inflammatory therapy.

Long-acting inhaled β_2-agonists (e.g. salmeterol and formoterol) have a bronchodilator action and protect against bronchoconstriction for more than 12 hours, and provide better symptom control (given twice daily) than regular treatment with short-acting β_2-agonists (four times daily).

- Formoterol has a more rapid onset of action than salmeterol and formoterol, but not salmeterol, is more effective as a reliever than short-acting β_2-agonists.
- Inhaled long-acting β_2-agonists may be added to low or moderate doses of inhaled corticosteroids if asthma is not controlled, and this is more effective than increasing the dose of inhaled corticosteroids.
- Long-acting inhaled β_2-agonists should be used only in patients who are taking inhaled corticosteroids, because these drugs have no anti-inflammatory action and are potentially dangerous without corticosteroids.
- Combination inhalers with a long-acting β_2-agonist and corticosteroid (fluticasone/salmeterol, budesonide/formoterol, budesonide beclomethasone dipropionate) are an effective and convenient way to control asthma
- Budesonide/formoterol is very effective as a reliever when added to maintenance treatment with the same drug (allowing single inhaler therapy).

Side effects

Unwanted effects result from stimulation of extra-pulmonary β-receptors. Side effects are uncommon with inhaled therapy, but more common with oral or IV administration (Table 4.3.1).

Table 4.3.1 Side effects of β_2-agonists

- Muscle tremor – direct effect on skeletal muscle β_2-receptors
- Tachycardia – direct effect on atrial β_2-receptors, reflex effect from increased peripheral vasodilatation via β_2-receptors
- Hypokalaemia – direct effect on skeletal muscle uptake of K^+ via β_2-receptors
- Restlessness
- Hypoxaemia – increased V/Q mismatch because of pulmonary vasodilatation

Safety

A recent large trial in the USA showed that salmeterol increased mortality in asthmatic patients, but this was mainly in poor patients who were not using concomitant inhaled corticosteroids. This provides a strong argument for only prescribing long-acting β_2-agonists in a combination inhaler.

Tolerance

Continuous treatment with an agonist often leads to tolerance (desensitisation), which may result from uncoupling and/or down-regulation of the receptor. Tolerance of non-airway β-receptor responses (e.g. tremor, cardiovascular and metabolic responses) is readily observed. Loss of bronchodilator action is minimal, but there is some loss of bronchoprotective effect against exercise. This is incomplete and not progressive, and is not a clinical problem.

Theophylline

Theophylline remains the most widely used anti-asthma therapy worldwide because it is inexpensive, but the greater incidence of side effects with theophylline and the greater efficacy of β-agonists and inhaled corticosteroids have reduced its use. It still remains a useful drug in patients with severe asthma. There is increasing evidence that low-dose theophylline (plasma concentration 5–10mg/L) has an anti-inflammatory or immunomodulatory effect and may be effective in combination with inhaled corticosteroids.

Mode of action

Theophylline is a bronchodilator only at high doses (>10mg/L) when side effects are common and its anti-asthma effect is more likely to be explained other effects (e.g. immunomodulation). Several modes of action have been proposed:

- Inhibition of phosphodiesterases, which break down cAMP leads to an increase in intracellular cAMP concentrations. This accounts for the bronchodilator action of theophylline, but also for the side effects of nausea and headaches.
- Adenosine receptor antagonism – adenosine is a bronchoconstrictor in asthmatic patients, via activation of mast cells (A2B receptors). Adenosine antagonism may account for some side effects of theophylline (e.g. seizures, cardiac arrhythmias, diuresis).
- Histone deacetylase activation – therapeutic concentrations of theophylline activate histone deacetylases in the nucleus, resulting in the switching off of inflammatory genes and enhancing the anti-inflammatory action of corticosteroids.

Clinical use

In patients with acute asthma, IV aminophylline (combination of theophylline and ethylenediamine) is less effective than nebulised β_2-agonists, and should therefore be reserved for the few patients who fail to respond to β-agonists. Theophylline is less effective as a bronchodilator than inhaled β_2-agonists and is more likely to have side-effects. Low doses (plasma concentrations of 5–10mg/L) may be useful when added to inhaled corticosteroids, particularly in more severe asthma.

Theophylline is readily and reliably absorbed from the gastrointestinal tract, but there are many factors affecting plasma clearance, and thereby plasma concentration, that make the drug relatively difficult to use (Table 4.3.2).

Side effects

Side effects are usually related to plasma concentration and occur when plasma levels exceed 20mg/litre, though many patients develop them at lower plasma concentrations. The severity of side effects may be reduced by gradually increasing the dose until therapeutic concentrations are achieved. The most common side-effects are nausea and vomiting, headache, abdominal discomfort and restlessness. The most severe side effects are cardiac arrhythmias and seizures.

Table 4.3.2 Factors affecting theophylline clearance

Increased clearance

* Enzyme induction (rifampicin, phenobarbitone, ethanol)
* Smoking (tobacco, marijuana)
* High-protein, low-carbohydrate diet
* Barbecued meat
* In children

Decreased clearance

* Enzyme inhibition (cimetidine, erythromycin, ciprofloxacin, allopurinol, zafirlukast)
* Congestive heart failure
* Liver disease
* Pneumonia
* Viral infection and vaccination
* High-carbohydrate diet

Anticholinergics

Atropine is a naturally occurring compound that was introduced for the treatment of asthma but, because of side effects (particularly drying of secretions), less soluble quaternary compounds (e.g. ipratropium bromide) were developed.

Mode of action

Anticholinergics are specific antagonists of muscarinic receptors and inhibit cholinergic nerve-induced bronchoconstriction. A small degree of resting bronchomotor tone is present because of tonic cholinergic nerve impulses, which release acetylcholine in the vicinity of airway smooth muscle, and cholinergic reflex bronchoconstriction may be initiated by irritants, cold air and stress. Although anticholinergics protect against acute challenge by sulphur dioxide and emotional factors, they are less effective against antigen, exercise and fog – they inhibit reflex cholinergic bronchoconstriction only and have no significant blocking effect on the direct effects of inflammatory mediators such as histamine and leukotrienes.

Clinical use

Ipratropium bromide and oxitropium bromide are administered three or four times daily via inhalation, whereas tiotropium bromide is given once daily.

* In asthmatics, anticholinergic drugs are less effective than β2-agonists and offer less protection against various bronchial challenges.
* Nebulised anticholinergics are effective in acute severe asthma, but less effective than β2-agonists. Anticholinergic drugs may have an additive effect with β2-agonists in acute and chronic treatment and should therefore be considered when control of asthma is inadequate, particularly when there are side-effects with theophylline or inhaled β-agonists.

Side effects

* Inhaled anticholinergic drugs are well tolerated, and systemic side-effects are uncommon because almost no systemic absorption occurs.
* Ipratropium bromide, even in high doses, has no detectable effect on airway secretions.
* Nebulised ipratropium bromide may precipitate glaucoma in elderly patients as a result of a direct effect of the nebulised drug on the eye; this is avoided by use of a mouthpiece rather than a face-mask.
* Paradoxical bronchoconstriction with ipratropium bromide, particularly when given by nebuliser, was largely explained by the hypotonicity of an earlier nebuliser solution and by antibacterial additives such as benzalkonium chloride; this problem is avoided with current preparations.

Corticosteroids

Corticosteroids are the most effective therapy available for asthma. Inhaled corticosteroids have revolutionised the management of chronic asthma and are now used as first-line therapy in all patients with persistent symptoms. By contrast they are poorly effective in COPD, cystic fibrosis and interstitial lung disease.

Mode of action

Corticosteroids enter target cells and bind to glucocorticoid receptors (GR) in the cytoplasm. Activated GR are transported to the nucleus, where they:

* Bind to specific sequences on the upstream regulatory element of certain target genes, resulting in increased or decreased transcription of the gene and increased or decreased protein synthesis.
* Inhibit proinflammatory transcription factors, such as nuclear factor-κB and activator protein-1, which regulate inflammatory gene expression by a non-genomic mechanism.
* Inhibit acetylation of core histones that results in increased inflammatory gene expression by recruiting histone deacetylase-2 to the transcriptional complex (Fig. 4.3.2). The mechanism of action of corticosteroids in asthma is most likely to be related to their anti-inflammatory properties. Corticosteroids have widespread effects on gene transcription, increasing transcription of anti-inflammatory genes and, more importantly, suppressing transcription of many inflammatory genes. They also have inhibitory effects on many inflammatory and structural cells that are activated in asthma (Fig. 4.3.4). The inhibitory action of inhaled corticosteroids on airway epithelial cells may be particularly important; this results in a reduction in airway hyper-responsiveness, though in long-standing asthma airway responsiveness may not return to normal because of irreversible structural changes in airways.

Clinical use

* Systemic corticosteroids are used in acute asthma and accelerate their resolution. There is no advantage to very high doses of IV corticosteroids (e.g. methylprednisolone 1g). Prednisolone (30–60 mg orally) has an effect similar to IV hydrocortisone and is easier to administer.
* Regular oral corticosteroids are reserved for patients whose asthma cannot be controlled on other therapy; the dose is titrated to the lowest that provides acceptable

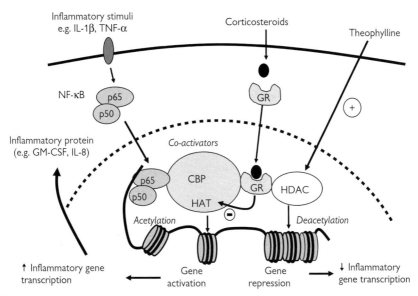

Fig. 4.3.2 Corticosteroids suppresses inflammation by switching off the transcription of multiple activated inflammatory genes. Inflammatory genes are switched on by inflammatory stimuli through the activation the transcription factor nuclear factor κB (NF-κB). NF-κB translocates to the nucleus and binds to specific recognition sites on inflammatory genes and also to coactivators, such as CREB-binding protein (CBP), which has intrinsic histone acetyltransferase (HAT) activity. This leads to acetylation of core histones, resulting in increased expression of genes encoding multiple inflammatory proteins such as cytokines. Glucocorticoid receptors (GR) after activation by corticosteroids also translocate to the nucleus and bind to coactivators to inhibit HAT activity directly and more importantly by recruiting histone deacetylase-2 (HDAC2), which reverses histone acetylation leading in suppression of these activated inflammatory genes. HDAC2 is markedly reduced in COPD, accounting for the corticosteroid resistance in this disease.

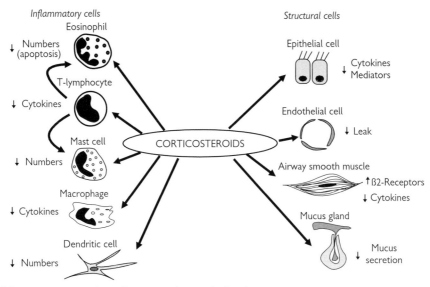

Fig. 4.3.3 Effect of corticosteroids on inflammatory and structural cells in the airways.

symptom control. Objective evidence of corticosteroid responsiveness should be obtained before maintenance therapy is instituted.

- Short courses of oral corticosteroids (prednisolone, 30–40 mg daily for 1–2 weeks) are indicated for exacerbations of asthma. The dose may be tapered over 1 week once the exacerbation is resolved.
- Inhaled corticosteroids are currently recommended as first-line therapy in all patients with persistent asthma. They may be started in any patient who needs to use a β2-agonist inhaler for symptom control more than twice a week. In most patients, inhaled corticosteroids are used twice daily.
- Some patients with severe asthma fail to respond to corticosteroids and may require oral corticosteroids.

Side effects

- Corticosteroids inhibit cortisol secretion by a negative feedback effect on the pituitary gland. Hypothalamo–pituitary–adrenal axis suppression is dependent on dose, and usually occurs when a dose of prednisolone of >7.5 mg daily is used. Significant suppression after short courses of corticosteroid therapy is not usually a problem, but prolonged suppression may occur after several months or years; corticosteroid doses after prolonged oral therapy must therefore be reduced slowly. Symptoms of 'corticosteroid withdrawal syndrome' include lassitude, musculoskeletal pains and occasionally fever.
- Side-effects of long-term oral corticosteroid therapy include fluid retention, increased appetite, weight gain, osteoporosis, capillary fragility, hypertension, peptic ulceration, diabetes, cataracts and psychosis. The incidence increases with age.
- Systemic side-effects, such as cataract formation and osteoporosis are reported but often in patients who are also receiving oral corticosteroids. There has been particular concern about growth suppression in children

using inhaled corticosteroids, but in most studies doses of 400mcg daily or less have not been associated with impaired growth, and there may even be a growth spurt because asthma is better controlled.

Tabl e 4.3.3 Side effects of inhaled corticosteroids

Local side effects
- Dysphonia
- Oropharyngeal candidiasis
- Cough

Systemic side effects
- Adrenal suppression
- Growth suppression
- Bruising
- Osteoporosis
- Cataracts
- Glaucoma
- Metabolic abnormalities (glucose, insulin, triglycerides)
- Psychiatric disturbances

- The fraction of corticosteroid inhaled into the lungs acts locally on the airway mucosa and may be absorbed from the airway and alveolar surface, thereby reaching the systemic circulation. The fraction of inhaled corticosteroid deposited in the oropharynx is swallowed and absorbed from the gut (Fig. 4.3.4). The absorbed fraction may be metabolised in the liver before it reaches the systemic circulation. Budesonide and fluticasone have a greater first-pass metabolism than beclomethasone dipropionate and are therefore less likely to produce systemic effects at high inhaled doses. The use of a spacer reduces oropharyngeal deposition, thereby reducing systemic absorption of corticosteroid
- Inhaled corticosteroids may have local side-effects caused by deposition of corticosteroid in the oropharynx, including dysphonia, oral candidiasis and dry cough.

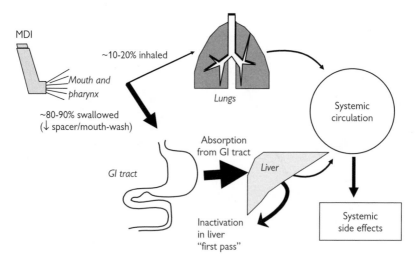

Fig. 4.3.4 Pharmacokinetics of inhaled glucocorticoids (GI = gastrointestinal).

Cromones

Cromones include sodium cromoglycate, and the structurally-related nedocromil sodium.

Mode of action

- Initial investigations suggested that cromoglycate acts as a mast-cell stabiliser, but this effect is weak in human mast cells. Cromoglycate blocks the early response to allergen, which is mediated by mast cells,
- Cromones also inhibit bronchoconstriction induced by sulphur dioxide, metabisulphite and bradykinin, which are believed to act through activation of sensory nerves in the airways.
- Cromones have variable inhibitory actions on other inflammatory cells that may participate in allergic inflammation, including macrophages and eosinophils and inhibits the late response to allergen.
- The molecular mechanism of cromone action is not understood; recent evidence suggests they may block a type of chloride channel that may be expressed in sensory nerves, mast cells and other inflammatory cells.

Clinical use

Cromones are prophylactic treatments and must be given regularly. They protect against indirect bronchoconstrictor stimuli such as exercise, allergen and fog. Cromones are poorly effective compared to low doses of inhaled corticosteroids as they have a very short duration of action and systematic reviews show that they provide little benefit in chronic asthma. Cromones are administered four times daily and may also be taken before exercise in children with exercise-induced asthma. There has been an increasing tendency to substitute low dose inhaled corticosteroids for cromoglycate in adults and children so they are now rarely used.

Side effects

Cromoglycate is one of the safest drugs available and side effects are extremely rare.

- The dry-powder inhaler may cause throat irritation, coughing and, occasionally, wheezing, but this is usually prevented by prior administration of a β-agonist inhaler.
- Very rarely, a transient rash and urticaria or pulmonary eosinophilia are seen as a result of hypersensitivity.
- Side effects are not usually a problem with nedocromil, though some patients have noticed a sensation of flushing after using the inhaler.

Anti-leukotrienes

Anti-leukotrienes (leukotriene receptor antagonists), such as montelukast and zafirlukast, are much less effective than inhaled corticosteroids in the control of asthma.

Mode of action

Elevated levels of leukotrienes are detectable in broncho-alveolar lavage fluid, exhaled breath condensate, sputum and urine of asthmatic patients. Cysteinyl-leukotrienes (cys-LTs) are generated from arachidonic acid by the rate-limiting enzyme 5-lipoxygenase (5'-LO)(Fig. 4.3.5). Cys-LTs are potent constrictors of human airways in vitro and in vivo, cause airway microvascular leakage in animals, and stimulate airway mucus secretion. These effects are all mediated in human airways via cys-LT1-receptors. Montelukast and zafirlukast are potent cys-LT1-receptor antagonists that markedly inhibit the bronchoconstrictor response to inhaled leukotrienes, reduce allergen-induced, exercise-induced and cold air-induced asthma by about 50–70%, and inhibit aspirin-induced responses in aspirin-sensitive asthmatics almost completely. 5'-LO inhibitors (e.g. zileuton) have a similar inhibitory and clinical effect but are not currently available outside the USA.

Clinical use

Anti-leukotrienes may have a small and variable bronchodilator effect, indicating that leukotrienes may contribute to baseline bronchoconstriction in asthma. Long-term administration reduces asthma symptoms and the need for rescue β_2-agonists, and improves lung function. However, their effects are significantly less than with inhaled corticosteroids

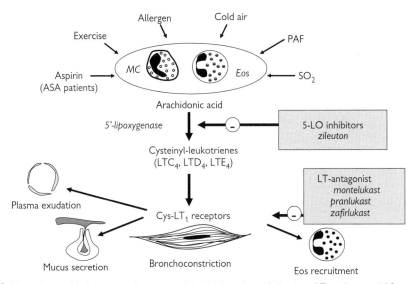

Fig. 4.3.5 Effects of cysteinyl-leukotrienes on the airways and their inhibition by anti-leukotrienes (LT = leukotriene; 5-LO = 5'-lipoxygenase; ASA = aspirin sensitive asthmatic).

in terms of symptom control, improvement in lung function and reduction in exacerbations. Anti-leukotrienes are not as effective as inhaled corticosteroids in the management of mild asthma and are not the preferred therapy. They may be useful in some patients whose asthma is not controlled on inhaled corticosteroids as an add-on therapy to inhaled corticosteroids, but are less effective in this respect than a long-acting β_2-agonist or low dose theophylline. They are effective in some but not all patients with aspirin-sensitive asthma. Patients appear differ in their response to anti-leukotrienes, and it is impossible to predict which patients will respond best.

A major advantage of anti-leukotrienes is that they are orally active, and this is likely to improve compliance with long-term therapy. However, they are expensive, and a trial of therapy is indicated to determine which patients will benefit most.

Side effects

- Montelukast is well tolerated.
- Zafirlukast may produce mild liver dysfunction, so liver function tests are needed.
- Several cases of Churg–Strauss syndrome (systemic vasculitis with eosinophilia and asthma) have been observed in patients on anti-leukotrienes, but this is likely to be because a concomitant reduction in oral corticosteroids (made possible by the anti-leukotriene) allows the vasculitis to flare up.

Anti-IgE therapy

Mode of action

Omalizumab is a humanised recombinant monoclonal antibody that binds to circulating IgE and thus blocks it from activating high affinity IgE receptors on mast cells and low affinity IgE receptor on other inflammatory cells. This results in reduced responses to allergens. Over time the blocking of IgE reduces its synthesis from B-lymphocytes results in a sustained reduction in IgE (Fig. 4.3.6).

Clinical use

Omalizumab reduces airway inflammation in patients with mild to moderate asthma, and reduces the incidence of asthma exacerbations with improved control of asthma in patients maintained on reduced doses of inhaled corticosteroids. Omalizumab is most useful in patients with severe asthma who are not controlled of maximal doses of inhaled therapy as it reduces exacerbations and improves asthma control. Only about 30% of patients show a good response and this is not predictable by any clinical features and therefore a trial of therapy over 4 months is indicated. Omalizumab should only given in patients with serum IgE levels of 20–700 IU/ml; above these levels it is not possible to give enough antibody to neutralise the IgE. The dose of omalizumab is determined by the serum IgE levels and is given either once or twice a month. Because of its high cost, only patients at steps 4 (severe) and 5 (very severe) of the BTS Guidelines who have frequent exacerbations (>5/year) are suitable for this therapy.

Side effects

- Occasionally local reactions occur at the injection sites and very rarely anaphylactic reactions have been seen.
- Immunosuppressive/corticosteroid-sparing therapy
- Immunosuppressive therapy has been considered in asthma when other treatments have been unsuccessful or when a reduction in the dosage of oral corticosteroids is required; it is therefore indicated in very few (<1%) asthmatic patients at present.

Methotrexate

Low-dose methotrexate, 15mg weekly, has a corticosteroid-sparing effect in some patients with asthma, but side effects are relatively common and include nausea (reduced if

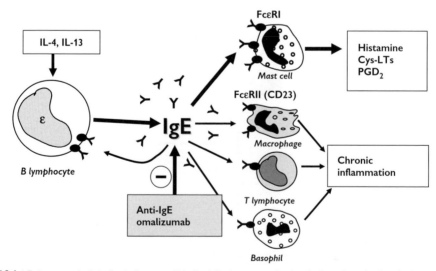

Fig. 4.3.6 IgE play a central role in allergic diseases and blocking IgE using an monoclonal antibody omalizumab is beneficial in some patients with severe asthma. IgE may activate high affinity receptors (FcβRI) on mast cells as well as low affinity receptors (FcβRII, CD23) on other inflammatory cells so that anti-IgE therapy inhibits mast cell mediated effects as well as reducing chronic inflammation. (IL = interleukin, cys-LT = cysteinyl-leukotriene, PG = prostaglandin).

methotrexate is given as a weekly injection), blood dyscrasia and hepatic damage. Careful monitoring (monthly blood counts and liver enzymes) is essential.

Gold

Gold has long been used in the treatment of chronic arthritis. A controlled trial of an oral gold preparation (auranofin) demonstrated some corticosteroid-sparing effect in chronic asthmatic patients maintained on oral corticosteroids, but side effects (skin rashes and nephropathy) are a limiting factor.

Cyclosporin A

Low-dose oral cyclosporin A in patients with corticosteroid-dependent asthma is reported to improve control of symptoms, but in clinical practice it is unimpressive and its use is limited by severe side effects (nephrotoxicity, hypertension).

Anti-tumour necrosis factor

Anti-TNF-α therapy (antibody or soluble receptor) is reported to improve symptoms or reduce exacerbations in patients with severe asthma, but large controlled studies have not so far shown efficacy, so that this treatment is not approved for asthma. Anti-TNF is ineffective in COPD patients.

Mucolytics

Several drugs have been shown to reduce mucus viscosity in vitro by breaking down disuphide bonds between mucus glycoproteins, but these drugs have been disappointing in clinical practice. The most widely used drug N-acetylcysteine (NAC) appeared to reduce exacerbations in meta-analyses, but a large placebo-controlled study in COPD showed no overall clinical benefit, although patients not on inhaled corticosteroids a reduction in exacerbations.

4.4 Asthma in pregnancy

Epidemiology

Asthma is the commonest respiratory disease occurring in pregnancy, affecting up to 12% of pregnant women. Approximately one fifth of pregnant asthmatics suffer exacerbations during pregnancy. The major risk to mother and fetus is due to uncontrolled, sub-optimally treated asthma. There is an associated mortality (Table 4.4.1).

Table 4.4.1 Maternal deaths in the UK from asthma, other respiratory disease and, for comparison, pulmonary embolism.

	1997–99	2000–2	2003–5
Asthma	5	5	5
Other	4	5	1
Pulmonary embolism	31	25	33

Source *'Saving Mothers' Lives 2003-2005'* Confidential Enquiry into Maternal and Child Health

Physiological changes during pregnancy

The major changes in respiratory physiology are outlined in Table 4.4.2. So-called physiological breathlessness is common in pregnancy, happening in up to three-quarters of pregnant women.

Table 4.4.2 Changes in respiratory physiology in pregnancy

pH	Mild alkalosis
PaO_2	Increased
$PaCO_2$	Reduced
Minute ventilation	Increased
Total lung capacity	Reduced/static
Functional residual capacity	Reduced
Tidal volume	Increased
DLCO supine	Reduced
Peak flow	No change
FEV_1	No change

Differentiating this from pathological breathlessness is important, requiring careful clinical assessment. Easily assessable features of potentially pathological breathlessness are listed in Table 4.4.3.

Table 4.4.3 Features of 'pathological breathlessness' in pregnancy

- Previous history of cardio-respiratory disease
- Sudden change in symptom of breathlessness
- Increased respiratory rate >20/minute
- Abnormal spirometry
- Abnormal total lung capacity
- Abnormal alveolar–arterial oxygen gradient

Pregnancy: effect on asthma (Table 4.4.4)

Table 4.4.4 Effects of pregnancy on asthma

		Proposed mechanisms
33%	No change	
33%	Improved	Rise in serum free cortisol
		Progesterone mediated smooth muscle relaxation
33%	Worsened	Cessation of maintenance therapy
		Reduced β_2 adrenoreceptor response
		Changes in immunological response
		Oesophageal reflux
		Female fetus

Asthma: effect on pregnancy

There is no effect for the majority; good medical management of asthma in pregnancy is important. Babies born to women with uncontrolled asthma with severe gestational exacerbation are at increased risk of low birth weight. Poorly controlled maternal asthma may be associated with higher incidence of pre-term labour, pre-eclampsia and Caesarean section.

Management of asthma in pregnancy

The importance of smoking cessation in pregnancy should be emphasised and support to stop offered.

Effective communication prior to conception and during pregnancy is important to allay fears about medication use in pregnancy. Asthma therapy is safe in pregnancy; poorly controlled asthma is not.

Close liaison between the physician and obstetrician involved in management is important

Long-term management

There is no evidence that standard asthma therapy, used appropriately, is unsafe in pregnancy. Management of chronic asthma in pregnancy should be aimed at maximising control and minimising the risk of acute exacerbation.

The use of leukotriene receptor antagonists (LTRAs) in pregnancy should be limited to those women already on them prior to conception whose asthma was not adequately controlled without them. LTRAs should not be started in pregnancy.

All other drugs for asthma are thought to be safe.

Self-monitoring and regular review are important to detect any changes and intervene early.

Acute exacerbations

Exacerbations affect some 20% of pregnant asthmatics. They are more common in mothers with severe, poorly controlled asthma and occur most commonly late into the second trimester. Acute severe asthma should be promptly managed in hospital as per standard guidelines for adult treatment of adults. Systemic steroids should not be denied pregnant women. Fetal monitoring should be available and maternal oxygen saturations kept at >95%.

Asthma in labour

Normal medication should be continued during labour where possible. The increased stress of labour theoretically increases the risk of hypoadrenalism in women taking regular corticosteroids. Hydrocortisone, 100mg IV 6-hourly, should be given to women in labour who have taken 7.5mg prednisolone or more daily for the preceding 2 weeks.

β-blockers, prostaglandin F2, and (in aspirin/NSAID-sensitive subjects) NSAIDs can cause bronchospasm and should be avoided.

Breastfeeding and asthma

The benefits of breastfeeding to baby and mother are well established. All drugs used to treat asthma appear safe. Asthma therapy need not be modified during breastfeeding.

Further reading

BTS/SIGN British Guideline on the Management of Asthma 2005 Update. www.brit-thoracic.org.uk

Murphy VE, Clifton VL, Gibson PG. Asthma exacerbations during pregnancy: incidence and association with adverse pregnancy outcomes. *Thorax* 2006; **61**: 169–176

Schatz M. Asthma and rhinitis during pregnancy. In Busse WM, Holgate ST (eds) *Asthma and Rhinitis*, 2nd edn. Oxford: Blackwells Scientific, 2000; pp. 1811–1826.

4.5 Acute asthma

There is no general agreement on the definition of an exacerbation of asthma, or on grading of severity. An increase in symptoms is an obvious component, but most definitions also include a measure of peak expiratory flow (PEF) because some patients remain relatively uncomplaining despite significant bronchoconstriction, and because this provides an objective measurement of severity.

- Some pharmacological studies have defined a severe exacerbation as a PEF level below 70% of that patient's best PEF, but most clinical guidelines require a lower value for an attack to be regarded as severe.
- The GINA guideline (2006) classifies a moderate exacerbation on the basis of symptom increase plus a PEF persistently below 80% best (or predicted) and a severe episode as one with PEF below 60%.
- The BTS/SIGN guideline uses thresholds of 75% for moderate and 50% for severe attacks; this guideline also incorporates the term 'life-threatening' asthma where PEF is less than 33%
- The principle that treatment intensity should be tailored to disease severity is more important than quibbles about precise thresholds.

Epidemiology

There are no reliable data on the frequency of exacerbations of asthma in the population, since there is no formal method of collecting information on minor or moderately severe episodes. We know that deaths from asthma in the UK have been falling since the late 1970s, as have hospital admissions, although the latter is more evident in children than adults. These changes have occurred against a background of high asthma prevalence, possibly increasing but certainly not falling, and imply that management of asthma has improved and that patients are less likely to have severe exacerbations. Nonetheless, most asthmatic patients will have exacerbations of some degree at some point in the course of their illness. In a large community study in the UK 12.5% of patients with asthma had required a course of oral steroids in the previous year.

A number of risk factors have been shown to increase the likelihood of a life-threatening episode of asthma, mostly of a behavioural or psychological nature. These include:

- non-compliance with treatment, monitoring or appointments;
- alcohol or other drug abuse;
- learning difficulties;
- employment or income problems;
- any severe domestic stress.

Clinical features

History

Most patients presenting with an acute asthma attack will already have a diagnosis of asthma, but in a few the acute attack will be the first presentation. In these patients it is usually possible to obtain a history suggesting the correct diagnosis (see Chapter 4.6), but in a few with severe dyspnoea the diagnosis will necessarily be based mainly on examination findings. Although other conditions can be confused with acute asthma, there is considerable overlap in the treatment of the various causes of acute wheeze, and it is almost always reasonable to treat suspected acute asthma as asthma and arrange confirmatory investigations when the patient has recovered.

> **AUTHOR'S TIP**
> Always question why an asthma attack has arisen, with particular attention to under-treatment and poor concordance.

In patients with known asthma, attempts should be made to understand why the attack has occurred.

- There is some evidence that viral (but not bacterial) infection is a common precipitant.
- It is important to explore whether regular control has been adequate (chronic under-treatment).
- Consider concordance.
- Ask about any recent change in medication (including asthma medication, but also any treatment for other conditions, e.g. NSAIDs).

Examination

Patients will exhibit some degree of tachypnoea and will usually have widespread wheeze. Features which should be particularly noted are:

- Pulse rate. This will increase with severity (bradycardia may develop *in extremis*, but by this stage the patient will be obviously critically unwell).
- Respiratory rate. Also increases with severity, and serial measurement is a useful, objective measure of improvement with treatment.
- Inability to complete sentences is a sign of a severe exacerbation.
- Auscultation will usually reveal widespread wheeze. A difference between the two sides of the chest should prompt consideration of additional pathology, particularly the possibility of pneumothorax.
- Quiet breath sounds indicate life-threatening asthma.

Factors such as cyanosis, exhaustion and confusion indicate life-threatening asthma but are fortunately rare. Hypotension is also associated with extreme severity, but attempts to measure pulsus paradoxus are unnecessary.

Investigations

PEF

An objective measurement of airway calibre is crucial to the assessment of severity of an attack, and in turn to decisions on management. In some regards, FEV_1 is a superior measurement, and its use is now becoming more frequent, but PEF retains the advantage of being more easily available, and of being measurable by the patient at home should they be in any doubt about the severity of an attack. Ideally patients should possess an Action Plan instructing them to start oral corticosteroids if their PEF drops to a pre-agreed level (usually set at about 75% of best PEF).

> **AUTHOR'S TIP**
> Always obtain an objective measure of airflow obstruction at an early stage in an acute asthma attack.

Pulse oximetry

Significant uncorrected hypoxia will contribute to end-organ damage and to death from asthma. Monitoring of oxygenation using pulse oximetry is mandatory in severe asthma attacks. The suggested target level is an oxygen saturation (SaO_2) of 94–98%.

Blood gases

Elevation of $PaCO_2$ does not occur in acute asthma until the attack is advanced; high $PaCO_2$ is one of the defining features of a life-threatening attack. However, blood gas measurement is painful, and performing this unnecessarily might discourage patients from seeking medical help in future exacerbation. Blood gases are not required if SaO_2 is 92% or better on room air and no other life threatening features are present.

Other blood tests

Once through the hospital door, 'routine' blood tests tend to be done irrespective of the illness causing admission. A full blood count can be justified since significant anaemia will reduce oxygen carriage despite satisfactory SaO_2. Treatment of acute asthma can lower serum potassium; both β-agonists (especially nebulised or IV) and corticosteroids can have this effect. It is therefore worth establishing whether the baseline is low. Corticosteroids and β-agonists can also elevate blood glucose levels.

CXR

A CXR is not necessary in all patients. One should definitely be performed if:

- there is any suspicion of additional pathology such as pneumothorax;
- there are any signs of life-threatening asthma;
- the patient fails to show an adequate response to treatment.

Treatment

The intensity of treatment must reflect the severity of the attack. Minor exacerbations of asthma can be treated at home with a temporary increase in use of short-acting bronchodilators with or without a course of oral corticosteroid. Asthma action plans facilitate this, and management need not necessarily involve a health care professional. Conversely, life-threatening asthma represents a medical emergency requiring urgent high dependency or ITU assessment.

The following forms of treatment may be required.

> **AUTHOR'S TIP**
>
> High flow O_2 should be given immediately to patients with: PEF <50% best; inability to speak full sentences; respiratory rate >25/min; pulse >110/min. It can be adjusted later when O_2 saturation results are available.

Oxygen

- Therapy can be guided by pulse oximetry, supplemented if necessary by blood gases (see Blood gases). If the measurement is not available, and the patient has any signs of severe asthma, hypoxaemia is likely and oxygen should be administered without waiting for oximetry.
- Treatment should be started with a high concentration of oxygen. An MC mask can be used to give an inspired oxygen concentration of 40–60%; a reservoir bag can be added if necessary.

- The aim should be to achieve an SaO_2 of 94–98%. Failure to achieve a level of 92% in any patient indicates either life-threatening asthma, or the presence of additional complicating pathology.

β-agonists

- β-agonists will usually relieve bronchospasm quickly, although repeat doses are often necessary for a variable period of time. In mild asthma, patients can treat themselves at home
- Traditionally β-agonists have been given in Accident & Emergency Departments, or to inpatients, using a nebuliser. However, there is good evidence that in most cases repeated activation of a metered-dose inhaler (MDI) with a large volume spacer works just as well, with a lower incidence of side-effects. This is particularly so in children, but the evidence is also convincing in adults. However, it should be noted that many of these studies have excluded those patients with the most severe attacks, and it is still preferable to use a nebuliser in these instances.

> **AUTHOR'S TIP**
>
> β-agonists work better by the inhaled route than intravenously, and using an MDI via a spacer is preferable to a nebuliser (except in life-threatening asthma).

- If nebulised bronchodilators are judged necessary, consideration should be given to continuous nebulisation. This technique uses a nebuliser designed to deliver a steady, constant dose of β-agonist (5–10 mg/hour). Studies have shown some advantages over conventional repeated bolus nebulisation. There are reports of 'continuous' nebulisation being misinterpreted as administration of a consecutive series of bolus nebulisations, one after the other without gaps; this is an abuse of the concept and increases the risk of significant side effects.
- In theory, IV β-agonists might be expected to have advantages where bronchospasm is so severe that airways are completely obstructed, preventing access of nebulised or inhaled agents. In practice, the majority of studies have failed to show any advantage of IV administration in severe asthma.

Ipratropium

- The addition of ipratropium to a β-agonist via a nebuliser has been shown to produce significantly greater bronchodilation than the β-agonist alone, and to reduce the length of hospital admission. In milder attacks, β-agonists alone are likely to produce close to the maximal possible bronchodilatation and the value of adding ipratropium is questionable. Even in the more severe attacks, it is not clear whether adding ipratropium is superior to simply increasing the dose of β-agonist; this comparison has not been made. A sensible strategy based on the available evidence is to add ipratropium during more severe attacks, or where there is a poor response to initial β-agonist therapy.
- Adding ipratropium to a β-agonist using a MDI plus spacer has also been studied and shown to be of value, but again the comparison with a higher dose of the β-agonist has not been made.

Corticosteroids

- Corticosteroids reduce mortality from acute attacks, expedite recovery and reduce the risk of relapse. Although not needed for minor exacerbations, BTS/SIGN guidelines recommend their use where PEF is below 75% predicted (or best recorded for that patient). In such circumstances they should be given as soon as possible during an attack.
- Corticosteroids take several hours to produce their effect, and tablets are well absorbed. Accordingly, there is no advantage to IV administration, unless there are concerns that the patient is at risk of vomiting.
- There are speculative reasons for suggesting that an inhaled steroid might be of benefit in addition to oral steroid, but no practical benefit of the combination has yet been shown in terms of outcome of exacerbations. However, it is good practice to continue the patient's regular inhaled steroid during an exacerbation in order to emphasise its importance in regular treatment.
- The practice of treating mild exacerbations of asthma with a temporary doubling of inhaled corticosteroid dose has not been shown to be effective.

> **AUTHOR'S TIP**
> Don't stop inhaled corticosteroids when patients are taking a booster course of prednisolone. This could give the patient the wrong impression of the importance of inhaled corticosteroids.

Intravenous aminophylline or magnesium

- Aminophylline offers acute bronchodilatation via a different mechanism than either β-agonist or ipratropium, and anecdotally, individual patients get clinically useful benefit from aminophylline despite having responded poorly to inhaled agents. However, it is difficult to demonstrate benefit from the addition of aminophylline in controlled studies, so such patients appear to be rare. Side effects are not uncommon, and use of aminophylline is therefore confined to those patients with life-threatening asthma who have not responded to initial treatment.
- The potential indications for IV magnesium are similar to those of aminophylline. Unlike aminophylline, intravenous magnesium given as a single bolus dose has been shown to be of benefit in acute severe asthma, and side effects appear less common. Benefit from magnesium is less obvious in adults than in children. Moreover, some of the studies showing benefit from magnesium are not of high standard, and benefit is not observed in all studies.
- Magnesium and aminophylline have not been compared directly against one another.

Other agents

- Antibiotics are often given to patients with an exacerbation of asthma who feel that the attack has been caused by an infection 'going to my chest'. Whilst infections are certainly implicated in acute asthma, these are almost always viral rather than bacterial. Routine prescription of antibiotics is therefore not indicated, and their use should be the exception rather than the rule.
- Heliox (helium/oxygen mixture containing 70–80% helium) improves the flow of an inspired breath because its decreased gaseous viscosity (compared to air) reduces turbulent flow. It may therefore help alleviate symptoms, although would not necessarily be expected to expedite recovery from an asthma attack. There is insufficient evidence to recommend routine use of heliox at this time.
- Leukotriene receptor antagonists are of proven benefit in the treatment of chronic asthma, and an IV preparation has been shown to produce bronchodilatation in acute asthma. At the time of writing the product is not licensed for use, and there is insufficient evidence to recommend it.

Differential diagnosis

In an adult with acute dyspnoea and wheeze the common diagnostic question is whether the patient has asthma or COPD. The younger the patient, the more likely is asthma. Absence of a significant smoking history also favours asthma. However, in neither case does the converse apply.

> **AUTHOR'S TIP**
> Antibiotics should not be given in an acute asthma attack unless there is a good reason for suspecting *bacterial* infection.

A detailed history and supplementary tests can usually make the distinction between asthma and COPD, but may not be possible in the acute situation. Fortunately, the acute treatment of the two conditions does not differ hugely. Corticosteroids and bronchodilators will help both, as will oxygen (although thresholds for measuring blood gases will differ between the two). Use of antibiotics is more likely to be of benefit in COPD.

Vocal cord dysfunction (VCD) can be difficult to distinguish from asthma. The astute physician may appreciate that wheezing is not generated from the lower airways in patients with VCD, and note the absence of hyperinflation on examination (or on the CXR if performed). However, distinction can be almost impossible without direct inspection of the vocal cords, something which should only be attempted by the experienced and which is rarely practical. It is safer to treat the patient as if dealing with asthma unless completely confident in the alternative.

Critical care unit

Any feature of life-threatening asthma should prompt immediate discussion with the critical care team, whether present on admission and failing to improve quickly, or if developing despite treatment. Such features are:

- deteriorating PEF;
- hypoxia which fails to improve;
- elevated CO_2;
- acidosis on blood gas analysis;
- exhaustion, drowsiness or confusion;
- respiratory arrest.

It is difficult to be dictatorial about the need for intubation since this depends to some degree on the time which therapy has had to work, and the rate of change of vital signs. The decision should be made by the most experienced available medical staff. However, the clear indications for intubation are development of type-2 respiratory failure and decreased consciousness.

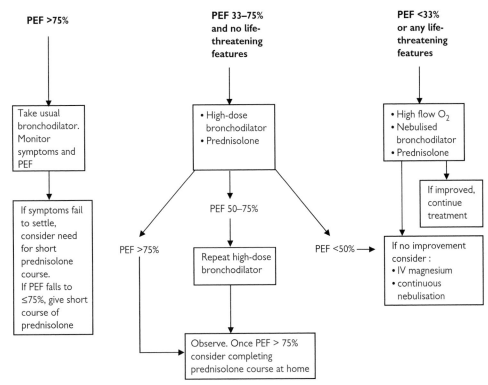

Fig. 4.5.1 Overview of the management of acute asthma attacks. Management is guided by symptoms and an objective measure of severity, usually PEF – decision to admit to hospital is influenced by a number of factors including symptom severity, PEF level, history of previous life-threatening attacks, and social ciircumstances.

Further reading

Anderson HR, Gupta R, Strachan DP, et al. Time trends in allergic disorders in the UK. Thorax 2007; **62**:85–90.

British Guideline on the Management of Asthma. Thorax 2003; **58** (Suppl 1): i1–i84.

Camargo CA, Spooner CH, Rowe BH. Continous versus intermittent beta-agonists in the treatment of acute asthma. Cochrane Database Syst Rev 2003; 4:CD001115.

Cates CJ, Crilly JA, Rowe BH. Holding chambers (spacers) versus nebulisers for beta-agonist treatment of acute asthma. Cochrane Database Syst Rev. 2006; **2**:CD000052.

Global strategy for asthma management and prevention, Global Initiative for Asthma (GINA) 2006. http://www.ginasthma.org

Harrison TW, Oborne J, Newton S, et al. Doubling the dose of inhaled corticosteroid to prevent asthma exacerbations: randomised controlled trial. Lancet 2004; **363**: 271–275.

Nicholson KG, Kent J, Ireland DC. Respiratory viruses and exacerbations of asthma in adults. Br Med J 1993; **307**:982–986.

Parameswaran K, Belda J, Rowe BH. Additions of intravenous aminophylline to beta2-agonists in adults with acute asthma. Cochrane Database Syst Rev 2000; **4**: CD002742.

Pauwels RA, Lofdahl C-G, Postma DS, et al. Effect of inhaled formoterol and budesonide on exacerbations of asthma. N Engl J Med 1997; **337**:140501411.

Rodrigo GJ, Castro-Rodriguez JA. Anticholinergies in the treatment of children and adults with acute asthma: a systematic review with meta-analysis. Thorax 2005; **60**:640-646.

Rowe BH, Bretzlaff JA, Bourdon C, et al. Magnesium sulfate for treating exacerbations of acute asthma in the emergency department. Cochrane Database of Syst Rev 2000; **1**: CD001490.

Travers A, Jones AP, Kelly K, et al. Intravenous beta2-agonists for acute asthma in the emergency department. Cochrane Database of Syst Rev 2001; **1**: CD002988.

Walsh LJ, Wong CA, Cooper S, et al. Morbidity from asthma in relation to regular treatment: a community based study. Thorax 1999; **54**:296–300.

4.6 Chronic asthma management

Overview

Between 10–15% of adults in Western societies have a diagnosis of asthma, and for the majority the disorder is chronic. This represents a significant burden on economic and healthcare resources. In the UK, it is estimated that asthma-management costs exceed £850 million per year to the health service and result in the loss of 12.5 million working days. Despite therapeutic advances, asthma-related mortality has failed to decline significantly and remains at approximately 1400 deaths per year. Confidential enquiries of asthma mortality suggest over 80% are preventable. Together, these statistics highlight both the impact of asthma as a chronic disease to society and the deficiencies that remain in its management.

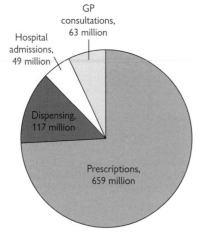

Fig. 4.6.1 Diagram of asthma economic costs.

Aims

The aims of management in chronic asthma are focused on both short- and long-term goals. These are:
- Controlling asthma symptoms (**short term**)
- Reducing the risk of future asthma exacerbations (**medium to long term**)
- Preventing accelerated lung function decline (**long term**)

The relationship between short- and longer-term goals is complex. There is a growing body of evidence that supports the importance of considering these goals independently, both in clinical practice and in the assessment of outcome measures in clinical trials.

Asthma symptoms

The clinical expression of asthma symptoms is frequently multifactorial and depends predominantly on the degree of physiological airflow obstruction and perception of this limitation, which has an important psychological element. Airflow obstruction is due to airway smooth muscle contractility and airway inflammation causing mucosal oedema. Chronic inflammation can lead to structural changes in the airway wall (remodelling) that may contribute to persistent airflow limitation. Symptoms lead to both physical and psychological morbidity if poorly controlled, predisposing

to anxiety and depression that can lead to a vicious cycle of deteriorating control.

Exacerbations

Exacerbations are defined as periods of poor asthma control manifest by an increase in symptoms and deterioration in lung function that are not adequately managed by the individual's usual therapeutic regimen. They are frequently precipitated by allergen exposure or viral infections. Severe exacerbations may lead to hospitalisation and are the major cause of asthma mortality. Although exacerbations may be precipitated by a number of different aetiologies, recent evidence suggests a close relationship between the future risk of a severe asthma exacerbation and present levels of eosinophilic airway inflammation. Moreover, controlling this inflammation with corticosteroids leads to a reduction in the exacerbation risk.

Lung function decline

Chronic asthma is associated with accelerated decline in lung function that is considered a function of persistent airway inflammation. Clinically important decrease in lung function is seen most commonly in those with severe childhood asthma that impacts upon lung development and manifests as fixed airflow obstruction in adulthood. An accelerated rate of decline in adults is seen with:
- severe, non-atopic disease;
- frequent exacerbations;
- smokers.

Although interventions preventing decline are poorly understood, it is likely that smoking cessation, early removal from occupational sensitisers and (possibly) optimisation of corticosteroid therapy are effective.

> **AUTHOR'S TIP**
> As with other chronic diseases, management options for asthma should be viewed in terms of whether they palliate symptoms only or whether they impact upon medium- and long-term goals and are therefore disease modifying.

Principles of asthma management

In common with other chronic diseases, the management of asthma requires a multidisciplinary approach that is patient-centred. An algorithm highlighting the general principles of asthma management is shown (Fig. 4.6.2).

Management interventions incorporate both pharmacological and non-pharmacological measures. Although pharmacotherapy forms the basis of care, non-pharmacological strategies can effectively complement this and in many cases, help avoid over-treatment. Management strategies should therefore be tailored to the individual and will depend primarily upon careful clinical assessment.

Patient assessment

This should address the following important areas:
- Assessing control of symptoms and asthma severity.
- Identifying aetiological factors that may confound or exacerbate asthma symptoms.
- Assessing future severe asthma exacerbation risk.

A careful history provides the most valuable information and will determine the plan of investigation and management to follow.

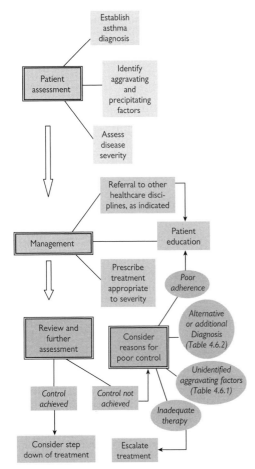

Fig. 4.6.2 Overview of the principles of asthma management.

Assessing control of symptoms
There are several well-validated questionnaire tools for measuring symptom control in asthma. The favoured clinical tool in the UK is the RCP 3 questions as it is concise and ideal for use in busy clinical practice.

RCP 3 QUESTIONS
1. Have you had difficulty *sleeping* because of asthma symptoms?
2. Have you had your usual asthma symptoms *during the day*?
3. Has your asthma interfered with your usual *daily activities*?

A positive response to any question indicates persistent symptoms and should prompt a management review.

Factors associated with poor control of symptoms
The consideration and identification of factors that can mimic or aggravate asthma symptoms is clearly important. These may be categorised as patient factors and disease factors, although considerable overlap exists.

Patient factors
- Exposure to triggers that precipitate and exacerbate airway inflammatory and bronchoconstrictor responses (Table 4.6.1).
- Poor adherence with recommended care.

Table 4.6.1 Common triggers aggravating asthma symptoms

Trigger	Comments
Cold air exercise	Altered osmolarity of the bronchial mucosa activates mast cell release of pro-inflammatory and bronchoconstrictor molecules
Aeroallergens	E.g. pollen, pet allergens HDM, fungal spores
Non-specific irritants	E.g. perfumes, cigarette smoke
Drugs	E.g. β-blockers, aspirin and NSAIDs, ACE inhibitors
Occupational agents	E.g. isocyanates (spray painting), flour, wood dust, gluteraldehyde/latex (healthcare), solder/colophony (welding and soldering)

Occupational asthma
It is estimated 10–15% of adult-onset asthma may be attributable in part to occupation. Mechanistically, occupational agents may be broadly subdivided into those causing hypersensitivity (90%) and those that are direct irritants (10%). The latter cause sudden symptoms at first exposure whereas hypersensitivity is predominantly IgE mediated and leads to symptoms that develop after a variable latent period of exposure. Early avoidance may prevent persistent disease and accelerated lung function decline. The diagnosis is suspected when there is a clear improvement in symptoms and peak flow measurements during a period away from work. Referral to a specialist is recommended in all cases.

> **AUTHOR'S TIP**
> Consider occupational asthma in all patients presenting.

Assessing adherence
Adherence problems with therapy are a generic problem in the management of chronic diseases. In asthma, adherence rates are estimated to range between 30–70%. Poor adherence is more frequently seen in:
- Younger and elderly patient groups.
- Frequent attenders at emergency departments.
- Patients with coexistent psychosocial morbidity.

Studies show a positive correlation between self-reported non-adherence and formal measurement of prescription collections. Patients should therefore be questioned about their adherence patterns. Further strategies for investigating adherence include:
- Monitoring frequency of prescription collections.
- Measuring plasma levels of medication (e.g. theophylline levels or prednisolone levels in conjunction with cortisol).
- Measuring levels of exhaled NO (see Exhaled NO, p. 84).

Disease factors
- Disorders that coexist with asthma and contribute to the clinical expression of asthma-like symptoms (Table 4.6.2)

- Disorders that may mimic asthma in their clinical expression (Table 4.6.2)

Table 4.6.2 Differential diagnosis of disease factors associated with poor control of clinical symptoms

Without airflow obstruction		With airflow obstruction
Normal spirometry	Restrictive spirometry	
Dysfunctional breathing*	Cardiac failure†	COPD*
Vocal cord dysfunction*	Pulmonary fibrosis	Bronchiectasis*† (including allergic bronchpulmonary aspergillosis)
Gastroesophageal reflux disease*		Churg–Strauss syndrome*
Pulmonary vascular disease		Inhaled foreign body†
Chronic cough syndromes		Obliterative bronchiolitis
		Large airway stenosis
		Sarcoidosis†

* These conditions may coexist with asthma
† These conditions may be associated with normal spirometry

> **AUTHOR'S TIP**
> As Table 4.6.2 highlights, the likely differential diagnosis of disease factors for patients with asthma and poorly controlled symptoms will depend upon whether there is evidence of airflow obstruction.

Evaluating future exacerbation risk – measuring eosinophilic airway inflammation
It has been traditionally presumed that exacerbation risk is closely related to symptom control. Although controlling symptoms effectively reduces the risk of exacerbations, several studies identify the level of underlying eosinophilic airway inflammation to be a powerful objective predictor of future exacerbation risk. In most instances, titrating therapy to control symptoms will control underlying eosinophilic inflammation. However, a disparity between symptoms and inflammation should be suspected in patients that have recurrent exacerbations on a background of good symptom control between episodes. These patients may have poor perception or under-report symptoms. The former will contribute to poorer therapy adherence and the latter to inadequate dosing.

Objective, non-invasive measurement of eosinophilic airway inflammation is now possible:

1. Sputum induction
This involves administering nebulised hypertonic saline to promote expectoration of bronchial sputum. The cellularity of obtained samples is studied microscopically (Fig. 4.6.3) and is representative of the inflammatory profile within the proximal lower airways.

2. Exhaled NO
A more recent technique is the measurement of NO in exhaled air. NO is a product of the inflammatory process and levels are closely related to the extent of eosinophilic airway inflammation. It is easily measured in clinical practice (Fig 4.6.3), though its place in asthma management is yet to be determined.

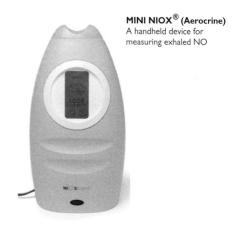

MINI NIOX® (Aerocrine)
A handheld device for measuring exhaled NO

Fig. 4.6.3 Measuring eosinophilic airway inflammation.

> **AUTHOR'S TIP**
> Patients with recurrent exacerbations requiring frequent oral corticosteroids may have uncontrolled eosinophilic airway inflammation. Optimising therapy in these patients may be facilitated by monitoring eosinophilic airway inflammation.

Identifying high-risk patients
Patients at high risk of severe exacerbations should be identified early in Primary Care as they contribute disproportionately to asthma mortality (Table 4.6.3). Prompt referral to a specialist respiratory physician for further assessment is recommended.

Table 4.6.3 Risk factors for asthma mortality

Major risk factors	Previous mechanical ventilation for asthma
	Previous admission to intensive care
	Recent exacerbation (<12 months) requiring hospital admission
Minor risk factors	Asthma requiring oral steroid or theophylline for control
	High short acting beta agonist consumtion
	Factors associated with poor compliance

Pharmacological management of asthma
Pharmacotherapy forms the mainstay of asthma management. Details of drug pharmacology are discussed elsewhere. Here we discuss the principles of their use in clinical practice. The efficacy of different asthma medications for achieving the major goals of asthma care is summarised in Table 4.6.4.

Stepwise algorithm for asthma pharmacotherapy
Present BTS guidelines recommend a stepwise approach to the titration of asthma therapy that is based upon achieving control of asthma symptoms (Fig. 4.6.4) at the lowest dose of therapy. Changes in therapy should be reviewed every 3 months until stability is achieved.

This algorithm assumes a close correlation between clinical symptoms and underlying disease activity. However, symptoms are often multifactorial and several studies have indicated dissociation between airway inflammation and clinical symptoms. Nevertheless, more than 80% of patients achieve satisfactory control in Primary Care.

Table 4.6.4 Effectiveness of different pharmacological treatments for achieving goals of asthma therapy

	Controlling symptoms	Preventing exacerbations	Preserving lung function
Corticosteroids	+++	+++	?
Long acting beta agonists	++	+(*)	–
Anti-leukotrienes	+	+	–
All bronchodilators	++	-	–

* Long-acting beta agonists are only efficacious at preventing exacerbations when used in conjunction with a corticosteroid

Combination therapy of inhaled LABA and corticosteroid

It is notable that step 3 of the treatment ladder advocates the addition of a LABA to low-dose inhaled corticosteroid. This strategy is preferred to the escalation of corticosteroid dose as studies have shown a comparable improvement in lung function and fall in exacerbation rate with this strategy at a lower dose of corticosteroid. There is also molecular evidence of synergy between the two drug classes. In clinical practice, this means that patients are likely to be co-prescribed both drugs at an early stage. Several combination inhalers have been developed to overcome the problem of multiple inhaler use for maintenance therapy that contributes to poor therapy adherence.

Single inhaler therapy

More recently, studies have shown the use of formoterol and budesonide in a single combination inhaler (Symbicort ®) for both symptoms relief and maintenance of asthma control is associated with significant improvements in lung function, reduction in exacerbation frequency and better control of symptoms, when compared with standard therapy. This approach exploits the association between symptoms and airway inflammation such that patients receive more frequent dosing with inhaled corticosteroids when symptoms are poorly controlled that may be sufficient to suppress worsening underlying eosinophilic airway inflammation and avert the onset of an exacerbation. Although a long-acting beta agonist, formoterol has a rapid onset of action comparable to salbutamol that permits its use as a reliever. Single inhaler therapy is theoretically attractive for its potential impact on improving therapeutic adherence. The combination inhaler of budesonide with formoterol has recently been granted a license for use in this way.

AUTHOR'S TIP

Single inhaler therapy with a combination inhaler of budesonide and formoterol may be tried in place of steps 3 and 4 of the BTS algorithm. It may be a particularly useful strategy in cases of suspected poor therapeutic adherence.

Leukotriene inhibitors

This class of drugs incorporates different mechanistic subgroups that inhibit the formation or function of

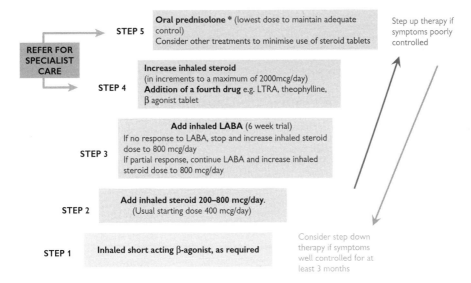

LABA: long acting β-agonist LTRA: leukotriene receptor antagonist

* Patients requiring maintenance or frequent courses of oral prednisolone should be referred for a bone mineral density scan and consideration given to bone protection therapy

Fig. 4.6.4 Stepwise algorithm for chronic asthma therapy in adults.

leukotriene mediators. These mediators are significantly elevated in the subgroup of asthma with aspirin intolerance and/or nasal polyps due to a constitutive deficiency in prostaglandin E_2 that is an important regulator of leukotriene production. The use of leukotriene inhibitors as add on therapy are therefore theoretically favourable in this clinical setting and have also been advocated for the management of exercise induced asthma. In practice however, clinical outcomes with the use of these agents have been disappointing.

Steroid-sparing therapies

Between 5–10% of patients have asthma that requires therapy at step 4 or above. Regular maintenance oral corticosteroid therapy or frequent short courses for exacerbations contribute to the iatrogenic burden of disease in these patients. Targeting corticosteroid therapy according to levels of underlying eosinophilic airway inflammation may help optimise corticosteroid dosing. However, the development of efficacious steroid-sparing agents is a major focus of pharmacological research in asthma.

Monoclonal antibody therapy and omalizumab
A number of monoclonal antibodies are being developed to target key pro-inflammatory mediators that are believed to be significant for perpetuating chronic airway inflammation in asthma. Of these, omalizumab (IgE receptor antagonist) is the first to receive a license for use in patients with uncontrolled allergic asthma. Monoclonal therapies may have limited side effects in view of their specificity. However, this limits their efficacy as heterogeneity in the clinical and pathophysiological expression of disease is increasingly recognised within the asthma population. It is likely that such therapies will only be effective in well defined subgroups.

Immunosuppressants and methotrexate
A number of different non-steroidal immunosuppressants have been trialled for their steroid-sparing properties in refractory asthma. Of these, methotrexate has the most convincing evidence of beneficial effect; a recent meta-analysis concludes methotrexate may have a modest steroid-sparing effect. The response in individual cases is however unpredictable and should be weighed up against potential treatment toxicity.

Non-pharmacological aspects of asthma management

Non-pharmacological measures play an important role in the management of asthma. The different commonly employed strategies and the role of allied healthcare professionals in the various aspects of care is summarised in Tables 4.6.5 and 4.6.6.

Patient education
A central principle in the long-term care of all patients with chronic disease is a patient-centred approach that gives patients a degree of control over their disease. The success of this approach relies on effective patient education, to which there are several components in asthma:

• Identifying and avoiding asthma triggers, most importantly smoking cessation.
• Understanding the role of prescribed therapies. This can improve adherence and forms a necessary pre-requisite for implementing an asthma action plan
• Ensuring correct inhaler technique
• Recording and monitoring peak flow measurements
• Following a personalised asthma action plan

Table 4.6.5 Effectiveness of different non-pharmacological tools for achieving goals of asthma therapy[†]

	Control of asthma symptoms	Prevention of exacerbations	Preservation of lung function
Patient education	++	+	
Trigger avoidance	++	+	*
Smoking cessation	+++	?	++
Breathing retraining techniques	++	?	

[†]It is notable that non-pharmacological measures are generally effective for improving asthma symptoms. Only smoking cessation has a significant disease modifying effect.
* Early identification and avoidance of *occupational* triggers can prevent the *onset* of chronic asthma and arrest decline in lung function.

Personalised asthma action plans
Previously known as self management plans, these programmes incorporate personalised information for patients, facilitating a successful patient-centred approach (Table 4.6.7) that includes:

• Structured education, reinforced with written plans.
• Specific advice about recognising loss of asthma control, assessed by symptoms, peak flow or both.
• Action to take if asthma deteriorates that is appropriate to clinical severity. This includes temporarily increasing inhaled steroids, commencing a rescue course of oral steroids or seeking emergency help.

Although asthma action plans vary in their detail, they are effective at improving asthma morbidity and reducing the frequency of hospitalisations and unscheduled doctor visits. Studies have shown symptoms and peak flow measurements to be similar in their efficacy for monitoring asthma control. However, peak flow monitoring may be more helpful in cases where patients exhibit poor perception of worsening of lung function.

> **AUTHOR'S TIP**
>
> All patients that are hospitalised for an asthma exacerbation should receive a personalised asthma action plan from an asthma healthcare specialist prior to discharge.

Table 4.6.6 Multidisciplinary approach to asthma care

Specialist asthma nurses	Review of potential asthma triggers
	Relevant advice about disease and treatment, including providing self-management plans
	Review of inhaler technique
Physiotherapy	Physical training and breathing retraining techniques
Pharmacist	Education and advice about therapies
	Adherence assessments
Dieticians	Avoidance strategies for identified food allergens, including salicylate-free diets for aspirin sensitive asthma
Smoking cessation service	

Table 4.6.7 Generic asthma action plan

Monitoring symptoms	Peak flow (% best or predicted)	Risk stratification	Recommended action
More frequent symptoms or new nocturnal symptoms requiring reliever use	60–75%	Mild to moderate exacerbation	Increased dose of inhaled steroids and continue higher dose until symptoms have settled for >1 week. Use reliever as needed. Effects of reliever should last >3 hours
Effects of reliever lasting <2 hours	50–60%	Moderate to severe exacerbation	Contact GP Commence oral steroids
No improvement with reliever or failing to improve with oral steroids after 2 days	<50%	Acute severe exacerbation	Call emergency services immediately

Further reading

British Guideline on the Management of Asthma: A national clinical guideline. British Thoracic Society and Scottish Intercollegiate Guidelines Network. Revised edition July 2007 `http://www.brit-thoracic.org.uk/c2/uploads/asthma_full-guideline2007.pdf`

Davies H, Olson L, Gibson P. Methotrexate as a steroid sparing agent for asthma in adults. *Cochrane Database Syst Rev* 2000; **2**: CD000391.

General Register Office collated in Office for National Statistics mortality statistics for England and Wales.

Green RH, Brightling CE, McKenna S, et al. Asthma exacerbations and sputum eosinophil counts: a randomised controlled trial. *Lancet* 2002; **360**(9347): 1715–1721.

Juniper EF, O'Byrne PM, Guyatt GH, et al. Development and validation of a questionnaire to measure asthma control. *Eur Respir J* 1999: **14**(4): 902–907.

Nathan RA, Sorkness CA, Kosinski M, et al. Development of the asthma control test: a survey for assessing asthma control. *J Allergy Clin Immunol* 2004; **113**(1): 59–65.

Newman Taylor AJ, Cullinan P, Burge PS, et al. BOHRF guidelines for occupational asthma. *Thorax* 2005; **60**(5): 364–366.

Powell H, Gibson PG. Options for self-management education for adults with asthma. *Cochrane Database Syst Rev* 2003; **1**: CD004107.

Rabe KF, Atienza T, Magyar P, et al. Effect of budesonide in combination with formoterol for reliever therapy in asthma exacerbations: a randomised controlled, double-blind study. *Lancet* 2006; **368**(9537):744–753.

Robinson DS, Campbell D, Barnes PJ. Addition of leukotriene antagonists to therapy in chronic persistent asthma: a randomised double-blind placebo-controlled trial. *Lancet* 2001; **357**(9273): 2007–2011.

Walker S, Monteil M, Phelan K, et al. Anti-IgE for chronic asthma in adults and children. *Cochrane Database Syst Rev* 2006; **2**: CD003559.

Chronic obstructive pulmonary disease

Chapter contents

5.1 COPD genetics and epidemiology

Background

The airflow obstruction in smoking-related COPD is the result of small airways disease (obstructive bronchiolitis) and alveolar destruction (emphysema). These are discrete pathological processes, each of which may make an independent contribution to the overall burden of airflow obstruction in an affected individual. Irreversible airflow obstruction may develop in a number of other respiratory disease including chronic asthma, bronchiectasis (and cystic fibrosis), obliterative bronchiolitis and sarcoidosis. These diseases have a different aetiology, pathology and natural history and therefore it is essential that they are considered as separate conditions to COPD.

Epidemiology

Cigarette smoking is the major environmental risk factor for the development of COPD. The exact prevalence of COPD is unknown as the disease may be asymptomatic in its early stages, however:

- In 1996 COPD accounted for more than 2 million deaths worldwide
- In 2004 more than 26,000 deaths in the UK were attributed to COPD
- The prevalence of COPD in the UK may be as high as 1 million.
- In the USA it is estimated that 6.6% of the adult population have spirometrically defined COPD.

The prevalence of COPD amongst women has risen because of the increased number of women who smoke. With the increased prevalence of cigarette smoking in China and developing countries it has been predicted that the global prevalence of COPD will increase so that by 2020 it will account for more than 4.5 million deaths, making it the third most common cause of death worldwide.

COPD and smoking

- Cigarette smoking is the single greatest risk factor for COPD.
- The relationship between cumulative smoking and forced expiratory volume in 1 second (FEV_1) is relatively weak within a population, with less than 10% of variation in FEV_1 explained by differences in pack years smoked (one pack year is equivalent to 20 cigarettes a day for a year).
- In their longitudinal study of middle age smokers, Fletcher and Peto identified a sub-group of smokers who showed an accelerated decline in FEV_1.
- These 'susceptible smokers' represented about 15% of the smoking population.
- This data is often misinterpreted as suggesting that the prevalence of COPD among smokers is 15%. This is not the case.
- The prevalence of spirometrically-defined COPD in older populations of smokers is significantly greater than 15%.
- The most susceptible individuals may have more advanced disease at an earlier age.

People who start to smoke in childhood may not achieve their maximum FEV_1 in adulthood and therefore may be susceptible to even a modest increase in rate of decline in FEV_1. Current evidence suggests that the increased risk of COPD

in later life amongst childhood smokers is mainly the result of extra pack years smoked.

The recognition that not all smokers are equally susceptible to the development of COPD and the identification of a subgroup of susceptible smokers means that other factors, environmental or genetic, must interact with cigarette smoke to predispose some individuals to developing COPD.

> **AUTHOR'S TIP**
>
> Smoking is the major risk factor for COPD but variation in susceptibility between smokers means other factors are important.

Environmental exposures

A number of environmental exposures other than smoking have been associated with a reduced FEV_1 or airflow obstruction. These include:

- occupational exposures (e.g. underground tunnel workers);
- domestic fuels;
- low birth weight;
- childhood exposure to passive smoking;
- viral respiratory tract infections;
- social economic class.

Several population-based studies have shown an inverse association between dietary antioxidants (found in fruit and vegetables), lung function and/or symptoms. It is postulated that these antioxidants may provide protection against harmful free radicals in cigarette smoke. However, there is no evidence to suggest that increasing intake of dietary antioxidants protects against smoking-related COPD. Compared to the effect of cigarette smoking, the effect of other identified environmental exposures is relatively weak and none of the currently identified environmental exposures adequately explains the variation in susceptibility to COPD seen amongst smokers.

Genetic factors

To date the only identified genetic risk factor for the development of COPD is deficiency of α1-antitrypsin (α1-AT). This is an important inhibitor of the enzyme neutrophil elastase, and homozygotes for α1-AT deficiency are at an increased risk of developing emphysema if they smoke. However, α1-AT deficiency accounts for only 1–2% of all cases of COPD seen in clinical practice. Studies which have recruited families through the identification of an individual with early onset COPD in the absence of α1-AT deficiency (referred to as a proband), have shown that smoking siblings of the proband have a 3–4-fold greater risk of COPD than unrelated smokers. The non-smoking siblings of these probands have relatively normal lung function, which suggest that it is not shared environment that is the cause of this familial clustering. The increased prevalence of COPD among smoking siblings of probands is independent of pack years smoked and supports the hypothesis that there are other, as yet unidentified, genes that predispose to the development of COPD. A large number of studies have aimed to identify genes that predispose to the development of COPD: the most common types of studies are candidate gene studies and linkage analysis.

AUTHOR'S TIP

α1-AT deficiency is currently the only proven genetic risk factor for COPD and can be screened for by blood levels.

Candidate gene studies

Candidate gene studies are popular because they are relatively simple to undertake. In brief, investigators identify a gene that they hypothesise may be important in the development of COPD and compare the prevalence of a mutation in this candidate gene in individuals with COPD with the prevalence in individuals without COPD. If a mutation or polymorphism is more prevalent in the COPD population, it supports the hypothesis that the gene may predispose to COPD. These studies rely on the identification of possible candidate genes. Most genes that have been studied have coded for proteins that are antioxidants, antiproteinases or mediators of inflammation, in keeping with current hypotheses on the mechanism of COPD pathogenesis.

Examples of candidate genes

Antioxidants

- *GSTP1, GSTM1.*
- *EPHX1.*
- *HMOX1.*

Protease/antiprotease

- *MMP1, 9 & 12.*
- *SERPIN A3.*

Inflammation

- *Tumour necrosis factor alpha (TNF-α).*
- *Transforming growth factor beta.*
- *Vitamin D binding protein.*
- *Interleukin 13.*

Glutathione S transferase (GST) and *microsomal epoxide hydrolase (EPHX)* genes code for enzymes that can detoxify the harmful substances in tobacco smoke whilst haem oxygenase-1 (HMOX) is an enzyme which results in the generation of anti-oxidants. Matrix metaloproteinases (MMP) are zinc dependant enzymes that degrade collagen, inactivate α1-AT and activate TNFα. MMP inhibitors are possible future therapeutic agents in the management of COPD.

There are a number of limitations to the candidate gene approach, not least of which is the ability to only study genes that have been previously identified, therefore eliminating the possibility of identifying novel genes that may predispose to the development of COPD. Ideally the studies would also use control subjects who are identical to the cases in every way (including smoking history and originating from the same population) except that they do not have COPD. This is rarely achieved and therefore it can be difficult to determine if positive associations are the result of selection bias. Consequently many of the positive associations of candidate genes described above have not been reproducable. Finally, studies often include many alleles

and genes, increasing the risk of a type I statistical error if a p value of 0.05 is used.

Linkage analysis

Linkage analysis is a more complex method of identifying areas of the genome that segregate with the disease phenotype within a population. This has been made possible through the identification of a large number of single nucleotide polymorphisms (SNPs) throughout the human genome. Linkage analysis studies have the advantage that they may allow the identification of previously unidentified genes that may be associated with COPD. For example, Silverman and colleagues identified linkage of FEV_1/FVC to a region on chromosome 2q. These studies may provide important future insights into the genetic basis of COPD.

Effect of phenotype definition

A limitation of current studies is that they usually define the COPD phenotype by the presence of irreversible airflow obstruction. COPD is itself a heterogeneous disease, in which airflow obstruction is the result of emphysema and small airways disease. If each of these components has a separate genetic predisposition then failure to adequately define the phenotype will reduce the power of the study to identify significant genes. The advent of high resolution CT scanning has enabled further refinement of the COPD phenotype by allowing quantification of emphysema. This refinement of the COPD phenotype may help in identifying susceptibility genes for emphysema and small airways disease.

Conclusion

Cigarette smoking is the major risk factor for developing COPD. There is however increasing evidence that there may be genetic susceptibility to COPD.

Further reading

British Thoracic Society 2003, The burden of lung disease. A statistics report from the British Thoracic Society.

Fletcher C, Peto R. The natural history of chronic airflow obstruction. *Br Med J* 1977; **1** (6077): 1645–1648.

Lomas DA, Silverman EK. The genetics of chronic obstructive pulmonary disease. *Resp Res* 2001; **2**(1): 20–26.

Lundbäck B, Lindberg A, Lindström M, et al. Not 15 but 50% of smoker develop COPD? Report from the Obstructive Lung Disease in Northern Sweden Studies. *Respir Med* 2003; **97**(2):115–122.

McCloskey SC, Patel D, Stephenson TJ, et al. Siblings of patients with severe COPD have a significant risk of airflow obstruction. *Am J Respir Crit Care Med* 2001; **164**(8 Pt 1): 1419–1424.

Murray CJ, Lopez, AD. Alternative projections of mortality and disability by cause 1990–2020: Global Burden of Disease Study. *Lancet* 1997; **349**(9064):1498–1504.

Patel BD, Coxson HO, Pillai SG, et al. Airway wall thickening and emphysema show independent familial aggregation in chronic obstructive pulmonary disease. *Am J Respir Crit Care Med* 2008; **178**; 500–505.

Silverman EK, Palmer LJ. Case-control association studies for the genetics of complex respiratory diseases. *Am J Respir Cell Mol Biol* 2000; **22**(6): 645–648.

Silvermann EK, Palmer L J. Genomewide linkage analysis of quantitative spirometric phenotypes in severe early-onset chronic obstructive pulmonary disease. *Am J Hum Genet* 2002; **70**(5): 1229–1239.

5.2 COPD pathophysiology

The pathological changes of COPD are complex and correlate poorly with the physiological abnormalities. COPD is an inflammatory disease with pulmonary and systemic effects. Physiologically it is characterised by airflow limitation, impaired gas exchange, hyperinflation and reduced efficiency of the respiratory muscles.

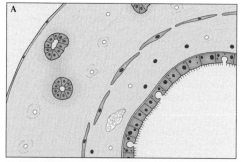

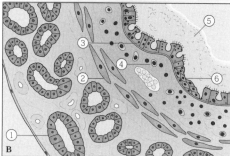

Fig. 5.2.1 Schema of a normal bronchial (A) and the changes seen in the airways in COPD (B) 1. Mucus gland hypertrophy. 2. Smooth muscle hypertrophy. 3. Goblet cell hyperplasia. 4. Inflammatory cell infiltrate. 5. Excessive mucus. 6. Squamous metaplasia. Reproduced with permission from Halpin DMG. Rapid Reference to COPD. Copyright © 2001 Mosby International Limited.

Pathological changes

Within the lungs COPD is associated with (Fig. 5.2.1):
- an increase in the volume and number of submucosal glands;
- an increase in the number of goblet cells in the mucosa;
- mucosal inflammation;
- emphysema (see below);
- loss of alveolar attachments to small airway;
- inflammatory exudate within airway lumens.

Emphysema

Emphysema is defined as 'abnormal, permanent enlargement of airspaces distal to the terminal bronchiole accompanied by destruction of their walls and without obvious fibrosis'.

Emphysema can be classified into:
- panacinar;
- centriacinar;
- paraseptal.

Centriacinar emphysema is commonest in the upper zones of both upper and lower lobes and has a closer relationship to cigarette smoking than panacinar disease.

In α-1 antitrypsin deficiency panacinar emphysema is generally maximal at the base.

The pattern of emphysema has no effect on the clinical symptoms it produces, but the two forms of emphysema have distinct mechanical properties and distinct peripheral airway involvement. Lung compliance is greater in panacinar than in centrilobular emphysema, leading to a greater contribution to airflow limitation from loss of elastic recoil.

Bullae are areas of emphysema larger than 1cm in diameter that are locally over distended.

Small airway obstruction

The airflow obstruction that characterises COPD is located primarily in the small peripheral airways. Pathologically, the changes in these airways are subtle but include:
- loss of alveolar attachments that act like guy ropes to hold open the airway;
- increased surface tension as a result of replacement of surfactant by inflammatory exudate;
- occlusion of the lumen by exudate;
- oedema and inflammation of the mucosa;
- bronchoconstriction.

Vascular and systemic effects

As well as the changes in the airways and lung parenchyma, there are changes in the pulmonary vessels, leading to pulmonary hypertension, and systemic effects leading to skeletal muscle dysfunction, weight loss, osteoporosis and cardiac disease.

In hypoxaemic patients with COPD characteristic changes occur in peripheral pulmonary arteries: the intima of small arteries develops accumulations of smooth muscle; and muscular arteries develop medial hypertrophy.

Cellular pathology

Inflammation in COPD is distinct from that in asthma and is characterised by a predominance of CD8+ cells at all airway levels, and in the lung parenchyma. Inflammatory changes are seen in the airways of young smokers before structural changes are present, but in general, there is a further enhancement of the inflammatory response with increasing severity of COPD.

Smoking cessation does not stop the inflammatory response in the airways, particularly in advanced COPD. The molecular mechanisms for this remain unclear but it has been proposed that transcription factor activation and chromatin remodeling, perhaps as a result of increased oxidative stress, might be responsible for perpetuating the inflammatory process.

Cellular changes seen in COPD

- Airway epithelial cells can be activated by cigarette smoke to produce inflammatory mediators, including TNFα, IL-1β, GMCSF and IL-8.
- Smoking and COPD are associated with infiltration of the airway wall by CD8+ T-lymphocytes.
- The number of CD8+ cells correlates with the degree of airflow limitation.
- Macrophages and neutrophils are found in the airway lumen.
- Cigarette smoke activates macrophages to release inflammatory mediators, including TNF α, IL-8 and other

chemokines, reactive oxygen species and proteases, including MMP-2, -9 and -12 and cathepsins K, L, and S.

- Macrophages appear to recruit neutrophils by releasing IL-8 and leukotriene B4.
- Neutrophils release proteolytic enzymes such as neutrophil elastase, cathepsins and matrix metaloproteinases, which may cause the tissue destruction seen in emphysema.
- Neutrophils move rapidly out of capillaries, through the airway wall and into the lumen. The number of neutrophils correlates with disease severity and reduction in FEV_1.
- Eosinophils are not present in the airway of patients with COPD but they do appear during exacerbations.

Mechanisms of lung damage in COPD
It appears that multiple mechanisms are responsible for the development of the complex pathology found in COPD. The three principal mechanisms that have been identified are protease–antiprotease balance, oxidative stress and apoptosis, but it is likely that interactions also occur between these mechanisms.

Protease–antiprotease imbalance
On the basis of studies of the pathogenesis of emphysema in patients with α-1 antitrypsin deficiency, protease–antiprotease imbalance, leading to the breakdown of connective tissue components, particularly elastin, has been proposed as the key mechanism in the pathogenesis of emphysema. Whilst there is evidence that smoking may partially inactivate α-1 antitrypsin and cause a partial 'functional' deficiency, and that the elastase burden could be increased in chronic smokers as a result of increases in the numbers of neutrophils and macrophages which release of proteases, it is clear that protease-antiprotease imbalance cannot account for all the changes seen in COPD.

As well as increased degredation as a result of protease action, abnormalities of elastin synthesis and repair may also be involved in the pathogenesis of emphysema.

Oxidative stress
In addition to imbalance in protease/antiprotease activity, there is now considerable evidence that increased oxidative stress is present in smokers and may lead to some of the changes seen in lungs in patients with COPD

Increased oxidative stress can cause direct lung injury through damage to proteins and DNA and it also induces indirect injury thorough activation of metabolic processes. Oxidative stress also affects the extracellular matrix and inhibits protective mechanisms, such as surfactant and antiproteases.

Oxidative stress also appears to lead to inflammation in the lungs by activating transcription factors such as nuclear factor-kappa B (NF-κB) and activator protein-1 (AP-1).

In patients with COPD the protective effects of intra- and extracellular antioxidant defence systems may be overwhelmed by oxidative stress.

Cigarette smoke is a complex mixture of many compounds, including high concentrations of free radicals and other oxidants. Components of the lung matrix (e.g. elastin and collagen) are damaged by oxidants in cigarette smoke and cigarette smoke has a detrimental effect on alveolar epithelial cell function that is, in part, oxidant mediated

Apoptosis
It is now thought that cigarette smoke may also induce emphysema by triggering alveolar cell apoptosis as a result of blockade of the vascular endothelial growth factor (VEGF) receptor.

Alpha-1 antitrypsin deficiency
In 1963 α-1 antitrypsin deficiency was identified and found to be associated with the early onset of severe lower zone emphysema. It should always be considered in these circumstances. It accounts for around 2% of cases of COPD. See Chapter 5.8, p.120 for more information.

Phsyiological abnormalities
Pulmonary abnormalities
Decreased maximal expiratory flow and impaired gas exchange are fundamental to the pathophysiology of COPD. The effects of static airway obstruction are exacerbated by the loss of lung recoil due to destruction of the lung parenchyma.

In clinical practice, airflow obstruction is usually assessed using spirometry (Fig. 5.2.2). The time volume curve shows a reduced FEV_1 and often a reduced FVC, but the characteristic feature is a reduced FEV_1/FVC ratio (less than 0.7). FEV_1, FVC and FEV_1/FVC ratios must be related to predicted values based on the individual's age, sex and height.

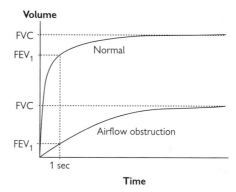

Fig. 5.2.2 Spirometry in a normal individual and a person with airflow obstruction due to COPD.

KEY ISSUES

In older patients the results of spirometry need to be interpreted with caution as there are age-related changes in lung structure which can lead to functional changes similar to those seen in COPD:

- Loss of elastic tissue leads to dynamic airway collapse.
- FEV_1/FVC ratio falls with age.
- FEV_1/FVC ratio less than 0.7 in:
  - 35% of healthy non smokers aged >70 yrs;
  - 50% of healthy non smokers aged >80 yrs.
- RV increases and alveolar walls disappear leading to what has been called 'senile emphysema'.

Increased resting lung volumes are another characteristic feature of COPD. The resting volume of the thorax is determined by the balance between the elastic recoil of the lungs and the chest wall. When the lung parenchyma is destroyed in emphysema the lungs are more compliant and thus there is less force to balance the recoil of the chest wall and thus the resting thoracic volume is increased. This is in part responsible for hyperinflation seen in COPD and the increase in functional residual capacity (FRC) (Fig. 5.2.3).

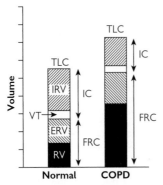

Fig. 5.2.3 Static lung volumes in a healthy individual and in a patient with COPD. RV residual volume, ERV expiratory reserve volume, VT tidal volume, IRV inspiratory reserve volume, TLC total lung capacity, FRC functional residual capacity, IC inspiratory capacity.

Loss of lung recoil also means that the airways collapse earlier in expiration (i.e. at larger lung volumes) increasing the amount of air trapped in the lungs and again increasing the FRC and RV.

Patients with COPD are said to be flow limited when unlike normal individuals they cannot increase the expiratory flow they generate during tidal breathing at any given lung volume (Fig. 5.2.4)

Expiratory flow limitation contributes to hyperinflation by preventing the exhalation of sufficient volume in the time

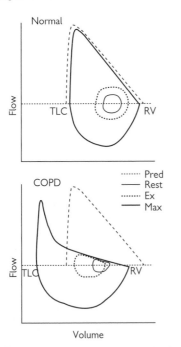

Fig. 5.2.4 Flow volume loops in a healthy individual and a patient with COPD showing how at rest and during exercise (Ex) expiratory flow is significantly reduced in people with COPD compared to the predicted value (Pred) and is limited by the maximum flow possible (Max).

available to allow the end expiratory lung volume (EELV) to fall to the relaxation volume determined by elastic recoil. EELV is dependent on both the degree of airflow limitation and the time available for exhalation and is thus dynamically determined.

Dynamic hyperinflation (DH) refers to acute and variable increase in EELV above its baseline value. DH occurs during exercise in flow-limited patients as inspired tidal volume increases and expiratory time decreases so that the lungs are unable to deflate fully prior to the next inspiration.

Development of dynamic hyperinflation can be assessed by measuring the inspiratory capacity (IC) and this correlates better with the degree of exercise limitation and dyspnoea than the FEV_1.

Respiratory muscles

Hyperinflation and the resultant increase in FRC greatly increase the work of breathing (Fig. 5.2.5). In COPD both the force of contraction generated by the inspiratory muscles and the mechanical load against which they are required to act are abnormal.

- The inspiratory load is increased as a result of the airway obstruction.
- The force of contraction is reduced as a consequence of: the effect of hyperinflation altering the mechanical advantage of the muscles (both intercostal and diaphragmatic), malnutrition and, in some cases, respiratory muscle fatigue.
- Inspiratory muscle dysfunction is central to the development of hypercapnia.

Gas exchange abnormalities

Pulmonary gas exchange abnormalites may arise as a result of:

- alveolar hypoventilation;
- impaired alveolar-capillary diffusion;
- ventilation-perfusion (V_A/Q) mismatching;
- shunting.

Although emphysema impairs alveolar–capillary diffusion, impaired ventilation–perfusion matching appears to be the major mechanism leading to impaired gas exchange in COPD.

Circulatory abnormalities

Pulmonary artery hypertension is an important complication of COPD and it is associated with a poor prognosis. The normal pulmonary circulation is a low-pressure low-resistance system with low vasomotor tone. The considerable increases seen in cardiac output with exercise do not lead to significant increases in pulmonary artery pressure because they are associated with recruitment of under-perfused vessels, particularly at the lung apex.

In hypoxaemic patients with COPD the structural changes in peripheral pulmonary arteries appear to be more important in the development of sustained pulmonary hypertension than hypoxic vasoconstriction. Pulmonary thrombosis may also develop, possibly secondary to small airway inflammation.

Ventilatory abnormalities

Patients with COPD may develop difficulty in excreting CO_2. This appears to be due to a combination of inspiratory muscle fatigue, ventilation perfusion mismatch and possibly alveolar hypoventilation.

- Some patients respond to the difficulty in excreting CO_2 by increasing the frequency and depth of their breathing to maintain a normal arterial partial pressure of CO_2 ($PaCO_2$).

- Other patients are unable to maintain adequate alveolar ventilation and there is an adaptive response in the control of breathing, with a reduced ventilatory response to the $PaCO_2$. This leads to a rise in the $PaCO_2$ and the arterial partial pressure of oxygen (PaO_2) becomes an important factor controlling breathing.
- Some, but not all, of these patients hypoventilate if given too much oxygen and it is these patients
- who are at risk of CO_2 narcosis and respiratory arrest

There is a very poor relationship between ventilatory capacity (i.e. FEV_1) and the development of ventilatory failure.

Exacerbations

Exacerbations are associated with increased airway inflammation which worsens airflow obstruction, and reduced V/Q matching and systemic inflammation which increases oxygen consumption and circulatory abnormalities.
- Worsening airflow limitation leads to increased static hyperinflation and the effects of this are increased by rapid breathing which leads to dynamic hyperinflation.
- These effects increase the work of breathing by forcing the respiratory muscles to operate on the flatter part of the pressure volume curve (Fig. 5.2.5).
- The additional work of breathing leads to recruitment of the accessory muscles.

During exacerbations the efficacy of respiratory muscles is affected by:
- additional elastic loading;
- reduced resting length in the diaphragmatic muscles as a result of worsening hyperinflation;

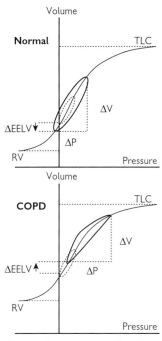

Fig. 5.2.5 Pressure-volume curves at rest (dotted) and on exercise (solid) in a normal individual and a person with COPD showing the higher residual volume (RV) and total lung capacity (TLC), differential change in end-expiratory lung volume (EELV) and the reduced changes in volume(ΔV) for a given transpleural pressure change (ΔP).

- hypoxia;
- acidosis.

These effects may precipitate ventilatory failure.

The consequences of worsening airflow limitation and DH during exacerbations are summarised in Fig. 5.2.6.

Hypoxaemia during exacerbations results from:
- worsening ventilation perfusion matching;
- reduction in mixed venous oxygen tension resulting from increased oxygen consumption.

The deterioration in ventilatory mechanics and gas exchange that occur during an exacerbation take approximately 10 days to recover.

Systemic effects

COPD is associated with important extra-pulmonary, or systemic effects. There is systemic as well as pulmonary inflammation in COPD and this together with systemic oxidative stress contributes to their development.
- Circulating levels of pro-inflammatory cytokines (including tumour necrosis factor α (TNFα) and interleukin 8 (IL-8)) and acute phase proteins, particularly C reactive protein (CRP) are elevated in patients with COPD.
- CRP levels are inversely related to disease severity as assessed by the FEV_1.
- There is increased systemic oxidative stress.
- There are increased numbers of circulating inflammatory cells which show evidence of activation.
- Exacerbations appear to increase the level of systemic inflammation.

The origin of systemic inflammation is not clear and a number of mechanisms may be responsible. It may be due to:
- systemic effects of tobacco smoke;
- spillover of pulmonary inflammation, with release of cytokines produced in the lungs into the systemic circulation;
- inflammation induced in systemic tissues by consequences of COPD such as hypoxia;
- an autoimmune process.

Whatever the origin, it appears that systemic inflammation is important in the development, at least in part, of some, if not all of the systemic effects of COPD.

Skeletal muscle dysfunction contributes to exercise limitation. There is a loss of muscle mass and a reduction in the proportion of type 1 fibres. Sedentarism, hypoxia, corticosteroid therapy, nutritional depletion and systemic inflammation contribute to its development.

Weight loss is another important effect. It is associated with a worse prognosis which changes with therapy and may be due to reductions in calorie intake, changes in intermediate metabolism and effects of systemic inflammation.

Cardiovascular disease is a frequent cause of death in COPD and coronary artery disease, left ventricular failure and arrhythmias are systemic effects of COPD as well as co-morbidities sharing a common aetiology. Exacerbations of COPD may increase the risk of coronary events by increasing the level of systemic inflammation.

Osteoporosis is more common in COPD (even after adjusting for corticosteroid usage) and may be due to a combination of inactivity and the effects of systemic inflammation.

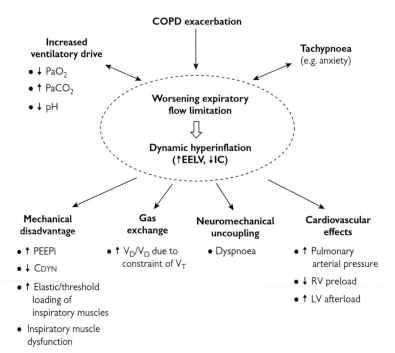

Fig. 5.2.6 The pathophysiological consequences of worsening airflow limitation and dynamic hyperinflation. Reproduced with permission from *Thorax* 2006; **61**: 354–361.

COPD is also associated with systemic endothelial dysfunction and central nervous system abnormalities (including depression) which may also be due to the effects of systemic inflammation.

Further reading

Agusti A. Thomas A. Neff lecture. Chronic obstructive pulmonary disease: a systemic disease. *Proc Am Thorac Soc* 2006; **3**(6): 478–481.

Barbera JA, Roca J, Ferrer A, et al. Mechanisms of worsening gas exchange during acute exacerbations of chronic obstructive pulmonary disease. *Eur Respir J* 1997; **10**(6): 1285–1291.

Gibson GJ. Pulmonary hyperinflation a clinical overview. *Eur Respir J* 1996; **9**(12):2640–2649.

Hogg JC, Macklem PT, Thurlbeck WM. Site and nature of airway obstruction in chronic obstructive lung disease. *N Engl J Med* 1968; **278**(25): 1355–1360.

Janssens JP, Pache JC, Nicod LP. Physiological changes in respiratory function associated with ageing. *Eur Respir J* 1999; **13**(1): 197–205.

Jeffery PK. Comparison of the structural and inflammatory features of COPD and asthma. Giles F. Filley Lecture. *Chest* 2000; **117** (5 Suppl 1): 251S–260S.

MacNee W, Wiggs B, Belzberg AS, et al. The effect of cigarette smoking on neutrophil kinetics in human lungs. *N Engl J Med* 1989; **321**(14): 924–928.

MacNee W. Pathophysiology of cor pulmonale in chronic obstructive pulmonary disease. Part One. *Am J Respir Crit Care Med* 1994; **150**(3): 833–852.

Magee F, Wright JL, Wiggs BR, et al. Pulmonary vascular structure and function in chronic obstructive pulmonary disease. *Thorax* 1988; **43**(3): 183–189.

Niewoehner DE, Kleinerman J, Rice DB. Pathologic changes in the peripheral airways of young cigarette smokers. *N Engl J Med* 1974; **291**(15): 755–758.

O'Donnell DE, Parker CM. COPD exacerbations. 3: Pathophysiology. *Thorax* 2006; **61**(4): 354–361.

Saetta M, Di Stefano A, Maestrelli P, et al. Airway eosinophilia in chronic bronchitis during exacerbations. *Am J Respir Crit Care Med* 1994; **150**(6 Pt 1): 1646–1652.

Saetta M, Turato G, Maestrelli P, et al. Cellular and structural bases of chronic obstructive pulmonary disease. *Am J Respir Crit Care Med* 2001; **163**(6): 1304–1309.

Shapiro SD. The macrophage in chronic obstructive pulmonary disease. *Am J Respir Crit Care Med* 1999; **160**(5 Pt 2): S29–S32.

Stockley RA. Neutrophils and protease/antiprotease imbalance. *Am J Respir Crit Care Med* 1999; **160**(5 Pt 2): S49–S52.

5.3 Investigations in COPD

Investigations in COPD confirm a diagnosis suspected on clinical grounds. Further investigations are used to define the level of physiological compromise associated with the condition and to define interventions to be considered as part of the management plan.

The following categories of investigation will be considered:
- lung function testing;
- imaging: plain radiology;
- cross sectional imaging;
- oxygen assessment;
- functional assessment & anthropometry;
- bloods;
- cardiac investigations.

Lung function testing

Diagnosis of COPD is suggested by a compatible symptom and exposure history and is confirmed by the presence of air-flow obstruction on lung function testing. Current UK Guidelines (NICE)[1] suggest performing lung function measurements in patients over the age of 35 who have smoked and who describe symptoms of regular cough, wheeze, sputum production, or exertional dyspnoea.

Spirometry

Airflow obstruction is confirmed by the presence of a FEV_1 of less than 80% predicted (defined using reference values based on a patients height, sex and age) and an FEV_1 to FVC ratio of 70% or less. Classification of disease severity in guidelines is based on patients FEV_1 – though this may not reflect degree of functional impairment. The severity stratification developed by GOLD is given in Table 5.3.1.

Table 5.3.1 MRC dyspnoea scale

Score	Definition
1	Not troubled by breathlessness except on strenuous exercise
2	Short of breath when hurrying or walking up a slight hill
3	Walks slower than contemporaries on the level because of breathlessness, or has to stop to catch breath when walking at own pace
4	Stops for breath after about 100m or after a few minutes on the level
5	Too breathless to leave the house, or breathless when dressing or undressing

Further investigations:

Where there is diagnostic uncertainty and asthma is being considered in the differential diagnosis a peak flow (PEF) diary showing greater than 20% variability in PEF may provide additional diagnostic information.

Where uncertainty still exists reversibility testing may be carried out using spirometry pre- and post-inhaled bronchodilator or steroid challenge (30mg prednisolone for 10 days). A positive test is one where FEV_1 improves by >15% and the magnitude of the change is at least 150ml.

Where the patient's symptoms are in excess of the measured spirometry detailed lung function measurements can be made. TLC, RV and FRC are all characteristically increased in COPD and are related to the degree of hyperinflation of the lungs.

The carbon dioxide transfer coefficient is also reduced in COPD and is a marker of the severity of emphysema.

Imaging

Radiological investigations are not required to make a diagnosis of COPD however all patients should have a CXR to exclude other pathologies. Typical appearances of COPD on the plain radiograph include hyper-inflated lung fields (>7 posterior ribs visible overlying the lung fields), flattening of the diaphragm, horizontal ribs and narrowing of the mediastinum. Bullae may be visible on some fields. Care must be taken not to misinterpret these as evidence of a pneumothorax (Fig. 5.3.1).

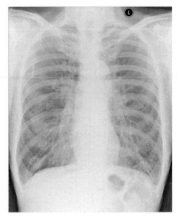

Fig. 5.3.1 CXR showing changes consistent with COPD.

High resolution CT scanning (Fig. 5.3.2) may also be considered. This permits identification of large bullae or upper zone predominant emphysematous changes which may be amenable to surgery.

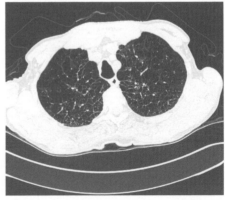

Fig. 5.3.2 Typical appearance of emphysema on HRCT.

Oxygen assessment

Routine measurement of arterial blood gases is not recommended and should be reserved for those with resting oxygen saturations, measured using pulse oximetry, of less than 93% or if carbon dioxide retention is suspected.

Arterial blood gases are required for assessment for long-term oxygen therapy. Mortality is improved by administration of oxygen for >15 hours per day at a rate sufficient to improve pO_2 to >8KpA in patients with chronic obstructive pulmonary disease with PaO_2 < 7.3 kPa when breathing air during a period of clinical stability or in patients with COPD with PaO_2 7.3–8 kPa in the presence of co-morbidities such as secondary polycythaemia, nocturnal hypoxia, peripheral oedema, pulmonary hypertension.

Ambulatory oxygen may also be considered in some patients. It is usually only appropriate for those with oxygen desaturations of more than 4% to below a saturation of 90% who experience an improvement in oxygenation and exercise capacity with supplementary oxygen. Due to the subjective nature of improved exercise capacity it is recommended that assessment for ambulatory oxygen be conducted in a blinded manner using air and oxygen cylinders.

Functional assessment

Selection for interventions such as pulmonary rehabilitation is based on an assessment of patients lung function and their functional capacity. The most commonly used tool is the MRC dyspnoea scale (Table 5.3.1).

Anthropometry

BMI is calculated as weight (Kg)/height^2(m). Low BMI (<25 kg/m^2) or a loss of >1 unit in BMI is associated with increased mortality whilst a >2kg weight gain following nutritional supplementation is associated with improved mortality.

Haematological investigation

Full blood count

The combination of hypoxia and carboxyhaemoglobin in COPD can lead to polycythaemia which is marked by an increased haemoglobin and haematocrit >60%. In subjects with headache, visual disturbance or other features of hyperviscosity symptoms can be improved by phlebotomy.

α-1 antitrypsin

In subjects with proven COPD aged <45 assay of α-1 antitrypsin should be considered. This is an anti-proteinase inhibitor inherited on chromosome 14. 70 variants have been identified. Normal variants are labelled M. The commonest abnormal variants are designated S and Z. Subjects inheriting 2 normal versions are designated PiMM. Abnormal subjects may be homozygous or heterozygous for the abnormal forms of the enzyme so enzyme activity is quoted when abnormal results are quoted. α-1 AT is also present in the liver so LFTs should be checked in abnormal subjects.

Cardiac investigations

Electrocardiography

A number of abnormalities may be noted on the ECG of subjects with severe COPD including right axis deviation (a mean electrical axis of the heart to the right of +90°), right bundle branch block (QRS width >120ms and rSR pattern in V1) or prominent p-waves (p-pulmonale – tall peaked p-waves in leads II, III and aVF).

Echocardiography

In subjects in whom cor-pulmonale is suspected the degree of pulmonary hypertension may be estimated by measurement of the velocity of the tricuspid regurgitant jet. Pulmonary hypertension is present when mean pulmonary artery pressure exceeds 25 mmHg at rest or 30 mmHg (4000 Pa) with exercise.

Further reading

Chronic obstructive pulmonary disease. National clinical guideline on management of chronic obstructive pulmonary disease in adults in primary and secondary care. *Thorax* 2004; **59** (Suppl 1): 1–232.

Prescott E, Almdal T, Mikkelsen KL, et al. Prognostic value of weight change in chronic obstructive pulmonary disease: results from the Copenhagen City Heart Study. *Eur Respir J* 2002; **20**(3): 539–544.

Schols AM, Slangen J, Volovics L, et al. Weight loss is a reversible factor in the prognosis of chronic obstructive pulmonary disease. *Am J Respir Crit Care Med* 1998; **157**(6 Pt 1): 1791–1797.

5.4 Pharmacological therapy (including cor pulmonale)

Pharmacological treatment plays a central role in COPD management but it is not the only treatment approach and should be used in conjunction with other therapies such as pulmonary rehabilitation.

The emphasis of treatment changes as the disease progresses and a more aggressive approach to symptomatic treatment is now recommended.

It is important to understand what treatment is designed to do and how effective it is likely to be. At present much therapy has relatively non-specific benefits on a range of clinical endpoints while the side effects experienced appear to be individual to the treatment used.

Classification of severity

Spirometric (Table 5.4.1) – the approach developed by GOLD and modified by the ATS/ERS and NICE is used. This defines the disease in terms of the severity of airflow limitation and comprises a threshold FEV_1/FVC less than 0.7 and a reduction in the percent predictive FEV_1. It is useful prognostically but does not describe symptom intensity or the degree to which health status is impaired.

Problem based (Fig. 5.4.1): This is the management approach adopted by NICE. It allows identification of patient-base problems and individualised treatment regimens to control these separately.

Types of treatment

Smoking cessation aids

Nicotine replacement therapy (NRT): these can be given by patch, gum and inhaler routes. Like other smoking cessation aids they should be used as part of a goal-directed smoking cessation programme. Quitting is more likely in patients with less nicotine dependence (longer time to first cigarette in day) and NRT approximately doubles quit rates in the general population.

Bupropion

This antidepressant drug increases quit rate above placebo and has been shown to benefit smoking cessation in COPD patients. It can provoke anxiety and insomnia. Perceived risks of cardiovascular complications have limited its use although it is difficult to be sure that this was a causal relationship.

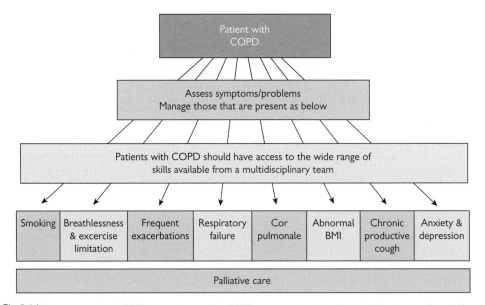

Fig. 5.4.1 Management of stable COPD. A general approach to COPD management based on the individual patient's problems. Although these are generally paralleled by the severity of airflow obstruction this relationship is not strong enough to base therapy solely on this measurement.

Table 5.4.1 Spirometric classification of COPD severity

I: Mild	$FEV_1/FVC < 70\%$ or lower limit of normal $FEV_1 > 80\%$ predicted
II: Moderate	$FEV_1/FVC < 70\%$ or lower limit of normal $50\% < FEV_1 < 80\%$ predicted
III: Severe	$FEV_1/FVC < 70\%$ or lower limit of normal $30\% < FEV_1 < 50\%$ predicted
IV: Very Severe	$FEV_1/FVC < 70\%$ or lower limit of normal $FEV_1 < 30\%$ predicted or $FEV_1 < 50\%$

Varencline

The most effective drug to date to augment quit rates in healthy subjects: This partial α-antagonist has not yet been tested in COPD although studies are on-going. It is well tolerated and was superior to bupropion in healthy subjects in previous randomised studies.

Bronchodilator drugs (Table 5.4.2)

Beta-agonists
- These can be given orally although this route is not recommended.
- They are most commonly administered as short-acting drugs with a duration of action of 3–4 hours (salbutamol, tearbutline) or as long-acting inhaled agents with a 12-hour duration of action (salmeterol, formoterol). Formoterol has a faster onset of action but the potential for improved symptom control in COPD has not been tested.
- All these drugs are available in dry powder form and salbutamol and salmeterol can also be used as CFC-free metered dose inhalers. All produce bronchodilation of modest degree (150–250ml depending on the patient population).
- The longer-acting agents improve exercise tolerance and reduce end-exercise breathlessness, decrease the likelihood of exacerbations and improve quality of life.

Table 5.4.2 Commonly used drugs in COPD management

Drug	Inhaler (mcg)	Solution for Nebuliser (mg/ml)	Oral	Vials for Injection (mg)	Duration of action (hours)
β₂-agonists					
Short-acting					
Salbutamol (albuterol)	100,200 (MDI & DPI)	5	5mg (Pill) Syrup 0.024%	0.1, 0.5	4–6
Terbutaline	400,500 (DPI)	-	2.5, 5 (Pill)	0.2, 0.25	4–6
Long-acting					
Formoterol	4.5–12 (MDI & DPI)			12+	
Salmeterol	25–50 (MDI & DPI)			12+	
Anticholinergics					
Short-acting					
Ipratropium bromide	20, 40 (MDI)	0.25–0.5			6–8
Oxitropium bromide	100 (MDI)	1.5			7–9
Long-acting					
Tiotropium	18 (DPI)				24+
Combination short-acting β₂-agonists plus anticholinergic in one inhaler					
Fenoterol/Ipratropium	200/80 (MDI)	1.25/0.5			6–8
Salbutamol/Ipratropium	75/15 (MDI)	0.75/4.5			6–8
Methylxanthines					
Aminophylline			200–600 mg (Pill)	240 mg	Variable, up to 24
Theophylline (SR)			100–600 mg (Pill)		Variable, up to 24
Inhaled glucocorticosteroids					
Beclomethasone	50–400 (MDI & DPI)	0.2–0.4			
Budesonide	100, 200, 400 (DPI)	0.20, 0.25, 0.5			
Fluticasone	50–500 (MDI & DPI)				
Triamcinolone	100 (MDI)	40		40	
Combination long-acting β₂-agonists plus glucocorticosteroids in one inhaler					
Formoterol/budesonide	4.5/160, 9/320 (DPI)				
Salmeterol/fluticasone	50/100, 250, 500 (DPI) 25/50, 125, 250 (MDI)				
Systemic glucocorticosteroids					
Prednisone			5–60 mg (Pill)		

These effects seem to relate to the longer duration of action.

- Nebulised salbutamol is the most widely used beta-agonist given by this route but there is no good evidence that this is superior to using this agent through a metered dose inhaler. It is widely used in high doses in exacerbations.
- Typical side effects are palpitations, tachycardia and increased somatic tremor. Previous concerns about cardiovascular safety of long-acting inhaled salmeterol have been resolved by the good safety profile of these drugs in the TORCH study.

Anti-cholinergic drugs

- Ipratropium is the typical short-acting agent (4–6 hours duration of action) while tiotropium produces sustained bronchodilatation for at least 24 hours after inhaling a single dose. The side-effect profile is similar with dry mouth the most common complaint. Ipratropium has a bitter taste and there is a potential for glaucoma and prostatism, although these problems are very infrequent.
- Tiotropium consistently increases FEV_1 by 150–300ml, improves exercise tolerance, reduces breathlessness, decreases the number of exacerbations and improves quality of life. Nebulised ipratropium is often used often used together with nebulised salbutamol in exacerbations although the evidence base for this is not strong.

Theophylline

Xanthine derivatives have been widely used as bronchodilators in COPD but have a narrow 'therapeutic window'. High doses can produce headache, nausea and vomiting with more toxic side effects such as ventricular tachycardia and convulsions possible. Lower doses may have an anti-inflammatory action and as monotherapy can have clinical benefits but good comparative studies with the agents above are currently lacking and theophylline remains a third-line supplementary treatment.

Corticosteroids

- Oral corticosteroids are not used in the management of stable disease. They are associated with significantly increased healthcare use and specifically with osteoporosis and skeletal muscle weakness.
- Inhaled corticosteroids: Fluticasone propionate and budesonide are the most widely used drugs although new longer acting formulations of beclomethasone are being developed. These agents are not licensed for monotherapy in COPD and do not modify airway histology in this disease despite their other anti-inflammatory properties. However, they do produce small but consistent improvements in post-bronchodilator FEV_1 and are associated with fewer clinical exacerbations and better health status.
- Previous concerns about the risk of progressive metabolic bone disease, skin bruising or eye complications have been down played after the TORCH trial although local hoarseness and weakness of the voice can be troublesome in individual patients.
- Physician diagnosed pneumonia is significantly more likely to occur in patients taking inhaled corticosteroids alone or in combination with other treatments. This does not translate into worse mortality or health status but these drugs do not reduce the frequency of hospitalisation.

Single inhaler combination treatments:

- Salbutamol + ipratropium: this combination treatment improves FEV_1 more than either drug alone but must be used four times daily and is being withdrawn because no CFC-free alternative can be formulated.

LABA/ICS (salmeterol, fluticasone SFC or budesonide formoterol BF):

- These drugs are available in dry powder form and in the case of SFC in metered dose inhalers as well. They are given twice daily. SFC can decrease airway inflammation in COPD. Both drug combinations are better than their individual components in improving FEV_1, reducing exacerbation treatment and sustaining improved health status.
- There is evidence of a reduction in mortality compared with placebo or inhaled steroid monotherapy when the SFC combination is given. Like LABA alone, hospitalisation was reduced in patients randomised to SFC in the TORCH study.

Agents with less evidence for efficacy

Leukotriene receptor antagonist: there are no good data to suggest these agents are beneficial.

Mucolytic/anti-oxidant drugs: maintenance drug use of a simple mucolytics such as bromhexol appears ineffective. Systematic reviews suggested a reduction in exacerbation frequency from using these drug classes, principally due to an effect of N-acetylcysteine. This drug has antioxidant properties and similar effects are likely with carbocysteine and erdosteine, the latter two being available in the UK. NAC reduced exacerbations in patients not receiving inhaled steroids in one adequate conducted randomised control trial. More data are needed before these can be confidently recommended. Erdosteine may enhance recovery from exacerbations treated with antibiotics and is currently licensed for this indication.

Maintenance antibiotics: this treatment is not currently recommended although it is the study of several clinical trials.

General treatment approaches

Smoking cessation

This is relevant at all stages of COPD but it is influenced by the degree of dependence on tobacco. Tobacco dependence is a relapsing and remitting condition and repeated attempts at quitting are required. Care is best delivered in conjunction with a smoking cessation councillor and a choice of treatment individualised to the patient's need.

Rescue therapy

This is commonly recommended for patients with acute symptomatic deterioration. This idea has been borrowed from asthma and has not been thoroughly tested in COPD. In general it is better to provide sustained bronchodilatation, as acute within day variation in airflow obstruction is not seen in COPD.

Bronchodilator therapy

> **AUTHOR'S TIP**
>
> Consider using long-acting inhaled bronchodilators in all patients with persistent exercise limitation/exercise-induced breathlessness on a daily basis and in those in whom pulmonary rehabilitation is used to augment physical activity.

There are no clear data about the relative benefits of long-acting beta-agonists and anti-cholinergics, although the latter tend to produce better results when used as monotherapy. It is important to ensure that patients complaining of exacerbations have long-acting bronchodilator therapy as a first-line treatment approach.

Supplementary inhaled corticosteroid
These are useful in patients who exacerbate despite adequate bronchodilator treatment. The addition of an inhaled corticosteroid to a long-acting beta-agonist seems to be preferred by patients to monotherapy with tiotropium and may be associated with a better quality of life. More data are needed before this distinction can be considered completely established. Combinations of bronchodilator and inhaled corticosteroid may improve exercise tolerance although whether this is greater than use of the bronchodilator than alone is not clear. Hospitalisation is reduced with this regimen.

Severe disease
Patient admitted to hospital should have maximal treatment as their risk of future exacerbations is greater and hospitalisation is associated with a worse outcome. The combination of a long-acting anti-cholinergic, beta-agonist and inhaled corticosteroid is likely to be the preferred maintenance regimen. There are some data which support the value to patients of this approach.

Prevention of exacerbations
All the long-acting inhaled bronchodilators and inhaled corticosteroids do this, as does the combination of these regimes. Treatment should also include routine administration of influenza vaccination and pneumococcal vaccination. There are good data to support the use of the latter as a way of decreasing pneumonias and hospitalisations. Whether the addition of other therapies will be synergistic or will address episodes not currently well prevented remains to be seen.

Assessing progress
Unlike bronchial asthma where symptom control can be readily assessed, treatment for COPD involves modification of persistent symptoms which do not always disappear. Treatment tends to be cumulative. Focused questions which identify specific activities that limit the patient and enquiry after episodes of symptomatic deterioration, even if they did not lead to a treatment change, provide the best way of clinically assessing progress. Assessing the risk to the patient of complications (largely based on a combination of baseline FEV_1, MRC breathlessness score and body mass index together with walking distance where available) should help stratify how intensive treatment may need to be and whether additional therapy should be used earlier.

AUTHOR'S TIP

Disease management is more like cardiovascular prevention than asthma control where treatment is given to obtain a long-term goal rather than an immediate symptomatic improvement. The relationship between early symptom improvement and reductions in subsequent complications has not been defined yet.

Co-morbidities
Co-morbidities are much commoner in COPD than previously realised.
- Occult cardiac disease is particularly common and a low FEV_1 is almost as predictive as raised cholesterol for its occurrence.

- Osteoporosis is seen in both men and women irrespective of their prior inhaled corticosteroid use and can affect around a third of patients with severe disease. A low threshold for starting bone protection in these patients is needed, particularly in those who have required courses of oral corticosteroids.
- Cataracts are frequent and not necessarily related to steroid use either. Awareness of visual impairment is relevant in patients over 65 years.
- Wasting of the peripheral muscle is important for prognosis and daily function. Reversing this is difficult and no specific drugs have been shown to augment muscle function yet.
- In patients with milder disease, obesity can be a complicating factor which requires specific advice and management.

Cor pulmonale
- This is a pathological term which describes right ventricular hypertrophy secondary to pulmonary circulatory disorders. COPD is the commonest cause of this but there is an impression that this is becoming less frequent, at least in the developed world. It can be diagnosed *in vivo* with cardiac MRI. The diagnosis is normally based on clinical assessment – ankle swelling and raised JVP in a patient with persistent hypoxemia together with ECG evidence of right heart strain and p-pulmonale with or without echocardiographic dysfunction.
- In COPD, hypoxemia is the major factor that leads to cor pulmonale and its correction is the most effective treatment. Although this does not lead to regression of severe pulmonary hypertension it can prevent its progression. Two randomised controlled trials reported over 25 years ago have shown that patients with a PaO_2 less than 7.3kPa live longer if given domiciliary oxygen. These changes are not necessarily correlated with physiological improvements in the pulmonary circulation. Oxygen is best delivered from an oxygen concentrator using a face mask or nasal prongs, whichever is complied with the better. Patients should be assessed when clinical stable to confirm the presence of persistent hypoxemia and that the prescribed oxygen concentration achieves a PaO_2 above 8.0kPa without producing hypercapnia. Careful explanation of the purposes of oxygen treatment is important. It is unlikely to improve exertional breathlessness and the patient should know this. Ambulatory oxygen should be provided for patients who are likely to leave their home or undertake significant amounts of exercise.
- Medical therapy has a limited role here. Diuretics are still used to reduce significant peripheral oedema while ACE inhibitors are widely prescribed and likely to be effective, although large clinical studies confirming this are absent. The use of other cardiac drugs, such as digoxin is not recommended unless the patient has atrial fibrillation. Vasodilators of whatever type including inhaled NO all worsen gas exchange significantly in cor pulmonale due to COPD. No studies have yet shown that giving these drugs has a beneficial effect on the natural history.

KEY FACT

Engaging the patient

Patients who comply with treatment, even when it is a placebo, do significantly better than those who do not. Persuading people to comply with their treatment regimen is likely to be one of the best therapies we can use. Identifying individuals with significant depression and anxiety is important and the severity of the symptoms should be treated on their own merits. Spending time explaining the nature of the disease to the patient, what it means and what their treatment is intended to achieve is always worthwhile, providing a realistic assessment of what can be done for them and when it is going to be done will help build confidence that all is not hopeless. Careful checks to ensure the patient can use inhaled therapy are necessary and require repetition. Advice specific to the device employed is mandatory. Tracking their adherence with prescribed medication is a useful guide as to those who may have more problems in future, particularly when less than 80% of the prescribed doses are taken.

Further reading

Calverley PM. Effect of corticosteroids on exacerbations of asthma and chronic obstructive pulmonary disease. *Proc Am Thorac Soc* 2004; **1**(3): 161–166.

Calverley PM, Anderson JA, Celli B, *et al.* Salmeterol and fluticasone propionate and survival in chronic obstructive pulmonary disease. *N Engl J Med* 2007; **356**(8): 775–789.

Celli BR, MacNee W. Standards for the diagnosis and treatment of patients with COPD: a summary of the ATS/ERS position paper. *Eur Respir J* 2004; **23**(6): 932–946.

National Institute for Clinical Excellence. Chronic obstructive pulmonary disease. National clinical guideline on management of chronic obstructive pulmonary disease in adults in primary and secondary care. *Thorax* 2004; **59** (Suppl 1): 1–232.

Rabe KF, Hurd S, Anzueto A, *et al.* Global strategy for the diagnosis, management, and prevention of chronic obstructive pulmonary disease: GOLD executive summary. *Am J Respir Crit Care Med* 2007; **176**(6): 532–555.

Srivastava P, Currie GP, Britton J. Smoking cessation. *BMJ* 2006; **332**(7553):1324–1326.

Wedzicha JA, Seemungal TA. COPD exacerbations: defining their cause and prevention. *Lancet* 2007; **370**(9589): 786–796.

5.5 Non-pharmacological management for COPD

In recent years it has become evident that COPD is a complicated systemic disease with consequences that go far beyond the damage to the airways. Pharmacological treatment for COPD is disappointing in comparison to its central role in asthma. No pharmacological treatment convincingly modifies the progress of the disease and the role of drug treatment is confined to amelioration of symptoms. The lack of effective pharmacological treatment has in the past resulted in a nihilistic attitude towards therapy that has only recently changed, alongside a greater understanding of the nature and development of disability in COPD. The content of this chapter will cover the relevant areas of non-pharmacological treatment. Other important areas of non-pharmacological treatment such as smoking cessation and lung volume reduction surgery are covered elsewhere in the book.

- The nature and assessment of disability in COPD.
- Formal pulmonary rehabilitation.
- Other forms of performance enhancement.
- Self-management programmes.

Nature and assessment of disability

Breathlessness resulting in activity limitation (disability) is a major feature of advanced COPD. In the early stages of the condition the mild airflow obstruction may have no impact. However as airflow obstruction or hyperinflation progresses, dyspnoea on exertion eventually becomes a significant feature of daily life. These effects may be delayed until loss of airway function is quite advanced. This is because people generally have a large reserve of pulmonary function that may not be required by a modern lifestyle. In addition, people with exertional dyspnoea can limit the sensation by avoiding the provoking stimulus. Subsequently the skeletal musculature may become de-conditioned as a consequence of activity avoidance and further compound the problem. Once disability ensues it can be compounded by loss of confidence, low mood and poor task performance.

The onset of disability is therefore a complicated picture of airway pathophysiology that is compounded by skeletal muscle dysfunction and psychosocial influences. To date, the nature of the muscle dysfunction is thought probably to be consequent upon the de-conditioning. There is an argument for a specific inflammatory myopathy in COPD but this is difficult to sustain when muscle groups other than the quadriceps appear immune. Nevertheless the muscles in COPD are also vulnerable to the effects of hypoxia, poor nutrition and steroid medication or other potential myopathic agents.

Assessing disability

The relationship between airway function (FEV$_1$) and disability is poor and non-predictive. The assessment of disability in COPD requires a specific approach. The options include dyspnoea scales, health status questionnaires and direct observation of exercise performance.

Dyspnoea scales

The MRC Dyspnoea Scale (Table 5.5.1) is the best known of simple rating scales. This was originally developed as part of a wider questionnaire but has become a useful and rapidly applicable tool for clinical staging of disability. It is really an activity scale rather than a dyspnoea scale. The format is simple with a 1 to 5 score. The modified scale that is used in the USA has a 0–4 scale.

Table 5.5.1 MRC Dyspnoea Scale

Grade	Degree of breathlessness related to activities
1	Not troubled by breathlessness except on strenuous exercise
2	Short of breath when hurrying or walking up a slight hill
3	Walks slower than contemporaries on the level ground because of breathlessness, or has to stop for breath when walking at own pace
4	Stops for breath after walking about 100m or after a few minutes on the level ground
5	Too breathless to leave the house, or breathless when dressing or undressing

Other simple scales such as the Oxygen Cost Diagram exist but are not widely used. The attraction of the MRC scale is the simplicity to which it can be applied to clinical interview and broad acceptance of its validity.

Health status

- Quality of life (health status) questionnaires all differ in their content and emphasis. However, most disease-specific questionnaires contain domains that relate to activity limitation or dyspnoea on exertion.
- The most well known questionnaires are the Chronic Respiratory Questionnaire (CRQ) and the St George's respiratory questionnaire (SGRQ). These are both validated and responsive questionnaires that have been used as outcome assessments for studies of therapeutic intervention.
- The CRQ is a predominantly responsive questionnaire while the SGRQ has both discriminative and evaluative qualities.
- Other disease-specific questionnaires that specifically examine physical functioning such as the pulmonary function scale and dyspnoea questionnaire (PFSDQ) exist but are not so widely used
- All these questionnaires have value as outcome measures in clinical trials. They can also be used for quality assurance purposes in a rehabilitation programme.
- Unlike the MRC scale they do not have any value in the management of the individual case.

Exercise tests

Objective assessment of exercise capacity is possible with field and laboratory examinations. Well-known field walking tests that have been applied to COPD are the 6-minute walk test (6MWT) and the shuttle walk tests.

6MWT

This simple self-paced walking test has been used extensively for evaluation. It has normal reference ranges and a defined minimally important clinical difference. Although the test is in widespread use it has some disadvantages as a performance measure because of its vulnerability to learning and encouragement effects. The physiological challenge of the 6MWT is also unpredictable.

The shuttle walk tests

These were developed as the field equivalents of the maximal capacity and submaximal (endurance) laboratory exercise tests. The incremental shuttle walk test (ISWT) involves walking around a coned 10m course at speeds that increase every minute. The endurance shuttle walk test (ESWT) involves walking at a constant speed around the cones. Both are externally paced and symptom limited. These tests are growing in popularity because they are less vulnerable to the influences of learning and encouragement and the physiological challenge is known. In contrast to the 6MWT, the ISWT has a graded physiological response. Recently a minimally clinical important difference has been defined.

Laboratory exercise testing

Metabolic laboratory exercise testing provides the most comprehensive description of disability but the technology may not be widely available. Usually the tests are conducted on a cycle ergometer for convenience though this may not be a natural mode of exercise for elderly people. Maximal incremental exercise tests can provide a measure of disability and an explanation of limitation. Endurance or constant workload tests, however, are a more sensitive reflection of change induced by therapeutic intervention.

Formal pulmonary rehabilitation programmes

Since disease modification cannot readily be achieved in COPD, the aims of therapy are to improve symptoms, functional status and quality of life. Secondary aims of treatment would include improvements in independence and reduction in health care burden. Once medical care has been optimised the aim of formal rehabilitation is to restore the individual to best possible social and physical functioning. Most of the evidence for the benefit of rehabilitation is derived from studies in patients with COPD but there is a growing realisation that similar benefits can be achieved in people with disability from a variety of chronic respiratory diseases.

Overall concept

Pulmonary rehabilitation programmes with similar structures have now become established in most countries. A formal rehabilitation programme is distinguished from self-management or activity promotion programme. It is also different from informal exercise classes of the type that may follow on from formal rehabilitation. In principle, a formal programme should address the needs of the individual patient by involvement of a multiprofessional team, the patient and their relatives. There are various options for settings but the stages of rehabilitation include assessment, core rehabilitation, re-assessment and maintenance. The content of a programme includes physical exercise training, disease education and self-management.

Assessment

The rehabilitation process aims to improve disability and promote independence so the appropriate individual assessments should include measures of physical function and health status. Lung function would not be expected to change. At a population level, rehabilitation has been shown to reduce impact on hospital admission and may even have an impact on survival.

Content

Physical exercise training/endurance

Individually prescribed, supervised, lower limb physical training is a mandatory component of the programme. Exclusion of physical training removes the benefit. Most programmes will offer a combination of lower limb endurance and strength training. Endurance training usually takes the form of cycling or brisk walking. Training schedules require a combination of intensity, duration and frequency. These principles are similar to exercise training in health. Patients with COPD can actually train at a higher relative proportion of their maximal oxygen uptake than healthy people. This is because the usual cardiovascular limit to exercise is pre-empted in many people with advanced COPD by a ventilatory limit imposed by dynamic hyperinflation. Opinions vary as the correct prescription intensity of endurance training. Higher intensity (>60% VO_2 peak) training produces better results, and genuine physiological training, than lower intensity training. However some health status benefits occur even with low intensity activity.

> ### AUTHOR'S TIP
> A key point is that the exercise prescription should be deliberate and incremented with time over duration of the training programme.

The method of setting a prescription for exercise intensity is often poorly understood. One method is simply to measure peak performance on a walking test or cycle and then to identify the speed or load to equate to the required relative workload (e.g 85% of peak predicted VO_2). The current recommendations for session duration (30 mins exercise per session) and course length suggest that at least three sessions of training are required per week for a period of at least 4 weeks to have an effect. Two of the weekly sessions need to be supervised and further home based sessions are desirable.

Strength training

Training for strength alone can also produce similar benefits in health status and exercise performance to endurance training. Most programmes will combine upper and lower limb strength exercises with the aerobic (endurance) programme. Strength (or resistance) training is performed on gym apparatus or uses free weights. In some severely disabled patients it may simply be lifting their body weight. Once again an attempt should be made to make a positive prescription for the training load. This is usually done on by the one repetition maximal (1RM) method where the prescription is set at 70% of the maximal possible contraction load. There are arguments for and against training on gym equipment and free weights. Obviously the multi-gym apparatus can provide greater precision and flexibility of exercises. On the other hand, patients cannot take the gym home with them so the free weights may be the more pragmatic solution.

Upper body exercise

Most of the described benefits of rehabilitation follow from lower limb exercise training. This is logical since upper limb strength is better preserved. However, there is some purpose in conducting upper limb training in order to improve activities of daily living. The literature on upper limb training alone suggests that upper limb training can improve task performance but does not have any carry over effects on general exercise performance or health status. Most programmes will therefore include upper limb training in addition to lower limb training. This training will take the form of supported arm exercise using an arm ergometer or other apparatus or unsupported exercises using free weights.

Respiratory muscle training

This remains a controversial subject that attracts supporters and detractors. Current opinion supports the view that respiratory muscle function is relatively well preserved in people with COPD and that specific respiratory muscle training is unlikely to have wider benefits. In fact the trial evidence suggests that respiratory muscle training can improve respiratory muscle strength and task associated dyspnoea but does not improve general exercise performance or health status. Supporters of respiratory muscle training argue that trials seldom use sufficient training loads or go on for long enough. When this is done there do appear to be some longer lasting benefits. For the present, the addition of respiratory muscle training adds little to the general training benefits.

Oxygen during training

This is an area of concern and interest for people involved in pulmonary rehabilitation. There are two facets to consider.

Firstly there is the aspect surrounding safety concerns in people who de-saturate on exercise and secondly the benefit of oxygen itself as a training adjunct

The safety profile of pulmonary rehabilitation is extremely good but it is difficult to feel comfortable about deliberately provoking hypoxaemia even if the patient is likely to do so at home.

The second point about whether oxygen can enhance physical training is perhaps more interesting. Some studies have shown that training on oxygen carries no additional benefit but other have demonstrated that training on oxygen permits a higher load that should theoretically result in more efficient training. In practice it is quite difficult to arrange oxygen for people while they are training, especially if it involves brisk walking.

AUTHOR'S TIP

From the safety perspective it is reasonable to offer oxygen to patients who de-saturate (SpO$_2$ <85%) during supervised treatment.

Disease education and self-management

Physical training is the major component of rehabilitation but it needs to be supported by an educational programme. This may take the form of lectures or discussion topics around aspects of lung disease and self-management. These sessions are provided by the relevant members of the multiprofessional team. It is important to encourage relatives and carers to attend these sessions so that they too have an understanding of the condition and the principles of rehabilitation. The education sessions offer an opportunity to select patients who have special specific needs. Continuing smokers, if willing, can be directed to the smoking cessation service. Smoking and rehabilitation are controversial areas. Some authorities recommend that current smokers should not be offered rehabilitation because they are known to have a higher drop out rate. However, smokers do derive exactly the same benefits from rehabilitation if they stick to the course. Our policy would be to accept current smokers but offer targeted smoking cessation. There are other groups that may require specific attention and referral. These include those with excessive sputum production who need physiotherapy advice.

Other patients to pick out would be those with clinical evidence of psychiatric illness or relationship difficulties where counselling may be appropriate.

Suggested education content (accompanied by written material)

- Disease management.
- Devices and oxygen.
- Relaxation.
- Benefits advice.
- Travel.
- Sexual relations.
- Smoking cessation.
- Energy conservation.

Specific psychological intervention

There is considerable evidence to suggest that anxiety and depression commonly co-exist with COPD. The literature describes a wide range of prevalence of psychiatric morbidity and in some cases does not make a distinction between low mood associated with chronic illness and a pathological state requiring specific treatment. Clearly pathological states merit identification and treatment on their own.

The evidence for including specific psychological interventions such as cognitive behavioural therapy in a rehabilitation programme is less convincing. It is possible that behaviour modification may have an effect on specific areas such as smoking cessation or dyspnoea. However, the rehabilitation process itself offers substantial mood enhancing and anxiety relieving benefits. This is mediated through the education sessions as well as the support provided by the group interactions.

Programme organisation and management

There are obvious differences between the delivery of a rehabilitation programme and the usual therapeutic interaction. The programme requires a continuing active commitment from the patient and the synchronised involvement of a number of health care professionals. It is a principle of rehabilitation that the diagnosis is secure and that the patient is on optimal medical treatment. It is not the role of the rehabilitation process to provide a diagnostic service or review medication.

The service is delivered by a team that generally includes a medical representative, physiotherapist, occupational therapist, dietician, pharmacist and others. These can be supplemented by volunteers or relatives. Some larger programmes may include a sports scientist or psychologist in their teams. There needs to be a specific role for a programme co-ordinator to manage timetabling.

Safety and quality assurance

Staffing ratios for rehabilitation classes are set to ensure efficiency and safety. A reasonable staffing level would be to ensure that there are at least one member of staff for eight patients in an exercise class or 1:16 for the education classes. For safety purposes it is recommended that there are at least two members of staff present at all times. There are no reports of adverse events associated with rehabilitation but it is sensible to take precautions with staff having current resuscitation skills and available equipment.

Quality assurance is an important component of any service delivery. In rehabilitation several parameters can be used to monitor programme quality. Individual patients will have assessments of functional capacity and health status on entry and completion. This data can be used to monitor the effectiveness of the programme. Other monitoring can be derived from patient satisfaction questionnaires and records of attendance and drop out.

Setting and accessibility

Successful rehabilitation programmes have been described in various settings. These include hospital outpatient, hospital inpatient, community centres and even within the patient's home. The choice of setting is not as important as the skills and enthusiasm of the staff. Accessibility for the patient is a critical determinant of uptake and continued commitment. In this case transport arrangements are often critical to the success of the programme. Careful choice in site of the programme and awareness of transport is a major consideration. So too is the timing of the sessions. People with COPD are not at their best first thing in the morning so a later start is welcome. Seasonal changes may also have influence since spontaneous physical activity is less in the winter. Ultimately the choice of venue may be determined by cost. At present, hospital outpatient rehabilitation is the most cost effective because of the availability of staff and infrastructure. However, the lack of capacity compared to demand for rehabilitation should lead to the development of active community based rehabilitation. Such programmes are likely to be as effective but must also adhere to the same principles of quality control.

Timing of rehabilitation

The best timing for entry in to a rehabilitation programme is when patients are in a stable phase and able to attend the programme without interruption. There are also other times when adapted forms of rehabilitation are appropriate. There have been successful reports of rehabilitation being delivered immediately after a hospital admission. Another occasion where intervention may be valuable is during the hospital admission itself where the inactivity associated with the enforced rest may be detrimental and could be offset by timely intervention.

Maintenance programmes

The purpose of rehabilitation is to induce a lifestyle change that maintains the improvement. These immediate benefits of rehabilitation may remain for 12–18 months and then diminish with disease progression. It is not known for certain whether maintenance programmes or repeated courses can retain the benefit for longer. The literature suggests that maintenance programmes or repeated programmes can have a short term effect but no prolonged effect can yet be demonstrated. Nevertheless patients do appear to enjoy post-rehabilitation exercise classes and these may be best considered as part of the self management approach to activity promotion.

Key features of a rehabilitation programme

- A rehabilitation programme must contain individually prescribed, physical exercise training together with lifestyle and self-management advice.
- The programme should be delivered by a multi-disciplinary team and include two supervised sessions per week for at least four weeks. Further home training should be encouraged.
- Individual progress should be assessed by the use of appropriate assessment and outcome measures (usually health status and functional exercise capacity).

- There should be evidence of programme quality control and improvement.

Other forms of performance enhancement

Transcutaneous electrical muscle stimulation

Physical training is the most popular form of muscular conditioning but other methods of improving muscle function exist. One method is transcutaneous electrical muscle stimulation which conditions muscles by means of superficial electrodes. These are generally available over the counter but have been used in trials of rehabilitation in COPD. At least three randomised controlled trials have shown improvements in muscle strength and walking distance that compare favourably with active physical training. The precise role of this type of muscular conditioning is uncertain but it is possible to see a role for these devices in immobile patients during exacerbation or those recovering on intensive care units.

Nutrition and pharmaceutical agents

- Patients with COPD who have nutritional depletion (BMI <19 or FFM <16) are greater risk of death than those who maintain their body weight and muscle mass.
- Nutritional support would be a logical therapy to improve prognosis but supplementation alone does not appear to be effective. This is likely to be because giving people nutritional supplements does not necessarily guarantee calorie supplementation.
- An alternative is to consider dietary supplementation during physical training to enhance the increase in muscle mass. This seems to work, as it does in athletes and in people with normal body weight. However, it does not have any effect on the target population who are depleted.
- It is possible that by this stage the nutritional changes are irreversible by anything but lung volume reduction or transplantation.
- In most rehabilitation programmes obesity is a bigger problem than nutritional depletion. In this case the dietician's advice must be tailored to the individual needs.
- There are a number of pharmaceutical agents that are reputed to enhance physical performance in athletes. It is reasonable to explore this route of pharmaceutical performance enhancement in patients with impaired mobility. Trials have been conducted with anabolic steroids and nutritional supplements such as creatine. Anabolic agents do appear to increase muscle bulk but this does not translate into improved physical performance or health status.
- Similarly, the benefits of nutritional supplements combined with physical training seem meagre. By contrast, training on long-acting anticholinergic bronchodilator therapy does appear to have an additive effect.

Walking aids

The provision of mobility aids to people with advanced disability seems quite natural in patients with neurological or orthopaedic disease but is often forgotten in those who are disabled by breathlessness. However, walking aids have been shown to be useful in patients with COPD. The use of rollators or wheeled walkers is associated with increased walking distance especially in the most disabled patients. In spite of improved performance, not everybody that improves their walking performance with the walking aid will subsequently continue to use the device. However, those that persevere, continue to find them useful.

Miscellaneous methods of improving dyspnoea

Surgical techniques to reduce dynamic hyperinflation (lung volume reduction and bullectomy) have a role in selected patients with heterogeneous emphysema and static hyper-inflation. These are dealt with elsewhere in this book.

Breathing retraining is not as effective in COPD as it is in dysfunctional breathing or asthma. In particular, there seems to be no role for teaching diaphragmatic breathing or similar techniques. However some patients with emphysema do learn to use pursed lip breathing as a method of reducing flow limitation by increasing end-expiratory airway pressure. Most patients develop this habit naturally but it is possible that they can be taught if necessary.

Distressing dyspnoea may also be helped by distractive stimuli or learnt behaviour. Disease education in the course of the rehabilitation programme may teach patients relaxation techniques or strategies to limit dyspnoea. Examples of dyspnoea-limiting techniques include resting against a wall while supporting the shoulder girdle or using the supermarket trolley to provide similar support whist shopping.

It is claimed that much of the benefit obtained from short burst oxygen in non-hypoxic patients may simply be the effect of air flowing on the face. This can be reproduced by a simple hand-held fan. Finally, the observation that joggers use portable music players while running has stimulated research to show that patients with COPD can get similar benefit from such distractive stimuli.

Self-management programmes

As with all chronic diseases a degree of self-management is likely to improve health outcomes. This is certainly true with asthma and would, for example, be fully accepted as part of the management of bronchiectasis and cystic fibrosis. However, the value of self-management programmes remains undetermined in COPD. In theory, a formal programme of remote supervision and disease education accompanied by action plans for exacerbations would be expected to produce obvious benefits. To date, the results suggest that they probably do marginally improve health outcomes and reduce health care consumption. This is a very important area of study because the future delivery of services for COPD will inevitably involve some form of educated self-management for the majority of patients with COPD. More severe patients will require more active case-management. One of the difficulties with the research data to date is that the reported self-management programmes have had different strategies. For example, the education components may comprise of verbally delivered information, written or other visual aids. The programme may also offer different levels of advice about physical activity and become confused with formal rehabilitation. These confounding approaches are probably responsible for some of the uncertainties. Future studies should clarify the situation.

Another area of potential confusion is the distinction between formal rehabilitation and the promotion of physical activity. Formal rehabilitation programmes are a specific course of therapy that has the aim of restoring physical functioning and well-being. These programmes are defined, structured, supervised and time limited. However, outside of the boundaries of the rehabilitation programme the promotion of physical activity is vital advice. In COPD, reduced physical activity is linked to mortality and hospital admission. Every opportunity should be taken to encourage the patient to remain active and challenge their breathlessness in order to retain their fitness. This advice should also be applied to people at the end of their rehabilitation programme so that they can more easily retain the benefit.

Further reading

Pulmonary rehabilitation. *Thorax* 2001; **56**: 827–834.

Chronic obstructive pulmonary disease. National clinical guideline on management of chronic obstructive pulmonary disease in adults in primary and secondary care. *Thorax* 2004; **59** (Suppl 1): 1–232.

Lacasse Y, Goldstein R, Lasserson TJ, *et al.* Pulmonary rehabilitation for chronic obstructive pulmonary disease. *Cochrane Database Syst Rev* 2006; **4**: CD003793.

Nici L, Donner C, Wouters E, *et al.* American Thoracic Society/European Respiratory Society statement on pulmonary rehabilitation. *Am J Respir Crit Care Med* 2006; **173**: 1390–1413.

Ries AL, Bauldoff GS, Carlin BW, *et al.* Pulmonary Rehabilitation: Joint ACCP/AACVPR Evidence-Based Clinical Practice Guidelines. *Chest* 2007; **131**: 4–42.

Troosters T, Casaburi R, Gosselink R, Decramer M. Pulmonary rehabilitation in chronic obstructive pulmonary disease. *Am J Respir Crit Care Med* 2005; **172**: 19–38.

5.6 Management of an exacerbation of COPD

Introduction
Exacerbations of COPD cause much of the morbidity, mortality and therefore health-care costs associated with this prevalent disease. In general, exacerbations become both more frequent and more severe as the severity of the underlying COPD increases. However, some patients appear more susceptible to these events than others and patients who experience frequent exacerbations (two or more courses of antibiotics and or corticosteroids per year) have a more rapid decline in lung function, poorer quality of life and higher mortality. It is particularly important to target these patients for the preventative therapies described below.

General management principles
1. Make the diagnosis. Exacerbation of COPD is a clinical diagnosis of exclusion – there is no diagnostic test. It is important to consider, and where appropriate exclude other possible causes of breathlessness in a patient with underlying COPD, for example pneumonia, pulmonary embolus, pneumothorax and cardiac failure.
2. Assess severity. Whilst there is no uniformly accepted method of assessing exacerbation severity, clinical assessment is important to judge the intensity of the treatment required, and the need for hospital care. In general, the presence of new onset respiratory failure, the need for treatment unavailable in the community, multiple co-morbidities or the absence of adequate social support all indicate the need for specialist assessment and possible hospital admission.
3. Institute treatment. Therapy is administered step-wise, described further below, and following the basic principles illustrated in Fig. 5.6.1 that includes disease-modifying treatments, interventions designed to support respiratory function until such disease-modifying treatments have had time to act, assessment and treatment of co-morbidities, and the institution of appropriate preventative strategies to reduce the risk of further exacerbation.

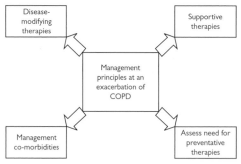

Fig. 5.6.1 Basic principles of therapy

Investigations
The purpose of investigations at exacerbation of COPD is to provide additional information in excluding other diagnoses, identifying co-morbidities and assessing exacerbation severity.

The following tests are usually appropriate in a hospital setting:
- FBC.
- U&Es.
- Blood glucose (steroid-associated hyperglycaemia).
- CRP. Whilst CRP is not useful in confirming diagnosis, it may help in monitoring the response to therapy.
- 12-lead ECG.
- CXR. This should be no different from a radiograph when the patient is stable, but may show features of underlying COPD such as hyper-expansion and pulmonary artery enlargement. The major reason to perform the radiograph is to exclude alternative causes of dyspnoea in a patient with underlying COPD.
- ABG.

The following tests are generally unhelpful:
- Sputum culture, as the presence of bacteria in sputum does not imply causation. Many patients have the same species of bacteria in sputum even when clinically stable, a phenomenon called 'bacterial colonisation'. The most common isolates are *Haemophilus influenzae*, *treptococcus pneumoniae* and *Moraxella catarrhalis*
- LFTs including serial peak-expiratory flow measurements, as the changes in individual patients are small, and the tests are difficult to perform in patients who are acutely dyspnoeic.

Therapy
Fig. 5.6.2 summarises the disease-modifying, and supportive aspects of therapy at exacerbation of COPD, described in further detail in later sections. It is important to emphasise the need for prompt therapy: this reduces exacerbation length which is one measure of exacerbation severity.

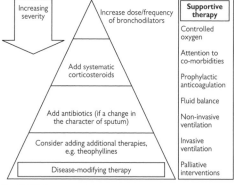

Fig. 5.6.2 Disease-modifying and supportive aspects of therapy

Disease-modifying therapy
Bronchodilators
- Some exacerbations will respond to an increased use of bronchodilators alone, including β_2-agonists and anti-cholinergic drugs, and this forms the basis of therapy in all exacerbations. These drugs target the additional

bronchoconstriction and hyperinflation present at exacerbation, which is presumed to result from increased airway inflammation.

- Short-acting β_2-agonists are preferred as they have a more rapid rate of action than short-acting anti-cholinergics.
- Although most guidelines suggest the use of both classes of drug together when the response to one or other is inadequate, there is in fact no evidence that this is superior to β_2-agonists alone.
- There is also no evidence that nebulisers are superior to administration via an inhaler and spacer. Nebulisation may be preferred in patients who are acutely dyspnoeic. The nebuliser driving gas should be prescribed, and is usually air with any additional oxygen administered separately.
- Long-acting bronchodilator drugs have no role acutely, but patients prescribed long-acting β_2-agonists when stable would normally continue on such therapy. It is not recommended that patients receive both long- and short-acting anti-cholinergics simultaneously but the benefits of one therapy over the other have not been reported.
- There is no evidence supporting the use of intravenous salbutamol at exacerbation of COPD.

Systemic corticosteroids

- These drugs should be added in all exacerbations not responding to an increase in bronchodilators alone. The rationale is to attenuate the additional airway inflammation that occurs during exacerbations, and which results in the symptomatic and physiological deterioration.
- The most robust evidence suggests that these drugs improve the rate of recovery of lung function, but effects on other outcome measures are more variable, and there is no evidence of a mortality benefit.
- Most guidelines recommend 30–40mg of prednisone for between 10–14 days, longer courses (and tapering the dose) are not of additional benefit and are associated with a greater chance of side-effects, especially hyperglycaemia.
- Nebulised budesonide appears equally effective to oral dosing but is more expensive.
- Inhaled corticosteroids have an important role in preventing exacerbations discussed below, and patients already prescribed these drugs would normally continue on this therapy during an exacerbation, but there is no role for initiating inhaled corticosteroids in the acute setting.

Antibiotics

- Pathogenic bacteria may be isolated in sputum from approximately 50% of patients with moderately-severe COPD at the time of exacerbation. Despite this, antibiotics are of limited efficacy. This, in part, reflects the presence of bacterial colonisation as already described. More recently it has been suggested that exacerbations result from change in the colonising strain, though the situation is complex as not all strain changes are associated with exacerbation, and not all exacerbations are associated with strain change.
- Respiratory viruses, particularly rhinoviruses, are also commonly isolated at the time of exacerbation and this is a further reason why antibiotics are of limited benefit.
- Sputum purulence is a reliable indicator of the presence of bacteria, and in general antibiotics are only indicated if there has been a change in the sputum volume or purulence.

- An aminopenicillin, tetracycline or quinolone would be a reasonable empiric choice, though local resistance patterns should be considered.
- Intravenous therapy is rarely required.
- 7–10 days of therapy is generally adequate.

Additional therapies

- Methyxanthines, usually IV aminophylline, may be used in patients not responding to the described measures, although evidence of benefit from these drugs is generally absent. Theophyllines are said to have a variety of effects on the respiratory, cardiovascular and immune systems which are of potential benefit during exacerbations. Against this, the narrow therapeutic index, side effects and drug interactions make administration difficult.
- The use of central respiratory stimulants has declined with the availability of non-invasive ventilation (NIV). Doxapram is still occasionally used as a holding measure prior to NIV, when NIV is inappropriate or unavailable, or (with specialist advice) in conjunction with NIV.
- There is currently no defined role for mucolytics at exacerbation of COPD.
- Sputum clearance techniques and nebulised saline are also not supported by available evidence and therefore not recommended routinely.
- There is no strong data to support the use of leukotriene receptor antagonists, intravenous magnesium or Heliox (helium and oxygen) at exacerbation of COPD.

Controlled oxygen

Oxygen therapy is indicated in all exacerbations associated with respiratory failure. This may be the result of a severe exacerbation in a patient with milder underlying disease, or be pre-existing in those with more advanced COPD. As a proportion of patients with COPD are at risk of developing hypercapnia with high-flow oxygen, oxygen should be administered at the minimum concentration able to maintain saturations at 90–92%. Failure to achieve this without a rise in $PaCO_2$ or fall in pH suggests the need for ventilatory support.

> **AUTHOR'S TIP**
>
> Attention to co-morbidities: Co-morbidities are common in COPD, and it is appropriate to consider and optimise co-existent medical conditions.

Prophylactic anticoagulation

In the absence of contra-indications it is our practice to administer prophylaxis against venous thromboembolism in patients at exacerbation of COPD. This in part reflects the risk of such complications developing, but also the potentially serious consequences of pulmonary embolus in a patient with already impaired gas exchange.

NIV

- NIV refers to the provision of ventilatory support via a nasal or full-face mask and the patients own upper airway, rather than an endotracheal tube.
- Primarily by reducing the complications associated with invasive ventilation, NIV is associated with reduced mortality, hospital stay and health-care costs. It may also be used earlier, intermittently, outside an intensive-care

environment (with trained staff) and facilitates patient communication, nutrition and physiotherapy.

- NIV is usually administered as pressure-cycled bi-level positive airway pressure.
- Instigation of NIV should be made with a clear plan of progression to invasive ventilation or palliation in the event of treatment failure.

Invasive ventilation

Patients with exacerbations of COPD do not have worse outcomes following invasive ventilation than those with respiratory failure from other causes. However, the decision to institute invasive ventilation can de difficult and should consider the prior functional status of the patient, the reversibility of the insult, the presence of co-morbidities and the wishes of the patient and their family.

Palliative interventions

For patients failing to improve on maximal therapy, or in whom escalation of therapy is inappropriate, a range of palliative measures may be instituted including benzodiazepine and opiate drugs for relief of terminal dyspnoea.

Preventative therapy

Following an exacerbation it is important to consider the introduction of interventions that may reduce the likelihood of a subsequent exacerbation. Such approaches to reduce the impact of exacerbations and hospitalisations in COPD are illustrated in Fig. 5.6.3. Not every treatment is appropriate for every patient.

Summary

- Exacerbations are important events in COPD.
- Exacerbation of COPD is a clinical diagnosis of exclusion.
- The principles of exacerbation therapy consist of supporting gas exchange while disease-modifying therapies have time to act, addressing co-morbidities, and considering appropriate interventions to reduce the likelihood of subsequent exacerbation.
- An increase in the dose of short-acting bronchodilators with oral corticosteroids form the basis of therapy for most exacerbations, with antibiotics added when there is a change in the character of the sputum.
- Oxygen is necessary for all patients in respiratory failure.
- NIV has revolutionised the management of hypercapnic respiratory failure.
- There are a number of evidence-based strategies able to reduce the risk of further exacerbation and hospitalisation in COPD including drugs, vaccines and pulmonary rehabilitation.

Further reading

Wedzicha JA, Martinez F (eds). *Chronic Obstructive Pulmonary Disease Exacerbations. Lung Biology in Health and Disease*, 2008. London: Informa Healthcare.

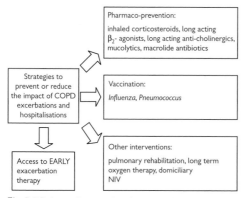

Fig. 5.6.3 Approaches to reduce the impact of exacerbations and hospitalizations.

5.7 Surgery for COPD

History

Surgical treatment of emphysema was first contemplated in the early 20th century. Costochondrectomies of the upper ribs in conjunction with transverse sternotomy as well as paravertebral thoracoplasty were performed until it was commonly accepted that the hyperinflated chest was the result of emphysema rather than its cause. Abdominal belts, phrenic nerve paralysis and pneumoperitoneum were aimed at restoring the curvature of the flattened diapahragm.

In 1954 in an attempt to treat the airway component of COPD, Nissen proposed tracheoplasty using prosthetic devices to support the membranous trachea. Each of these procedures was ultimately found to be ill-advised, and surgical morbidity outweighed by far their clinical benefits.

Brantigan and colleagues at the University of Maryland/Virginia have to be credited with the introduction of basic principles of lung volume reduction surgery (LVRS) in 1957. They postulated that surgically reducing hyperinflation of the emphysematous lung would restore radial traction on terminal bronchioles, improve respiratory airflow obstruction and diaphragmatic movement. The modern concept of LVRS was introduced by J. Cooper in 1993, performing bilateral stapled wedge resections on patients with heterogeneous emphysema and evidence of hyperinflation. In his early series of 20 patients the objective improvement in FEV_1 6 months after surgery was reported to be 82%.

Between 1997 and 2002 the National Emphysema Treatment Trial (NETT) randomised 1218 patients to undergo LVRS or continued medical care. The outcomes published in 2003 together with the results of a number of case controlled series and smaller randomised trials are best available evidence for the choice of emphysema patients to be considered for surgery.

Pathophysiology

The typical physiologic change of COPD is progressive expiratory airflow limitation caused by chronic inflammation. Following remodelling and obstruction of the small airways a loss of alveolar attachment and decreased elastic recoil of the lung parenchyma sets in.

A decrease in the FEV_1 ratio to FVC is a first indicator of developing airflow limitation. Small airflow obstruction is revealed by severe reduction in the forced expiratory flow in the 25–75% range. The reduction in diffusion capacity for carbon monoxide (DLCO) reflects the degree of parenchymal destruction.

In advanced disease, hypoxemia is mainly caused by a combination of airway obstruction, parenchymal involvement and changes in the ventilation/perfusion (V/Q) ratio as a consequence of pulmonary vascular abnormalities. Severe V/Q mismatch, increased dead space ratio, alveolar hypoventilation and inspiratory muscle dysfunction potentially lead to exertional and/or resting hypercapnia.

Radiographic signs of diaphragmatic flattening, increased retrosternal air space, and increased lucency of the lung fields, go along with the physiologic changes mainly consisting of hyperinflation.

Surgical management

Treatment of bullous emphysema (giant bullous lung disease)

Bullae are defined as air-flilled spaces within the lung parenchyma, lined by a fibrous wall and trabeculated by remnants of alveolar septae. These air-filled spaces can develop as a result of generalised emphysema or in the setting of a normal underlying parenchyma. In 1989 Morgan introduced the concept of bullae representing areas of parenchymal weakness being ventilated preferentially, in disagreement with the check valve concept of bullae formation which had been adopted until then.

Patient selection

DeVries and Wolfe subdivided patients with bullous emphysema in four groups based on the anatomy of the bulla and the quality of the underlying parenchyma taking into account their surgical prognosis:

- Group I: large single bulla/normal underlying lung.
- Group II: multiple bullae/normal underlying lung.
- Group III: multiple bullae/diffusely emphysematous underlying lung.
- Group IV: multiple bullae/underlying lung with other diseases.

The principles of surgery in the context of bullous disease are based on the concept of re-expanding compressed normal lung parenchyma and restoring physiological chest wall excursions rather than focusing on the resection of areas of dead space ventilation.

Good functional results are therefore more likely to be achieved in deVries Groups I and II, whereas the role of surgery in Groups III and IV remains controversial.

Surgical indications

Inclusion criteria (modified Greenberg et al. criteria):

- Incapacitating dyspnoea related to single/multiple bulla/ae (included in NICE guidelines for COPD).
- Bulla/ae occupying at least one-third of hemithorax.
- Complications related to bulla/ae (pneumothorax, infection, haemoptysis, cancer).
- CT chest/V/Q scan confirming deVries Groups I or II.
- 6MWT of >600 feet.

Preoperative preparation

To include:

- Pulmonary function testing (PFT), with gas transfer and ABG analysis.
- CT chest.
- V/Q scan.
- Pulmonary rehabilitation (not mandatory).
- Smoking cessation >6 months.
- Maximal medical treatment of associated airway disease and nutritional deficits.

Surgical technique

Three surgical techniques have emerged:

- Video assisted thoracoscopy (VATS) with stapled excision of bullous parenchyma. *Advantages*: minimal invasive access, rapid postoperative convalescence, good cosmetic result.
- Open bullectomy with excision of bullous parenchyma through (anterior) thoracotomy. *Advantages*: suitable for

patients not tolerating one-lung ventilation, technically less challenging procedure compared to VATS.
- Intracavitary drainage (modified Monaldi procedure) adopting rib resection and direct drainage of bulla with Foley catheter. *Advantages*: suitable for high-risk patients not tolerating one-lung ventilation and/or excisional procedures, and for selected patients in deVries Groups III and IV.

Factors predicting outcome
Better results are anticipated for:
- Bulla/ae occupying >50% hemithorax with normal underlying lung.
- Younger patients with no comorbidity, no weight loss and rapidly progressing dyspnoea.
- Normal and slightly decreased FVC.
- FEV_1 >40% predicted.
- Normal DLCO and ABG analysis.

Results
- Perioperative mortality ranging from 0% to 8%.
- Morbidity primarily related to prolonged air leaks.
- Postoperative clinical and symptomatic improvements may be better than reflected by PFT results.

LVRS
LVRS provides an opportunity for palliation of symptoms and improvement of quality of life for patients with severe end-stage emphysema, and since 2005 its use is supported by NICE.

LVRS implies resection of target areas of emphysematous lung and aims at:
- Improving V/Q matching by allowing compressed lung to re-expand.
- Restoring outward traction on small airways.
- Restoring physiological chest wall and inspiratory muscle excursions by reducing hyperinflation.
- Natural history studies of emphysema have shown that 50% of patients with a FEV_1 of <30% predicted will die within 3–4 years. The Kaplan–Meier estimate of survival after LVRS at 5 years published by Cooper *et al.* in 2003 was 68%, with an in-hospital mortality of 4.8%.

Patient selection
As in NICE guidelines for COPD:
- Incapacitating dyspnoea due to severe COPD despite maximal medical therapy (incl. rehabilitation).
- Upper lobe predominant emphysema.
- FEV_1 >20% predicted.
- DLCO >20% predicted.
- $PaCO_2$ <55 mm Hg

The inclusion criteria published by Cooper *et al.* emphasize the importance of radiographic patient evaluation and in summary turn out to be less restrictive than the NICE guidelines:
- Incapacitating dyspnoea despite rehabilitation.
- Marked emphysema, airflow obstruction and hyperinflation.
- Heterogeneous distribution of emphysema with target zones of poorly perfused lung.
- DLCO <50% predicted and >10% predicted.
- $PaCO_2$ <60 mm Hg.
- Essentially normal cardiac ejection fraction with mean pulmonary artery (PA) pressure of <35 mmHg.

Preoperative preparation
See Treatment of bullous emphysema, p. 116.
In addition:
- 6MWT.
- Completion of questionnaires assessing dyspnoea and quality of life.

Surgical technique
The most common LVRS procedure is a bilateral stapled resection of emphysematous lung parenchyma, performed by
- median sternotomy;
- bilateral VATS or;
- unilateral staged VATS.

The NETT trial has confirmed that there is no significant difference in the incidence of complications as well as outcome after LVRS by VATS or median sternotomy.

Unilateral staged VATS requires two anaesthetics and creates an 'unbalanced mediastinum' during the interval between procedures, explaining why it is currently the least preferred of these three surgical approaches.

Factors predicting outcome
NETT (RCT) findings:
- Upper lobe disease/low exercise capacity → improvement in survival, exercise tolerance, quality of life (compared to medical group).
- Upper lobe disease/high exercise capacity → improvement in exercise tolerance and quality of life; no difference in survival.
- Non-upper lobe disease/low exercise capacity → improvement in quality of life; no difference in survival and exercise tolerance
- Non-upper lobe disease/high exercise capacity → higher risk of death.
- Overall exercise tolerance in 2 years after LVRS nearly back to base-line level, whilst progressive decline in medical group.
- Negative prognostic factors: low FEV_1 (<20%) in combination with either DLCO <20% or homogeneous pattern of emphysema.

Findings of Cooper *et al.* (prospective controlled consecutive case series):
- Improvement in FEV_1, residual volume (RV), DLCO and quality of life sustained for 5 years in majority of patients when compared to preoperative values.
- Improvement in 6MWT and dyspnoea score maintained for 3 years.
- Negative prognostic factors: advanced age, male gender, low FEV_1, reduced 6MWT, $PaCO_2$ >50 mmHg, lower lobe disease.

Results
- Perioperative mortality ranging from 4–6%.
- Prolonged air leaks most common complication (45%), with overall re-exploration rate of 4.5%.
- Cost-effectiveness (NETT): incremental cost per quality-adjusted life-years (QALY) gained with LVRS relative to medical therapy after 3 years of treatment 190,000 USD.
- To tie this in with potential costs borne by the society: about 1% of estimated two million patients with emphysema in the US were potentially considered eligible for LVRS by Ramsey in 2003, this being called a conservative estimate.

Endoscopic lung volume reduction

The concept of removing hypoventilated and non-functional areas of lung and the favourable results of the NETT have led to the development of various bronchoscopic techniques to provide alternative means of achieving the results of LVRS.

Concepts:
- To promote atelectasis in emphysematous lung (using endobronchial valves, fibrin-based glue or fibrin-hydrogel and thrombin).
- Radiofrequency-induced fenestrations in segmental bronchi to enhance expiratory airflow.

Wan et al. have recently published the results of a multicentre trial including 98 patients after insertion of a silicone-based one-way endobronchial valve (Fig. 5.7.1). They report improvements in FEV_1, FVC, RV and exercise tolerance at follow-ups 90 days after the procedure. 8% of their patients had serious perioperative complications.

The Endobronchial Valve for Emphysema Palliation Trial (VENT) is ongoing in the US.

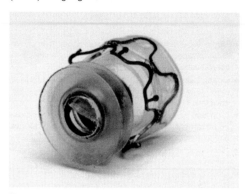

Fig. 5.7.1 The Emphasys Medical endobronchial valve.

The other techniques mentioned are currently either trialled at animal level or as Phase I studies.

Lung transplantation

More than 8000 lung transplantations were performed worldwide between 1995 and 2001, and emphysema was the main indication for these procedures.

Patient selection

As in NICE guidelines for COPD:
- Incapacitating dyspnoea due to severe COPD despite maximal medical therapy.
- Considerations to include age, FEV_1, $PaCO_2$, homogeneous distribution of emphysema, elevated PA pressure with progressive deterioration.

Further reading

Brantigan O, Mueller E, Kress M. A surgical approach to pulmonary emphysema. *Am Rev Respir Dis* 1959; **80**: 194–202.

Ciccone AM, Myers BF, Guthrie TJ, et al. Long-term outcome of bilateral lung volume reduction in 250 consecutive patients with emphysema. *J Thorac Cardiovasc Surg* 2003; **125**: 513–125.

Cooper JD, Trulock EP, Triantafillou AN, et al. Bilateral pneumonectomy (volume reduction) for chronic obstructive pulmonary disease. *J Thorac Cardiovasc Surg* 1995; **109**: 106–119.

Greenberg JA, Singhal S, Kaiser L. Giant bullous lung disease: evaluation, selection, techniqes and outcomes. *Chest Surg Clin N Am* 2003; **13**: 631–649.

Maxfield RA. New and emerging minimally invasive techniques for lung volume reduction. *Chest* 2004; **125**: 777–783.

National Emphysema Treatment Trial Research Group. A randomized trial comparing lung-volume-reduction surgery with medical therapy for severe emphysema. *N Engl J Med* 2003; **348**: 2059–2073.

National Institute for Clinical Excellence. Chronic Obstructive Pulmonary Disease; *NICE Clinical Guideline* 2004; **12**.

Ramsey SD. Cost effectiveness of lung volume reduction surgery. *Chest Surg Clin N Am* 2003; **13**: 727–738.

Wan IY, Torna TP, Geddes DM, et al. Bronchoscopic lung-volume-reduction for end-stage emphysema. *Chest* 2006; **129**: 518–526.

5.8 Alpha-1-antitrypsin deficiency

The most important genetic factor in the development of COPD is α_1-antitrypsin (AAT) deficiency. It is found in 1–2% of affected individuals. AAT is an acute phase glycoprotein that is synthesised in the liver and secreted into the plasma where it is the most abundant circulating protease inhibitor. Its primary role is to inhibit neutrophil elastase.

Severe AAT deficiency (defined as a plasma level <0.5g/l) is an autosomal co-dominant condition that results from point mutations in the AAT gene.

Molecular epidemiology

The Z variant (Glu342Lys) accounts for 95% of cases of severe AAT deficiency. Homozygotes (PI*Z) have plasma AAT levels that are 10–15% of those seen in individuals with normal M alleles (PI*M). Approximately 4% of Northern Europeans are heterozygous for the Z allele (PI*MZ) with 1 in 1600–2000 being homozygotes. Other rare variants of AAT that are associated with severe plasma deficiency are AAT Siiyama (Ser53Phe) in Japan, AAT Mmalton (del 52Phe) in Sardinia and the rare Null variants that have no detectable AAT in the plasma. The S allele (Glu264Val; PI*MS) is found in 28% of southern Europeans but is infrequently associated with clinical disease as plasma levels in homozygotes are 60% of normal.

Pathophysiology of COPD

Cigarette smoking is the most important environmental factor for accelerated decline in lung function in individuals with AAT deficiency. Several pathways are recognised to predispose to early onset panlobular emphysema in the Z AAT homozygote (Fig. 5.8.1).

- The retention of AAT within hepatocytes reduces the AAT that is available to protect the lungs from uncontrolled proteolytic digestion by neutrophil elastase.
- The Z AAT that enters the lung is 5-fold less effective at inhibiting neutrophil elastase than is normal M AAT.
- Monomeric Z AAT spontaneously forms polymers within the alveoli thereby inactivating AAT as a proteinase inhibitor.
- Polymeric Z AAT is chemotactic for human neutrophils. This proinflammatory effect of polymers may explain the progression of lung disease and airway obstruction after smoking cessation in PI*Z individuals.

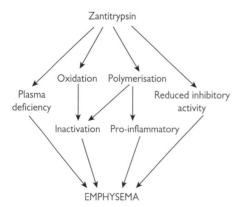

Fig. 5.8.1 Mechanisms for the pathogenesis of emphysema.

- Oxidants in cigarette smoke can inactivate AAT as an inhibitor of neutrophil elastase.

PI*Z individuals have marked variability in the severity of COPD suggesting that factors other than smoking are important in the development and progression of airflow obstruction. The PI*MZ phenotype is associated with variably increased risk of lung disease in smokers.

Clinical features

Symptomatic COPD usually presents between 30–40 years of age in smokers and is rare before the third decade. The symptoms are similar to those of non-AAT deficient COPD and may include:

- Episodic wheeze and dyspnoea suggestive of asthma. The prevalence of asthmatic features is higher in severe AAT deficiency and symptoms occur early in the development of airway disease.
- Allergic rhinitis which may precede airway obstruction.
- Fatigue.

No one physical sign is specific for detecting the AAT-deficient individual. Exacerbations occur more frequently in individuals with chronic bronchitis and more severe disease and are associated with a greater degree of inflammation than in those with COPD without AAT-deficiency. There is little evidence that airway hyper-responsiveness is more prevalent in this group

> **AUTHOR'S TIP**
> The presence of bronchiectasis in AAT-deficient individuals is well recognised but remains controversial. It may be a consequence of emphysema in PI*Z patients rather than a primary effect. The AAT phenotype distribution and gene frequencies are not different between patients with bronchiectasis and control subjects.

Extra pulmonary manifestations

- Liver disease – the Z mutation allows one AAT molecule to lock into a second which then extends to form chains of pathogenic loop-sheet polymers (Fig. 5.8.2a and 5.8.2b). These accumulate within the endoplasmic reticulum of hepatocytes as PAS positive inclusions (Fig. 5.8.2c) that are associated with neonatal hepatitis, cirrhosis and hepatocellular carcinoma. Z AAT deficiency is the most common genetic indication for liver transplantation in childhood. Only a subpopulation of AAT-deficient individuals develop significant liver injury and these appear to have inefficient intracellular degradation mechanisms for the removal of retained Z AAT protein.
- Panniculitis that is characterised by painful red nodules on the thighs or buttocks. It results from uncontrolled proteolysis within the skin.
- ANCA positive systemic vasculitis and Wegener's granulomatosis are rare complications.
- Nephropathy with membranoproliferative glomerulonephritis especially in children and young adults. This may be a consequence of the associated liver disease.

Investigations

PI*Z AAT deficiency is suspected where plasma AAT levels are abnormally low (< 0.5g/l) in individuals with associated diseases. The diagnosis is confirmed by identifying abnormal AAT phenotypes by isoelectric focusing. Genotyping offers diagnosis at the molecular level.

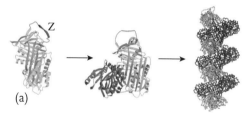

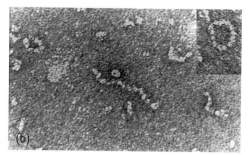

Fig. 5.8.2a Mutants of AAT (left) cause the protein to link together as dimers (middle) that extend to form chains of polymers that are retained within hepatocytes.

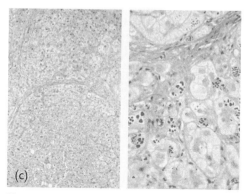

Fig. 5.8.2b Polymers of Z AAT that are retained within hepatocytes.

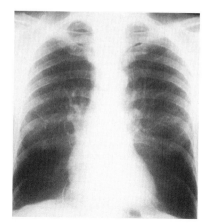

Fig. 5.8.3 Emphysema with basal radiolucency.

Lung function tests
- Spirometry, static lung volumes, ABG analysis and gas transfer should be measured at baseline and generally mirror abnormalities seen in 'usual' COPD except in being out of proportion to the smoking history.
- FEV_1 is the most important predictor of survival.
- There is a wide variation in bronchodilator response which may explain why some cases of AAT-deficient COPD are diagnosed as asthma.
- Some individuals have discordant physiology with marked emphysema and little airway disease or *vice versa* for reasons that remain unclear.

Natural history

Liver dysfunction represents the major clinical problem before the third decade while lung function is preserved. Lung dysfunction begins thereafter. A more rapid rate of FEV_1 decline is associated with:
- male sex;
- age between 30 to 44 years;
- current smoking;
- FEV_1 between 35–60% predicted;
- bronchodilator response (asthmatic features);
- chronic bronchitis;
- previous episodes of pneumonia.

Severe AAT deficiency is associated with shortened life expectancy and survival falls exponentially as FEV_1 declines to <35% predicted. Median life expectancy for smokers is between 40–49 years and 65–69 years for never smokers. Emphysema and cirrhosis are the most common causes of death (72% and 10% respectively) and account for the excess mortality.

Fig. 5.8.2c The accumalation of Z AAT causes cirhosis (left) and cherry red PAS positive inclusions (right).

Radiology
- The CXR is normal in early disease. Hyperinflation, diaphragmatic flattening and increased lower lung radiolucency may be evident in advanced disease (Fig. 5.8.3).
- HRCT is more sensitive for detecting emphysema in AAT deficiency. It allows assessment of the severity of associated bullous disease and bronchiectasis.

AUTHOR'S TIP

Cirrhosis in adults is more commonly the underlying cause of death in non smokers which is consistent with cirrhosis affecting survivors over the age of 50 years.

Management and treatment

Preventing the development of COPD is solely dependent on early smoking cessation and limiting exposure to environmental pollutants. The prevalence of smoking in PI*Z adolescents who are aware of their diagnosis is half that of age-matched peers.

Guidelines for treatment of 'usual' COPD are applicable to individuals with AAT-deficient lung disease including bronchodilators, oxygen, pulmonary rehabilitation, nutritional advice, influenza vaccinations and surgery (bullectomy and transplantation). Lung volume reduction surgery offers only short-term benefits in AAT deficiency emphysema and is generally not recommended. Liver transplantation remains the only treatment for liver cirrhosis.

Augmentation therapy

The IV administration of pooled plasma purified AAT has been the mainstay of treatment for severe AAT deficiency in a limited number of countries since 1987. A protective threshold above 0.5g/l of AAT is thought to limit proteolytic lung injury and so guard against the development of emphysema. Exogenous doses are administered once a week to achieve a trough level above this threshold but the interval can be extended to 14 or 21 days to achieve adequate concentrations. There is good evidence that IV augmentation therapy raises serum levels above the protective threshold and AAT is detectable in bronchoalveolar lavage fluid. The largest studies looking for evidence of clinical efficacy have been observational cohort studies which indicate a lower overall mortality and a slower rate of annual decline in FEV_1 in recipients with moderate COPD (FEV_1 of 35–65% predicted). In addition IV AAT use has been associated with a reduction in the frequency of respiratory tract infections, a significant decline in sputum markers of inflammation and relatively few serious side effects. The only randomised control trial of IV augmentation therapy showed no significant difference in the rate of FEV_1 decline or the rate of loss of lung density as defined by CT densitometry although there was a trend in favour of the active treatment group.

Analyses of IV AAT therapy suggests an incremental cost effectiveness ratio of £103,400 per quality of life-years for treatment until FEV_1<35% when the costs of other general COPD treatments are included.

Aerosolised delivery of recombinant AAT has been developed for daily administration but is of unproven efficacy.

Novel strategies

Novel therapeutic approaches include strategies using:

- All-trans retinoic acid to initiate the growth of new alveoli in emphysematous lungs. Rat studies have demonstrated encouraging results and human trials are ongoing.
- Identifying small molecules capable of preventing the polymerisation of AAT within hepatocytes or rescuing misfolded AAT protein (chaperone therapy).
- Adeno-associated viral vectors to deliver and express AAT in the liver and other tissues.
- Transplantation of hepatocytes as an alternative to whole liver transplantation.

Support groups and useful websites:

- Alpha-1 UK (www.alpha1.org.uk).
- Alpha-1 Foundation (www.alphaone.org).
- Alpha-1 National Association (www.alpha1.org).
- British Liver Trust (www.britishlivertrust.org.uk).

Further reading

ATS/ERS statement: Standards for the diagnosis and management of individuals with AAT deficiency. *Am J Respir Crit Care Med* 2003; **168**: 818–900.

DeMeo DL, Sandhans RA, Barker AF, *et al*. Determinants of airflow obstruction in severe alpha-1-antitrypsin deficiency. *Thorax* 2007; **62**: 806–813.

Lomas DA, Mahadeva R. α_1-Antitrypsin polymerization and the serpinopathies: pathobiology and prospects for therapy. *J Clin Invest* 2002; **110**: 1585–1590.

Needham M, Stockley RA. α_1-Antitrypsin deficiency. 3: Clinical manifestations and natural history. *Thorax* 2004; **59**: 441–445.

Perlmutter DH, Brodsky JL, Balisteri WF, *et al*. Molecular pathogenesis of Alpha -1- Antitrypsin deficiency- associated liver disease: A meeting review. *Hepatology* 2007; **45**: 1313–1323.

Stoller JK, Aboussouan LS. α_1-antitrypsin deficiency. *Lancet* 2005; **365**: 2225–2236.

Oxygen

Chapter contents

6.1 Home oxygen therapy

Since the two landmark clinical trials of long-term oxygen therapy (LTOT) that reported in the early 1980s, there have been considerable advances in the understanding, prescription and provision of home oxygen therapy. The purpose of home oxygen therapy is to correct hypoxaemia and not primarily as a therapy for breathlessness. LTOT is an important therapy as to date it is one of the few interventions that can improve survival in patients with COPD and chronic respiratory failure.

There are three main types of oxygen therapy that can be prescribed for home use and these will be discussed in this article. Home oxygen therapy may also in used in infants and children but paediatric prescription is relatively small and this article will concentrate on home oxygen in adults.

LTOT is prescribed for patients for continuous use at home usually through an oxygen concentrator. These patients will have chronic hypoxaemia (PaO$_2$ at or below 7.3kPa, (55mmHg)), though LTOT may also be indicated in patients with a PaO$_2$ between 7.3 and 8kPa (55 to 60 mmHg), if they have evidence of pulmonary hypertension, secondary hypoxaemia, oedema or significant nocturnal arterial oxygen desaturation. There is no benefit in the use of LTOT in COPD patients with a PaO$_2$ above 8kPa. Once started, this therapy is likely to be life long.

Ambulatory oxygen therapy

> **KEY FACT**
> LTOT is usually given for at least 15 hours daily, to include the overnight period, as arterial hypoxaemia worsens during sleep.

Ambulatory oxygen therapy refers to the provision of oxygen therapy with a portable device during exercise and daily activities. It is usually prescribed in conjunction with LTOT, though a small group of normoxaemic patients may benefit from ambulatory oxygen of they have significant arterial oxygen desaturation on exercise.

Short-burst oxygen therapy (SBOT) refers to the intermittent use of supplemental oxygen at home usually provided by static cylinders and normally for periods of about 10–20 minutes at a time to relieve dyspnoea. Although considerable amounts of SBOT is used in the UK, the evidence for benefit of SBOT is weak and other treatments for dyspnoea should be used.

Indications for LTOT (Table 6.1.1)

Table 6.1.1 Indications for LTOT

- COPD
- Severe chronic asthma
- Interstitial lung disease
- Cystic fibrosis
- Bronchiectasis
- Pulmonary vascular disease
- Primary pulmonary hypertension
- Pulmonary malignancy
- Chronic heart failure

There are three main indications for the prescription of long term oxygen therapy:

1 chronic hypoxaemia;
2 nocturnal hypoventilation;
3 palliative use.

Chronic hypoxaemia

As already discussed identification of patients with chronic hypoxaemia is important, as LTOT is one of the few treatments that can improve prognosis in patients with COPD. Chronic hypoxaemia, with or without carbon dioxide retention, can occur in several respiratory and cardiac disorders, including COPD, chronic severe asthma, interstitial lung disease such as fibrosing alveolitis and asbestosis, cystic fibrosis and pulmonary hypertension. Chronic hypoxaemia leads to an increase in pulmonary arterial pressure, secondary polycythaemia and neuropsychological changes, and these complications can be improved with LTOT.

Patients who have daytime hypoxaemia may develop further arterial oxygen desaturation at night during nocturnal hypoventilation and this will contribute to the observed rise in pulmonary artery pressure. Thus LTOT is always prescribed to include the night-time as it will reduce the nocturnal hypoxia episodes and thus reduce the peaks of pulmonary hypertension.

LTOT has been shown to improve survival in hypoxaemic patients, to reduce secondary polycythaemia and increase sleep quality. Chronic hypoxaemia is related to poor health status (Fig. 6.1.1), anxiety and depression and these parameters will improve with LTOT. It is also possible that LTOT may reduce the severity of COPD exacerbations as hypoxaemic patients, who are not taking LTOT, have been shown to be at increased risk for hospital admission.

Patients with severe cardiac failure may also develop arterial hypoxaemia, caused mainly by ventilation perfusion inequalities. However there are few studies of LTOT in cardiac failure and large studies with appropriate outcome measures are required.

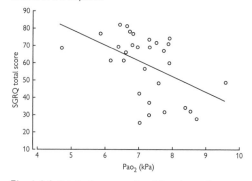

Fig. 6.1.1 Relation between quality of life and arterial hypoxaemia COPD patients. Reproduced from Okubadejo AA *et al., Thorax* 1996; **51**: 44–47.

Patients with chest wall or neuromuscular diseases .who develop hypercapnic respiratory failure usually require ventilatory support with NIV rather than LTOT. Use of LTOT in these patients may lead to a potentially dangerous rise in PaCO$_2$.

However if chronic hypoxaemia persists while the patient is on ventilatory support, then LTOT should be prescribed but to start at a low oxygen flow rate e.g. 1l/minute.

Patients on home oxygen should stop smoking as the use of oxygen in the presence of smoking is can cause burns and is a fire hazard. Any patient who persists in smoking despite using any form of home oxygen must be warned of the potential risks.

Benefits of LTOT are listed in Table 6.1.2.

Table 6.1.2 Benefits of LTOT

- Increased survival
- Increased quality of life
- Prevention of deterioration of pulmonary haemodynamics
- Reduction of secondary polycythaemia
- Neuropsychological benefit with reduction in symptoms of anxiety and depression
- Improved sleep quality
- Reduction in cardiac arrhythmias
- Increase in renal blood flow

Nocturnal hypoventilation

LTOT may also be used in patients with PaO_2 above 7.3kPa but who have evidence of nocturnal hypoventilation. This patient group will include those with chest wall disease caused by obesity, chest wall or neuromuscular disease. LTOT may also be used in conjunction with continuous positive airway pressure (CPAP) for obstructive sleep apnoea. though LTOT is not first-line therapy for sleep apnoea. Prescription of LTOT in these situations will require referral to a physician with a specialist interest in these disorders as specialist investigation is required. Although LTOT is usually given life-long for patients with COPD, in the case of some chest wall disorders and sleep apnoea, LTOT will be prescribed for a temporary period, perhaps till the respiratory failure improves with ventilatory support or weight reduction in the case of sleep apnoea patients has been successful.

Palliative use

LTOT may also be prescribed for palliation of severe dyspnoea in patients with lung cancer and other causes of disabling dyspnoea such as is found in patients with severe end-stage COPD or neuromuscular disease.

Assessment for LTOT

It essential that all patients who may have require LTOT undergo a full assessment in a specialist centre. The purpose of assessment is to confirm the presence of hypoxaemia and to ensure that the correct oxygen flow rate is provided to adequately correct the hypoxaemia. Assessment for LTOT depends on measurement of ABGs. Either blood gases from a radial or femoral artery or arterialised ear-lobe capillary blood gases can be used for assessments. The advantages of ear-lobe gases are that samples can be performed by various health care professionals. Prior to LTOT assessment and prescription, it is essential that there has been optimum medical management of the particular condition and clinical stability. Patients should not be assessed for LTOT during an acute exacerbation of their disease. As exacerbation recovery may be prolonged, hypoxaemia can persist after exacerbation and thus assessment should occur no sooner than at around 5–6 weeks after exacerbation. It is usual to start with a supplemental oxygen

flow rate of 2 l/minute via nasal cannulae, or from a 24% controlled oxygen face mask, and to aim for a PaO_2 value of at least 8kPa.

Blood gases must be measured, rather than SaO_2 with a pulse oximeter, as assessment of hypercapnia and its response to oxygen therapy is required for safe prescription of LTOT. Pulse oximetry has also poor specificity in the crucial PaO_2 range for LTOT prescription and thus is unsuitable when used alone for assessment. However, oximetry may prove valuable in screening patients with chronic respiratory disease and selecting those patients who require further blood gas analysis. Patients on LTOT require formal assessment after prescription to ensure that there is adequate correction of hypoxaemia and that they are adherent to the treatment.

Indications for ambulatory oxygen therapy

Patients with chronic lung disease especially those with COPD or interstitial lung disease show increased arterial hypoxaemia when they exercise. Ambulatory oxygen can correct this exercise hypoxaemia, and this has been shown to also reduce breathlessness and increase exercise capacity though responses to ambulatory oxygen are variable amongst patients. As for LTOT, the purpose of ambulatory oxygen is to correct exercise hypoxaemia and not as a therapy with the sole aim of reduction in dyspnoea. However most of the studies of the effects of ambulatory oxygen are relatively short-term studies and there is less evidence that ambulatory oxygen improves quality of life over the longer term.

Ambulatory oxygen can be prescribed in three broad groups of patients:

- Grade 1. Some patients on LTOT are already housebound and unable to leave the home. In this group ambulatory oxygen will be used for short periods only and intermittently. These patients will generally use ambulatory oxygen at the same flow rate as with their LTOT.
- Grade 2. Patients on LTOT, who are mobile and need to or can leave the home on a regular basis. In this patient group assessment will need to include a review of activity and oxygen flow rate required to correct hypoxaemia.
- Grade 3. Patients without chronic hypoxaemia (PaO_2> 7.3kPa), who are not on LTOT, but who show evidence of arterial oxygen desaturation on exercise, with a fall of SaO_2 of at least 4% below 90%. Ambulatory oxygen should only be prescribed if there is evidence of exercise de-saturation that is corrected by the proposed device.

Ambulatory oxygen therapy is indicated in a number of respiratory conditions, with COPD being the most common. Ambulatory oxygen is not indicated in patients with no evidence of arterial hypoxaemia and is not indicated in patients with chronic heart failure. The other indications are listed in Table 6.1.3:

Table 6.1.3 Indications for ambulatory oxygen

- COPD
- Severe chronic asthma
- Interstitial lung disease
- Cystic fibrosis
- Pulmonary vascular disease
- Primary pulmonary hypertension
- Chest wall disease e.g. kyphoscoliosis

Assessment for ambulatory oxygen

The type of ambulatory oxygen assessment will depend on the patient's grade and thus on the patient's activity and ability to leave the home (Table 6.1.4). Traditionally assessments for ambulatory oxygen therapy use short-term response to supplemental oxygen therapy during an exercise test (e.g. 6MWT) . However it is now recognised that short-term responses do not predict benefit over a longer period of time and thus the short-term response cannot be used to select patients for ambulatory oxygen. In some cases the weight of the ambulatory device has been shown to negate the benefit of the therapy on the short-term response. Thus the ambulatory oxygen assessment should be used as an opportunity to assess the patient's activity, to set the optimal oxygen flow rate and introduce the patient to the ambulatory device. The assessment should ideally be performed after a course of exercise training as part of a pulmonary rehabilitation programme. The initial assessment should be followed by a review after approximately 2 months of oxygen usage and ambulatory oxygen withdrawn if unhelpful.

Table 6.1.4 Ambulatory oxygen therapy – patient assessment

GRADE 1 OXYGEN REQUIREMENTS – same flow rate as for static source
GRADE 2 OXYGEN REQUIREMENTS – evaluate oxygen flow rate to correct exercise SaO$_2$ above 90% using exercise test e.g. 6MWT
GRADE 3 OXYGEN REQUIREMENTS – exercise test required, performed on air and oxygen. Require evidence of exercise desturation and improvement with oxygen

There is little information on compliance with ambulatory oxygen therapy, though when assessed, compliance has been found to be generally poor, with most patients only using it occasionally to go out of the house or into their gardens and much less than instructed by their healthcare professionals. Thus appropriate education should be provided with prescription of the ambulatory equipment.

Before prescription of ambulatory oxygen, it is important to determine the level of outside activity that the patient is likely to perform, so that the most effective and economic device is provided for the patient. Most ambulatory oxygen is provided with lightweight portable cylinders, though small cylinders provide oxygen for a short duration and oxygen-conserving devices may be useful in prolonging oxygen availability. However, patient responses to these conserving devices vary due to varying inspiratory flow rates and patients should to be assessed on the same equipment that they will eventually use when at home. Liquid oxygen systems can provide a longer period of ambulatory oxygen usage but are expensive to provide and not so widely available.

SBOT

Despite extensive prescription of short burst therapy, there is no evidence available for benefit of this oxygen modality and other interventions should be used for control of dyspnoea. SBOT has traditionally been used for pre-oxygenation before exercise, recovery from exercise and control of breathlessness at rest. It has been also used in palliative care to relieve disabling dyspnoea though patients in this condition usually require a source of LTOT at home. SBOT has also been used after a COPD exacerbation when a patients has not yet recovered form hypoxaemia, though in that case, temporary LTOT would be more appropriate.

Further reading

Clinical component for the home oxygen service in England and Wales, accessed www.brit-thoracic.org.uk

Domiciliary Oxygen Therapy Services. Clinical Guidelines and Advice for Prescribers. A report of the Royal College of Physicians. 1999

Medical Research Council Working Party. Long term domiciliary oxygen therapy in chronic hypoxic cor pulmonale complicating chronic bronchitis and emphysema. *Lancet* 1981; **1**: 681–686.

Nocturnal Oxygen Therapy Trial Group. Continuous or nocturnal oxygen therapy in hypoxaemic chronic obstructive lung disease. *Ann Intern Med* 1980; **93**: 391–398.

Diffuse parenchymal lung disease

Chapter contents

7.1 Usual interstitial pneumonia

Epidemiology

Limited data is available and most of the studies pre-date the new ATS/ERS re-classification of IIPs (idiopathic interstitial pneumonias). Data from computerised UK general practice records suggest that the 12-month period prevalence of the previously used unclassified term, cryprogenic fibrosing alveolitis, (CFA) is 15 to 18 per 100,000 person years. Median survival of newly diagnosed patients with CFA is 3 years, a figure which is similar to that currently reported for patients with UIP. The median age of presentation of CFA is 70 years, with the disease uncommon below the age of 50 years. It is more common in men with a male:female ratio of 1.5–2.0:1. There is an increased risk of developing lung cancer in these patients.

Clinical approach

Key points

- Natural history of the condition to date? Typically gradual onset of breathlessness.
- Presence of any respiratory risk factors/aetiological agents?
- Severity of symptoms?

Examination: key points

- Finger clubbing is suggestive of UIP (49–66% of patients) particularly in men.
- Fine, basal 'velcro-like' inspiratory crackles are characteristic of UIP (>90% cases).
- Additional added sounds (squeaks or wheeze) are suggestive of alternate or co-existing diagnoses.
- Cyanosis reflects relatively severe hypoxaemia. Pulse oximetry can readily detect less severe hypoxaemia.
- Physical signs of pulmonary hypertension and right ventricular failure which may reflect hypoxia from severe pulmonary fibrosis for example in UIP.

Investigation

Lung function

- A restrictive defect with reduced gas transfer is characteristic of UIP.
- Severe lung function impairment is associated with poor outcome.
- A gas transfer of less than 35–40% predicted has 80% sensitivity and specificity for predicting death within 2 years and serves as the main basis for a proposed distinction between 'advanced' and 'limited' disease in IPF.
- A 10% reduction in FVC, or 15% change in DLCO is needed to identify a true change in disease severity (as opposed to measurement variation).
- Serial FVC is likely to be more sensitive to change than serial DLCO, particularly important in advanced disease where identifying 15% change may be impractical.
- Oxygen saturations are often reduced particularly on exercise.
- The 6MWT is reproducible in UIP patients and desaturation to 88% during or at the end of the test may be a more powerful predictor of mortality than resting lung function tests.

Chest radiography

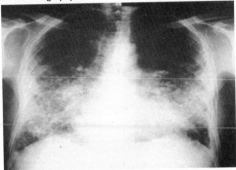

Fig. 7.1.1 CXR showing bilateral diffuse alveolar shawoing obscuring heart border.

Peripheral and basal reticular shadowing are characteristic but can be normal in biopsy proven cases.

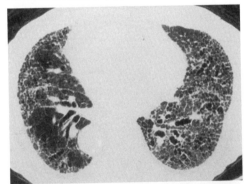

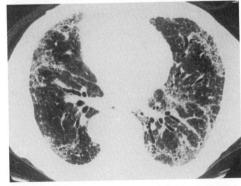

Fig. 7.1.2 CT scans showing reticular shadowing particularly in the subpleural regions with secondary bronchial dilatation and some honeycombing.

HRCT
HRCT features from ATS/ERS guidelines:
- HRCT is a very sensitive, but not 100%, technique for the diagnosis of UIP with a low false-positive rate.
- Typical HRCT appearances of UIP by expert radiologists are correct in the majority (>90%) of cases.
- HRCT may be useful in providing an explanation in patients in whom there is a sudden and unexpected deterioration in clinical status.
- It provides useful information on the distribution of disease that may be used to guide subsequent BAL, transbronchial biopsy or surgical lung biopsy if being considered.

> **AUTHOR'S TIPS**
> - Beware of false positive interpretation of CXR in obese patients.
> - Increasing use of HRCT has led to situations in which limited features are seen in patients in whom the clinical significance is uncertain but probably limited.

BAL and TBB
- BAL and TBB have only a limited role in the diagnosis of UIP. If the clinical and HRCT findings are characteristic of UIP it adds little.
- The decision to perform BAL, TBB or both is also informed by the likely differential diagnosis and patient fitness, but also on availability of local expertise in differential BAL cell count.
- The optimal BAL technique has been addressed in several guidelines.
- Traditionally, BAL has been performed in one lobe, either the right middle lobe or one of the basal segments of the right lower lobe. Whilst single, site BAL has been considered to be representative of the lung as a whole, based largely on studies comparing the same lobe in either lung, there is some evidence that this is not the case. BAL may be more useful if targeted to a segment most affected, as identified by HRCT.
- Similarly the optimum site for TBLB should be informed by the HRCT appearance.
- Where the HRCT appearance suggests fibrosis with a UIP-like pattern, then the BAL cell count does not differentiate between fibrotic NSIP and UIP either diagnostically or prognostically.
- BAL neutrophils, which are strongly linked to the extent of disease on HRCT and the severity of functional impairment, mainly reflect disease severity.
- It may be useful in patients with a sudden deterioration or exacerbation to exclude infection or malignancy.
- There is insufficient evidence to support the routine use of BAL cell counts to determine need for treatment in UIP.
- Transbronchial biopsies do not allow a specific diagnosis of UIP.

Open lung biopsy
Surgical biopsy confirmation, when clinical and HRCT features are typical of UIP, cannot easily be justified.

Management and treatment
Overview
In the majority, UIP will progress over a period of months and years towards a terminal phase. At the time of diagnosis patients often show relief that they are not suffering from lung cancer. In patients with UIP, a general management approach comparable to that of patients with inoperable lung cancer is appropriate. This includes providing patient information and support, palliative treatment of symptoms and complications of the disease and best supportive care; both for young patients with IPF awaiting lung transplant, patients in clinical trials of novel therapy and patients with advanced disease facing-end-of life issues. Further, drawing on the analogy with lung cancer, this general management approach may be best delivered in a multidisciplinary setting with appropriate input from palliative care medical and nursing specialists.

> **AUTHOR'S TIPS**
> *Communicating the diagnosis*
> - The long-term prognosis is little different than that of many malignancies leading to patients with advanced IPF receiving sub-optimal care.
> - Patients should be offered tailored but clear and accurate information regarding the diagnosis, very limited treatment options and prognosis.

Smoking cessation
There is a 10-fold increased risk of developing lung cancer whether they smoke or not, increasing to 200 in a 20/day smoker. There are reports in the literature that patients with IPF who smoke have a better prognosis than those who do not smoke. This is almost certainly due to the co-existence of COPD leading to an earlier presentation of IPF and these reports should not discourage the use of smoking cessation services.

Treatment of symptoms and complications of UIP
Breathlessness
- Breathlessness in UIP is exacerbated by exercise and cough. When accompanied by hypoxaemia, domiciliary and/or ambulatory oxygen should be prescribed to relieve this symptom. It is reasonable to titrate oxygen therapy according to resting oxygen saturations, but augmented flow may be required immediately following exercise. Patients may therefore need both an oxygen concentrator and a cylinder. However, there is no evidence that administration of oxygen influences long-term survival or improves quality of life.
- Oral opiates may be effective in relieving distress from breathlessness. Liaison with palliative care services, if available, may lead to a more holistic approach to symptom relief.
- Pulmonary rehabilitation programmes have not been evaluated in IPF but are likely to contribute to overall well-being.

Cough
- Cough is a frequent and troublesome symptom. In current or ex-smokers productive cough may arise from co-existent chronic bronchitis. Gastro-oesophageal reflux disease (GORD) may be associated with cough. Whilst the role of GORD in the pathogenesis and progression of IPF remains uncertain, symptomatic patients should be treated with a proton pump inhibitor.
- Conventional anti-tussive agents, such as oral codeine, are widely used, but there is no evidence of efficacy. Oral opiates may be used for intractable cough particularly in end-stage disease.

Pneumothorax

Spontaneous pneumothorax or pneumo-mediastinum is a recognised complication of IPF and should be suspected when a patient complains of a sudden increase in breathlessness. Pleurodesis is not a contra-indication to future lung transplantation. Pneumothorax can be a late complication of IPF and cause severe breathlessness. In such cases the lung may fail to re-expand after insertion of an intercostal drain because of altered lung compliance and palliative care may be more appropriate.

Lung cancer

IPF predisposes to non-small cell and small cell lung cancer. Diagnosis and staging should be undertaken as for any other patient, although poor lung function from co-existing pulmonary fibrosis makes the possibility of curative treatment less likely.

Potential disease modifying

UIP as the most common form of IIP has/is being studied in more recent trials with recruitment of a virtually homogenous population of patients, albeit at varying stages in the natural history of the disease. Three of these have reported, interferon-gamma 1β, pirfenidone and N-acetylcysteine, the latter as an adjunct to prednisolone and azathioprine, others will follow including endothelin-1 antagonists and TNF-α blockade.

Steroid monotherapy

More recent studies do not support the use of corticosteroids in IPF. A meta-analysis concluded that there was no evidence that steroids prolonged survival or improved quality of life in this condition. High-dose steroids should not be given (0.5–1mg/kg).

Steroids and azathioprine

There is not substantial evidence for treatment benefit but some clinicians still use this regimen (see BTS guidelines).

Cyclophosphamide

There is no evidence that oral or pulsed cyclophosphamide is of any long-term benefit in terms of survival or quality of life for patients with IPF and it has a significant side effect profile.

Pirfenidone

Pirfenidone is a pyridone which inhibits fibroblast proliferation and collagen synthesis in vitro and ameliorates bleomycin-induced pulmonary fibrosis in animals. A placebo (2:1) controlled, double-blind phase 2 study of pirfenidone therapy in 107 Japanese patients with moderate IPF has recently been reported. Planned for 1 year, the study was prematurely stopped at 9 months due to significantly greater acute exacerbations in the placebo group. Patients receiving pirfenidone also had significantly smaller decline in VC and a small but significant improvement in degree of desaturation following a 6MWT at 9 months. Further randomised trials of Pirfenidone in IPF are ongoing.

Interferon-gamma 1β

Interferon gamma is a Th1 cytokine which down-regulates collagen gene expression and suppress products/effects of pro-fibrotic growth factors. This led to the hypothesis that it might prevent progression of pulmonary fibrosis initially.

A prospective double-blind placebo controlled trial of interferon-gamma-1β in 330 patients reported no significant affect on lung function at any time point. There were more deaths in the placebo group (17%) than those treated with interferon-gamma 1β (10%), but this trend did not reach statistical significance (p=0.08). The hypothesis that interferon-gamma-1β may confer a survival benefit, particularly in patients with milder disease, remains unproven and the results of ongoing randomised controlled studies are awaited.

N-acetylcysteine (NAC)

A number of in vitro and animal model experiments led to the suggestion that a redox imbalance may contribute to the development of IPF. The subsequent clinical observation that lung epithelial lining fluid from IPF subjects was deplete of reduced glutathione laid the foundation for clinical trials of NAC.

A 12 month double-blind study to assess the affects of NAC (600 mg tds) in patients with a confident UIP diagnosis analysed 155 receiving prednisolone (tapering from 0.5 mg/kg a day) and azathioprine (2 mg/kg a day). 80 patients received NAC and 75 patients placebo. VC was 9% and DLCO 24% higher in the NAC group but no significant differences in mortality were found. However, patients in whom the standard regimen with prednisolone and azathioprine was contraindicated or 'not justified' were excluded from the study and 40% of participants were recruited within 6 months of diagnosis.

Key recommendations

- Steroid monotherapy should not be given.
- If treatment with azathioprine/prednisolone therapy is given, patients should also receive N-acetylcysteine (600mg tds).
- Treatment should be given within multi-centre trials where possible.

Lung transplantation

- A multi-variable analysis from a single centre study of 46 patients with IPF accepted for transplantation (28 successfully transplanted, 16 died awaiting transplantation) suggested that lung transplantation reduced the risk of death by 75%.
- Transplant should be considered in those patients below who fulfil established selection criteria for transplant, thus generally excluding those over the age 65 and/or those with significant co-morbidity.
- Definite UIP (clinico-radiologically or a pathological diagnosis) should be discussed with a transplant centre.
- Advanced UIP (DLCO<39% predicted), or progressive disease (10% or greater decline in FVC during 6 months of follow up) should be referred to a transplant centre for assessment.

AUTHOR'S TIP
Don't miss the transplant window.

Further reading

American Thoracic Society/European Respiratory Society International Multidisciplinary Consensus Classification of the Idiopathic Interstitial Pneumonias. Am J Respir Crit Care Med 2002; **165**: 277–304.

Azuma A, Nukiwa T, Tsuboi E, et al. Double blind, placebo-controlled trial of pirfenidone in patients with idiopathic pulmonary fibrosis. Am J Respir Crit Care Med 2005; **171**: 1040–1047.

Bradley B, Branley HM, Egan J J, *et al.* Interstitial lung disease guideline: the British Thoracic Society in collaboration with the Thoracic Society of Australia and New Zealand and the Irish Thoracic Society. *Thorax* 2008; **63**: (Suppl 5) VI–58.

BTS Interstitial lung disease guidelines. *Thorax* 2008; **63**: v1–v58.

Crockett AJ, Cranston JM, Antic N. Domiciliary oxygen for interstitial lung disease. *The Cochrane Database of Systematic Reviews* 2001, Issue 3. Art. No.: CD002883. DOI: 10.1002/14651858. CD002883.

Flaherty KR, King TE Jr, Raghu G, *et al.* Idiopathic interstitial pneumonia: what is the effect of a multidisciplinary approach to diagnosis? *Am J Respir Crit Care Med* 2004; **170**: 904–910.

International guidelines for the selection of lung transplant candidates. The American Society for Transplant Physicians (ASTP)/American Thoracic Society (ATS)/European Respiratory Society(ERS)/International Society for Heart and Lung Transplantation(ISHLT). *Am J Respir Crit Care Med* 1998; **158**(1): 335–339.

Katzenstein AA, Myers JL. Idiopathic pulmonary fibrosis, clinical relevance of pathologic classification. *Am J Respir Crit Care Med* 1998; **157**: 1301–1315.

Raghu G, Brown KK, Bradford WZ, *et al.* A placebo-controlled trial of interferon gamma-1β in patients with idiopathic pulmonary fibrosis. *N Engl J Med* 2004; **350**: 125–133.

Wells AU, Desai SR, Rubens MB, *et al.* Idiopathic pulmonary fibrosis: a composite physiologic index derived from disease extent observed by computed tomography. *A J Respir Crit Care Med* 2003; **176**: 962–969.

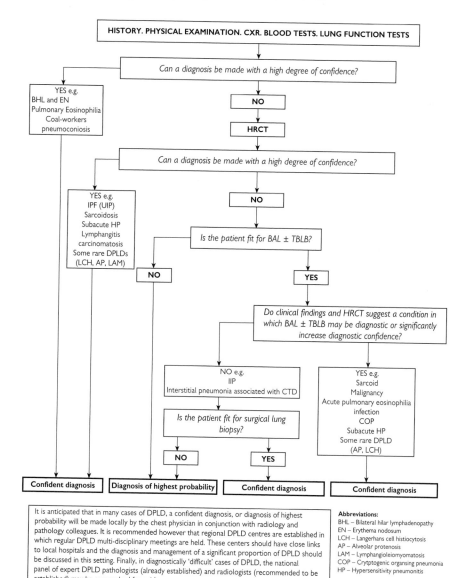

Fig. 7.1.3 Generic algorithm for DPL.

7.2 Non-specific interstitial pneumonia

Introduction

NSIP is a specific histological entity within the classification of IIPs. NSIP was first highlighted by Katzenstein and Fiorelli in a histological review of 110 biopsies taken from patients with interstitial lung disease. It was recognised that a minority of these biopsies did not reflect the pattern of UIP. The term 'non-specific interstitial pneumonia' was applied, acknowledging that these biopsies may represent 'sampling errors' from patients with alternative diagnosis such as extrinsic allergic alveolitis.

Key points

Whether NSIP represents 'early' UIP remains uncertain.

- The survival of patients with advanced fibrotic NSIP defined as a DLCO > 35% mirrors that of UIP.
- UIP could represent a final common pathway of NSIP.
- In contrast, NSIP is frequently associated with connective tissue diseases.

In a retrospective study of 476 patients with systemic sclerosis:

- 80 patients with clinically and radiologically evidence of fibrosing alveolitis associated with systemic sclerosis underwent surgical biopsy.
- 77.5% had the histological pattern of NSIP.

In a retrospective analysis by Kinder et al.:

- 88% of patients with biopsy proven idiopathic NSIP meet the criteria for undifferentiated connective tissue disease.
- NSIP may represent a specific pulmonary manifestation of undifferentiated connective tissue disease.

Epidemiology

- The precise incidence and prevalence of NSIP are unknown.
- The prevalence of NSIP could range from 1–3/100,000 of the general population.
- In a highly selected case series of 193 suspected cases of NSIP only 67 (37%) were confirmed as having NSIP after multidisciplinary review.

Clinical characteristics and lung function

Many of the clinical features of NSIP are comparable to IPF. Cough and shortness of breath with impaired exercise tolerance are the major symptoms and usually evolve over several months or years. Clubbing can also be present but is less frequent when compared to IPF patients. Crackles on auscultation are often detected. The average age at diagnosis is 52 years, which compares to 63 years for IPF patients. 67% are women and 69% have never smoked.

Pulmonary function studies show a restrictive pattern in 69% of patients with impaired gas exchange. A DLCO of less than 35% predicted is associated with early mortality defined as death within 2 years. A change in FVC (10% and more) is associated with disease progression.

Radiographic findings

The chest radiograph often only shows a subtle increase in opacity, typically at the lung bases. In 10% of the patients the chest radiograph is normal.

On HRCT examination the predominant findings are bilateral ground glass opacities associated with a moderate reticular pattern and traction bronchiectasis (Fig. 7.2.1). Patchy consolidation can also be present. Honeycombing is rarely seen and when present is thought to represent the 'fibrosing' pattern (see Pathologic findings) of NSIP.

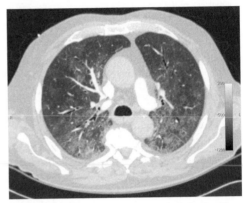

Fig. 7.2.1 HRCT of the lungs shows at the level of carina diffuse ground glass opacities and septal lines are not a major finding.

> **AUTHOR'S TIP**
> A diagnostic algorithm for interpreting HRCT including the anatomical distribution, the presence of honeycombing or reticular lines and extent of ground glass opacities can be used to discriminate between NSIP and UIP.

In this algorithm the presence/absence of honeycombing is initially evaluated. Honeycombing with a basilar distribution indicates 'Definitive UIP' while honeycombing with no basilar distribution suggests 'Probable UIP'. If honeycombing is not present the detection of septal lines is then evaluated. If septal lines are not a major feature this would lead to the diagnosis of 'Definitive NSIP'. If septal lines are a major feature, then the distribution of ground glass opacities is evaluated. A basilar distribution of ground glass opacities with septal lines and no honeycombing is categorised as 'Intermediate' probability of UIP or NSIP. The presence of diffuse or central distribution of ground glass opacities indicates 'Possible NSIP'. However the interpretation of HRCT in cases of NSIP can still be difficult. In a study by Aziz et al. the accuracy of interpreting HRCT in diffuse parenchymal lung disease was found to be variable. The inter-observer accuracy for the diagnosis NSIP between different 11 thoracic radiologists was only modest ($\kappa = 0.48$).

Pathologic findings

In a patient with a suspected interstitial pneumonia, to determine the specific pattern of pulmonary fibrosis a sizeable lung biopsy is required .Therefore transbronchial biopsies are not helpful. Minimal invasive VATS is the optimal method for diagnosis by providing adequate histological material and should be obtained from at least two sites from different lobes.

NSIP can be subdivided into either fibrosing or a cellular pattern. Fibrosing NSIP occurs in 84% of the cases and the cellular pattern occurs in 16%. The hallmark of the NSIP is the temporal homogeneity and the absence of fibroblast foci, granulomas and eosinophilic granulocytes. (Figs. 7.2.2 and 7.2.3). However, it can be difficult to distinguish the fibrosing NSIP from UIP.

Fig. 7.2.2 Low magnification of a biopsy with temporal uniformity, the absence of honeycombing and airspace remodelling (hematoxilin and eosin staining, magnification: x 2.)

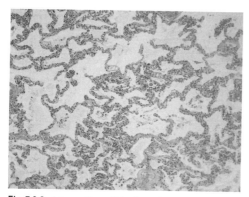

Fig. 7.2.3 Advanced interstitial collagen deposition with low cellularity, which resemble fibrotic NSIP. (Masson–Trichome staining, magnification: x10.)

Fibrosing NSIP shows dense or loose interstitial fibrosis with chronic inflammation. However, histopathologic variability between different biopsied lobes may be observed. For example Flaherty et al. have evaluated three histological permutations of NSIP and UIP. Firstly, 'concordant UIP' was defined when UIP pattern was exclusively observed in different lobes. Secondly, 'discordant UIP' was defined when both UIP and NSIP patterns were found in different lobes. Thirdly, 'concordant NSIP' was defined when only histological changes of NSIP were detected. These groupings appear to influence the clinical outcome. A survival analysis showed a significantly better survival for those patients with concordant NSIP compared to patients with mixed UIP and NSIP patterns or concordant UIP findings. The risk of mortality was 16.8 times greater in patients with discordant UIP and 24.4 times greater in patients with

concordant UIP compared to the patients with concordant NSIP. These findings underline the importance to obtain biopsies of at least two sites from different lobes.

Cellular NSIP is characterised by a mild to moderate uniform chronic inflammation with lymphocytes and type II pneumocyte hyperplasia in the setting of preserved lung architecture. The differential diagnosis for cellular NSIP includes hypersensitivity pneumonitis. Cellular NSIP may also represent the cellular form of the term 'cryptogenic fibrosing alveolitis'(CFA). When first described by Scadding, CFA contained a subgroup of patients who were younger, female and had a cellular pattern on biopsy. These patients were also thought to be steroid responders. In hindsight 'cellular NSIP' probably matches 'cellular CFA'.

Survival

The natural history of the NSIP is uncertain because of the absence of prospective studies, however, the survival of NSIP patients is generally thought to be superior to those patients with IPF. Combining the diagnostic techniques of HRCT and histology can be helpful for estimating survival in NSIP. Flaherty et al. identified a superior survival in patients with both radiologic evidence and histologic evidence of NSIP (median survival >9 years) compared to patients with NSIP on HRCT but UIP pattern in the biopsy (median survival 5.76 years).

Management and treatment

Patients with NSIP may benefit from immunosuppressive treatment. However, appropriate clinical trials have not been performed to date. Based on the close association between NSIP and connective tissue diseases, the standard of care would include corticosteroids and immunosuppressants. A recent double-blind, randomised, placebo-controlled trial of oral cyclophosphamide was performed in 158 patients with scleroderma-related lung disease. In this study pulmonary disease in patients with limited or diffuse systemic scleroderma was defined as the presence of active alveolitis in bronchoalveolar lavage (neutrophilia >3 %, eosinophilia >2% or both) or ground glass opacities on HRCT or a decreased FVC (45–85% predicted) and increased Mahler dyspnoea index. Patients with history of smoking within preceding 6 months or clinically significant pulmonary arterial hypertension requiring drug therapy were excluded. The patients in the cyclophosphamide group had a significant but modest beneficial effect on lung function compared to the patients in the placebo group. A mean absolute difference in adjusted 12-month FVC predicted of 2.53% was observed (95% confidence interval, 0.28 to 4.79% (P <0.03)). Six patients died in each group and none death was related to the cyclophosphamide. There was also an improvement in the dyspnoea index and quality of life was achieved in the cyclophosphamide group for a period up to 2 years. Among the patients in the cyclophosphamide group adverse events as hematuria, leukopenia, neutropenia, anemia and pneumonia were more common.

A retrospective study by Kondo et al. was performed in 12 patients with fibrosing NSIP and 27 IPF patients. The treatment of these patients included steroids in combination with cyclophosphamide. After 1 year, 8 NSIP patients had an improvement in their vital capacity (VC predicted 56.7% versus 77.2%, p <0.001) and the other 4 remained stable. The improvement was sustained in 5 patients with long term follow up (mean 91.8 months, range 60–148). One patient died and 2 patients experienced disease progression.

However, the toxicity associated with the cyclophosphamide therapy was significant: 21% of the patients had serious adverse effects including haemorrhagic cystitis, leucopenia, myelodysplastic syndrome and one patient died because of an opportunistic infection.

Therefore less toxic immunosuppressive combinations including steroids with azathioprine or steroids with mycophenolate mofetil may be an attractive option for the treatment of NSIP. However, little data exist supporting these strategies. Novel therapies, which address cellular targets of inflammatory responses or fibrogenic cytokines may be promising agents for the future. For example, the application of TNF-α antibody therapy may be a reasonable approach in NSIP based on the association with connective tissue disorders. However, there is no specific data to support this approach. Ultimately in patients with advanced and progressive disease the surgical treatment of lung transplantation should be considered.

Futher reading

American Thoracic Society/European Respiratory Society International Multidisciplinary Consensus Classification of the Idiopathic Interstitial Pneumonias. *Am J Respir Crit Care Med* 2002; **165**: 277–304.

Aziz ZA, Wells AU Hansell DM, *et al*. HRCT diagnosis of diffuse parenchymal lung disease: inter-observer variation. *Thorax* 2004; **59**: 506–511.

Bouros D, Wells AU, Nicholson AG, *et al*. Histologic subsets of fibrosing alveolitis in patients with systemic sclerosis and their relationship to outcome. *Am J Respir Crit Care Med* 2002; **165**: 1581–1586.

Chang AC, Yee J, Orringer MB, *et al*. Diagnostic thoracoscopic lung biopsy: an outpatient experience. *Ann Thorac Surg* 2002; **74**: 1942–1946.

Costabel U, Du Bois RM, Egan JJ. Diffuse parenchymal lung disease. *Progress in Respiratory Research* 2007; **36**: 160–174, Karger Switzerland.

Egan JJ, Martinez FJ, Wells AU, *et al*. Lung function estimates in idiopathic pulmonary fibrosis: the potential for a simple classification. *Thorax* 2005; **60**: 270–273.

Flaherty KR, Thwaite EL, Kazerooni EA, *et al*. Radiological versus histological diagnosis in UIP and NSIP: survival implications. *Thorax* 2003; **58**: 143–148.

Flaherty KR, Travis WD, Colby GB, *et al*. Histopathologic variability in usual and non-specific interstitial pneumonias. *Am J Respir Crit Care Med* 2001; **164**: 1722–1727.

Hartman T, Swensen D, Hansell D, *et al*. Non-specific interstitial pneumonia: variable appearances at high-resolution chest CT. *Radiology* 2000; **217**: 701–705.

Jegal Y, Kim DS, Shim TS, *et al*. Physiology is a stronger predictor of survival than pathology in fibrotic interstitial pneumonia. *Am J Respir Crit Care Med* 2005; **171**: 639–644.

Katzenstein AL, Fiorelli RF. Nonspecific interstitial pneumonia/fibrosis. Histologic features and clinical significance. *Am J Surg Pathol* 1994; **18**: 136–47.

Kinder BW, Collard HR, King TE, *et al*. Idiopathic non-specific interstitial pneumonia: lung manifestation of undifferentiated connective tissue disease? *Am J Respir Crit Care Med* 2007; **176**: 691–697.

Kondo Y, Taniguchi H, Yokoi T, *et al*. Cyclophosphamide and low dose prednisolone in idiopathic pulmonary fibrosis and fibrosing non-specific interstitial pneumonia. *Eur Respir J* 2005; **25**: 528–533.

Latsi PI, du Bois RM, Nicholson AG, *et al*. Fibrotic idiopathic interstitial pneumonia: The prognostic value of longitudinal functional trends. *Am J Respir Crit care Med* 2003; **168**: 538–542.

MacDonald S, Rubens M, Hansell D, *et al*. Non-specific interstitial pneumonia and usual interstitial pneumonia: comparative appearances at and diagnostic accuracy of thin section CT. *Radiology* 2001; **221**: 600–605.

Tashkin DP, Elashoff R, Clements PJ, *et al*. Cyclophosphamide versus placebo in scleroderma lung disease. *N Engl J Med* 2006; **354**: 2655–2666.

Travis WD, Colby TV, Koss MN, *et al*. Non-Neoplastic Disorders of the Lower Respiratory Tract, Atlas of Nontumour Pathology. 2002 American Registry of Pathology and the Armed Forced Institute of Pathology Washington DC.

Travis WD, Hunninghake G, King TE, *et al*. Idiopathic non-specific interstitial pneumonia report of an ATS Project. *Am J Respir Crit Care Med* 2008 Apr 3; [Epub ahead of print]

7.3 Respiratory bronchiolitis-associated interstitial lung disease

Introduction

Respiratory bronchiolitis-associated interstitial lung disease (RBILD) is a smoking-induced diffuse interstitial lung process. RBILD is best conceptualised as an exaggerated form of respiratory bronchiolitis, a very common incidental finding in cigarette smokers, consisting of an accumulation of pigmented macrophages within respiratory bronchioles and adjacent alveoli. It is now generally accepted that the spectra of histologic abnormalities in respiratory bronchiolitis and RBILD are identical. However, whereas respiratory bronchiolitis is usually asymptomatic, RBILD, by definition, manifests as a clinically significant diffuse lung disease, resulting in cough, shortness of breath and pulmonary function impairment.

Relationship to smoking

Respiratory bronchiolitis and RBILD are both almost invariably associated with smoking. In the large biopsy series of Fraig, typical respiratory bronchiolitis was seen in all the current smokers and in half of the former smokers but was never present in non-smokers. Based on this and other smaller series, it can be argued that respiratory bronchiolitis represents a highly specific physiologic response to smoking, with no convincing reports of typical respiratory bronchiolitis in non-smokers. RBILD is also strongly linked to smoking with all patients being current smokers in dour clinical series containing a total of 65 patients, apart from a single non-smoker heavily exposed to solder fumes.

Histological features

- The cardinal histological feature of both respiratory bronchiolitis and RBILD is the accumulation of alveolar macrophages in respiratory bronchioles, with variable extension into the neighbouring alveoli. Macrophages are characterised by brown, finely granular pigmentation (representing constituents of cigarette smoke).
- A chronic inflammatory cell infiltrate is often present in bronchiolar and surrounding alveolar walls. Peribronchial alveolar septal thickening by collagen deposition, radiating from the involved bronchiole, is more variable.
- The pulmonary parenchyma distant from involved respiratory bronchioles is normal except when there is smoking-related emphysema.
- These features do not vary substantially with the global severity of the process and, thus, distinctions between respiratory bronchiolitis and RBILD should not be made histologically, but are wholly based upon symptoms, pulmonary function impairment and HRCT abnormalities.
- A surgical biopsy may be useful when other disease processes require exclusion, but should not be used, in isolation, to diagnose RBILD.

Imaging features

- Chest radiographic abnormalities are absent or limited in respiratory bronchiolitis but tend to be more obvious in RBILD, with bronchial wall thickening, patchy ground-glass attenuation and reticulo-nodular opacities in most cases.
- RBILD can not be diagnosed with confidence on chest radiography. Frequent HRCT abnormalities in healthy smokers, representing respiratory bronchiolitis, include profuse, ill-defined parenchymal micronodules, areas of ground-glass attenuation and dependent areas of decreased attenuation, with occasional background emphysema.
- The spectrum of HRCT appearances in RBILD is exactly that of respiratory bronchiolitis.
- Based on the largest HRCT series of patients with a clinico-pathologic diagnosis of RBILD, the most frequent HRCT features are central or peripheral bronchial wall thickening, centrilobular nodules and areas of ground-glass opacity.
- Emphysema is also common.
- Areas of hypoattenuation ('mosaic attenuation') are seen in a minority of RBILD cases on inspiratory CT, but are frequent on expiratory CT in both respiratory bronchiolitis and RBILD.
- In essence, the limited HRCT abnormalities due to respiratory bronchiolitis in smokers are similar but more extensive in RBILD.

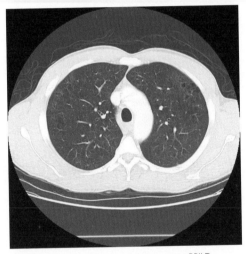

Fig. 7.3.1 CT scan of patient with biopsy-proven RBILD showing typical features with profuse, ill-defined parenchymal micronodules, areas of ground-glass attenuation and dependent areas of decreased attenuation (Courtesy of Dr Fergus Gleeson).

Pulmonary function tests

Despite the fact that RBILD is bronchiolocentric, restrictive and obstructive pulmonary function abnormalities have both been documented. A mixed, predominantly restrictive ventilatory defect is usual and the carbon monoxide diffusing capacity (DLCO) is generally mildly to moderately reduced. The severity of pulmonary function impairment is crucial in distinguishing RBILD from respiratory bronchiolitis.

Coexistent centrilobular emphysema is a frequent confounder in the interpretation of pulmonary function tests in RBILD, probably explaining the fact that DLCO levels were disproportionately reduced in over half the patients with RBILD in the two largest clinical series. However, emphysema may also accompany limited respiratory bronchiolitis. Thus, the distinction between respiratory bronchiolitis and RBILD on severity grounds requires the integration of clinical, pulmonary function and HRCT data. RBILD can be diagnosed when the combined severity of pulmonary function impairment, HRCT findings and symptoms is indicative of a clinically significant interstitial lung disease.

Clinical presentation, natural history and treated course

RBILD usually presents between the third and sixth decades with insidious exertional dyspnoea and persistent cough. However, RBILD may be diagnosed in asymptomatic patients based upon the severity of functional impairment and chest radiographic or HRCT abnormalities. Bilateral end-inspiratory crackles, which may be predominantly basal, are common, but clubbing is rare. In RBILD and respiratory bronchiolitis alike, a characteristic brown pigmentation of macrophages has been consistently observed at BAL, and in RBILD there are increases in macrophage numbers, and lower percentages of other percentages components. A BAL neutrophilia or eosinophilia is rare in RBILD.

AUTHOR'S TIP

RBILD is a relatively benign disorder, compared to IPF or fibrotic NSIP. In most cases, there is functional improvement or stability, provided that smoking cessation is achieved. However, the paucity of longitudinal data, including treatment data, in RBILD should be stressed. Accumulated anecdotal experience indicates that a significant functional improvement following smoking cessation or treatment in RBILD is confined to a minority of patients.

It is not yet clear how often residual functional impairment after cessation of smoking represents residual RBILD as opposed to other smoking-related processes such as emphysema. Although inflammation in RBILD may abate with time, a fibrotic component may result in significant residual functional impairment.

Diagnosis and management

The formulation of a diagnosis of RBILD requires: (a) that the disease presents as a clinically significant diffuse lung disease (as opposed to asymptomatic or mildly symptomatic respiratory bronchiolitis); and (b) that other diffuse lung diseases with similar presentations are excluded. Symptoms, clinical signs and the pattern and level of functional impairment are highly non-specific (except in distinguishing between RBILD and respiratory bronchiolitis) and, thus, HRCT findings most often provide discriminatory information.

HRCT findings typical of RBILD exclude most other diffuse lung diseases, including the predominantly fibrotic idiopathic interstitial pneumonias (IPF, fibrotic NSIP). The distinction between RBILD and sub-acute hypersensitivity pneumonitis on HRCT is sometimes difficult, as widespread poorly formed nodular abnormalities and areas of hypoattenuation may co-exist in both diseases. However, the smoking history (RBILD occurs exclusively in smokers, hypersensitivity pneumonitis is rare in smokers) and BAL profile (lymphcytosis in hypersensitivity pneumonitis, excess of pigmented macrophages in RBILD) are usually diagnostic in this context.

The management of RBILD is largely driven by the severity of pulmonary function impairment. Smoking cessation is essential. In mild disease, observation without treatment is appropriate. In more severe disease, a trial of corticosteroid, with or without immunosuppressive drugs, is usual, especially if there is no regression after smoking cessation. However, the risk–benefit ratio of prolonged treatment (with attendant side effects) is a key consideration. Early withdrawal of treatment in non-responders is usually appropriate.

Further reading

Fraig M, Shreesha U, Savici D, et al. Respiratory bronchiolitis: a clinicopathologic study in current smokers, ex-smokers, and never-smokers. *Am J Surg Pathol* 2002; **26**: 647–653.

Moon J, du Bois RM, Colby TV, et al. Clinical significance of respiratory bronchiolitis on open lung biopsy and its relationship to smoking related interstitial lung disease. *Thorax* 1999; **54**: 1009–1014.

Myers JL, Veal CF (Jr), Shin MS, et al. Respiratory bronchiolitis causing interstitial lung disease: a clinicopathological study of six cases. *Am Rev Respir Dis* 1987; **135**: 880–884.

Nicholson AG, Colby TV, du Bois RM, et al. The prognostic significance of the histologic pattern of interstitial pneumonia in patients presenting with the clinical entity of cryptogenic fibrosing alveolitis. *Am J Respir Crit Care Med* 2000; **162**: 2213–2217.

Park JS, Brown KK, Tuder RM, et al. Respiratory bronchiolitis-associated interstitial lung disease: radiologic features with clinical and pathologic correlation. *J Comput Assist Tomogr* 2002; **26**: 13–20.

Portnoy J, Veraldi KL, Schwarz MI, et al. Respiratory bronchiolitis-interstitial lung disease: long-term outcome. *Chest* 2007; **131**: 664–671.

Remy-Jardin M, Remy J, Boulenguez C, et al. Morphologic effects of cigarette smoking on airways and pulmonary parenchyma in healthy adult volunteers: CT evaluation and correlation with pulmonary function tests. *Radiology* 1993; **186**: 107–115.

Veeraraghavan S, Latsi PI, Wells AU, et al. Bronchoalveolar lavage findings in idiopathic UIP and NSIP. *Eur Respir J* 2003; **22**: 239–244.

Wells AU, Nicholson AG, Hansell DM. Challenges in pulmonary fibrosis. 4: smoking-induced diffuse interstitial lung diseases. *Thorax* 2007; **62**: 904–910.

Yousem SA, Colby TV, Gaensler EA. Respiratory bronchiolitis-associated interstitial lung disease and its relationship to desquamative interstitial pneumonia. *Mayo Clin Proc* 1989; **64**: 1373–1380.

7.4 Desquamative interstitial pneumonia

The term desquamative interstitial pneumonia (DIP) was originally coined to reflect the belief that the intra-alveolar accumulation of cells, characteristic of the disease, represented desquamated epithelium. It has since become apparent that these cells represent intra-alveolar macrophages laden with brown tobacco-smoke related pigment. Indeed smoking is strongly associated with DIP, as it is with RBILD and it may be that both conditions form part of a spectrum of smoking-related ILDs.

> **AUTHOR'S TIP**
> DIP is probably part of a spectrum of smoking-related ILDs which includes RBILD and Langerhans cell histiocytosis.

Epidemiology

- DIP is a rare disease.
- The condition occurs almost invariably in current or recent ex-smokers. There is considerable circumstantial evidence indicating that cigarette smoke is a causative factor. Only occasionally is the condition seen in those that have never smoked; drugs, connective tissue disease or other inhaled irritants have been implicated, and there are reports of 'idiopathic' DIP.
- DIP is diagnosed most commonly in patients aged 40–60 years.

Clinical and radiological features

- Patients typically present with breathlessness and unless there is co-existing chronic bronchitis, a non-productive cough. Most will have inspiratory crepitations and in one study a quarter of 26 reported cases were clubbed.
- The plain CXR appearances are non-specific. The most common pattern is bilateral often diffuse, occasionally patchy ground-glass opacities and/or reticulo-nodular opacities and in some cases the CXR is virtually normal.
- Normal, restrictive and mild obstructive patterns of lung function have all been described in DIP
- HRCT scan invariably reveals ground-glass changes that are usually basal and peripheral and sometimes extensive (Fig. 7.4.1). The presence of centrilobular ground-glass nodules may reflect associated smoking-related RBILD.

Co-existing emphysema may also be present (Fig. 7.4.2). Importantly, peripheral honeycomb cysts are rare, distinguishing DIP from a characteristic usual interstitial pneumonia (UIP) pattern of disease. However architectural distortion and minor scarring in the form of linear inter- and intralobular septal thickening and minor bronchiectasis or bronchiolectasis may be seen and when associated with ground-glass change is consistent with DIP.

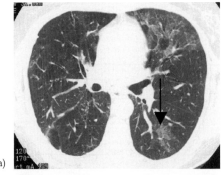

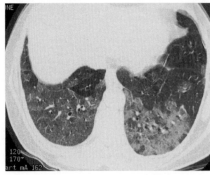

(a)

(b)

Fig. 7.4.1 65-year-old man with DIP. (a) At the level of the lower pole of hila there are patchy areas of ground glass opacification (arrowed). (b) Lower down at the lung base the ground glass spacification is much more extensive.

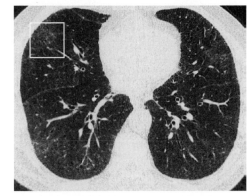

Fig. 7.4.2 Patchy predominantly peripheral ground glass attenuation due to DIP with associated centilobular emphysema (boxed area).

Diagnosing DIP

- The clinical and HRCT features described in a middle-aged smoker may be suggestive of DIP, but are in no way specific. There are no features on TBB or BAL to reliably distinguish DIP from other ILDs, in particular NSIP, which may present in an identical manner.
- Surgical lung biopsy is therefore always required to make a confident diagnosis of DIP.

> **AUTHOR'S TIP**
> DIP can only be confidently diagnosed by surgical lung biopsy.

Treatment and prognosis of DIP

- There are no controlled studies on which to make evidence-based recommendations on treatment. All current smokers should receive smoking cessation advice.
- In patients with only mild functional impairment, smoking cessation alone will often lead to resolution of DIP.
- In those with more significant impairment, there should be a low threshold for introducing a trial of corticosteroid therapy since treatment is associated with improvement, if not complete resolution, in up to 75% and stability in a further 10%.
- The dose and duration of corticosteroid therapy should be tailored to the individual; prednisolone initially at 0.5–0.75 mg/kg/day for 4–8 weeks with dose reduction thereafter depending on clinical response is a reasonable regimen. Relapse is not uncommon, sometimes occurring many months or years after resolution. Higher corticosteroid doses are justified in the occasional patient with severe disease. Other immunomodulatory therapies have been used with varied success.
- DIP is associated with overall good outcome, far better than is associated with IPF or fibrotic NSIP. However, death due to lung fibrosis and progressive respiratory failure is reported in DIP.

AUTHOR'S TIP

Smoking cessation is the critical therapeutic intervention, but unless the disease is mild, treatment with corticosteroids is also recommended.

Further reading

Akira M, Yamamoto S, Hara H, *et al*. Serial computed tomographic evaluation in desquamative interstitial pneumonia. *Thorax* 1997; **52**(4): 333–337.

Carrington CB, Gaensler EA, Coutu RE, *et al*. Natural history and treated course of usual and desquamative inter-stitial pneumonia. *N Engl J Med* 1978; **298**: 801–809.

Hartman TE, Tazelaar HD, Swensen SJ, *et al*. Cigarette smok-ing: CT and pathologic findings of associated pulmonary diseases. *Radiographics* 1997; **17**: 377–390.

Nicholson AG, Colby TV, du Bois RM, *et al*. The prognostic signifi-cance of the histologic pattern of interstitial pneu-monia in patients presenting with the clinical entity of cryptogenic fibros-ing alveolitis. *Am J Respir Crit Care Med* 2000; **162**: 2213–2217.

Tubbs RR, Benjamin SP, Reich NE, *et al*. Desquamative interstitial pneumonitis. Cellular phase of fibros-ing alveolitis. *Chest* 1977; **72**: 159–165.

Wells AU, Nicholson AG, Hansell DM. Challenges in pulmonary fibrosis 4: Smoking-induced diffuse interstitial lung diseases. *Thorax* 2007; **62**(10): 904–910.

7.5 Acute interstitial pneumonia

Introduction

Acute interstitial pneumonia (AIP) is a rapidly progressive form of diffuse lung disease, first described by Hamman and Rich over 50 years ago. AIP is characterised by a histological pattern of diffuse alveolar damage (DAD), indistinguishable from appearances in the acute respiratory distress syndrome (ARDS) and best conceptualised as the idiopathic form of that disorder. There is no gender predilection and the age range is wide, peaking in the sixth decade. Although the aetiology is uncertain, there is indirect evidence to suggest that lung injury results from viral infection or other toxic insults in some cases. However, histological appearances are similar in some patients with autoimmune disease or acute exacerbations of IPF, prompting the hypothesis that AIP represents a fulminant variant of IIPs that more typically present as chronic fibrotic disease.

Presentation

- In typical cases, dyspnoea progresses inexorably over days to weeks, often in association with distressing cough.
- In some cases, there is no obvious prodrome but more commonly, the illness begins with symptoms suggestive of viral infection, including fever, myalgia and malaise.
- The clinical findings at presentation do not distinguish between AIP and ARDS of known cause. Inspiratory crackles are usual but clubbing has not been reported.
- Pulmonary function data have yet to be reported (due to the rapidly progressive nature of the presentation).
- In most cases, there is the highly non-specific finding of a neutrophilia at BAL.

High resolution CT

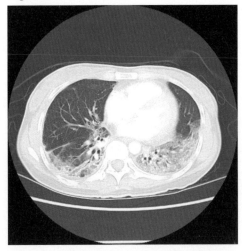

Fig. 7.5.1 CT scan of patient with AIP showing widespread ground glass shadowing with some consolidative changes typically in a sub-pleural distribution (Courtesy of Dr Fergus Gleeson).

- On CT, ground-glass attenuation is almost always the most prominent abnormality and tends to be extensive, although often patchy, and variably associated with anatomical distortion and traction bronchiectasis.

- Ground-glass is indicative of early proliferative diffuse alveolar damage when the airways are normal, whereas the presence of bronchiectasis is a cardinal feature of advanced proliferative or fibrotic diffuse alveolar damage.
- Other frequent CT findings include nodular opacities, interlobular septal thickening and, especially, consolidation, which is present in over two-thirds of cases, often in a sub-pleural distribution.
- Septal thickening on CT is believed to represent limited alveolar collapse when located within areas of ground-glass. Honeycombing is not a cardinal feature of AIP and should prompt suspicion of an acute exacerbation of underlying IPF.
- Outcome is linked to the morphologic extent of disease, with more extensive ground-glass or consolidation linked to a higher mortality, especially in patients with prominent traction bronchiectasis.

Diagnosis

For definitive diagnosis, a typical clinical and CT presentation should be associated with the absence of an overt cause and the presence of DAD at a diagnostic surgical biopsy. However, disease is often too extensive at presentation to allow a biopsy to be performed and in many cases, BAL to exclude underlying infection with confidence may not be realistic. In reality, the diagnosis is often based on clinical and CT features and the differential diagnosis can be subdivided into other forms of diffuse lung disease (considered below) and heart failure, infection or drug-induced lung disease. The combination of extensive ground-glass attenuation and traction bronchiectasis on CT is strongly indicative of AIP. However, it should not be forgotten that both infection and drug toxicity may result in DAD. Furthermore, even when it is clear that heart failure is not the primary problem, the possibility of supervening heart failure due to hypoxia should be kept in mind.

Prognosis

The average survival rate is probably less than 20%, based upon a reported range of 10–50%, but with advances in intensive care practice this may be an underestimate. In approximately half of survivors, pulmonary function is either normal or stable but impaired in the long term. In the remaining cases, there is slow progression of underlying pulmonary fibrosis with recurrent acute respiratory failure in occasional patients. This has caused some to argue that AIP is sometimes an initial presentation of IPF, whether de novo or in a setting of hitherto unsuspected chronic disease.

Management

> **AUTHOR'S TIP**
> Because AIP is a rare disease, there are no controlled treatment data and it is not known whether therapeutic intervention is beneficial. It is usual to give high doses of corticosteroids (e.g. IV methyl prednisolone) and IV cyclophosphamide is occasionally employed. Because disease stabilises or resolves in half of survivors, an aggressive initial approach is warranted, including the use of mechanical ventilation in patients without major co-morbidity. In this regard, AIP should be distinguished from acute exacerbations of IPF, a disorder in which admission to the intensive care unit is virtually never appropriate

Other diffuse lung diseases with an AIP presentation

Acute exacerbations of IPF

It is increasingly recognised at least 10% of IPF patients develop a precipitous course, in which an episode of acute deterioration follows a period of relative stability. The term 'acute exacerbation of IPF' is currently reserved for episodes in which the aetiology is uncertain. Major variations in case definitions between clinical series have prompted a recent consensus statement in which it is recommended that diagnostic criteria should include:

* a previous or concurrent diagnosis of IPF;
* unexplained worsening or development of dyspnoea over 30 days;
* bilateral ground-glass abnormalities and/or consolidation superimposed on a background reticular or honeycomb pattern compatible with IPF on CT;
* no evidence of pulmonary infection, based on endotracheal aspirate or BAL;
* exclusion of alternative disorders including left heart failure, pulmonary embolism and identifiable causes of lung injury.

The risk of an acute exacerbation does not, in general, appear to be linked to underlying disease severity in IPF (as judged by the severity of lung function impairment). However, disease severity may be important in episodes developing after diagnostic surgical lung biopsy, which is believed to be a precipitating factor in some cases. This may explain a post-operative mortality of 15% in group of IPF patients with average gas transfer levels of approximately 30% of predicted.

Hypoxia is usual, and early respiratory failure is common. There are no diagnostic laboratory findings, with the typical BAL neutrophilia also expected in AIP. Diffuse groundglass is generally present on chest radiography and is prominent on CT, with or without consolidation. The key diagnostic CT feature, not seen in AIP, is the presence of typical IPF findings (predominantly bibasal sub-pleural reticular abnormalities or honeycombing). DAD in combination with usual interstitial pneumonia is almost always found at surgical biopsy, although organising pneumonia is occasionally seen in the absence of DAD.

The history of recent deterioration and presence of extensive ground-glass on HRCT in a setting of known IPF usually makes the diagnosis obvious. However, heart failure, opportunistic infection and drug-induced lung disease may all result in extensive ground-glass on CT in a setting of IPF and may all benefit from correct management. In typical disease, characterised by hypoxia and extensive ground-glass on CT, in-hospital mortality is 80–90% despite treatment. As in AIP, high dose corticosteroid therapy tends to be instituted, in the absence of controlled treatment data. Although non-invasive ventilatory support may be useful in selected patients, both as a bridge to transplantation and for palliation, invasive ventilation is not appropriate, because of the poor outcome associated with underlying IPF. In the small subset of patients presenting with milder disease, outcomes are more variable, but this may reflect major differences in diagnostic criteria. When ground-glass on CT is focal and limited, the short term outcome with corticosteroid therapy is relatively good. However, it is not clear that this CT picture is a precursor of typical extensive disease and nor is it clear that the better outcome in these patients can be ascribed to treatment.

Acute exacerbations of NSIP

A clinical and CT presentation of acute exacerbation, indistinguishable from that seen in IPF, is increasingly recognised in patients with idiopathic NSIP, and also in the setting of connective tissue disease. Although total numbers of reported cases are low, the treated outcome tends to be good, even when disease is extensive, except in rheumatoid arthritis (in which an underlying histological pattern of usual interstitial pneumonia is more likely). Underlying NSIP, which is, itself, characterised by prominent groundglass, tends to be more difficult than IPF to detect on CT, in the setting of an acute exacerbation. Pending further data, it appears reasonable to adopt a more aggressive management algorithm for acute exacerbations in known NSIP than in IPF, including mechanical ventilation in carefully selected cases.

Fulminant cryptogenic organising pneumonia (COP)

Very infrequently, COP is devastatingly severe at presentation and may progress to death, in the absence of overt pulmonary fibrosis. Fulminant COP has been described in a small series and number of case reports and has a variable but often good treated outcome. This clinical presentation with a picture resembling ARDS may be indistinguishable from AIP, clinically and on CT. However, the combination of traction bronchiectasis, interlobular septal thickening and intralobular reticular abnormalities tends to be more prominent on CT in AIP. In this lifethreatening disorder, the outcome may be critically dependent on ventilatory support and aggressive therapy with IV corticosteroids.

Further reading

Akira M, Hamada H, Sakatani M, et al. CT findings during phase of accelerated deterioration in patients with idiopathic pulmonary fibrosis. AJR Am J Roentgenol. 1997; **168**: 79–83.

Collard HR. Diseases: other entities of the idiopathic interstitial pneumonias. In Costabel U, du Bois RM, Egan JJ (eds): Diffuse Parenchymal Lung Disease. Cape Town: Karger, 2007; pp. 181–184.

Collard HR, Moore BB, Flaherty KR, et al. Idiopathic Pulmonary Fibrosis Clinical Research Network Investigators. Acute exacerbations of idiopathic pulmonary fibrosis. Am J Respir Crit Care Med 2007; **176**: 636–643.

Hamman L, Rich AR. Acute diffuse interstitial fibrosis of the lungs. Bull Johns Hopkins Hosp 1944; **74**: 177–212.

Ichikadu K, Suga M, Muller NL, et al. Acute interstitial pneumonia: comparison of hig-resolution computed tomography findings between survivors and non-survivors. Am J Respir Crit Care Med 2002; **165**: 1551–1556.

Kondoh Y, Taniguchi H, Kitaichi M, et al. Acute exacerbation of interstitial pneumonia following surgical lung biopsy. Respir Med 2006; **100**: 1753–1759.

Nizami IY, Kissner DG, Visscher DW, et al. Idiopathic bronchiolitis obliterans with organizing pneumonia. An acute and life-threatening syndrome. Chest 1995; **108**: 271–277.

Park IN, Kim DS, Shim TS, et al. Acute exacerbation of interstitial pneumonia other than idiopathic pulmonary fibrosis. Chest 2007; **132**: 214–220.

Utz JP, Ryu JH, Douglas WW, et al. High short-term mortality following lung biopsy for usual interstitial pneumonia. Eur Respir J 2001; **17**: 175–9.

Vourlekis JS, Brown KK, Cool CD, Y et al. Acute interstitial pneumonitis: case series and review of the literature. Medicine 2000; **79**: 369–378.

7.6 Lymphoid interstitial pneumonia

Definition

Lymphoid interstitial pneumonia (LIP) is a rare clinico-pathological entity first described by Liebow and Carrington in 1966. Some cases previously described as LIP have been re-evaluated as non-Hodgkin's low-grade B cell MALT (mucosa-associated lymphoid tissue) lymphoma. LIP is now considered a histological variant of diffuse pulmonary lymphoid hyperplasia although its pathogenesis remains unknown. Idiopathic and secondary forms of LIP are recognised. Idiopathic LIP is one of seven IIPs in the new ATS/ERS re-classification.

Epidemiology

Incidence and prevalence are unknown. Patients may present at any age (mean 48 years). LIP is more common in women with a male: female ratio of 1:2.2. The typical delay between symptom onset and presentation ranges from 1 month to 12 years (mean of 29 months).

Clinical approach

History: key points

- Breathlessness – typically progressive over several months.
- Cough – usually dry, productive in 20%.
- Additional symptoms – fever, malaise, weight loss, pleuritic pain and arthralgia less common.
- Symptoms of specific autoimmune disease or immunodeficiency states.

Examination: key points

- Basal inspiratory crackles in around 60% of patients; become more prominent as the disease progresses.
- Finger clubbing is uncommon (10% cases), unless advanced fibrotic disease is present.
- Examination may be unremarkable.
- Peripheral lymphadenopathy and splenomegaly are uncommon and suggest an alternate or co-existing diagnosis.
- Features of underlying autoimmune disease or systemic manifestations of immunodeficiency in 50% of cases.

Causes

Underlying associations

- LIP is associated with underlying collagen vascular diseases, particularly Sjögrens' syndrome (approximately 25% of cases) and up to 1% of patients with Sjögrens's syndrome will acquire LIP at some time.
- LIP is also associated with the following conditions: systemic lupus erythematosus, rheumatoid arthritis, pernicious anaemia, autoimmune haemolytic anaemia, Hashimoto's thyroiditis, chronic active hepatitis, primary biliary cirrhosis, myasthenia gravis, common variable immunodeficiency (CVID) – high incidence of conversion to malignancy.
- Drug-induced LIP may occur with phenytoin and captopril.
- Rarely associated with bone marrow transplantation, legionella pneumonia and Castleman's disease.
- Epstein–Barr viral has been isolated in some cases.
- Once systemic disease has been excluded, LIP may be termed idiopathic.

> **AUTHOR'S TIP**
> Idiopathic LIP is rare. All cases must be thoroughly investigated for underlying cause or associations such as collagen vascular disease and immunodeficiency.

LIP and HIV infection

- LIP is seen in 16–50% of HIV affected children and is an AIDS-defining illness in the <13 years age group.
- Can be diagnosed by symptoms and radiographic appearances alone.
- Usually occurs when the CD4+ T-lymphocyte count is within the normal range.
- Is rare in adults with HIV (<5%).

Investigations

Lung function

- There is a restrictive defect with reduced gas transfer.
- Airways obstruction has occasionally been reported.
- Levels of hypoxaemia are variable.

Serological tests

- A mild anaemia and raised ESR are often present.
- Over 80% of patients have dysproteinaemias – most commonly polyclonal elevation of IgG and IgM.
- Hypogammaglobulinaemias (~20% of all patients) and monoclonal gammopathies (IgG or IgM) are less frequent.

> **AUTHOR'S TIP**
> Check serum immune electrophoresis in all patients with LIP. A monoclonal gammopathy or hypogammaglobulinaemia suggest lymphoproliferative malignancy.

Chest radiography (Fig. 7.6.1)

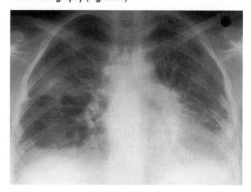

Fig. 7.6.1 Typical CXR features of LIP.

- Bibasal, reticulonodular opacities, with or without septal lines, are common.
- There may be nodules merging with patchy, multifocal consolidations which are occasionally transient.
- In severe disease honeycombing can develop.
- Pneumothorax is a rare presenting feature.

HRCT thorax (Fig. 7.6.2)

- Ground glass attenuation with poorly defined centrilobular (and often sub-pleural) nodules is common.
- Thickening of bronchovascular bundles and interlobular septa are seen in > 80% cases.
- Cystic airspace shadowing and lymphadenopathy occur in 68% cases.
- Pleural effusions are rare, except in HIV-related LIP and may represent underlying lymphoproliferative disease.

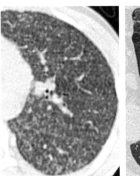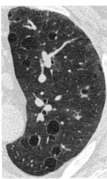

Fig. 7.6.2 Some of the different HRCT changes seen in LIP (images courtesy of Prof David Hansell).

- Thin-walled, perivascular cysts ranging from 1–30mm in size are seen in 68–82% of cases.
- CT differential diagnosis includes: hypersensitivity pneumonitis, DIP, NSIP, sarcoidosis and lymphangitis.

> **AUTHOR'S TIP**
> Demonstration of mediastinal or hilar lymphadenopathy necessitates exclusion of other diagnoses, e.g. lymphoma.

Surgical lung biopsy
- Allows definitive diagnosis in >90% cases.
- Procedure of choice if patient fit enough and able to tolerate intended therapy.

Histopathology
- Benign-looking, predominantly T lymphocytes expand the interstitium and compress alveolar spaces.
- There are perilymphatic and bronchial lymphoid aggregates of polyclonal B cells.
- There is type II cell hyperplasia and interstitial giant cells. Non-caseating granulomata may be seen.
- Perivascular and paraseptal amyloid deposition may occur.
- Pathological findings must be differentiated from: B-cell lymphoma, follicular bronchiolitis, lymphomatoid granulomatosis, hypersensitivity pneumonitis, NSIP, UIP and EBV-associated infections.

> **AUTHOR'S TIP**
> In immunocompromised patients, histochemical stains to exclude *Pneumocystis jirovecii* and Epstein–Barr virus must be performed as these conditions mimic LIP.

Management and treatment
Overview
- No formal controlled trials
- Current therapeutic regimens are based on anecdotal experience from small case series.
- Decisions regarding treatment should take into account the patient's symptoms, physiological variables, fitness and desire for therapy.
- Exclude infections such as *Mycobacterium tuberculosis* and fungi before commencing steroid therapy.

Corticosteroid monotherapy
- Corticosteroids are used in >90% of cases

- Unproven effect on the natural history of the condition.
- Optimum dose and duration of therapy uncertain.
- Similar treatment regimens as recommended for COP have been utilized:
  - Prednisolone 0.75–1mg/kg/day for 8 to 12 weeks or until maximum improvements in lung function/radiology
  - Subsequent slow dose tapering to 0.25mg/kg/ day for 6 to 12 weeks
- Most patients with HIV-related LIP treated with corticosteroids exhibit a good response.

Anti-retroviral therapy
- Symptoms improve with a reduction in viral load and increase in the CD4+ count.
- Single agent (Zidovudine) and triple therapy with nucleoside analogues have resulted in clinico-radiological resolution in some HIV-positive patients.

Other treatments
- There are anecdotal reports of clinical response to other immunosuppressive agents outlined in Prognosis.
- Case reports on CVID-related LIP have improved with cyclosporin (which inhibits CD4 +ve Th2 lymphocyte activation) and IV immunoglobulin.

Prognosis
- In a recent observational study of 15 patients the median survival was 11.5 years.
- Survival in HIV-positive patients is similar to those without LIP.
- Prognosis is better in younger patients and those with non-idiopathic LIP.
- Combining five studies of 52 patients all treated with corticosteroids alone or with additional chlorambucil, cyclophosphamide, colchicine, azathioprine or methotrexate: 35% had a dramatic improvement, 15% had some improvement, 27% remained stable and 23% died (from progressive pulmonary fibrosis, respiratory failure, infection from immunosuppression or transformation to lymphoma).

Malignant transformation
Malignant transformation to a low grade B-cell lymphoma occurs in <5% of patients and has a favourable outcome.

Lung transplantation
Single lung transplantation should be considered in patients who deteriorate despite therapy. Referral criteria are broadly similar to those for patients with UIP.

Further reading
Cha S-I, Fessler MB, Cool CD, *et al.* Lymphoid interstitial pneumonia: clinical features, associations and prognosis. *Eur Respr J* 2006; **28**: 364–369.

Davies CWH, Juniper MC, Gray W, *et al.* Lymphoid interstitial pneumonitis associated with common variable hypogammaglobulinaemia treated with cyclosporin A. *Thorax* 2000; **55**: 88–90.

Johkoh T, Muller NL, Pickford HA, *et al.* Lymphocytic interstitial pneumonia: thin-section CT findings in 22 patients. *Radiology* 1999; **212**: 567–572.

Nicholson AG, Wotherspoon AC, Diss TC, *et al.* Reactive pulmonary lymphoid disorders. *Histopathology* 1995; **26**: 405–412.

Swigris JJ, Berry GJ, Raffin TA, *et al.* Lymphoid Interstitial Pneumonia: a narrative review. *Chest* 2002; **122**: 2150–2164.

7.7 Cryptogenic organising pneumonia

The terms cryptogenic organising pneumonia (COP) is preferred to bronchiolitis obliterans organising pneumonia (BOOP) since the former better reflects the clinico-pathological entity of organising granulation tissue within the alveolar ducts and sacs that sometimes, but not always, extends into the small bronchioles. There are a number of causes of, or associations with, organising pneumonia that must be considered before a diagnosis of *cryptogenic* OP can be made (Table 7.7.1).

> **AUTHOR'S TIP**
> The presentation of COP is often indistinguishable from community acquired pneumonia; failure to respond to antibiotic therapy and migratory CXR changes should always raise the possibility of COP.

Table 7.7.1 Is it cryptogenic? Some causes of secondary organising pneumonia

Infective pneumonia	*Streptococcus pneumoniae, Mycoplasma pneumoniae, Legionella sp*, oppourtunistic organisms, viruses
Radiation	Post breast-cancer radiotherapy
Connective tissue disease	Rheumatoid arthritis, dermatomyositis/polymyositis, systemic sclerosis, systemic lupus erythematosus
Drugs	Bleomycin, amiodarone, methotrexate and others
Inflammatory bowel disease	Crohn's, ulcerative colitis
Neoplasms	In vicinity of bronchial carcinoma, in association with haematological malignancies.

Epidemiology

The incidence of COP is not known and has not been extensively studied. Whilst often considered a rare condition, most chest physicians will have experience of seeing patients with COP and indeed the condition may be more common than generally considered. COP occurs with equal frequency in men and women and is probably more common in smokers than non-smokers.

Typical COP

Clinical and radiological features

Most cases of COP present with symptoms, clinical signs and chest radiography that are largely indistinguishable from community acquired pneumonia, a far commoner condition. A diagnosis of COP is often first considered when there is failure to respond to empirical antibiotic therapy.

• Typical symptoms of COP are dry cough, breathlessness, fatigue and anorexia. Sputum production is uncommon and haemoptysis is rare.

• Fever with unilateral/bilateral crackles or clear chest are common examination findings. Bronchial breathing, even in the presence of radiographic evidence of consolidation, is rarely reported.

• Lung function tests play little or no role in diagnosing or monitoring COP. Airflow obstruction is uncommon despite the apparent 'bronchocentric' pattern of disease.

• Blood tests usually reveal mild neutrophilia and raised inflammatory markers (CRP, ESR)

• Chest radiography typically features unilateral or bilateral patchy non-segmental consolidation, without a particular zonal predilection. Presentation with a single area of lobar consolidation is far less common. Migratory or 'flitting' radiograph changes over a period of weeks or months is suggestive of COP (Fig. 7.7.1). Pleural effusion is rarely visible on CXR. Occasionally COP presents as a solitary lung nodule.

• The HRCT scan aids in the distinction of COP from fibrotic ILDs, in particular IPF, but the distinction from other IIPs or from hypersensitivity pneumonitis is less reliable. There are no pathognomic features on HRCT to distinguish COP from infection. Air-space consolidation, which is often peripheral and/or peribronchial, is present on CT in 90% of patients with COP (Fig. 7.7.2).

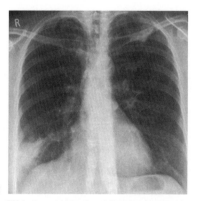
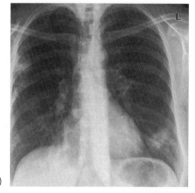

(a)   (b)

Fig. 7.7.1 40-year-old female with fitting consolidation due to COP.
(a) Right lower and left upper zone consolidation.
(b) Three months later there is consolidation lateral to left heart border, medially at the right base and laterally in the right mid zone.

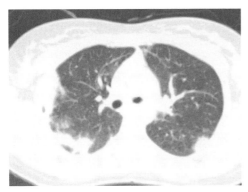

Fig. 7.7.2 HRCT scan of COP. Patchy peripheral consolidation with limited ground glass attenuation.

Typically the consolidation seen on HRCT is accompanied by diffuse ground-glass opacification and there may also be multiple small nodules not necessarily obvious on the plain chest radiograph. Another common finding is bronchial wall thickening and bronchial dilatation in involved areas. 20–30% patients are found to have small unilateral or bilateral pleural effusions on CT. Sub-pleural reticulation is seen occasionally.

Making a diagnosis of COP

> **AUTHOR'S TIP**
> The diagnosis of COP is dependent upon integrating clinical, radiological and wherever possible histological evidence. COP should never be diagnosed on the basis of histology alone.

- A confident diagnosis of COP requires integration of clinical, radiographic and histological evidence. Typical COP may be diagnosed with reasonable confidence on clinical and radiological grounds alone if infection can be excluded and a subsequent brisk response to corticosteroids is observed. In general however, lung tissue biopsy should be sought whenever possible before treating COP.
- Transbronchial lung biopsy may be sufficient to make a histological diagnosis of organising pneumonia, but a surgical lung biopsy should be sought if the diagnosis remains uncertain.
- The diagnosis of COP should <u>never</u> be made on histological basis alone because the histological pattern of organising pneumonia can occur in other settings. For example, it is quite common to find OP in the vicinity of lung cancer.

Treating typical COP and significance of relapses

- Corticosteroids are the mainstay of therapy in COP, although there are no randomised controlled studies upon which to base recommendations.
- Prednisolone at initial doses of 0.75–1mg/kg/day, with continued therapy for up to 1 year are often cited in the literature, but in practice, the precise dose and length of treatment should be judged on each individual case, taking into consideration the severity of the disease, patient co-morbidity and likelihood of steroid side-effects.

- Relapses, both on and off treatment are quite common, and may be more common with short-course (3–6 months) compared to extended-course (12 months) steroid therapy. However relapses in typical COP are; (i) not associated with increased mortality; (ii) not associated with progressive lung fibrosis; and (iii) as responsive to corticosteroids as the initial presentation.
- On this basis, a suggested regimen, that may be modified to suit the individual case, is oral prednisolone as follows:
  - 0.75mg/kg for 4 weeks;
  - 0.5mg/kg for 4 weeks;
  - 20mg daily for 4 weeks;
  - 10mg daily for 6 weeks;
  - 5mg daily for 6 weeks then stop.
- Relapses can be treated by re-instigating the regimen either with the initial dose, or with the lowest dose at which the disease was previously controlled.
- On occasion, COP can relapse and remit radiologically with few or no associated symptoms and without a change in therapy. Thus relapses of COP do not *always* require treatment.

Other manifestations of organising pneumonia
Acute fulminant COP

- Occasionally COP presents with widespread CXR infiltrates and acute respiratory failure, in a syndrome that overlaps with AIP and ARDS. The usual scenario is that such cases are initially misdiagnosed as severe community acquired pneumonia on the high dependency or intensive care unit, but fail to respond to conventional antibiotic therapy.
- BAL plays an important role in excluding infection (nosocomial, antibiotic resistant bacteria or opportunistic organisms) in this setting, but a confident diagnosis of COP again requires transbronchial or preferably surgical lung biopsy.
- The diagnosis of acute fulminant COP is important since there is the prospect of recovery with high dose corticosteroid therapy (e.g. methylprednisolone, 500–1000mg per day for 3 consecutive days followed by prednisolone 1–1.5mg/kg/day or equivalent).

Post-radiotherapy organising pneumonia

- A well-recognised form of OP occurs in association with radiotherapy, particularly tangential field radiotherapy for breast cancer.
- Post-radiotherapy OP is different to classic (sporadic) post-radiotherapy pneumonitis in that it generally occurs later (9–12 months, as opposed to 1–2 months following radiotherapy), involves non-radiated areas of lung, and does not progress to lung fibrosis.
- Post-radiotherapy OP is therefore very like the cryptogenic form of the disease and should be treated in the same way.

Organising pneumonia and fibrotic interstitial lung disease

- It is likely that a very small subgroup of COP is associated with treatment unresponsive disease and progression to lung fibrosis.
- Some cases of 'fibrosing organising pneumonia', whether cryptogenic or secondary to connective tissue diseases, are likely to represent 'overlap' syndromes. For example, radiological and histological features of organising

pneumonia are sometimes seen in cases in which the otherwise dominant lesion is a UIP or fibrotic NSIP.

• The outcome with corticosteroid therapy in organising pneumonia overlapping with fibrotic ILD is far less certain than for typical COP, but in general the prognosis is determined by the dominant co-existing interstitial lung disease.

AUTHOR'S TIP

The initial dose and duration of corticosteroid therapy should be tailored to the individual case; the risks and consequences of relapse in typical COP may be less serious than the risk of prolonged corticosteroid therapy.

Further reading

Cohen AJ, King TE Jr, Downey GP. Rapidly progressive bronchiolitis obliterans with organizing pneumonia. *Am J Respir Crit Care Med* 1994; **149**: 1670–1675.

Cordier JF. Cryptogenic organising pneumonia. *Eur Respir J* 2006; **28**: 422–446.

Davison AG, Heard BE, McAllister WA, *et al.* Cryptogenic organizing pneumonia. *Q J Med* 1983; **52**: 382–394.

Katzenstein AL, Zisman DA, Litzky LA, *et al.* Usual interstitial pneumonia: histologic study of biopsy and explant specimens. *Am J Surg Pathol* 2002; **26**: 1567–1577.

Lazor R, Vandevenne A, Pelletier A, *et al.* Cryptogenic organizing pneumonia. Characteristics of relapses in a series of 48 patients. The Groupe d'Etudes et de Recherche sur les Maladles 'Orphelines' Pulmonaires (GERM'O'P).*Am J Respir Crit Care Med* 2000; **162**: 571–577.

Lee KS, Kullnig P, Hartman TE, Muller NL. Cryptogenic organizing pneumonia: CT findings in 43 patients. *Am J Roentgenol* 1994; **162**: 543–546.

Nambu A, Araki T, Ozawa K, *et al.* Bronchiolitis obliterans organizing pneumonia after tangential beam irradiation to the breast: discrimination from radiation pneumonitis. *Radiat Med* 2002; **20**: 151–154.

Romero S, Barroso E, Rodriguez-Paniagua M, *et al.* Organizing pneumonia adjacent to lung cancer: frequency and clinico-pathologic features. *Lung Cancer* 2002; **35**: 195–201.

Yousem SA, Lohr RH, Colby TV. Idiopathic bronchiolitis obliterans organizing pneumonia/cryptogenic organizing pneumonia with unfavorable outcome: pathologic predictors. *Mod Pathol* 1997; **10**: 864–871.

7.8 Extrinsic allergic alveolitis

Epidemiology

The most common types of extrinsic allergic alveolitis (EAA) are bird fancier's lung from a pet bird in the home or the sport of pigeon racing, farmer's lung due to fungi in mouldy hay or straw and various types of humidifier lung due to fungi or bacteria in water aerosols in the home or workplace. A recent international study showed that 61% of cases of EAA were due to birds, 21% to farming and 12% to various fungi encountered in the home or workplace.

In 1.5% of cases the source of the antigen was not identified

In the UK one million homes have a pet bird, 2% of the population work in agriculture and there are approximately 85,000 registered pigeon fanciers. Only a small %age of those exposed to an antigen of EAA develop the disease. It is estimated that 3.4% of budgie fanciers, 8% of pigeon fanciers and 4.5% of farmers develop EAA but the prevalence varies according to the circumstances of antigen exposure. In Japan summer-type EAA is the most common type and is due to fungal moulds in the home. Work-related EAA accounts for about 6% of occupational lung disease with approximately 500 cases reported to the UK surveillance scheme over a decade, mainly involving workers in agriculture, foresting and fishing. As work practices change, some classic causes of EAA have faded but new syndromes emerge. Thus mushroom worker's lung and cork worker's lung are less common nowadays but metal working fluid EAA is now an important cause of EAA in workers in car manufacturing plants from contamination of fluid used to cool and lubricate metal.

> **AUTHOR'S TIP**
> Focus on the work, home and recreational environment.

Classification and course

EAA is a complex dynamic disease which varies in its presentation and clinical course (Fig. 7.8.1). Traditionally it is classified into acute, subacute and chronic forms, but patients don't always fit neatly into this classification and different patterns emerge over time and depend on the population studied.

- Sensitisation is the development of antibody and cellular responses as part of an antigen-processing mechanism, but only a few sensitised individuals progress to develop EAA.
- Acute EAA presents as fever, malaise, cough and dyspnoea 4–8 hours after antigen exposure, resolving within 48 hours. This is common amongst pigeon fanciers who have high intensity exposure to 100–200 racing pigeons. Many have acute mild stable symptoms which they manage themselves in the community without medical attention. More severe acute EAA presents to hospital with alveolitis and hypoxaemia, which usually resolve quickly, but may recur on further antigen exposure.
- Chronic EAA presents insidiously with progressive dyspnoea and fibrosis. This pattern is more common where there is low-grade protracted antigen exposure, such as occurs when pet birds are kept in the home.
- Subacute EAA is characterised by progressive dyspnoea and alveolitis with some acute symptoms after antigen exposure.

Acute or recurrent EAA does not usually progress to chronic fibrotic EAA and the outcome is usually good with only mild residual impairment of lung function. However, a small proportion of patients with EAA develop progressive fibrosis – even after stopping antigen exposure – which behaves like IPF. Chronic bronchitis, airways obstruction, and emphysema may occur as part of the spectrum of EAA. Factors influencing the onset and progression of EAA

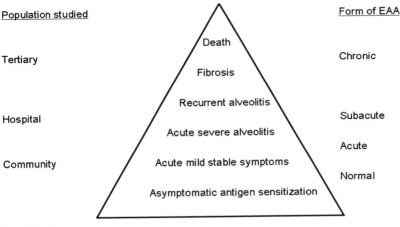

Fig. 7.8.1 EAA.

are poorly understood but include the circumstances of antigen exposure and individual susceptibility in terms of human leucocyte antigen (HLA) type, cytokine gene polymorphisms and T-regulatory cell function.

Investigation and diagnosis

Because EAA is so diverse and dynamic no single test is diagnostic, investigations should be adapted to the clinical circumstances, and the diagnosis is established from a combination of features and exclusion of alternative diagnoses.

- Suspicion of an association between symptoms and contact with a provoking antigen is the first step in diagnosis.

Table 7.8.1 Diagnosing extrinsic allergic alveolitis

1 Identify a provoking antigen
2 Demonstrate an immune response
3 Relate symptoms to antigen exposure
4 Measure impairment of lung function
5 Define the radiographic abnormalities
6 Consider the need for lung biopsy and lavage
7 Consider an antigen challenge study
8 Exclude alternative diagnoses

- Demonstration of an antibody or cellular response to the antigen is essential, but not sufficient for diagnosis since many asymptomatic exposed subjects show similar immune responses. At least 85% of patients with farmer's lung or bird fancier's lung have antibodies to the provoking antigen. Difficulties in detecting an antibody response may occur when the precise antigen is unknown or if exposure has now ceased although the patient has developed chronic disease. Antibody-negative EAA is unusual and the diagnosis then requires persuasive evidence from other tests. Lymphocyte stimulation tests may confirm the immune nature of the disease but these assays are not widely available and are not well validated since many of the antigens of EAA can provoke non-specific immune stimulation.
- Lung function tests typically show reduced lung volumes, impaired gas transfer and hypoxaemia.
- The chest radiograph usually shows diffuse parenchymal infiltrates but is normal in 20% of cases of acute EAA. HRCT is more sensitive and is probably always abnormal in active EAA. In acute EAA there is often a characteristic appearance of diffuse airway centred micronodules with patchy ground-glass shadowing and areas of hyperlucency on expiration due to bronchiolotis and air-trapping (Fig. 7.8.2).
- In chronic EAA the HRCT appearances may be similar to IPF with reticulation, secondary bronchial dilatation and honeycombing (Fig. 7.8.3).
- BAL typically shows a lymphocytosis with a predominance of CD_8 T-cells, but a neutrophil alveolitis occurs after antigen exposure and also in chronic fibrotic EAA. Furthermore asymptomatic exposed subjects may also have lymphocytosis so that it reflects a cellular immune response rather than disease. BAL also helps to exclude infection.
- The histopathology of EAA is distinctive but not pathognomonic and diagnosis requires compatible clinical features. In acute EAA transbronchial biopsy may provide supporting evidence of lymphocytic inflammation, foamy macrophages, giant cells with cholesterol clefts and

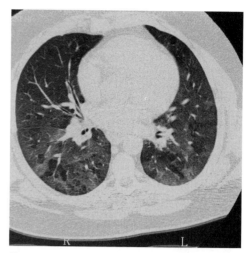

Fig. 7.8.2 Acute EAA showing airway centred nodules and ground glass shadowing with areas of hyperlucency.

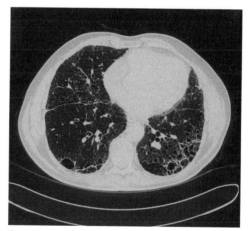

Fig. 7.8.3 Chronic EAA showing reticularious, secondary bronchial dilatation and honeycombing.

granulomas. Granulomas are most characteristic but are present in only 66% of cases. In chronic fibrotic EAA surgical biopsy may show the histological patterns of UIP, NSIP or COP. The prognosis is worse for patients with UIP but there can be considerable difficulty in determining whether this histopathological pattern has arisen from EAA or from IPF.

- Laboratory-based antigen challenge tests can be helpful in the context of research, particularly where new antigens are identified but for most forms of EAA there is a lack of standardised antigens and it can be difficult to differentiate EAA from other reactions such as inhalation fevers or organic dust toxic syndrome. A natural challenge may be helpful in clinical practice whereby the clinical features are monitored when the patient is removed from and then re-exposed to the suspect environment in the workplace or home.

Treatment

- Avoidance of further contact with the provoking antigen is the main treatment of EAA.
- Some patients have had mild stable symptoms for several years but have not consulted doctors because they fear that their livelihood is at stake in the case of farmers or that their commitment to their sport will not be appreciated in the case of pigeon fanciers. They may be reluctant to stop antigen exposure. Several long-term studies show a favourable outcome in such patients despite continued antigen exposure, indicating the complexity of the host–antigen interaction in EAA. Pigeon fanciers can be encouraged to spend less time in the loft, to avoid activities where there is a high level of antigen, such as 'scraping out', and to wear a loft coat and hat that are removed on leaving the loft so as to avoid continuing contact with antigen carried on clothing or hair. Farmers can use silage rather than hay for foddering animals and adopt modern practices with drying systems which reduce the moisture and mould content of hay.
- Respiratory protection masks have been shown to improve symptoms and prevent a reaction to antigen challenge.
- In acute severe EAA prednisolone 40 mg/day, tapering over 8 weeks to zero, hastens the rate of recovery of lung function but does not alter the longterm outcome.
- In chronic fibrotic EAA further antigen contact is not advisable. Many of these patients improve on prednisolone particularly when biopsy shows a NSIP or COP pattern. Patients with a UIP pattern respond poorly to steroids and they are usually treated in the same way as patients with IPF.
- Management of occupational EAA involves management of both the individual and the affected industry in order to reduce the risk to other workers.

Patients' FAQ: do I have to give up my work/birds?
Answer. stopping exposure is the safest advice, and is essential if you have severe or progressive EAA. If EAA has been mild and stable you may choose to continue exposure using respiratory protection and antigen avoidance but you should have medical supervision to ensure that progressive lung damage isn't developing.

Further reading

Bourke SJ, Banham SW, Carter R, et al. Longitudinal course of extrinsic allergic alveolitis in pigeon breeders. Thorax 1989; **44**: 415–418.

Bourke SJ, Dalphin JC, Boyd G, et al. Hypersensitivity pneumonitis: current concepts. Eur Respir J 2001; **18**(Suppl 32): 81s–92s.

Cormier Y, Brown M, Worthy S, et al. High resolution computed tomographic characteristics in acute farmer's lung and in its follow-up. Eur Respir J 2000; **16**: 55–60.

Dawkins P, Robertson A, Robertson W et al. An outbreak of extrinsic alveolitis at a car engine plant. Occup Med 2006; **56**: 559–565.

Erkinjuntti-Pekkanen R, Kokkarinen J, Tukiainen HO, et al. Longterm outcome of pulmonary function in farmer's lung: a 14 year follow-up with matched controls. Eur Respir J 1997; **10**: 2046–2050.

Fink JN, Ortega HG, Reynolds HY et al. Needs and opportunities for research in hypersensitivity pneumonitis. Am J Respir Crit Care Med 2005; **171**: 792–798.

Kokkarinen JS, Tukianen HO, Terho EO. Effect of corticosteroid treatment on the recovery of pulmonary function in farmer's lung. Am Rev Respir Dis 1992; **145**: 3–5.

Lacasse Y, Selman M, Costabel U et al. Clinical diagnsosis of hypersensitivity pneumonitis. Am J Respir Crit Care Med 2003; **168**: 952–958.

McDonald JC, Chen Y, Zeveld et al. Incidence by occupation and industry of acute work-related respiratory diseases in the UK, 1992–2001. Occup Environ Med 2005; **62**: 836–842.

Ohtani Y, Saiki S, Kitaichi M et al. Chronic bird fancier's lung: histopathological and clinical correlation. An application of the 2002 ATS/ERS consensus classification of the idiopathic interstitial pneumonias. Thorax 2005; **60**: 665–671.

7.9 Sarcoidosis

Sarcoidosis is a chronic multisystem disorder of unknown aetiology characterised by formation of granulomata within affected organs and consequent distortion of their normal architecture. Typically, these are non-caseating epithelioid granulomata involving organised collections of activated macrophages and T lymphocytes. Pulmonary involvement is most common followed by eyes, lymph nodes, skin and liver.

Presentations

- Asymptomatic: (10–20%); discovered during routine CXR screening.
- Acute: (20–40%); develops over 1–2 weeks with fever, malaise, polyarthralgia, anorexia, cough, chest discomfort, occasionally night sweats and weight loss.
- Lofgrens syndrome: acute onset with erythema nodosum, polyarthritis and bilateral hilar lymphadenopathy on CXR.
- Heerfordt syndrome: acute onset fever, parotid enlargement, anterior uveitis and facial nerve palsy.
- Insidiuous onset: (40–70%); this group tends to develop chronic sarcoidosis with gradual fibrotic remodelling of involved organs with eventual irreversible damage.

Organ involvement

- Lungs: 90% have abnormal findings at some point during the course of the disease. Around 50% develop permanent abnormalities including background parenchymal scarring and/or persistent mediastinal lymphadenopathy. 5–15% exhibit progressive disease with interstitial fibrosis, large airways involvement and/or pleural effusion (1–5%); pneumothorax is rare.
- Lymph nodes: lymphadenopathy (paratracheal, hilar, mediastinal commonest).
- Skin: erythema nodosum, plaques, maculopapular eruptions (Fig. 7.9.1), subcutaneous nodules, lupus pernio, infiltration of new/existent scars and keloid formation.

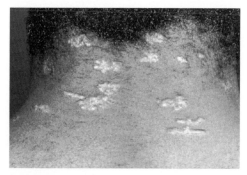

Fig. 7.9.1 Typical sarcoid cutaneous lesions on nape of neck. (See Plate 1.)

- Eye: anterior and posterior uveitis with secondary complications of glaucoma and cataract and blindness, retinopathy, conjunctival nodules (Fig. 7.9.2), optic nerve involvement, papilloedema, keratoconjunctivitis sicca.

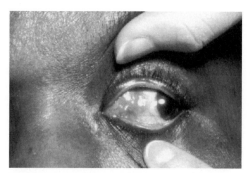

Fig. 7.9.2 Conjunctival sarcoid nodules. (See Plate 2.)

- Upper respiratory tract: involvement of nasal mucosa, larynx, epiglottis.
- Liver: granulomatous hepatitis, asymptomatic elevation of liver enzymes, hepatomegaly, intrahepatic cholestasis; portal hypertension is rare.
- Heart: restrictive cardiomyopathy, pericarditis, arrhythmias, conduction defects including complete heart block, sudden cardiac death, congestive cardiac failure, cor pulmonale.
- Musculoskeletal: polyarthritis, myopathy and myositis, bone lesions and dactylitis (Fig. 7.9.3).

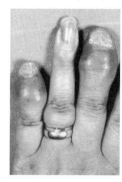

Fig. 7.9.3 Extensive hand digit distortion with bone cyst formation and associated dactylitis in sarcoidosis. (See Plate 3.)

- Nervous system: unilateral facial nerve palsy, multiple cranial nerve palsies, space-occupying lesion, aseptic meningitis, hypothalamic–pituitary axis involvement, seizures, cerebellar ataxia, spinal cord involvement, peripheral neuropathy; presentations can mimic multiple sclerosis.
- Haematology: peripheral lymphopaenia and splenomegaly, occasionally eosinophilia; bone marrow infiltration can cause anaemia, neutropaenia and thrombocytopaenia at presentation.
- Endocrine and metabolic: diabetes insipidus secondary to involvement of hypothalamic–pituitary axis, hypopituitarism, hypoadrenalism, hypercalcaemia (secondary

to overproduction of 1–25 dihydrocholecalciferol by acti-vated macrophages) with nephrocalcinosis and nephrolithiasis. Hypercalciuria can occur in the absence of hypercalcaemia.

- Exocrine glands: enlarged parotid and lacrimal glands.

Aetiology

- Cause is unknown.
- Various infectious and non-infectious agents implicated but no specific agent identified.
- There is heightened cellular response to unidentified antigens in individuals genetically predisposed.

Epidemiology

- Usually manifest in the 20–40 year age group.
- More usual in temperate than in tropical climates.
- Prevalence rates difficult to establish as disease is often asymptomatic; UK incidence is 10–20 in 100,000 population; frequency is higher in Ireland.
- More prevalent and chronic in black population, who have higher risk of non-pulmonary manifestations.

Differential diagnosis

Hilar lymphadenopathy

Tuberculosis, lymphoma, infectious mononucleosis, leukaemia, bronchogenic carcinoma, metastases, enlarged pulmonary arteries.

Hilar lymphadenopathy with pulmonary infiltrates

Tuberculosis, pneumoconiosis, lymphangitis carcinomatosa, idiopathic pulmonary haemosiderosis, pulmonary eosinophilia, alveolar cell carcinoma, histiocytosis X.

Diffuse pulmonary infiltration

Previous lists + chronic beryllium disease, idiopathic interstitial pneumonias, rheumatoid lung, Sjogren's disease, extrinsic allergic alveolitis.

Non-caseating granulomata

Tuberculosis and other mycobacterial infections, leprosy, syphilis, cat-scratch disease, berylliosis, hypersensitivity pneumonitis, foreign body reactions, lymphoma, carcinoma, primary biliary cirrhosis, Crohn's disease, hypogammaglobulinaemia, granulomatous vasculitis, parasitic and fungal infections.

Symptoms

- Asymtompatic.
- Dyspnoea: commonly on exertion.
- Cough: usually non-productive.
- Chest discomfort: intermittent sharp pains.
- Fatigue, malaise, weight loss, fever.
- Symptoms of other organ involvement and complications.

Investigations

Blood tests

Haematology: lymphopaenia, mild eosinophilia, raised ESR.

Biochemistry: raised serum angiotensin converting enzyme in 2/3 of acute patients, hypercalcaemia, hypercalciuria (may have normal serum calcium), hypergammaglobulinaemia, other abnormalities secondary to different organ involvement.

Chest radiograph

90% have abnormal chest radiographs; classic patterns are shown in radiological clinical staging.

Other abnormalities include nodular infiltrates and con-glomerate masses especially in a mid and upper zone bilateral distribution; rarely cavitating lesions, pleural effusions and atelectasis.

HRCT scan of chest

Upper lobe pre-dominance; parenchymal granulomatous load may be reflected as small nodules in peribronchovascular distribution (subpleural, septal and fissural) producing a characteristic 'beading' appearance and scattered patches of ground glass opacities or large conglomerate masses occasionally with presence of air - bronchograms.

ECG

Arrhythmias, bundle branch block pattern in some patients.

Pulmonary function tests

Can be entirely normal despite widespread radiographic abnormalities, or may show significant physiological dysfunction with clear lung fields. The classical abnormality in established pulmonary sarcoidosis is a restrictive defect with reduced lung volumes and diffusion capacity. Occasionally there may be airflow obstruction; in patients who have a history of asthma, airflow patterns may become fixed.

BAL

May be helpful adjunct to diagnosis; many patients with 'active' sarcoidosis show lavage lymphocytosis (Fig. 7.9.4); as fibrosis develops, an increase in neutrophils occurs.

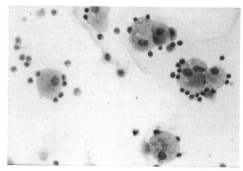

Fig. 7.9.4 A cytospin of sarcoid bronchoalveolar lavage showing lymphocytosis; a classical rosette pattern of lymphocytes in close proximity to alveolar macrophages is also seen.

Histology

Commonly performed on lymph nodes, lung tissue, skin, liver; classical well formed tightly knit non-caseating granulomata (Fig. 7.9.5).

Special situations may call for the following: gallium-67 scans (often positive in sarcoidosis); radioactive [201]Tl (taken up by sarcoid tissue and by ischaemic myocardium); MRI may be particularly useful in unusual or difficult diagnostic circum-stances such as neurosarcoidosis; opthalmological assess-ment should include slit lamp examination and if necessary fluorescein angiography in patients with associated ocular symptoms.

Course of disease

The clinical expression, natural history and prognosis of sarcoidosis are highly variable with a tendency to wax and wane, either spontaneously or in response to therapy.

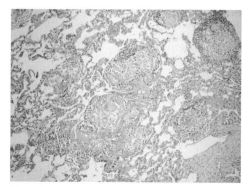

Fig. 7.9.5 Histological appearances of tightly knit, well formed granulomata formation. (See Plate 4.)

Spontaneous remissions: 70% patients within 1 year of presentation; the course is chronic or progressive in the rest.

Incidence of clinically significant extrapulmonary involvement increases with disease progression and can be influenced by background ethnicity.

Death (1–5%) is rare; when it occurs is typically secondary to respiratory failure, myocardial or central nervous system involvement.

Radiological clinical staging

Stage 0: normal chest (5–10%).

Stage I: bilateral hilar lymphadenopathy (50%) (Fig. 7.9.6).

Stage II: bilateral hilar lymphadenopathy and pulmonary infiltrates; paratracheal nodes may be enlarged (25%).

Stage III: parenchymal infiltrates only (15%).

Stage IV: established pulmonary fibrosis with parenchymal remodelling and lung volume loss, especially in upper lobes.

Treatment

Pulmonary sarcoidosis is usually benign and can resolve within 1 year of presentation.

Corticosteroids

There is so far limited data on the role of corticosteroids in the management of sarcoidosis.

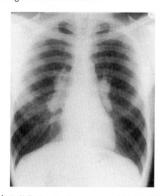

Fig. 7.9.6 A CXR showing the presence of bilateral hilar lymphadenopathy (sarcoid stage I).

Currently held view is that patients with stage I disease do not require treatment with oral steroids.

Patients with Stage II and Stage III may benefit from steroid treatment and show radiological improvement (Fig. 7.9.7).

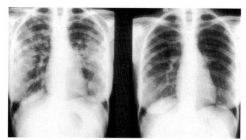

Fig. 7.9.7 CXRs of same patient at presentation with predominant mid-zone peripheral interstitial shadowing, which in this case has resolved following steroid treatment.

There is little documented evidence that treatment with oral steroids has a beneficial effect on lung function; in practice resolution of radiological granulomatous load is associated with lung function improvement.

There is limited evidence that oral steroids can alter clinical progression or that early treatment alters disease outcome.

Clinically, steroids may be helpful in controlling symptomatic manifestations of extrapulmonary sarcoidosis.

Inhaled steroids (with less systemic side effects) may be used in endobronchial sarcoidosis and bronchial hyperresponsiveness manifested by chronic troublesome cough although there are no published randomised trials.

Criteria for steroid use in sarcoidosis

Following consensus recommendations from the American Thoracic Society, European Respiratory Society and World Association of Sarcoidosis and Other Granulomatous Disorders:

- Progressive symptomatic pulmonary disease.
- Asymptomatic pulmonary disease with persistent infiltrates or progressive loss of lung function.
- Cardiac disease.
- Neurological disease.

Suggested steroid dosage

Prednisolone 30 mg daily for 4 weeks; reduced by 5 mg every month to 15 mg daily if patient improves; reduced by 2.5 mg every 1–2 months to 10 mg daily if patient stable; reduced gradually, aiming to stop after completing 12 months of continuous treatment if sarcoid activity in remission.

Methylprednisolone can be used in neurosarcoidosis and other cases of complicated extrapulmonary sarcoidosis.

Contraindications: uncontrolled hypertension, diabetes mellitus, infection, severe osteoporosis.

Relapses: treated by increased dose; patients with objective evidence of 2 or more relapses may need long-term low dose prednisolone alone or in combination with other agents.

Immunosuppressants and immunomodulatory agents used in sarcoidosis:
- Methotrexate.
- Chloroquine and hydroxychloroquine.
- Azathioprine.
- Infliximab.
- Thalidomide.
- Leflunomide.

Methotrexate, hydroxychloroquine and azathioprine are currently the preferred agents in pulmonary sarcoidosis.

Methotrexate and azathioprine can be used as steroid sparing agents. Methotrexate can be particularly useful in troublesome uveitis; recently proposed to be first-choice immunosuppressant in steroid resistant neurosarcoidosis.

Leflunomide is an analogue of methotrexate, effective in sarcoidosis with less pulmonary toxicity than methotrexate.

Antimalarial drugs chloroquine and hydroxychloroquine (less oculotoxicity than chloroquine) are more effective in skin and mucosal disease.

Thalidomide might be particularly suitable for lupus pernio.

Infliximab is a chimeric monoclonal antibody against soluble and membrane bound TNF-α and recently proved effective in refractory sarcoidosis.

Key points in sarcoidosis
- Spontaneous remission in ~2/3 of patients.
- Acute onset and Stage I disease have best prognosis.
- Serum ACE level is more useful for treatment follow-up than diagnosis.
- Often disparity between physiological and radiological parameters.
- There is still limited evidence on 'when to treat'.
- Some patients with repeated relapses may need long term steroids.

Recommended clinical evaluation in sarcoidosis
- Thorough history taking with emphasis on occupational and environmental exposure.
- Physical examination with emphasis on lungs, liver, eye, skin and heart.
- Pulmonary function tests: spirometry and diffusing capacity as a minimum.
- HRCT lung scan to document extent of parenchymal and nodal involvement and guide need for biopsy.
- Histological confirmation essential if diagnosis not clear cut or if clinical condition progresses; biopsy (usually lymph nodes, lungs, skin, liver or target affected organ), special stain and culture to exclude TB, fungi and other infectious agents.
- Ophthalmologic evaluation especially with slit-lamp.
- Full biochemical evaluation including serum calcium and 24-hour urinary calcium.
- Relevant tests as clinically appropriate to exclude other extrapulmonary disease.

Follow-up
- Especially in the first 2 years from presentation.
- Close monitoring for resolution or progression of disease and for new organ development.
  - 3–4-monthly checks with blood/urine tests and lung function.

if no change in symptoms or decline in lung function, CXR should be repeated within 6 months.
  Where possible repeat HRCT scan within 18 months.
- Referral to subspecialists if disease progression or new organ involvement.
- Multidisciplinary approach.

> **AUTHOR'S TIPS**
> - Serum ACE levels are elevated in 2/3 patients with sarcoidosis.
> - 5% patients have false –positive tests seen in a variety of conditions including asbestosis, silicosis, berylliosis, fungal infections, granulomatous hepatitis, hypersensitivity pneumonitis, leprosy, lymphoma and tuberculosis.

> **AUTHOR'S TIPS**
> - For young patients presenting with hilar/mediastinal lymphadenopathy, it is important that lymphoma and TB is excluded by mediastinoscopy and biopsy; if a biopsy is not performed at presentation, to follow these patients in their first year; then if clinical picture changes → early alert for biopsy.
> - Endobronchial biopsies can provide diagnosis in ~ 40% patients especially when there is characteristic visible cobblestone appearance.

> **AUTHOR'S TIPS**
> - Because of sarcoid centrilobular distribution, unlike IIPs; TBBs have a high diagnostic yield in pulmonary sarcoidosis (~4 biopsies are necessary for stage II disease).
> - TBB is also useful in diagnosing other granulomatous disease, metastatic disease, infections, pulmonary alveolar proteinosis and eosinophilic pneumonias.
> - Endobronchial biopsies can provide diagnosis in ~ 40% patients especially when there is characteristic visible cobblestone appearence.

Further reading
Costabel U, Hunninghake GW. ATS/ERS/WASOG statement on sarcoidosis. *Eur Respir J* 1999; **14**: 735–737.
Grutters JC, van den Bosch JMM. Corticosteroid treatment in sarcoidosis. *Eur Respir J* 2006; **28**: 627–636.
Newman LS, Rose CS, Maier LA. Sarcoidosis. *N Eng J Med* 1997; **336**: 1224–1234.
Paramothayan NS, Lasserson TJ, Jones PW. Corticosteroids for pulmonary sarcoidosis (review). *Cochrane database of systematic reviews* 2005.
Paramothayan NS, Lasserson TJ, Walters EH. Immunosuppressive (and cytotoxic) therapy for pulmonary sarcoidosis (review)). *Cochrane database of systematic reviews* 2005.

7.10 Pulmonary manifestations of connective tissue disorders

Connective tissue disorders (CTDs) by definition can affect any organ system including the lung. This chapter deals mainly with specific lung complications but it is critical to remember lung problems that are not CTD specific but may be more common in these subjects e.g. infection, COPD, bronchiectasis.

> **AUTHOR'S TIP**
> CTD patients can have COPD, bronchiectasis, community acquired pneumonia, ischaemic heard disease, and heart failure: *consider* but *do not assume* a specific CTD-related diagnosis in a breathless patient.

Non-CTD specific diagnosis

- *Smoking related lung disease.* Some CTD conditions such as rheumatoid disease can lead to significant physical limitation and discomfort. Smoking is common in these patients and COPD may present late due to physical inactivity. A typical presentation is following joint replacement when the cardiorespiratory system suddenly becomes the limiting factor.
- *Infection.* Many forms of CTD lead to relative immunocompromise either due to the condition itself e.g lymphopenia in SLE (systemic lupus erythematosus) or therapies used. If therapies are overtly cytotoxic this will be obvious but small doses of steroids in an elderly patients can be overlooked as a cause of either recurrent or opportunistic infection. Treatments are described in Chapter 9.1.
- *Bronchiectasis.* This may occur in many forms of CTD at least in part related factors described above. It is particularly a problem in RA and Sjogren's disease. Treatment is described in Chapter 10.2 with the additional recognition of potential relative immunocompromise.
- *Pleural effusion.* This is most commonly associated with rheumatoid disease. It may resolve with systemic treatment but may be an isolated presentation. Specific treatment is discussed in Chapter 14.8.

CTD: specific diagnosis

CTDs differ in the frequency with which specific lung complications occur. Certain common principles apply in terms of investigation and diagnosis, especially where ILD is concerned.

- Many of the principles described in other chapters for the general management of the ILD also apply to connective tissue disease associated ILD in particular relating to lymphocytic interstitial pneumonia (Chapter 7.6) and obliterative bronchiolitis (Chapter 7.7)
- Rheumatoid arthritis is the commonest of the CTDs to be associated with ILD, but data on treatment are limited.
- Systemic sclerosis (SSc) is much less prevalent than rheumatoid arthritis but is more commonly complicated by ILD and the evidence base is much more extensive.
- Not all the recent advances in understanding of the natural history of the IIPs can be extrapolated to their CTD-associated counterparts.

Presentation

Patients typically present with breathlessness and/or cough. Greater awareness of the pulmonary complications of CTD in the rheumatology field has led to an increase in presentation of asymptomatic patients with clinical findings e.g. basal crepitations.

Investigations

- FBC and differential. Anaemia, neutropenia or lymphopenia can be key issues in breathlessness or infection.
- Physiology. Lung volumes and gas transfer are essential. 6MWT and exercise oximetry both for monitoring change and particularly in cases of disproportionate breathlessness. In cases where any clinical suggestion of muscle weakness, then lying and standing VC and inspiratory and expiratory mouth pressures should be undertaken.
- Radiology. CXR may be normal. HRCT and diaphragm screening may be useful.
- ECG and echocardiography. Evidence of right heart abnormalities on ECG should be promptly followed with echocardiography. Evidence of pulmonary hypertension should be followed up promptly as described in Chapter 12.2.

HRCT and histological findings in CTD-associated ILD

- The histological entities of the ATS/ERS classification for IIP can all be associated with the connective tissue diseases.
- The prevalence of individual histological patterns differs strikingly between CTD and non-CTD related IIP.

> **AUTHOR'S TIP**
> The range of HRCT appearances from ground glass to reticular does not translate into corresponding differences in outcome in SSc and is unproven in other CTDs.

- In the only large study of lung histology in SSc, there was a high prevalence of NSIP (62/80, 75%) and a very low prevalence of UIP (6/80, 8%). The HRCT features of lung disease in SSc can range from predominant ground-glass attenuation to a predominant reticular pattern and are broadly similar to the range seen in idiopathic NSIP. Coarse reticulation and honeycombing are more unusual.
- Overall outcome differs little between UIP and NSIP in SSc, even after adjustment for baseline disease severity
- UIP in SSc has a better outcome than IPF, perhaps reflecting a lower profusion of fibroblastic foci in UIP in CTD in general or earlier diagnosis of the lung disease.
- NSIP is the predominant histological diagnosis in CTDs, with the possible exception of RA,
- HRCT reflects this to some extent but there tend to be particular HRCT profiles associated with specific CTD.
- Other than for SSc, data on treatment outcomes in relation to HRCT pattern have yet to emerge in suitably large series.

Management principles

No formal placebo-controlled trial has been performed in lung disease in CTD current management is based on anecdotal and inconclusive retrospective data. The decision to treat must be largely based on the likelihood, in individual patients, that the risk of therapy (drug toxicity) will be outweighed by the benefit (protection against progression of disease). Apart from a minority of patients with predominantly HRCT inflammatory appearances, therapy is aimed at slowing or preventing progression, rather than in the hope of a striking short term response. Early lung involvement in PM/DM is an important exception to this rule (see below)

Treatment issues, including the question of which patients to treat and the selection of therapeutic agent, have been most widely explored in SSc, perhaps because IIP is most prevalent in that disease. In SSc, the threshold for introducing treatment is reduced when:

- The duration of systemic disease is short (<4 years), indicating a higher risk of progression of lung disease
- Disease is severe, as judged by pulmonary function tests and the extent of fibrosis on HRCT. TLCO provides a stronger prediction of mortality and correlates better with the extent of disease on HRCT than other lung function variables.
- There is evidence of recent deterioration, as judged by symptomatic worsening and/or, a decline in serial pulmonary function tests. Ongoing deterioration in treated patients is more predictive of mortality than any clinical feature at presentation.
- HRCT appearances are strongly suggestive of predominantly inflammatory disease (seen in a minority of cases)
- BAL remains contentious, with opposing views that a BAL neutrophilia identifies greater risk of progression or merely greater disease severity at the time of sampling.
- In the absence of a strong evidence base, these broad considerations may be applied to other CTD.

Treatment in SSC

- Outcome in the IIP of SSc is substantially better than outcome in IPF, after adjustment for baseline disease severity. Complete remission as judged by serial HRCT is rare. Even with aggressive therapy, severe interstitial fibrosis remains a major poor prognostic feature.
- High dose corticosteroid should not be used as it is associated with renal crises.
- Current treatment recommendations (initial low dose corticosteroid therapy (e.g prednisolone 10mg daily) and an immunosuppressive agent, usually oral cyclophosphamide (1.0–1.5mg/kg)) are based on open observational data and retrospective comparisons of serial clinical data between treated and untreated. In a recent large multicentre study in SSc-associated IIP (relatively mild disease) the difference in lung function, whilst statistically significant was modest and given the potential long term toxicity, does not justify the routine use of oral cyclosphamide in unselected patients with SSc.
- Pulsed intravenous cyclophosphamide (500–1000mg at dose intervals of 2–4 weeks) has been evaluated and open therapy was associated with evidence of partial regression of IIP, based upon serial PFT or HRCT and treatment was well-tolerated. Placebo-controlled trials comparing oral with IV cyclophosphamide are awaited.

- Other immunosuppressive agents such as azothiaprine have been used but data are limited.

Treatment in RA

- There is an extreme paucity of data for the management of IIP in RA.
- IIP in RA may result from the disease itself or as a consequence of its treatment e.g. methotrexate (MTX)-induced pneumonitis, the two sometimes being indistinguishable. A smoking history of >25 pack years increases risk.
- Current treatment recommendations are based on anecdote.
- Oral prednisolone 0.5mg/kg/day for 1–3 months, weaned to 10mg/day or 20mg/alternate days if there is improvement.
- Immunosuppressant treatment such as cyclophosphamide, azathioprine, D-penicillamine, MTX and cyclosporin-A have been used in cases of treatment failure or progression.
- Anti-tumour necrosis factor (TNF)-alpha therapy has been reported to induce both both benefit and exacerbation of RA-associated IIP.
- Cyclophosphamide can also be useful for the treatment of MTX-induced pneumonitis, which has not responded to the usual management of MTX withdrawal, oxygen therapy and/or corticosteroids.
- Cryptogenic organising pneumonia (COP) in RA is highly likely to respond to corticosteroids.

Treatment in PM/DM

- Acute fulminant disease may require high-dose IV methylprednisolone (1.0g daily for 3 days)
- Less severe disease oral prednisolone 0.75–1.0mg/kg per day (or equivalent) followed by gradual weaning.
- In patients with a suboptimal response or adverse effects from corticosteroids, consideration should be given to second-line therapies with either immunosuppressant or cytotoxic agents as described for RA.
- Prognosis is good with early treatment. Short-term improvement is seen in greater than 90%. Patients with elevated CK levels have a 3-fold better response. In the longer term, response rates are resolution occurs in >70% and is reflected in long term survival.

CTD- associated pulmonary hypertension

Pulmonary hypertension had been most intensively studied in SSc where its relationship to the underlying CTD as a lone pulmonary vasculopathy has been recognised. This has led to clear cut investigation (including annual echocardiography) and treatment pathways as described in Chapter 12.2.

The advances in understanding of PHT in SSc cannot necessarily be extrapolated to other CTDs. The presence of pulmonary hypertension in other CTDs, often in the presence of other pulmonary pathology, e.g. COPD, IIP is not well characterised. Conventional treatment of associated lung pathology and correction of hypoxaemia must be undertaken as initial steps and may correct 'simple' hypoxaemic pulmonary vasoconstriction. Further investigation and management can be considered as described in Chapter 12.2.

CTD-associated muscle weakness

Muscle weakness of the respiratory muscles and diaphragm alone can lead to breathlessness without any intrinsic lung involvement and are most common in PM/DM.

A number of the CTDs can lead to isolated uni or bilateral diaphragm palsy whether directly or due to phrenic nerve palsy (Fig. 7.10.1)

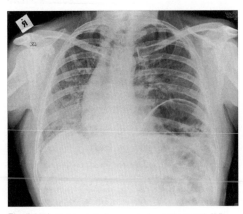

Fig. 7.10.1 Unilateral diaphragm palsy in a patients with SLE.

SLE is the characteristic condition in which 'shrinking lung' occurs and controversy continues as to whether this is due to a combination of muscle weakness and resultant underlying lung disease or intrinsic lung pathology/microembolic phenomenon.

Treatment is of the underlying CTD and recovery can occur. Diaphramatic pacing has been relatively unsuccessful.

Further reading

Pulmonary Manifestations of Systemic disease 2005; **10**: Monograph 34. *Thorax* 2008, DPLD guidelines in press.

7.11 Pulmonary manifestations of systemic diseases

Overview

Many systemic diseases can present with symptoms and signs of lung involvement. Pulmonary manifestations may also develop during the course of a large number of long term conditions. However, lung disease is common and its association with systemic disease may be casual rather than causal. Occasionally, lung disease may arise as a complication of treatment.

This chapter will give an account of pulmonary manifestations of systemic diseases not considered elsewhere in this handbook – gastroenterological, liver, endocrine, renal, haematological, cardiac and neurological diseases.

Gastroenterological diseases

Upper airway and oesophagus

Pharyngeal pouch and abnormalities of the upper airway
Post-deglutition aspiration occurs in the majority of larger pouches but is uncommon in small pouches. Video-fluoroscopy allows assessment of significant aspiration – an overlooked cause of recurrent pneumonia for which surgery is occasionally needed (Fig. 7.11.1). Tracheo-oesophageal fistula is a rare but important cause of recurrent aspiration pneumonia.

Investigation

Contrast swallow radiography

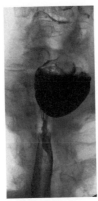

Fig. 7.11.1 A frontal projection from a contrast swallow examination shows a large contrast medium filled pharyngeal pouch in its characteristic location. There is no aspiration of contrast medium into the trachea

Gastro-oesophageal reflux (GORD)

GORD is common, affecting up to one third of people, in the presence and absence of hiatus hernia. The role of GORD in cough and asthma is reviewed in the relevant sections (see Chapters 4 and 5). GORD and recurrent aspiration is seen in oesophageal dysmotility in scleroderma or in neurological disorders such as motor neuron disease (MND) and multiple sclerosis. Ambulatory oesophageal pH monitoring and endoscopy have a relatively poor sensitivity and a therapeutic trial of proton-pump inhibitors is considered to be a reasonable initial diagnostic step. Aspiration is a significant risk factor for pneumonia in the intensive care environment (Fig 7.11.2).

Investigation
Chest radiography

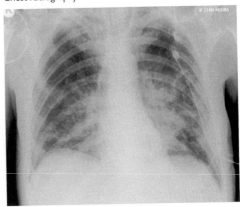

Fig. 7.11.2 Chest radiograph in a critical care patient performed following an acute respiratory deterioration shows extensive bilateral consolidation. This is most marked in the perihilar regions and lower zones corresponding to the most dependent portions of the lungs (apical and posterior segments of the lower lobes)

Pancreatitis

Acute pancreatitis is associated with acute lung injury, pneumonitis and hypoxaemia that may develop into ARDS. Patients with pancreatitis may have pleural effusion which is more commonly left sided. A grossly raised pleural fluid amylase is diagnostic. Pleural effusion is associated with poor prognosis.

Inflammatory bowel disease

One-third of patients with inflammatory bowel disease have significant extra-colonic manifestations. Pulmonary manifestations are being increasingly recognised as an important accompaniment of inflammatory bowel disease with as many as two thirds of patients having at least one respiratory symptom. Minor abnormalities in lung function are common and bronchial hyper-responsiveness occurs in 40% patients. Lung disease is usually related to disease activity and may affect any part of the lungs. It may develop years after the onset of bowel disease.

Tracheo-bronchitis and airway hyperresponsiveness

Changes in inflammatory and pro-inflammatory mediators in the airway, coupled with alteration in vascular permeability have confirmed that the lung is a target organ in inflammatory bowel disease. Cough and wheeze and occasionally large airway ulceration/mass can be presenting symptoms of Crohn's disease and ulcerative colitis.

Bronchiectatasis

The observation of bronchiectasis developing a short interval after colectomy for inflammatory bowel disease has led to further research and understanding of this important association (Fig. 7.11.3; see Chapter 11).

Investigations
Lung function
- Airways obstruction (including small airways obstruction).
- Air-trapping.
- Reduction in transfer factor.

CT radiography
- Air-trapping.
- 'Ground glass' appearance, indicating alveolitis.
- Obliterative bronchiolitis.
- Bronchiectasis.

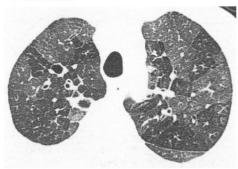

Fig. 7.11.3 Expiratory image of HRCT in a patient with ulcerative colitis shows widespread bronchiectasis with air trapping in keeping with small airways obstruction.

> **AUTHOR'S TIP**
> Early recognition of lung involvement in bronchiectasis is important as the disease is often strikingly steroid-responsive in early stages.

Treatment and complications
Aminosalicylates
Aminosalicylates such as sulphasalazine may be associated with a pneumonitis that can progress to pulmonary fibrosis. Peripheral blood eosinophilia is seen in 50% cases. The chest radiogarph may show pulmonary infiltrates.

Anti-TNF 2 alpha treatment
Humanised monoclonal antibodies against tumour necrosis factor (TNF) 2 alpha are effective in the treatment of Crohn's disease. Anti-TNF 2 alpha treatment is associated with a 4-fold increased risk of reactivation of tuberculosis, the majority of cases presenting within 12 weeks of starting therapy. Patients should be assessed for risk and for the presence of latent tuberculosis before starting treatment, in accordance with British Thoracic Society guidelines.

Liver diseases
Overview
Patients with liver disease are more susceptible to respiratory infection, particularly pneumococcus.

Unexplained refractory hypoxaemia and impaired lung function is commonly seen in advanced liver disease. Characteristically, lung function will show a substantially reduced transfer factor for carbon monoxide. Significant impairment of lung function is often asymptomatic but can present management difficulties when patients are considered for transplantation.

Pulmonary arterio-venous malformations – the hepatopulmonary syndrome
Multiple microscopic (and occasionally macroscopic) shunts occur between the small pre-capillary pulmonary arteries and veins in about 20% patients. The explanation for this vascular remodelling is not fully understood but may involve the local overproduction of nitric oxide. Hepatopulmonary syndrome is associated with substantially increased mortality.

Symptoms and signs
- Finger clubbing/signs of severe liver disease.
- Cyanosis can reflect severe hypoxaemia.
- Normal breath sounds.

Investigation
Lung function
- Reduced SpO$_2$.
- Reduced gas transfer (with normal spirometry and lung volumes).
- Demonstrable right-to-left shunt.

Chest radiography
A diffusely abnormal chest radiograph is seen in approximately 50% cases.

Porto-pulmonary shunting
In severe portal hypertension anastomoses may develop between the portal and pulmonary circulation.

Pulmonary hypertension
Rarely, severe pulmonary hypertension complicates cirrhosis of the liver.

Pleural effusion
Pleural effusion is a common consequence of hypoalbumeniaemia. Communications between the peritoneal and pleural cavities may account for pleural effusions seen patients with ascites.

Fulminant hepatic failure and ARDS
Fulminant hepatic failure is associated with failure of all functions of the liver with impairment of synthetic function leading to hypoalbuminaemia, coagulopathy and the hepatorenal syndrome. Fulminant hepatic failure causes changes to the permeability of the alveolar-capillary network leading to increased lung water, pulmonary oedema and ARDS.

> **AUTHOR'S TIPS**
> - Hypoxaemia is common in liver disease – full lung function testing should be performed in all patients with significant liver disease. An unexplained isolated reduction in transfer factor is likely to reflect pulmonary micro-arteriovenous shunting.
> - Consider occult respiratory infection as a precipitating factor in fulminant hepatic failure – CT scan of the lung may be highly informative.

Endocrine diseases
Obesity
Breathlessness is a common symptom in obesity and insulin resistance. This is due to several factors – reduced lung function, reduced aerobic capacity and impaired respiratory muscle and diaphragmatic function. Waist circumference may be a better predictor of reduction in lung function than body mass index.

Investigation
Lung function
Mild obesity:
- Reduced FEV$_1$.
- Reduced VC.
- Reduced static lung volumes.

Severe obesity:
- Reduced FEV_1.
- Reduced VC.
- Reduced transfer factor.
- Obstructive sleep apnoea.
- Type 2 respiratory failure.

Weight reduction is associated with a reduction in self assessed breathlessness and improved 6MWT.

Diabetes mellitus

Diabetes mellitus is associated with minor abnormalities of ventilatory control and lung function. Diabetic alveolar microangiopathy and respiratory autonomic neuropathy are both well recognised. With the exception of gross hyperventilation (Kussmaul's respiration) – a feature of diabetic ketoacidosis – pulmonary involvement in diabetes is almost always sub-clinical and is rarely the presenting complaint.

Better understanding of the natural history and pathophysiology of diabetic alveolar microangiopathy is of relevance to the emerging use of inhaled insulin.

Thyroid disease

Breathlessness, a common symptom in hyperthyroidism, may result from increased central respiratory drive. Respiratory muscle weakness is due to the metabolic effect of hyperthyroidism on the diaphragm and other respiratory muscles. These features all reverse with treatment.

Large thyroid goitre can cause progressive breathlessness (and occasionally stridor) due to tracheal displacement and compression. Tracheal compression is usually extrathoracic but may also extend into the thorax. Thyroid goitre may be a major factor in obstructive sleep apnoea with occasionally dramatic response to thyroidectomy.

Symptoms and signs

- Thyroid goitre ? extending retrosternally.
- Tracheal displacement.
- Stridor.

Investigation

Lung function

- Airflow obstruction.
- Proportionately a larger reduction in PEF than FEV_1.
- Characteristic flow-volume loop.
- Abnormal sleep study.

Chest radiography

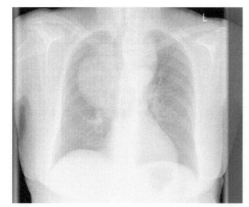

Fig. 7.11.4 Chest radiograph demonstrates a large superior mediastinal mass extending to both sides of the midline and deviating the trachea but not compromising its lumen.

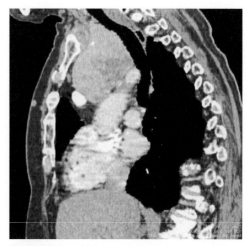

Fig. 7.11.5 Saggital CT reconstruction confirms the anterior mediastinal location and contiguity with the thyroid gland in the neck. The appearance is typical of a large thyroid goitre.

> **AUTHOR'S TIP**
> Consider thyroid disease and goitre in patients with unexplained breathlessness or obstructive sleep aponea.

Acromegaly

Patients with acromegaly have a 3-fold increased mortality and respiratory conditions are thought to account for around 25% of this increased risk.

Symptoms and signs

- Nasal polyps.
- Voice changes.
- Obstructive sleep apnoea syndrome (>50% patients with acromegaly).
- Pneumomegaly – an increase in the number of alveoli.

Renal diseases

Peritoneal dialysis

The incidence of hydrothorax, or pleural leak, in peritoneal dialysis is unclear. Acute hydrothorax leading to a massive pleural effusion is rare – a high sugar level in the effusion can be used to confirm that the pleural fluid is dialysate.

Peritoneal dialysis affects intravascular volumes and will alter lung mechanics. All patients undergoing dialysis may experience changes in lung water, that may occasionally present as flash pulmonary oedema – the accumulation of fluid into the pulmonary interstitium over a matter of minutes or hours.

Investigation

Lung function

- Reduced FEV_1 and FVC.
- Reduced transfer factor, that may persist after renal transplant.

Renal artery stenosis

May present as flash pulmonary oedema.

Chronic anaemia

Breathlessness in chronic renal failure is common and partly accounted for by chronic anaemia, which reduces the oxygen carrying capacity of blood and will limit tissue oxygen delivery. Erythropoietin improves self-assessed breathlessness and exercise capacity.

Haematological disorders

Lymphoma

The lung parenchyma may be involved in approximately 10% patients with lymphoma at presentation and approximately 30% have lung involvement at some stage. Hodgkin's disease can occasionally present with discrete masses in the lung in the absence of generalised lymphadenopathy. The major differential diagnosis is often opportunistic infection, diffuse alveolar haemorrhage or drug reaction. Pleural effusions occur in approximately 30% patients with lymphoma and, again, the major differential diagnosis is infection.

Hilar and mediastinal lymphadenopathy is common. Occasionally, giant mediastinal lymph nodes compress or invade larger airways with progressive breathlessness and the development of stridor. Emergency airway management with careful intubation may be required. The use of the very low density gas helium mixed with oxygen – given alone or in association with non-invasive ventilation – can be life-saving, by reducing the work of breathing. Mediastinal lymphadenopathy can compress the great veins, producing superior vena cava syndrome.

Investigation

CT radiography

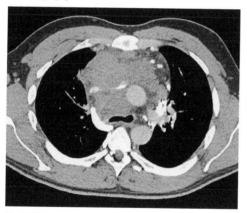

Fig. 7.11.6 CT image at the level of the carina shows extensive medistinal lymphadenopathy with encasement of the ascending aorta and superior vena cava with narrowing of both main bronchi.

Leukaemia

Leukaemic pulmonary infiltrates may occur which may be alveolar, interstitial, peribronchial or perivascular. Occult pulmonary haemorrhage can also occur. Opportunistic infection is the major important differential diagnosis, with aspergillus and cytomegalovirus amongst the most common infective agents. *Pneumocystis carinii* is uncommon if the patient has received correct prophylaxis.

Lung biopsy may be valuable in distinguishing non specific lung injury due to pulmonary toxic chemotherapy, infection, obliterative bronchiolitis or leukaemic infiltrates.

Bone marrow transplantation

Early non-infectious complications typically include:
• Pulmonary oedema.
• Upper airway complications.
• Diffuse alveolar haemorrhage.
• Pleural effusion.

Late non-infectious complications:
• Bronchiolitis obliterans.
• Graft versus host disease.
• Radiation induced lung injury.

Drugs

The lung has a susceptibility to injury with a large number of chemotherapeutic agents. Bleomycin and busulphan are amongst the more common.

Bleomycin causes severe lung disease early after treatment - 10% patients who have received 500mg of bleomycin or more will develop fatal pulmonary fibrosis. Pulmonary toxicity is rare below a cummulative dose of 150mg.

Busulphan, the first cytotoxic drug to be linked with pulmonary toxicity, causes hyperplasia of the type 2 pneumocyte. Chronic exposure, particularly when combined with other cytotoxic drugs, is associated with the development of pulmonary fibrosis.

Cardiac diseases

Lung water is increased if left atrial pressure is greater than plasma oncotic pressure. Increased lung water manifests as acute or chronic pulmonary oedema, peri-bronchial fluid or as transudative pleural effusion, which may be unilateral. Acute elevation in left atrial pressure can also be associated with pulmonary haemorrhage and significant haemoptysis.

Chronic elevation of left atrial pressure, as seen in mitral valve disease or refractory left ventricular failure, produces a chronic elevation of pulmonary venous pressure and remodelling of the pulmonary vasculature. This is best seen in mitral stenosis where lung function abnormalities are:
• Reduced FEV_1.
• Reduced VC.
• Reduced transfer factor.
• Bronchial hyperresponsiveness.

Amiodarone

Amiodarone, used in the treatment of both supraventricular and ventricular arythmias is recognised cause of drug-induced lung disease, Amiodarone-induced lung toxicity is usually seen in patients who have received larger doses (>200mg/day) over prolonged periods. Approximately 6% of patients taking more than 400mg amiodarone for 2 months or more will develop pulmonary toxicty. The mechanism is both immunologically mediated and through a direct toxic effect. Symptoms are of cough, breathlessness and occasionally pleritic pain. The major differential diagnosis is worsening cardiac failure or infection. Advanced age and pre-existing lung disease are risk factors. The disease is reversible if treatment is stopped early but the long half life of amiodarone (28 days) confers slow resolution. CT appearances commonly seen include high attenuation pleural and parenchymal lesions, pleural thickenting and non-specific infiltrates. High attenuation of the liver reflects the iodine content of the drug (Fig. 7.11.7).

Investigation

CT radiography

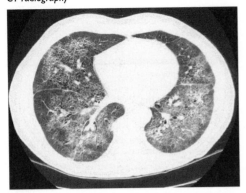

Fig. 7.11.7 HRCT image at the level of the inferior pulmonary veins in a patient with progressive breathlessness, one month following commencement of amiodarone therapy. There is extensive bilateral ground glass opacity and fine reticulation. This resolved following cessation of amiodarone and corticosteroid therapy.

Neurological diseases

Neurological disease can manifest as bulbar and laryngo-pharyngeal problems leading to aspiration pneumonia. Neurological disease also commonly affects the respiratory muscle pump – leading to hypoventilation and the development of type 2 respiratory failure.

Stroke

Following significant stroke the majority of patients will aspirate with foodstuffs when this is assessed by videofluoroscopy and in almost one half this may be silent aspiration (i.e. without choking). Tests of swallowing supplemented by videofluoroscopy are essential. Swallowing musculature is bilaterally represented in both motor cortices and many patients regain a safe swallow over a relatively short period. Dysphagia, however, confers a 7-fold increased risk of aspiration pneumonia and is an important predictor of increased mortality.

MND

MND frequently is associated with death within 5 years of diagnosis. The use of positive pressure non-invasive ventilation has been shown to improve survival and rate of decline of lung function. It may be offered to patients whose VC has fallen to below 50% of predicted value. Each individual patient will need to be involved in this decision along with the palliative care team. Ventilatory support is not suitable for all patients with MND but experience has shown that in 30% it is associated with improvement in quality of life.

> **AUTHOR'S TIPS**
> - Measurement of VC provides the best generally available bedside test for serial assessment of the respiratory muscle pump.
> - Peak expiratory flow rate (PEFR) – a test that measures flow for 0.01 seconds is a poor test of the respiratory muscle pump.

Further reading

Arguedas MR, Abrams GA, Krowka MJ, et al. Prospective evaluation of outcomes and predictors of mortality in patients with hepatopulmonary syndrome undergoing liver transplantation. *Hepatology* 2003; **37**(1): 192–197.

Dakin J, Kourteli E, Winter R. Making Sense of Lung Function. Arnold 2003.

Gaines DI, Fallon MB. Hepatopulmonary syndrome. *Liver Int* 2004; **24**(5): 397–401.

Gastro-oesophageal reflux treatment for prolonged non-specific cough in children and adults. *Cochrane Database Syst Rev* 2006; **18**(4): CD004823

Joint Tuberculosis Committee of the British Thoracic Society. Recommendations for assessing risk and for managing Mycobacterium tuberculosis infection and disease in patients due to start anti-TNF-α treatment. *Thorax* 2005; **60**: 800–805.

Kadhim AL, Sheahan P, Timon C. Management of life-threatening airway obstruction caused by benign thyroid disease. *J Laryngol Otol* 2006; **120**(12): 1038–1041. Epub 2006 Sep 25.

Mackle T, Meaney J, Timon C. Tracheoesophageal compression associated with substernal goitre. Correlation of symptoms with cross-sectional imaging findings. *J Laryngol Otol* 2007; **121**(4): 358–61.

Mahadeva R, Walsh G, Flower CD, et al. Clinical and radiological characteristics of lung disease in inflammatory bowel disease. *Eur Respir J* 2000; **15**(1): 41–48.

Poelmans J, Tack J. Extraoesophageal manifestations of gastro-oesophageal reflux. *Gut* 2005; **54**(10): 1492–1499.

Raghu MG, Wig JD, Kochhar R, et al. Lung complications in acute pancreatitis. *JOP* 2007; **8**(2): 177–185.

Infection

Chapter contents

8.1 Community-acquired pneumonia: diagnosis and clinical features

Epidemiology

Data from population studies have reported an incidence of CAP diagnosed in the community of 5–11 per 1000 adult population. The incidence of CAP requiring hospital admission has been reported at 1–4 per 1000 population. Of those admitted to hospital in the UK, around 5% are managed in a critical care setting. Mortality rates for patients treated in the community are very low (<1%) while average mortality rates for hospitalised patients range from 6–14%, rising to >30% in patients with severe CAP. Incidence and mortality rates are highest in the elderly.

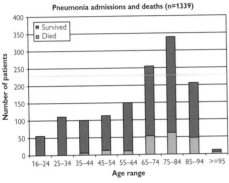

Pneumonia admissions and deaths (n=1339)

Fig. 8.1.1 Pneumonia admissions to 5 hospitals in a 1 year period.

Microbiology

Patients seen in the community (UK):

- *Streptococcus pneumoniae* (36%).
- Viruses (13%, mostly influenza A).
- *Haemophilus influenzae* (10.2%).
- *Mycoplamsa pneumoniae* (1.3%).

Patients seen in hospital (UK):

- *Streptococcus pneumoniae* (39%).
- *Chlamydophila pneumoniae* (13%).
- Viruses (12%, mostly influenza A).
- *Mycoplamsa pneumoniae* (11%).
- *Haemophilus influenzae* (5%).
- *Legionella pnemophilia* (3.6%).
- *Chlamydophila psittaci* (2.6%).

Diagnosis

A CXR is required to make a confident diagnosis of CAP. In one UK community study of adults with symptoms of a lower respiratory tract infection and focal chest signs, only 39% had CXR evidence of pneumonia.

Differential diagnosis

- Organising pneumonia.
- Bronchoalveolar cell carcinoma.
- Eosinophilic pneumonia.
- Vasculitis, e.g. Wegener's granulomatosis.
- Allergic bronchopulmonary aspergillosis.

- Pulmonary haemorrhage.
- Pulmonary embolism.
- Pulmonary oedema.

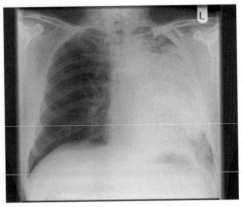

Fig. 8.1.2 Bronchoalveolar cell carcinoma presenting as extensive consolidation on CXR.

Clinical features

In the elderly, mental confusion and the lack of fever at presentation are more common than in younger patients. Pleuritic chest pain is more common in younger patients and has been associated with a good prognosis.

Unusually, patients with *Mycoplasma pneumoniae* infection may display extra-pulmonary features, e.g. erythema multiforma or other skin rashes in 25%, neurological signs in around 5%.

No combination of clinical features allows a confident prediction of the microbiological aetiology. Infection with *Mycoplasma pneumoniae*, *Legionella* spp., *Chlamydophila psittaci* or *Coxiella burnetii* generally involves younger patients.

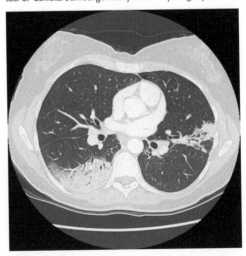

Fig. 8.1.3 Organising pneumonia presenting as consolidation.

AUTHOR'S TIP
- Hotel stay in last 14 days – *Legionella* sp infection?
- Lambing or calving season – Q fever?
- Pet bird at home – *Chlamydophila psittaci*?
- Flu-like illness initially – *Staphylococcus aureus*?
- Travel to East Asia, very ill - *Burkholderia pseudomallei*?
- Necrotising pneumonia, very ill – *Staphylococcus aureus*?
- Underlying structural lung disease – *Pseudomonas aeruginosa*?
- Cluster of cases – outbreak?

Investigations

CRP

A raised level of CRP is a more sensitive marker of pneumonia than a raised white cell count. In one study, all patients with CAP had a CRP of >50mg/l. Failure of the CRP to fall by 50% within 4 days suggests treatment failure or the development of complications.

Microbiological tests

A full range of microbiological tests should be performed on patients admitted to hospital with severe CAP. This includes:

- Blood for culture and sensitivity.
- Sputum for culture and sensitivity.
- Urine for pneumococcal antigen.
- Urine for legionella antigen.
- Blood for serological tests for *Mycoplasma pneumoniae*, *Chlamydophila* spp. *Legionella* spp. *Coxiella burnetti*.

Preferably, all samples for culture and sensitivity should be collected prior to administration of antibiotics.

In patients with non-severe CAP, the yield from routine microbiological tests including blood and sputum cultures has been found to be low (<15%). Evidence of an improvement in clinical outcome consequent on microbiological testing in patients with non-severe CAP and no co-morbid illness is lacking. Therefore, microbiological testing in non-severe CAP should be guided by patient and health resource characteristics.

AUTHOR'S TIP
Legionella and pneumococcal urinary antigen tests may remain positive for many weeks following infection.

Radiological tests

There are no features on CXR that allow a confident prediction of the microbiological aetiology. Nevertheless, certain patterns have been described:

- Multilobar involvement in bacteraemic pneumococcal infection (more commonly than in non-bacteraemic pneumococcal infection).

- Cavities, pneumatoceles, pneumothoraces in *Staph aureus* infection.
- Right upper lobe involvement with a bulging interlobar fissure in *Klebsiella pneumoniae* infection.
- Mediastinal lymphadenopathy in *Mycoplasma pneumoniae* infection.

CT scanning is more sensitive than CXR for detecting the presence of consolidation. However, the clinical significance of CT abnormalities consistent with pneumonia in patients with a normal CXR is unclear.

Complete resolution of the CXR changes of pneumonia occurred in 73% of cases at 6 weeks in one study. Resolution is generally slower in older patients, those with multilobar involvement and in legionella pneumonia.

Further reading

BTS Guidelines for the Management of Community Acquired Pneumonia in Adults. *Thorax* 2001; **56** Suppl 4: IV1–64.

Campbell SG, Marrie TJ, Anstey R, et al. The contribution of blood cultures to the clinical management of adult patients admitted to the hospital with community-acquired pneumonia: a prospective observational study. *Chest* 2003; **123**(4): 1142–50.

Jokinen C, Heiskanen L, Juvonen H, et al. Incidence of community-acquired pneumonia in the population of four municipalities in eastern Finland. *Am J Epid* 1993; **137**(9): 977–988.

Lim WS, Macfarlane JT, Boswell TC, et al. Study of community acquired pneumonia aetiology (SCAPA) in adults admitted to hospital: implications for management guidelines. *Thorax* 2001; **56**(4): 296–301.

Loeb M. Pneumonia in the elderly. *Curr Opin Infect Dis* 2004; **17**(2): 127–30.

Marston BJ, Plouffe JF, File TM, Jr., et al. Incidence of community-acquired pneumonia requiring hospitalization. Results of a population-based active surveillance Study in Ohio. The Community-Based Pneumonia Incidence Study Group. *Archives of Internal Medicine* 1997; **157**(15): 1709–1718.

Mittl RL, Jr., Schwab RJ, Duchin JS, et al. Radiographic resolution of community-acquired pneumonia. *Am J Respir Crit Care Med* 1994; **149**(3 Pt 1): 630–5.

Morgan M. *Staphylococcus aureus*, Panton-Valentine leukocidin, and necrotising pneumonia. *Bmj* 2005; **331**(7520): 793–4.

Smith RP, Lipworth BJ. C-reactive protein in simple community-acquired pneumonia. *Chest* 1995; **107**(4): 1028–1031.

Woodhead MA, Macfarlane JT, McCracken JS, et al. Prospective study of the aetiology and outcome of pneumonia in the community. *Lancet* 1987; **1**(8534): 671–674.

8.1 – *continued* Community acquired pneumonia: severity assessment and antibiotic management

Severity assessment

An accurate assessment of disease severity is fundamental to the management of CAP. The 2 most widely studied and used severity assessment tools in CAP are the Pneumonia Severity Index (PSI) and the CURB65 score. Both these tools stratify patients according to risk of mortality.

The PSI requires the calculation of an index (range 70–300) from 20 parameters derived from patient demographics, clinical findings and investigations.

The practical simplicity of the CURB65 score is its main advantage over the PSI.

CURB65 score – score 1 point for each parameter present:

- Confusion (mini-mental score <8 out of 10).
- Urea > 7mmol/l.
- Respiratory rate ≥30/min.
- Blood pressure: systolic <90mmHg or diastolic ≤60mmHg.
- Age ≥ 65 years.

CURB65 score	Risk of death (%)
0	0.7
1	2.1
2	9.2
3 to 5	15 to 40

- CURB65 score 0–1: patient may be suitable for home treatment.
- CURB65 score 2: patient may require short hospital stay.
- CURB65 score of 3 or more: patient should be managed in hospital as having severe CAP.
- Clinical judgement must always be exercised in all cases.

> **AUTHOR'S TIP**
> The 3 main reasons for admission to hospital other than disease severity are:
> - social needs;
> - worsening of other co-existing illness; eg. heart failure;
> - patient's preference.

Antibiotic management

- Initial treatment of CAP is usually empirical.
- Empirical therapy is primarily directed at *Streptococcus pneumoniae*.
- Newer generation fluoroquinolones with enhanced Gram-positive action are active against both *S. pneumoniae* and the atypical pathogens.
- Fluoroquinolones have a high bioavailability when taken orally.
- Administration of the first dose of antibiotic should occur as early as possible in view of some evidence that this confers in a survival benefit in the context of CAP.

Antibiotic resistance

- Antibiotic resistance of *S. pneumoniae* is a world-wide concern. Rates are relatively low in the UK.

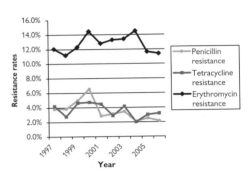

Fig. 8.1.4 Pneumococcal resistance rates to penicillin, erythromycin and tetracycline in England – data derived from invasive pneumococcal isolates from >44,000 patient episodes reported to the HPA Centre for Infections (1997 to 2006).

- Infection by *S. pneumoniae* exhibiting low to moderate levels of penicillin resistance (MIC <4mg/L) does not alter CAP outcomes provided appropriate antibiotics (ie. beta-lactams) at adequate doses are used.
- Resistance rates of *S. pneumoniae* to the tetracyclines and fluoroquinolones remain low in the UK.
- Beta-lactamase production in *Haemophilus influenzae* ranges from 2–17% in the UK.

CAP treated in the community

- Antibiotic cover for atypical pathogens (*Mycoplasma pneumoniae*, *Legionella* spp. and *Chlamydophila* spp.) has not been found to confer any clinically significant benefits except in cases of proven legionella pneumonia.
- For the majority of patients, beta-lactam based monotherapy is usually adequate (eg. amoxicillin 500 mg TDS PO).

Non-severe CAP treated in hospital

- Antibiotic cover for atypical pathogens is indicated.
- This may involve beta-lactam and macrolide combinations or monotherapy with a new generation fluoroquinolone.

Severe CAP treated in hospital

- Adequate empirical antibiotic cover against *S. pneumoniae* and *Legionella* spp. should be ensured in all patients.
- Some data indicate that in bacteraemic pneumococcal pneumonia, combination therapy (beta-lactam + macrolide) is associated with lower mortality than beta-lactam monotherapy.
- Empirical combination IV antibiotics are therefore usually indicated (e.g. beta-lactamase stable beta lactam + macrolide, or beta-lactam + fluoroquinolone).
- In selected patients, empirical therapy may need to be modified to embrace other pathogens such as MRSA, *Pseudomonas aeruginosa*, *Burkhoderia psuedomallei* etc.
- Once clinical stability is evident, antibiotics can be switched from IV to oral therapy.

Duration of antibiotic

The optimal duration of antibiotic therapy in CAP has not been established. In general, the following apply:

• Non-severe CAP: 5–7 days.
• Severe CAP: 10 days.
• *Legionella*, staphylococcal or Gram-negative enteric bacilli pneumonia: 14–21 days.

Other treatments

Steroids

• Moderate doses of steroid (hydrocortisone 300mg per day), given to patients with septic shock who do not mount an appropriate cortisol response to stimulation, have been shown in some studies to improve clinical outcome. Patients with CAP comprised a large proportion of patients studied.
• There is continued debate regarding patient selection and steroid dose.

Non-invasive ventilation (NIV)

• A randomised controlled trial demonstrated that the use of NIV in patients with severe CAP who did not require immediate intubation but who were hypoxaemic or in respiratory distress led to a 25% reduction in the need for intubation. The benefit was largely confined to the subgroup of patients with underlying COPD.
• The use of NIV has been shown to lead to a delay in intubation of some patients with CAP.
• Patients who require intubation following a long period of 'failed NIV' have poorer outcomes.

AUTHOR'S TIPS

• A trial of NIV should only be considered in severe CAP where there is a clear plan in place regarding what to do in the event of failure.
• There is no good evidence that patients without COPD benefit from NIV in the context of severe CAP.
• Clinical response to a trial of NIV should be assessed within 1 hour of NIV. If an inadequate response is observed, intubation should not be further delayed.

Further reading

Annane D, Bellissant E, Bollaert PE, et al. Corticosteroids for severe sepsis and septic shock: a systematic review and meta-analysis. *Bmj* 2004; **329**(7464): 480.

Antonelli M, Conti G, Moro ML, et al. Predictors of failure of noninvasive positive pressure ventilation in patients with acute hypoxemic respiratory failure: a multi-center study. *Intensive Care Med* 2001; **27**(11): 1718–1728.

Confalonieri M, Potena A, Carbone G, et al. Acute respiratory failure in patients with severe community-acquired pneumonia. A prospective randomized evaluation of noninvasive ventilation. *American Journal of Respiratory & Critical Care Medicine* 1999; **160** (5 Pt 1): 1585–1591.

Fine MJ, Auble TE, Yealy DM, et al. A prediction rule to identify low-risk patients with community-acquired pneumonia [see comments]. *New England Journal of Medicine* 1997; **336**(4): 243–250.

Lim WS, van der Eerden MM, Laing R, et al. Defining community acquired pneumonia severity on presentation to hospital: an international derivation and validation study. *Thorax* 2003; **58**(5): 377–382.

Marrie TJ, Wu L. Factors influencing in-hospital mortality in community-acquired pneumonia: a prospective study of patients not initially admitted to the ICU. *Chest* 2005; **127**(4): 1260–1270.

Meehan TP, Fine MJ, Krumholz HM, et al. Quality of care, process, and outcomes in elderly patients with pneumonia [see comments]. *JAMA* 1997; **278**(23): 2080–2084.

Mills GD, Oehley MR, Arrol B. Effectiveness of beta lactam antibiotics compared with antibiotics active against atypical pathogens in non-severe community acquired pneumonia: meta-analysis. *Bmj* 2005; **330**(7489): 456.

Roson B, Carratala J, Dorca J, et al. Etiology, reasons for hospitalization, risk classes, and outcomes of community-acquired pneumonia in patients hospitalized on the basis of conventional admission criteria. *Clin Infect Dis* 2001; **33**(2): 158–165.

Yu VL, Chiou CC, Feldman C, et al. An international prospective study of pneumococcal bacteremia: correlation with in vitro resistance, antibiotics administered, and clinical outcome. *Clin Infect Dis* 2003; **37**(2): 230–237.

8.1 – *continued* Community acquired pneumonia: other management issues

Time to clinical stability

Two-thirds of patients attain the following criteria for clinical stability within 3 days of hospital admission:

- temperature ≤37.8°C;
- heart rate ≤100/min;
- respiratory rate ≤24/min;
- systolic BP ≥90mmHg;
- oxygen saturation ≥ 90%;
- ability to maintain oral intake;
- normal mental status.

The median time to stability for heart rate and systolic BP is 2 days. For respiratory rate, oxygen saturation and temperature it is 3 days.

Non-resolving CAP

A lack of an adequate response to empirical therapy has been reported to occur in up to 15% of patients admitted with CAP. This is mostly evident within the first 72 hours. These patients have a longer length of hospital stay and increased mortality compared to patients who respond adequately.

The risk of treatment failure is associated with the presence on the admission CXR of:

- pleural effusions;
- multilobar involvement;
- cavitation.

Parapneumonic effusions occur in up to 57% of hospitalised patients with CAP. It is an important cause of a delay in resolution despite antibiotics.

Nosocomial infections account for a fifth of 'non-resolving CAP' and has been found to be independently associated with increased mortality.

Causes of non-resolving CAP: 'CHAOS'

- Complication – empyema; lung abscess; endocarditis; nosocomial infection particularly *Clostridium difficile* infection.
- Host – immunocompromised host.
- Antibiotic – inadequate dose; poor oral absorption; drug hypersensitivity.
- Organism – resistant organism (eg. high level (≥4mg/L) penicillin resistant *Streptococcus pneumoniae*); unexpected organism not covered by empirical antibiotics.
- Second diagnosis – pulmonary embolism; underlying cancer; organising pneumonia.

Procedures to consider in cases of delayed resolution include

- extended microbiological tests;
- CT scanning;
- pleural fluid sampling;
- bronchoscopy.

In one series of patients with 'non-responding CAP', a systematic approach including invasive techniques enabled a specific diagnosis to be made in 73%, of which over half were infectious causes.

> **AUTHOR'S TIP**
> In the elderly and those with chronic lung disease, improvement may be slower than expected.

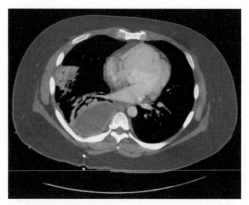

Fig. 8.1.5 Loculated parapneumonic effusion resulting in delay in resolution despite antibiotics.

Discharge from hospital

Based on the criteria for clinical stability (stated in Time to clinical stability), a prospective cohort study of 680 patients reported that in patients fulfilling all the criteria on the day of discharge, death or readmission subsequently occurred in 10.5% of patients compared to 46.2% of patients in whom ≥2 criteria were not met.

No real benefit has been found in delaying discharge by 24 hours following a switch from IV to oral antibiotics once clinical stability has been attained.

Follow up

Follow up at 6 weeks following hospital discharge is routinely practiced to:

- ensure full or on-going resolution;
- detect previously undiagnosed conditions predisposing to pneumonia, in particular lung cancer.

This practice is currently not evidence-based.

CXR at follow up

- In one study of CAP treated in the community, underlying lung cancer was detected on follow up CXR in 4% of 236 patients.
- In hospitalised patients, underlying lung cancer is usually identified during the admission episode.
- Lung cancer was detected in less than 1% of patients on follow up CXR in a study of 1011 hospitalised patients.

Prevention

Smoking is associated with an increased risk of CAP, pneumococcal bacteraemia and legionella infection. Smoking cessation advice should be offered to all current smokers.

Influenza vaccination of persons aged 65 years and above is effective in preventing respiratory illness, admission to hospital and death.

Pneumococcal polysaccharide vaccination is effective at preventing invasive pneumoncoccal disease in persons aged 65 years and above (efficacy 44–75%, decreasing with age).

- Pneumococcal polysaccharide vaccination can be safely given at the same time as influenza vaccination.
- Re-immunisation within 3 years is contraindicated due to the risk of severe reactions.
- A second dose 5 years or more later has been shown to be safe, with only slightly more local reaction compared to the first dose.
- The safety or value of a third dose has not been demonstrated.
- Currently, conjugate pneumococcal vaccines are available for children but not for adults.

Further reading

Arancibia F, Ewig S, Martinez JA, et al. Antimicrobial treatment failures in patients with community-acquired pneumonia: causes and prognostic implications. *Am J Respir Crit Care Med* 2000; **162**(1): 154–160.

Gibson SP, Weir DC, Burge PS. A prospective audit of the value of fibre optic bronchoscopy in adults admitted with community acquired pneumonia. *Respir Med* 1993; **87**(2): 105–109.

Halm EA, Fine MJ, Kapoor WN, et al. Instability on hospital discharge and the risk of adverse outcomes in patients with pneumonia. *Arch Intern Med* 2002; **162**(11): 1278–1284.

Halm EA, Fine MJ, Marrie TJ, et al. Time to clinical stability in patients hospitalized with community-acquired pneumonia: implications for practice guidelines. *JAMA* 1998; **279**(18): 1452–1457.

Jackson LA, Neuzil KM, Yu O, Benson P, et al. Effectiveness of pneumococcal polysaccharide vaccine in older adults. *N Engl J Med* 2003; **348**(18): 1747–1755.

Menendez R, Torres A, Zalacain R, et al. Risk factors of treatment failure in community acquired pneumonia: implications for disease outcome. *Thorax* 2004; **59**(11): 960–965.

Nuorti JP, Butler JC, Farley MM, et al. Cigarette smoking and invasive pneumococcal disease. Active Bacterial Core Surveillance Team [see comments]. 2000; **342**(10): 681–689.

Ramirez JA, Srinath L, Ahkee S, et al. Early-switch from intravenous to oral cephalosporins in the treatment of hospitalized patients with community-acquired pneumonia [see comments]. *Arch of Intern Med* 1995; **155**(12): 1273–1276.

Ramirez JA, Bordon J. Early switch from intravenous to oral antibiotics in hospitalized patients with bacteremic community-acquired Streptococcus pneumoniae pneumonia. *Arch Intern Med* 2001; **161**(6): 848–850.

Woodhead MA, Macfarlane JT, McCracken JS, et al. Prospective study of the aetiology and outcome of pneumonia in the community. *Lancet* 1987; **1**(8534): 671–674.

8.2 Hospital-acquired pneumonia: epidemiology and diagnosis

Definition

Hospital-acquired pneumonia (HAP) is broadly defined as pneumonia occurring 48 hours after hospital admission in the absence of any relevant symptoms or signs of infection at the time of admission.

HAP includes the 3 following subgroups:

- Ventilator-associated pneumonia (VAP)
- Health-care-associated pneumonia (HCAP)
- Hospital-acquired pneumonia in non-intubated patients.

VAP

- This is defined as pneumonia occurring more than 48 hours after endotracheal intubation.
- The vast majority of data on HAP is derived from studies of VAP.

HCAP

- The recognition of the specific subgroup of HCAP is relatively new.
- HCAP refers to pneumonia occurring in any of the following groups of patients:
  - (a) Was hospitalised in an acute care hospital for 2 or more days within 90 days of infections.
  - (b) Resided in a nursing home or long-term care facility.
  - (c) Received recent IV antibiotic therapy, chemotherapy, or wound care within the past 30 days of the current infection.
  - (d) Regularly attends a hospital or haemodialysis clinic.
- The main bulk of evidence that nursing home-acquired pneumonia (NHAP) should be managed differently from CAP arises from the United States. The only study of NHAP in the UK did not demonstrate any clinically relevant differences from CAP in the microbiological aetiologies implicated.
- Data specific to HCAP are relatively limited.

HAP in non-intubated patients

- Although this subgroup of patients is the largest, there are relatively few studies specific to this area.
- In the only prospective study using advanced methods to determine microbiological aetiology in these patients, the frequency of pathogens identified shared similarities with both CAP and VAP studies – *Streptococcus pneumoniae* was the most common pathogen identified (10% of cohort) following by *Legionella* spp. (4%), Enterobacteria (4%), *Pseudomona aeruginosa* (4%), and *Acinetobacter* spp. (4%).
- Non-intubated patients with severe HAP are often managed in an ICU. Management of these patients according to principles laid down for VAP is often appropriate.

> **AUTHOR'S TIP**
> When applying recommendations relating to 'HAP in general' to patients with 'HAP other than VAP', be aware of the patient groups from which the primary data were derived.

Epidemiology

HAP

- HAP affects 0.5 to 1.7% of patients admitted to hospital.
- It increases length of stay (LOS) by 7 to 9 days and is the most common nosocomial infection contributing to death.

- In the ICU setting, HAP accounts for 25% of all infections.

VAP

- VAP occurs in 9–27% of all intubated patients. The wide range in incidence rates reflects differences in the definition of pneumonia used to identify VAP.
- Half of all cases of VAP occur within 4 days of intubation.
- Patients with VAP have a mortality rate of 20–55%.
- VAP increases LOS by a mean of 6 days.

Diagnosis

Diagnostic criteria for HAP

The diagnosis of HAP is difficult. There are no diagnostic criteria for HAP that have both high (>90%) sensitivity and specificity.

The following criteria are offered by the 2008 British Society of Antimicrobial Chemotherapy HAP Guidelines to identify patients in whom HAP should be considered:

- New or persistent radiographic infiltrate which is unexplained.
- Fever (>38°C).
- Leucocytosis (>12 x 10^3/mm^3)/leucopenia (<4 x 10^3/mm^3).
- Purulent respiratory secretions.
- Increased oxygen requirements.

Specificity for the diagnosis of HAP may be enhanced if microbiological criteria in addition to clinical criteria are required to establish the diagnosis. Acquiring the relevant microbiological data necessitates microbiological testing (often invasive) from the time of clinical suspicion of HAP. This may lead to a delay in confirming the diagnosis and to institution of antibiotics.

The 2005 ATS/IDSA guidelines recommend that when HAP is suspected on clinical criteria, empirical antibiotics are commenced unless there is both (a) a low clinical suspicion for pneumonia and (b) negative microscopy of a lower respiratory tract sample. The diagnosis of HAP should be reviewed within 72 hours in the light of microbiological test results and the clinical response to empirical treatment.

> **AUTHOR'S TIP**
> Negative microbiology may be the due to antibiotic treatment in the preceding 72 hours. Therefore in patients who have recently received antibiotics, the suspected diagnosis of HAP cannot be refuted based on negative microbiology.

Microbiological diagnosis

- Most of the data are from VAP.
- Differentiating between colonisation and infection is difficult. Colonisation of the trachea precedes pneumonia in almost all cases of VAP.
- Quantitative cultures of lower respiratory tract samples have been used to define both pneumonia and the pathogen involved. Specialised laboratory skills are necessary.
- Different techniques (protected specimen brushing, BAL) have different thresholds for diagnosing infection (as opposed to colonisation). Diagnostic accuracy varies widely.

- Blind lavage is a simple and effective method to obtain LRT samples and to identify potential pathogens.
- Endotracheal aspirates are not recommended for the diagnosis of VAP due to low specificity.

Microbiology

In early-onset HAP (ie. occurring less than 5 days from admission), the predominant organisms implicated are:

- *Streptococcus pneumoniae*
- *Haemophilus influenzae*
- Methicillin-sensitive *Staphylococcus aureus* (MSSA)
- Antibiotic sensitive Gram-negative pathogens such as *Klebsiella pneumoniae*, *Escherichia coli*, *Enterobacter* spp., *Proteus* spp., *Serratia marcesens*.
- In late-onset HAP (occurring 5 days after admission), multi-drug resistant (MDR) pathogens are common.

Viral and fungal pathogens are uncommon as causes of HAP in immunocompetent patients.

MDR pathogens

- HAP caused by MDR pathogens is associated with increased mortality compared to pneumonia caused by non-MDR pathogens.
- Risk factors for infection by MDR pathogens in general include prior use of antibiotics, an immunocompromised state, and late-onset HAP.
- *Pseudomonas aeruginosa*, Methicillin-resistant *Staph aureus* (MRSA), *Acinetobacter baumannii* and Extended Spectrum Beta Lactamase (ESBL) producing *Klebsiella pneumoniae* are the main pathogens.
- One study found that up to 57% of patients with VAP had 'potentially resistant' pathogens. However, these figures cannot be generalised as resistance patterns vary between units.

MDR Gram-negative pathogens

- *Pseudomonas aeruginosa* is the commonest MDR pathogen in many units.
- Risk factors for acquiring *Ps aeruginosa* infection include the presence of ARDS, underlying COPD, prolonged mechanical ventilation and extended stay on ICU.
- Some isolates of *Ps aeruginosa* are susceptible only to polymyxin B (ie. resistant to aminoglycosides, cephalosporins, fluoroquinolones and antipseudomonal penicillins).
- Risk factors for *Acinetobacter* spp. infection include recent head trauma or neurosurgery, presence of ARDS and large-volume aspiration.

- *MDR Klebsiella, Serratia, Enterobacter* and *Acinetobacter* spp. often retain susceptibility to carbapenams.

MDR Gram-positive pathogens

- MRSA is an enlarging problem in many ICUs. Within ICUs in the US, MRSA is identified in up to 59% of patients with nosocomial *Staph. aureus* infection.
- Most MRSA isolates remain susceptible to vancomycin and linezolid although resistance to these antibiotics has been described.

Further reading

Baraibar J, Correa H, Mariscal D, *et al.* Risk factors for infection by Acinetobacter baumannii in intubated patients with nosocomial pneumonia. *Chest* 1997; **112**(4): 1050–4.

Craven DE. Epidemiology of ventilator-associated pneumonia. *Chest* 2000; **117**(4 Suppl 2): 186S–187S.

Chastre J, Trouillet JL. Problem pathogens (Pseudomonas aeruginosa and Acinetobacter). *Semin Respir Infect* 2000; **15**(4): 287–98.

Fabregas N, Ewig S, Torres A, *et al.* Clinical diagnosis of ventilator associated pneumonia revisited: comparative validation using immediate post-mortem lung biopsies. *Thorax* 1999; **54**(10): 867–73.

Guidelines for the management of adults with hospital acquired, ventilator-associated, and healthcare-associated pneumonia. *Am J Respir Crit Care Med* 2005; **171**(4): 388–416.

Guidelines for the management of hospital-acquired pneumonia in the UK: Report of the working Party as Hospital-Acquired Pneumonia of the British Society for Antimicrobial Chemotherapy. *JAC* 2008; **62**: 5–34.

Lim WS, Macfarlane JT. A prospective comparison of nursing home acquired pneumonia with community acquired pneumonia *Eur Respir J* 2001; **18**: 362–368.

Luna CM, Blanzaco D, Niederman MS, *et al.* Resolution of ventilator-associated pneumonia: prospective evaluation of the clinical pulmonary infection score as an early clinical predictor of outcome. *Crit Care Med* 2003; **31**(3): 676–82.

National Nosocomial Infections Surveillance (NNIS) System Report, data summary from January 1992 through June 2004, issued October 2004. *Am J Infect Control* 2004; **32**(8): 470–85.

Safdar N, Dezfulian C, Collard HR, *et al.* Clinical and economic consequences of ventilator-associated pneumonia: a systematic review. *Crit Care Med* 2005; **33**(10): 2184–93.

Sopena N, Sabria M. Multicenter study of hospital-acquired pneumonia in non-ICU patients. *Chest* 2005; **127**(1): 213–219.

8.2 – *continued* Hospital-acquired pneumonia: prevention and treatment

Prevention

How does HAP arise?

HAP to occur microbial pathogens first need to enter and then colonise the lower respiratory tract (LRT). Host defences must then be overcome before invasion and infection can ensue.

Aspiration of oropharyngeal pathogens represents the main route by which bacteria enter the LRT. Oropharyngeal colonisation by Gram-negative pathogens upon hospital admission is an independent risk factor for the development of HAP.

General strategies to prevent HAP

Most of the strategies that have been studied relate to VAP.

- Avoid intubation and mechanical ventilation. Consider non-invasive ventilation.
- In intubated patients, reduce the likelihood of aspiration of oropharyngeal pathogens by (a) maintaining endotracheal tube cuff pressures between 25–30cm water and (b) limiting the use of sedatives and paralytic agents which depress cough.
- Avoid nursing the patient in a supine position. In one RCT, the risk of HAP was decreased 3-fold when ICU patients were managed in the semi-recumbent position (30°–45°) compared to the supine position.
- Encourage oral feeding whenever possible. Enteral feeding increases the risk of aspiration of gastric contents although a clear association with HAP has not been demonstrated.
- If nutritional supplementation is required, enteral feeding carries fewer risks than parenteral feeding.

> **AUTHOR'S TIP**
> A high standard of infection control (e.g. hand washing) is as important as other measures through reducing environmental sources of infection and the transfer of pathogens between staff and patients.

Stress bleeding prophylaxis and HAP

Antihistamines and antacids are associated with an increased risk of HAP in patients managed on ICUs. Sucralfate, which does not decrease intragastric acidity nor alter gastric volume, has been associated in some trials with a lower incidence of VAP compared to antacids or antihistamines. In one large trial, sucralfate was associated with an increased risk of clinically significant gastrointestinal bleeding compared to antacids or antihistamines.

- Where stress ulcer prophylaxis is indicated, sucralfate is prefered to reduce the risk of VAP , but sucralfate should only be used in patients with low to moderate risks of bleeding.

Antibiotics and selective decontamination

The use of antibiotics for the selective decontamination of the digestive tract (SDD) has been associated with decreased rates of HAP and increased ICU survival. In ICUs with endemically high levels of antibiotic resistance,

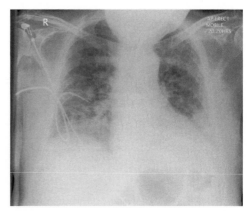

Fig. 8.2.1 MRSA pneumonia in a patient on ICU.

SDD has been less effective. Many units remain concerned regarding the selection of MDR pathogens through the routine adoption of SDD.

Antibiotic treatment: principles

- Antibiotic choices are based on the likelihood of MDR pathogens causing the episode of HAP being treated and not based on the severity of disease.
- Locally relevant microbiological data relating to (a) the range of potential pathogens and (b) antimicrobial resistance patterns are essential to guide local empirical antibiotic choices.
- A 7-day course of antibiotics is usually adequate unless the patient is not responding to treatment.

Importance of optimal empirical treatment

Inappropriate empirical antibiotic therapy in ICU patients with nosocomial pneumonia has been shown to be associated with increased mortality in various studies. This excess mortality is evident despite antibiotic switching according to microbiology results, emphasising the importance of optimal treatment *from the outset* in these already critically ill patients. Advocates of broad spectrum combination antibiotics as first-line empirical therapy, instead of second-line therapy as traditionally employed cite reasons related to:

- increasing antibiotic resistance; and
- the recognition of the importance of optimal (ie. appropriate and early) empirical therapy.

Combination therapy: effect on resistance

- Animal studies report less emergent antibiotic resistance in *Pseudomonas aeruginosa* using combination antibiotic therapy.
- There are limited data from human clinical trials demonstrating this effect.

Combination therapy: effect on efficacy

No clinical trial has demonstrated an improved prognosis with combination empirical antibiotic therapy versus monotherapy.

Antibiotic duration and emerging resistance

The emergence of MDR pathogens in the ICU is associated with the volume of antibiotics used. Optimising the duration of antibiotic treatment (and hence antibiotic volume) helps limit antibiotic resistance.

In a large prospective study of patients with VAP in 51 ICUs in France randomised to 8 versus 15 days of antibiotics:

• No significant differences were noted in (a) 28-day mortality (18.8% vs 17.2% respectively) or (b) microbiologically documented recurrent pulmonary infection (28.9% vs 26% respectively, 2.9% difference; 90% confidence interval (CI) −3.2 to 9.1).

• MDR pathogens were implicated less frequently when recurrent infection occurred (42% vs 62% respectively, p=0.038).

• In a subgroup of patients with *Pseudomonas aeruginosa* infection (a third of patients in each arm), recurrent pulmonary infection was more common in the 8-day group compared to the 15-day group (40.6% vs 25.4% respectively, p=0.09).

Which antibiotic to choose?

Early-onset HAP, no risk factors for resistance

In HAP caused by non-MDR pathogens, monotherapy with a limited spectrum antibiotic directed against the most likely pathogens is adequate:

• no prior antibiotics − consider co-amoxilas or cefuroxime;

• prior antibiotics − consider cefotamine, ceftriacene, a flurosamine or pipenacillin/tazobactam.

Late-onset HAP, risk factors for resistance

• MDR pathogens are likely to be implicated but the range of pathogens and their susceptibility patterns are highly variable.

• Antimicrobial choice should be based on local data of prevalent pathogens.

• Wherever possible antibacterial manotherapy should be used instead of combination therapy.

• In most instances, antimicrobials used should be active against *Pseudomonas aeruginosa*.

• If MRSA infection is suspected, either vancomycin or linezolid should be added.

AUTHOR'S TIPS

• Empirical antibiotic treatment should be reviewed after 48–72 hours in the light of microbiology results and patient progress. Narrow spectrum antibiotics should be used as soon as appropriate.

• Avoid using an antibiotic the patient has been exposed to recently.

• Ideally, avoid using the same class of antibiotic as other patients in the same unit.

• Individualising empirical antibiotic treatments leads to increased antibiotic heterogeneity within a unit which may in turn reduce pressure on emergent resistance within a unit.

• Linezolid has antitoxin properties as well as antibacterial properties. In comparison to vancomycin in MRSA pneumonia, it has also been shown in one analysis to offer significantly higher clinical cure rates (59% vs 35.5% respectively, p<0.01) and higher survival rates (80% v 63.5% respectively, p=0.03)

Further reading

Bonten MJ, Bergmans DC, Ambergen AW, *et al.* Risk factors for pneumonia, and colonization of respiratory tract and stomach in mechanically ventilated ICU patients. *Am J Respir Crit Care Med* 1996; **154**(5): 1339–46.

Chastre J, Wolff M, Fagon JY, *et al.* Comparison of 8 vs 15 days of antibiotic therapy for ventilator-associated pneumonia in adults: a randomized trial. *Jama* 2003; **290**(19): 2588–98.

Cook D, Guyatt G, Marshall J, *et al.* A comparison of sucralfate and ranitidine for the prevention of upper gastrointestinal bleeding in patients requiring mechanical ventilation. Canadian Critical Care Trials Group. *N Engl J Med* 1998; **338**(12): 791–7.

de Jonge E, Schultz MJ, Spanjaard L, *et al.* Effects of selective decontamination of digestive tract on mortality and acquisition of resistant bacteria in intensive care: a randomised controlled trial. *Lancet* 2003; **362**(9389): 1011–6.

Drakulovic MB, Torres A, Bauer TT, *et al.* Supine body position as a risk factor for nosocomial pneumonia in mechanically ventilated patients: a randomised trial. *Lancet* 1999; **354**(9193): 1851–8.

Driks MR, Craven DE, Celli BR, *et al.* Nosocomial pneumonia in intubated patients given sucralfate as compared with antacids or histamine type 2 blockers. The role of gastric colonization. *N Engl J Med* 1987; **317**(22): 1376–82.

Gastinne H, Wolff M, Delatour F, *et al.* A controlled trial in intensive care units of selective decontamination of the digestive tract with nonabsorbable antibiotics. The French Study Group on Selective Decontamination of the Digestive Tract. *N Engl J Med* 1992; **326**(9): 594–9.

Guidelines for the management of adults with hospital-acquired, ventilator-associated, and healthcare-associated pneumonia. *Am J Respir Crit Care Med* 2005; **171**(4): 388–416.

Neuhauser MM, Weinstein RA, Rydman R, *et al.* Antibiotic resistance among gram-negative bacilli in US intensive care units: implications for fluoroquinolone use. *Jama* 2003; **289**(7): 885–8.

Wunderink RG, Rello J, Cammarata SK, *et al.* Linezolid vs vancomycin: analysis of two double-blind studies of patients with methicillin-resistant Staphylococcus aureus nosocomial pneumonia. *Chest* 2003; **124**(5): 1789–97.

8.3 Aspiration syndromes

Definition
Aspiration is the inhalation of material into larynx, lower airways, or lungs and typically requires a defect in swallow or protective airways defences. Consequences are influenced by volume and nature of material aspirated. Not all aspiration will result in pneumonia.

Epidemiology
Incidence of aspiration pneumonia is unknown as cases classified as CAP may result from silent or unwitnessed aspiration. Estimates suggest aspiration accounts for 5–10% of CAP and up to 20% of pneumonias in care home residents.

KEY FACTS

A high index of suspicion is required in cases of community and hospital acquired pneumonia.

Diagnosis of aspiration has implications for acute treatment and management of future risk.

Pathophysiology
Radionucleotide studies have suggested that up to half of healthy adults have micro-aspiration during sleep without apparent adverse effect. Development of pathological consequences is influenced by:

- integrity of protective upper airways defences: cough reflex, mucocillary transport;
- integrity of host immune response: cellular immunity, nutritional status;
- nature and volume of material aspirated;
- extent of lung affected;
- colonisation of aspirate and bacterial virulence.

Aspiration of saliva may have significant pathological consequences as colonisation of the oropharynx by virulent bacteria is common in hospitalised or elderly institutionalised patients.

Specific factors increasing risk of aspiration
- Neurological: reduced GCS including alcohol and drug intoxication, sedating drugs and general anaesthesia; impaired swallow post stroke; motor neurone disease with bulbar involvement.
- Gastrointestinal: vomiting; gastro-oesophageal reflux; gastric distension, gastroparesis with residual volumes ≥150ml; oesophageal malignancies; upper gastrointestinal surgery.
- Mechanical: physical defences bypassed by tracheostomy or endotracheal intubation.
- Increasing age: swallowing reflex is prolonged; gastro-oesophageal junction incompetence increases.
- Bacterial virulence of oral secretions: poor oral hygiene, periodontal infections, bronchiectasis.

Diagnosis of aspiration
May be problematic when aspiration is not witnessed as presentations are varied and there is no universally applicable test to confirm diagnosis. A high index of suspicion is essential particularly in those at increased risk.

Persistent throat clearing, hoarseness and problems chewing food may be useful signs. Cough while eating or drinking is not a sensitive symptom, as it is often the lack of such protective reflexes which predisposes to aspiration. Bedside assessment of swallow as performed by speech and language therapists has high sensitivity and specificity.

Videofluoroscopy facilitates dynamic assessment as well as allowing identification of structural lesions seen with more traditional contrast swallowing studies. Technicium labelled colloids may be instilled down nasogastric (NG)/gastrostomy (PEG) feeding tubes to demonstrate reflux and aspiration. However all of these techniques are limited by the fact that aspiration may not occur consistently.

Various tests have been used to identify gastric contents in sputum: food dyes; glucose dipsticks after high sugar feeds; amylase and lipid laden macrophages. Of these methylene blue dye added to NG or PEG feeds has found most widespread use. Distinction of aspiration from mere gastro-oesophageal reflux may be difficult without bronchoscopic sampling. Mucosal oedema or erythema at bronchoscopy are further pointers to gastric aspiration.

Certain presentations should increase the suspicion of aspiration, including indolent anaerobic pneumonias, lung abscesses and recurrent pneumonias.

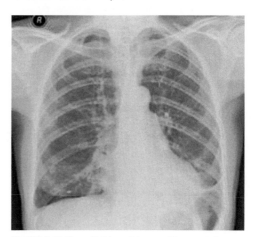

Fig. 8.3.1 Middle and left lower lobe consolidation in patient with systemic sclerosis. Videofluoroscopy demonstrated 'silent' aspiration without protective cough reflex.

Radiological distribution is in dependant parts of the lung. After the age of 15 the right main bronchus is more vertical, but until this age both lower lobes are equally affected by aspiration. If aspiration occurs when patients are recumbent, then superior segments of the lower lobes or posterior segment of upper lobes may be affected.

Aspiration pneumonias are frequently polymicrobial, reflecting the spectrum of pathogens found in oropharyngeal secretions. Anaerobic bacteria are rarely identified in sputum due to difficulties with their culture, but the presence of *Staphylococcus aureus* or Gram-negative bacilli should heighten suspicions of aspiration. *Streptococcus pneumoniae* may be present in oropharyngeal secretions, so its identification in CAP does not exclude the possibility of aspiration.

Aspiration syndromes

Aspiration may lead to various syndromes depending on the substance aspirated; whether inert, caustic, particulate or contaminated with pathogenic organisms.

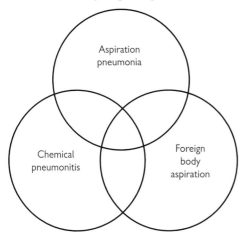

Fig. 8.3.2 Aspiration syndromes.

Distinction may be made between the inflammatory response seen with a chemical pneumonitis, the infective response to introduction of pathogens and the mechanical effect of foreign body aspiration. These processes are not mutually exclusive but represent a spectrum of lung injury and may evolve with time. Although difficult, distinction between syndromes may prompt manoeuvres to clear particulate matter from airways or permit avoidance of unnecessary antibiotics.

Chemical pneumonitis

- Aspiration of gastric contents, often witnessed and usually sterile, dispersed and rapidly neutralised.
- Gastric contents rapidly incite an inflammatory response causing atelectasis, peribronchial haemorrhage and oedema within minutes and CXR changes within 2 hours.
- Hypoxaemia exacerbated by reflex bronchospasm, impaired surfactant activity and VQ mismatch cause intrapulmonary shunting.
- Fever/leucocytosis may be present in absence of infection.
- Severity related to volume (>20 ml) and pH (<2.5).

Management

- Immediate suction of airways.
- Supportive measures including ventilatory support with high PEEP; avoidance of fluid overload.

No evidence of benefit from:

- Corticosteroids – may increase risk of secondary infection.
- Large volume lavage – as acid is promptly neutralised.
- Bronchoscopy – unless aspirate heavily contaminated with particulate matter.

Antibiotics are not mandatory. Data suggests prophylaxis does not reduce the risk of subsequent superadded bacterial infection (tends to occur after 2–5 days) and may increase selection of resistant organisms. However distinction between inflammatory response and infection is difficult so most clinicians give empirical antibiotics. These should be stopped if patient improves rapidly.

The majority of patients show prompt and complete resolution. Deterioration may be due to development of secondary infection in 25% or ARDS. Fibrosis or bronchiectasis may complicate long term recovery.

Foreign body aspiration

Consequences are influenced by size of particles, volume and composition of foreign matter aspirated. Even when not directly toxic to the lungs damage may occur through airways obstruction:

- Particles large enough to cause proximal obstruction may result in asphyxiation and rapid death (café coronary syndrome).
- Smaller particles may cause lobar/(sub)segmental collapse or atelectasis. Partial obstruction may result in gas trapping which is only visible on expiratory radiographs.
- Still smaller particles may result in formation of interstitial granulomata. These may mimic miliary tuberculosis, cause hypercalcaemia and progress to pulmonary fibrosis.
- Aspiration of vegetable or mineral oil (as in laxatives) may cause lipoid pneumonia with persistent consolidation or irregular mass lesions mimicking lung cancer.
- Large volume fluids may cause asphyxia due to laryngospasm (near drowning). Reflex bronchospasm and fleeting hypoxaemia may progress to pulmonary oedema.

Management

- Immediate airways clearance manoeuvres involving subdiaphragmatic abdominal thrusts (Heimlich) back blows or tracheal suction.
- Secondary bacterial infection may occur particularly if clearance is delayed. Recovery may be complicated by localised bronchiectasis.

Aspiration pneumonia

- Aspiration of colonised oropharyngeal and gastric secretions may result in pneumonia.
- Pneumonia may develop acutely after an infected aspiration; a secondary pneumonia may complicate inflammation or obstruction by non-infected aspirates.
- Likelihood of infection is influenced by volume aspirated and degree and virulence of bacterial contamination; more virulent pathogens require smaller aspirates.
- Less virulent organisms produce an indolent infection typified by gradual onset, non-specific systemic symptoms of malaise and weight loss, low grade fever and anaemia. CXR may show a rounded area of consolidation, demonstrate cavitation or pleural involvement at presentation.
- Misdiagnosis of lung cancer can occur, particularly if there is mediastinal lymphadenopathy, indeterminate bronchoscopic or sputum cytology, when further invasive investigation are limited by poor performance status.

KEY FACTS

- Anaerobes are difficult to culture by standard means. Their presence in aspiration pneumonias should be assumed.
- Clinical deterioration after 24–48 hours may suggest development of secondary infection. Broadening spectrum of antibiotics to cover *Staphylococcus* (MRSA) and Gram-negative bacilli should be considered.

Microbiology

- Spectrum of pathogens is wide and influenced by poor dental hygiene (so edentulous patients at less risk), previous antibiotic use and hospitalisation.
- Aspiration in hospitalised patients more frequently involves Gram-negative organisms and *Staphylococcus aureus*.
- Gastric contents rendered less acidic by proton pump inhibitors or NG feeding are at increased risk of colonisation by enteric bacilli.
- Anaerobes such as *Bacteriodes*, *Peptostreptococcus* and *Fusobacterium*, though difficult to culture, are thought to be implicated in over half of cases of aspiration pneumonia. These are more likely when there is foul sputum, parenchymal necrosis and abscess formation.

Management

- Antibiotics; choice influenced by probable spectrum of pathogens and risk of antibiotic resistance.
- Historically, high-dose penicillin had good activity against anaerobes, but resistant organisms are increasingly seen, hence combination with beta-lactamase inhibitors (e.g. co-amoxyclav).
- Metrondazole has activity against certain anaerobes, but should not be used as monotherapy because of its lack of activity against microaerophilic streptococci.
- Clindamycin has rapid action and low failure rates. Its use is limited by frequency of development of *Clostridium difficile* diarrhoea particularly in the aspiration-prone elderly.
- Newer quinolones (levofloxacin, moxifloxacin) currently still have broad spectrum including good anaerobic cover. Restricted use of chloramphenicol due to risk of serious haematological side effects is likely to help maintain bacterial sensitivity to this potent antibiotic.
- The increasing prevalence of MSRA and pseudomonas in hospital acquired aspiration requires further extension of antibiotic coverage. Combination therapy is increasingly appropriate.
- Optimum duration is unclear – typically 7–10 days is used, but longer courses needed for more aggressive pathogens or complications such as lung abscess or empyema.

KEY FACT

Enteral feeding offers many advantages but does not protect against aspiration of oral secretions

---

Prevention

- Education and counselling of patient and carers is essential.
- Foreign body aspiration is a leading cause of accidental death of infants in the home; restricting access to such items is key. Diagnosis can be difficult if the inhaled object is not radio-opaque.

- Body position: elevation of head of bed, ensuring sitting position while feeding and for 2 hours subsequently.
- Compensatory feeding strategies and training in chewing and swallowing manoeuvres to modify risk. Liquid thickeners reduce risk in those with neurogenic aspiration.
- Minimise sedation and optimise anti-epileptic medications
- Enteral tube feeding is often used to reduce risk of aspiration, but feed can still be aspirated if gastro-oesophageal reflux occurs. More importantly it offers no protection against aspiration of oropharyngeal secretions.
- NG tube position should be regularly reassessed. Gastric residual should be checked during feeding (4-hourly with rate reduced if residual >50ml).
- NG tubes impair lower oesophageal sphincter (LOS) function. Prokinetics (e.g. metoclopramide) stimulate gastric emptying and increase LOS tone. Despite theoretical benefits, trials have not shown clinical advantage of continuous over bolus feeding, of jejunal over gastric feeding, or of small bore tubes over large.
- Oral hygiene measures: aggressive oral care, treatment of dental infections, avoidance of dehydration. There is no benefit from medications which dry up secretions such as anticholinergics and antihistamines.
- Angiotensin converting enzyme inhibitors (ACEi) inhibit breakdown of substance P causing both increase cough sensitivity (potential benefit rather than annoying side-effect) and improved swallowing reflex in the elderly. Reduced pneumonia in stroke patients treated with ACEi, suggests benefit particularly in silent aspirators.
- If aspiration is severe and persistent, laryngectomy to separate tracheobronchial tree and GI tract may be necessary.

Further reading

Johnson LJ, Hirsch CS. Aspiration pneumonia: recognising and managing a potentially growing disorder. *Postgraduate Medicine* 2003; **113**: 99–102.

Marik PE, Kaplan D. Aspiration pneumonia and dysphagia in the elderly. *Chest* 2003; **124**: 328–336.

Sasaki H, Sekizawa K, Uania M, *et al.* New Strategies for Aspiration Pneumonia. *Internal Medicine* 1997; **36**: 851–855.

8.4 Lung abscess

Epidemiology
Since the introduction of penicillin in the 1940s the incidence has declined and the prognosis has improved. There remains a subgroup of elderly and immunocompromised patients in whom there is still significant morbidity and mortality. Male predominance (2:1) with a peak incidence in the 4th and 5th decades. Incidence twice as common in immunocompromised patients.

Aetiology
This can be split into the following main groups:
- Aspiration:
  (a) impaired consciousness (excess alcohol, epilepsy, anaesthesia);
  (b) neuromuscular disease;
  (c) oesophageal pathology (stricture, hiatus hernia, achalasia).
- Bronchial obstruction (malignancy, inflammation, foreign body).
- Pneumonia (e.g. Klebsiella pneumoniae, Staphylococcus aureus).
- Blood-borne infection.
- Immunosuppressive states.

Microbiology
Most lung abscesses are polymicrobial. Historically, with aspiration being the commonest aetiological factor, anaerobic bacteria are the predominant organisms isolated.

The spectrum of aetiological agents may however be evolving. A recent study noted the presence of anaerobes in only 31% of patients, with aerobes (in particular Klebsiella pneumoniae 33%) being most common. This may be partly due to taxonomic changes, but predominantly reflects the changing patient demographics with a growing number of immunosuppressed patients.

Infectious causes of lung abscess
- Bacteria

(a) anaerobe	fusobacteria	
	Gram-negative bacilli	
	(e.g. Prevotella)	
	Gram-positive cocci	
	(e.g. Peptostreptococcus)	
(b) aerobes	Gram-negative	
	(e.g. Klebsiella, Pseudomonas)	
	Gram-positive	
	(e.g. Staphylococcus aureus)	

  (c) Legionella pneumophila
  (d) Pseudomonas pseudomallei
- Fungal Coccidioidomycosis, Mucormycosis, Sporotrichosis, Cryptococcosis, Histoplasmosis, Blastomycosis, Aspergillosis
- Amoebic.
- Mycobacteria.
- Actinomycocis/Nocardiosis.
- Echinococcosis.

Clinical features
Symptoms
Depending on the aetiology of the abscess, symptoms can vary from being very acute (abrupt, short duration) to a more insidious or chronic picture. The most common symptoms are: cough (90%), fever (83%), putrid sputum (59%), chest pain (54%), weight loss (54%), night sweats (45%), and haemoptysis (31%).

Examination
Often unhelpful. Findings may be similar to those of pneumonia or pleural effusion, with dullness to percussion and bronchial breathing if the abscess is close to the pleural surface. Clubbing is sometimes noted.

Differential diagnosis
- Neoplastic (lung cancer or metastases).
- Vasculitis (Wegener's granulomatosis).
- Rheumatoid nodule.
- Pneumoconiosis (PMF, Caplans syndrome).
- Pulmonary infarction.
- Bullae, cysts or sequestration.
- Localised saccular bronchiectasis.
- Gas fluid level in oesophagus, stomach or bowel.

Investigations
Radiology
- Plain chest radiograph usually raises the possibility of a lung abscess.
- More common in right lung (60–75% vs 25–40%)
- Involves those segments dependent in recumbency i.e. posterior segments of upper lobes and superior segments of lower lobes.
- CT scanning can aid diagnosis and differentiate between empyema and abscess.
- Abscesses typically have an irregular wall, indistinct outer margin, oval or round shape, make an acute angle with the chest wall and show no evidence of compression of the lung.
- Radiological studies of cavity behaviour reveal that 13% will be gone in 2 weeks; 44% in 4 weeks; 59% in 6 weeks; and 70% in 3 months.

Blood sampling
Raised inflammatory markers are often present with a leukocytosis. Blood cultures may be useful. If chronic, anaemia is frequently present.

Microbiological sampling
The polymicrobial nature of these infections and the variations in antimicrobial susceptibility means that knowledge of the pathogens can optimize the choice of antibiotic. However it can be difficult to obtain a reliable specimen.

Sputum sampling
- Low diagnostic accuracy.
- Contamination by normal flora in upper airways.

Transtracheal aspiration
- Old studies showed reported high accuracy (80%).
- Relied on concept of sterile bronchial tree beyond vocal cords.
- Elevated concentrations of bacteria in lower airways, without clinical signs of infection, has cast doubt on its use.

Fibreoptic bronchoscopy.
- Can rule out tumour, foreign bodies & other diagnoses.
- Underlying bronchial carcinoma (7–17.5%).
- Risks of sample contamination reduce accuracy.

Percutaneous lung aspiration
- Can be guided by Fluoroscopy, ultrasound or CT.
- High accuracy depending on modality (79–94%).
- Changes antibiotic regimen in up to 47% patients.
- Commonest complication pneumothorax (14%).

Treatment

Antibiotics

It is reasonable to proceed with empiric antibiotic therapy without prior diagnostic investigations in those patients who have a classical clinical and radiographic presentation.
- Penicillin alone probably ineffective.
- Metronidazole not effective alone (50% response).
- Clindamycin has been reported superior to penicillin.
- Beta lactam/beta lactamase inhibitor combinations are effective.
- Other options include cephalosporins, macrolides, chloramphenicol, amoxicillin/metronidazole, imipenem and antipseudomonal penicillins.
- Published experience with newer antibiotics is limited.

Patients should be treated for a period of 4–6 weeks although there have been no formal trials to support this. The final decision on duration should be made according to clinical and radiological response.

Drainage

- Antibiotic therapy and physiotherapy are mainstays of treatment for most patients.
- Many spontaneously drain during the course of therapy via communication with the tracheobronchial tree.
- Complicated abscesses may require tube drainage, and timing depends on the clinical status of the patient.

Intervention more likely to be required if:
- Large cavity (>6cm).
- Necrotising pneumonia (multiple small abscesses).
- Elderly or immunocompromised patient.
- Bronchial obstruction.
- Aerobic bacterial pneumonia.

Drainage can be achieved by:
- Bronchoscopy:
  - Debate about role.
  - Value limited by the risk of spillage of abscess contents into the unaffected bronchial tree.
- External percutaneous drainage:
  - Preferred option, surgery frequently avoided (84%), marked improvement in sepsis indicators within 48 hours of drainage.
  - Variety of imaging techniques reported (fluoroscopy, ultrasound and CT scanning).
  - Ultrasound provides more precise spatial localisation, real-time images and no radiation dose.
  - CT scanning is frequently used, provides better visualisation of intrathoracic structures and is familiar with operators.
  - Complication rate low (bronchopleural fistula, haemorrhage, empyema).

Surgery

Surgery is now seldom required in the management of lung abscess (<10%).

Suggested indications for surgery:
- haemoptysis
- malignancy
- chronicity (6–8 weeks without clear progress)
- persisting sepsis after 2 weeks despite antibiotics
- radiological signs of inadequate healing
- complications - bronchopleural fistula, empyema

Post-operative complications include empyema (10–29%) and a mortality rate (11–16%).

Outcome

- On appropriate antibiotic therapy fever usually disappears within days (4–8 days).
- Persistence beyond 2 weeks is unusual and suggests inadequate drainage.
- Conservative medical therapy proves effective in 80–90% of patients.
- Despite the introduction of modern techniques overall mortality still remains at up to 10% (compared with pre-antibiotic era of 30–40%).
- Mortality rates vary depending on the aetiology e.g. 0–2% in non-immunocompromised patients vs 8% in immunocompromised patients. AIDS patients have been reported to have mortality rates of 28% and cure rates of only 36%.

Markers of poor outcome include:
- advanced age/debilitation/malnutrition;
- HIV (and other immunosuppressive states);
- malignancy;
- large cavity size (>6cm);
- duration of symptoms > 8 weeks.

Complications

- Recurrent abscess (8%).
- Empyema (4%).
- Life threatening haemorrhage (4%).
- Embolic cerebral abscess very rare.
- Longer term complications include aspergilloma and saccular bronchiectasis.

Further reading

Davis B, Systrom DM. Lung abscess: pathogenesis, diagnosis and treatment. *Curr Clin Top Infect Dis* 1998; **18**: 252–273.

Hirshberg B, Sklair-Levi M, Nir-Paz R et al. Factors predicting mortality of patients with lung abscess. *Chest* 1999; **115**: 746–750.

Mansharamani N, Balachandran D, Delaney D et al. Lung abscess in adults: clinical comparison of immunocompromised to non-immunocompromised patients. *Resp Med* 2002; **96**: 178–185.

Mwandumba HC, Beeching NJ. Pyogenic lung infections: factors for predicting clinical outcome of lung abscess and thoracic empyema. *Curr Opin Pulm Med* 2000; **6**: 234–239.

Wang J-L, Chen K-y, Fang C-T et al. Changing bacteriology of adult community-acquired lung abscess in Taiwan: *Klebsiella pneumoniae* vs anaerobes. *Clin Infect Dis* 2005; **40**: 915–22.

Wiedemann HP, Rice TW. Lung abscess and empyema. *Sem Thor Card Surg* 1995; **7**: 119–128.

8.5 Nocardia and actinomycosis

Nocardia

Nocardia species are aerobic actinomycetes, branching beaded filamentous bacteria which usually stain weakly acid fast. Nocardiosis results from opportunistic infection due to a variety of *Nocardia* spp. Infection is limited to the skin (subcutaneous or lymphocutaneous) in about 20% of cases. More invasive disease occurs in 80%, predominantly pulmonary infection (40%), but also systemic disease with frequent cerebral abscess formation.

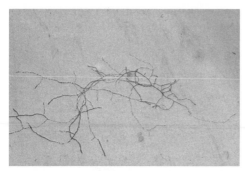

Fig. 8.5.1 Smear preparation of *Nocardia asteroides*. (See Plate 5.)

Epidemiology

Nocardia spp. are ubiquitous bacteria found in soil, water and vegetable matter. Infection usually occurs by inhalation, aspiration into the lung, direct inoculation of the skin or possibly from contaminated food via gastrointestinal tract. Hospital transmission has occurred in transplant and oncology units. Globally, the *N. asteroides* complex accounts for up to 90% of pulmonary and disseminated infections. *N. brasiliensis* is a common cause of skin mycetomas. *N. farcinica*, linked to hand transmission by anaethestists, has been associated with sternotomy wound infection. Incidence has been estimated as 500–1000 cases a year in the USA with a steady increase due to the increased number of immunocompromised individuals. Significant under-reporting is likely. Infection is three times more common in men.

History and examination

Clinical presentation varies widely and depends both on the site of infection and host response. Pulmonary nocardiosis may present as an acute pyogenic infection mimicking pneumonia or as a chronic insidious disease mimicking pulmonary tuberculosis, lung cancer or more rarely, aspergillosis and actinomycosis. Systemic infection and CNS involvement occur more frequently in those with severe immunocompromise. Infection also occurs in those with intact immunity and is usually focal such as following an inoculation injury of the skin.

> **AUTHOR'S TIP**
> *Consider nocardiosis if unexplained infiltrates/infection in:*
> - HIV infection.
> - Solid organ transplant recipients.
> - Lymphoreticular malignancy.
> - Other causes of immunocompromise – high dose corticosteroid use, alcoholism and diabetes.
> - Alveolar proteinosis.

Investigations

Imaging

Plain and CT chest imaging of pulmonary nocardiosis is protean and may show:
- Mild subtle infiltrates.
- Reticular nodular shadowing – patchy or diffuse.
- Lobar or multilobar consolidation.
- Diffuse alveolar infiltrates, especially in severe immunocompromise (HIV with CD4 <200).
- Abscess formation.
- Irregular nodules.
- Cavitary disease.
- Effusions and empyema.
- Pulmonary TB-like appearance with calcified lesions.

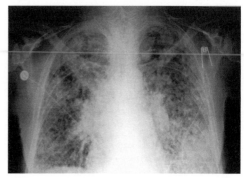

Fig. 8.5.2 CXR showing overwhelming pulmonary nocardiosis.

Microbiology

Sputum, BAL or other samples should be sent for prolonged culture. Specific molecular tests can be employed to distinguish species, particularly *N. farcinia*, a species associated with disseminated disease which may be resistant to co-trimoxazole.

Pathology

Biopsy material is usually suppurative with numerous polymorphonucleocytes, but can be granulomatous with an absence of epithelioid cells but multinucleate giant cells can be found.

Management

Patient's management must be individualised and take into account clinical presentation and *in vitro* antibiotic sensitivities. Empirical treatment prior to laboratory results should include trimethoprim-sulphamethoxazole (with a second agent in those with significant immunocompromise or systemic/ CNS involvement). Other agents include: carbapenems, amikacin, minocycline, cephalosporins or linezolid.

Prognosis

Outcome is determined by the site of infection and coexistent co-morbidity. Cutaneous infection is the most benign. Even uncomplicated pulmonary nocardiosis has a mortality of 10%. Patients with advanced immunocompromise have a worse outcome.

Key points
- Consider nocardiosis if spread to CNS or contiguous structures with soft tissue swellings or fistulas.
- Culture samples require prolonged incubation – alert laboratory if nocardiosis possible.
- Species identification in a Reference Laboratory will assist antibiotic choice.

Actinomycosis

Definition
An uncommon chronic suppurative infection caused by the genus, *Actinomyces*. These are slow-growing branching Gram-positive bacteria which form mycelia (mass of branching, thread-like hyphae) similar to fungi. Unlike *Nocardia* spp., they are not acid fast. Characteristically they invade locally, forming external sinuses which discharge sulphur granules.

Epidemiology
Actinomyces are common non-virulent oral saprophytes frequently found in association with dental infection. Spread may occur by local invasion through damaged mucosa or following surgery or trauma.

Sites of infection include:

Cervicofacial (direct invasion)	55%
Thorax (aspiration)	15%
Abdomen (ingestion)	20%
Other organs – bone, brain, skin	10%

Thoracic actinomycosis

History and examination
- Common – cough, fever, and chest pain.
- Less frequently – breathlessness, haemoptysis, weight loss, and night sweats.

Imaging
- Diagnostic triad
  - **(1)** Effusion and pleural thickening.
  - **(2)** Adjacent lung involvement.
  - **(3)** Periosteal rib involvement.
- Solid or patchy consolidation.
- Lower lobe predominance – perhaps due to aspiration.
- Mediastinum may be involved.
- May mimic lung cancer with either single lesions or bilateral ill-defined pulmonary opacities indistinguishable from lung neoplasia.

Other investigations
- Leukocytosis.
- Culture from sputum, bronchial washings or biopsy material (needs anaerobic culture).
- Histology from lung biopsy or resected lung.

Pathology
- *Actinomyces israelii* commonest cause.
- See chronic inflammatory and granulation tissue.
- Occasional multinucleate giant cells containing sulphur granules.
- Untreated disease may progress to:
  - Multiple abscesses.
  - Draining sinuses.

Management
- Penicillin is the treatment of choice but can also use ceftriaxone or a carbapenem.
- Treatment duration of 10 days with recent infections but need longer if fibrosis present. Consider co-infection.

Key points
- Despite forming mycelia, not a fungus and treated with penicillin.
- May *mimic* lung cancer or any abscess-forming organism.
- May *co-exist* with lung cancer or any abscess-forming organism.
- May see sinus formation with purulent discharge of sulphur granules.

Further reading

Beaman BL and Beaman L. Nocardia species: host-parasite relationships. *Clin Microbiol Rev.* 1994; **7**: 213–264.

CDC Division of Bacterial and Mycotic Diseases. Nocardiosis www.cdc.gov/NCIDOD/DBMD/diseaseinfo/nocardiosis_t.htm

Menendez R, Cordero PJ, Santos M. Pulmonary infection with Nocardia species: a report of 10 cases and review. *Eur Respir J* 1997; **10**: 1542–1546.

Menendez R, Cordero PJ, Santos M, *et al.* Differentiating Thoracic Actinomycosis From Lung Cancer. *Infect Med* 2000; **17**: 695-698.

Hsieh MJ, Liu HP, Chang JP, Chang CH. Thoracic actinomycosis. *Chest* 1993; **104**: 366–370.

Kwong JS, Muller NL, Godwin JD, *et al.* Thoracic actinomycosis: CT findings in eight patients. *Radiology* 1992; **183**: 189–192.

8.6 Viral infections of the respiratory tract

Despite medical advances in the control of most infectious diseases in the developed world, acute respiratory tract infections continue to impose substantial morbidity and mortality among the elderly and those with underlying chronic medical conditions.

Aetiology and epidemiology

Over 200 viruses are known to infect the respiratory tract, although many are recognised for their systemic manifestations, e.g. measles.

- 'Respiratory virus' typically refers to a pathogen whose major manifestations are respiratory in nature (Table 8.6.1).
- The number and diversity of viruses capable of infecting or re-infecting the respiratory tract explains the high incidence of community-acquired respiratory infection in all populations.
- The frequency of viral respiratory illness in populations varies by age; with highest incidence in children under 4 years of age, parents exposed to children, and the elderly.
- This age-related pattern reflects the crucial role that children play in virus transmission by acquisition of infection at school or nurseries and subsequent introduction into their homes.

Table 8.6.1 Viruses causing respiratory syndromes

Family	Species and subtype
RNA viruses	
Picornaviridae	Rhinovirus (>120 serotypes)
	Enteroviruses
Coronaviridae	Coronaviruses 229E, OC43
	SARS coronavirus
Orthomyxoviridae	Influenza A and B
Paramyxoviridae	Parainfluenza (PIV) 1–4
Metapneumoviridae	Respiratory syncytial virus A&B
	Human metapneumovirus
Bunyaviridae	Sin nombre
DNA viruses	
Adenoviridae	Adenovirus
Herpesviridae	HSV, CMV, VZV

Assessing the specific causes of acute respiratory infections is important to determine priorities for control.

However, diagnosis is challenged by

- Diversity of virus pathogens giving spectrum of clinically indistinguishable illness.
- Frequency of co-circulating pathogens.
- Difficulties in culturing certain rhinoviruses and coronaviruses.
- Relatively insensitive antigen detection assays and complement fixation tests used in serological diagnosis.
- Poor quality of diagnostic nasal samples and variable virus shedding reduces diagnostic yields.

Advances in molecular diagnostics permit rapid, specific and sensitive detection of respiratory viruses although these tests remain mainly a research tool.

Variation in specific at-risk groups

Although all respiratory viruses have the potential to cause illness there are specific features among at-risk populations.

Children

- Respiratory syncytial virus (RSV) is a common cause of broncholitis in infants and may be associated with development of asthma. Most children are infected before the age of 3 years, but immunity is incomplete and re-infection can occur later in life. Peak attack rates occur in infants aged below 6 months.
- Influenza is increasingly recognised as a significant cause of hospitalisations and attendances particularly in those aged under 12 months, whereas rhinovirus infections are frequent throughout childhood.
- Parainfluenza (PIV) is more associated with croup and laryngitis than other viruses.

Elderly

- As 30% of elderly people suffer from at least one respiratory infection per winter, even low rates of morbidity have significant impact.
- Limitations in physiological reserves, age-related decline in immune responses and chronic underlying medical conditions are associated with increased morbidity in the elderly.
- Residential or nursing homes facilitate transmission of respiratory viruses and outbreaks can be severe with high attack rates and fatality rates.
- Although influenza is responsible for considerable morbidity and mortality, RSV, PIV, and rhinoviruses are increasingly understood as causes of serious lower respiratory tract illness in aging populations.

Chronic pulmonary disease

- Acute respiratory infection is a leading cause of hospitalisation in those with underlying chronic medical conditions.
- Exacerbations of chronic airways disease have been linked to respiratory virus infections, with studies suggesting an association with up to two-thirds of exacerbations.

Immunocompromised patients

- Patients with myelosuppression, and bone marrow or solid organ transplant recipients are at risk of severe disease due to community or hospital-acquired respiratory viruses
- Disease may result from reactivation of latent adenovirus infection
- Dual pathogens are frequently identified.
- Pneumonia and death may complicate up to 80% and 50% of infections respectively, with greater morbidity for RSV and PIV than other viruses.

Seasonality of respiratory viruses

- Respiratory viruses exhibit seasonal patterns, but nosocomial outbreaks can occur year-round.
- In temperate areas, enveloped viruses including influenza and RSV circulate during winter, whereas rhinoviruses predominate in spring and summer.

- Reduced ventilation, indoor crowding, and improved survival of aerosolised virus at lower temperature and higher humidity have been suggested as factors that contribute to seasonality of winter outbreaks.

Transmission of respiratory viruses

- Transmission to a susceptible individual can occur as a result of virus-laden large droplets or small particle aerosols generated by an infected person during sneezing and coughing.
- Nosocomial transmission is often due to direct contact with the virus itself either by hand-to-hand contact, or transfer from contaminated fomites.

Pathogenesis of respiratory virus infection

The extent of virus shedding generally correlates with disease severity, although in the immunocompromised and children, prolonged shedding may continue after recovery.

- Generally, infection begins in the upper tracheobronchial respiratory tract then spreads down the airways.
- Viral replication destroys the epithelium and induces cytokine release that contributes to clinical symptoms, in addition to aiding viral clearance.
- Typically, rhinovirus and coronavirus are limited to upper airways, whereas influenza, RSV, PIV and adenovirus are capable of lower respiratory tract infection.
- SARS targets pneumocytes causing extensive and diffuse alveolar damage in the lower airways.
- Virus infection of the respiratory tract may alter bacterial flora, increase bacterial adherence to epithelial cells and disrupt mucociliary clearance leading to secondary bacterial invasion.
- The spread of highly pathogenic avian influenza H5N1 in poultry has been associated with >380 human cases worldwide. The determinants that confer virulence of highly pathogenic influenza viruses are unclear, but the ease with which the H5 haemagglutinin is cleaved is a major factor. Induction of excessive inflammatory responses (so called cytokine storm) exacerbates and sustains tissue injury.

Clinical features of respiratory virus infection

Influenza has been associated with the most severe illness, but as diagnostic techniques improve, other viruses have been shown to cause clinically indistinguishable disease.

Respiratory virus infections may be subclinical or cause symptoms ranging from mild upper respiratory illness to life-threatening pneumonia.

Infections cause overlapping syndromes that correspond to the site of infection.

- Upper respiratory tract: low-grade fever, nasal congestion and discharge, otitis media and sinusitis.
- Laryngopharyngitis: sore throat and hoarseness.
- Tracheobronchitis: wheeze, cough, dyspnoea, substernal chest pain and sputum production.
- Lower respiratory tract: exacerbations of airways disease, pleuritic chest pain, productive cough and crackles on auscultation.

Clinical characteristics of common respiratory viruses

Rhinovirus and coronavirus

- Prominent symptoms of the 'common cold' syndrome in healthy adults include sore throat, stuffy nose, sneezing and malaise.

- In a study of rhinovirus-infected elderly patients attending day care in the US, the majority had evidence of lower tract involvement including sputum (58%), crackles (48%) and dyspnoea (36%).

Influenza A and B

- Influenza A is characterised by an unproductive cough, nasal discharge, stuffiness and sore throat. Fever is prominent peaking at the time of systemic features and lasting for 1–5 days. Up to 80% of infected patients develop systemic features including myalgia, chills, headache, and malaise.
- Influenza B predominates every 3–5 years, typically produces a milder infection than H3N2 but may impose a significant burden on school-age children.

RSV

- RSV is a well known cause of lower respiratory tract disease among children in early life. As bronchiolitis progresses, tachypnoea, intercostal recession and cough are prominent features.
- In adults, fever is generally lower than seen in influenza but RSV is more frequently accompanied by wheeze and crackles on examination. RSV and PIV display the greatest morbidity in the immuno-compromised, particularly among bone marrow transplant recipients, and are associated with high fever, cough and lower respiratory symptoms.

Adenovirus

- In young military recruits, adenoviruses have been identified as dominant pathogens affecting up to 80% of new recruits within months of residence in camps.
- Adenovirus infection is more frequently associated with fever and conjunctivitis, than other pathogens.

Avian influenza

- Human H5N1 infections generally occur in younger adults or children exposed to infected poultry.
- Unlike human influenza viruses which bind predominantly to upper airway epithelial cells, avian influenza viruses are capable of binding to cells that are present deep in the lung tissue.
- Case-fatality rates in H5N1 infection exceed 60%.
- Infection is associated with high fever, bilateral lung infiltrates and rapid progression to respiratory failure.
- Gastrointestinal symptoms are prominent.
- Lymphopenia and thrombocytopenia are poor prognostic indicators.

SARS

- Severe multilobar pneumonia is frequent with 25% of symptomatic patients, particularly older persons, requiring ICU support.
- Diarrhoea and vomiting are prominent features.
- Clinical findings are non-specific including wheeze, crackles, and bronchial breath sounds over the involved lungs.
- Prolonged virus shedding and high infectivity of secretions after presentation require good infection control to prevent extensive nosocomial transmission.

Pulmonary complications of respiratory viruses

A chest radiograph should be obtained in all patients with suspected pneumonia for evidence of cavitations, effusion and consolidation. The presence of unilateral, bilateral or multilobe changes may be helpful in clinical management although radiological appearance does not allow differentiation between pathogens.

- Host factors influencing the incidence and outcome of respiratory virus-associated pneumonia include age, pre-infection immunity, and presence of chronic medical conditions as well as properties of the infecting virus.
- The interval between onset of symptoms and signs of pneumonia is variable.
- Two major patterns of pneumonia are recognised: primary viral and secondary bacterial pneumonia.
- Pneumonia is usually accompanied by fever, cough, dyspnoea, substernal and pleuritic chest pain.
- Viral pneumonia is generally considered to be radiologically and clinically indistinguishable from bacterial infections.

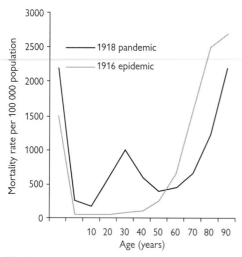

Fig. 8.6.1 Age-specific pneumonia and influenza mortality, 1916 and 1918.

Viral pneumonia
- During the 1918 Spanish H1N1 pandemic, the incidence of pneumonia and mortality was unusually high in those aged 20–40 years compared to earlier influenza epidemic years (Fig. 8.6.1).
- Clinical and post-mortem descriptions of influenza virus pneumonia have followed pandemic outbreaks. In the 1918 influenza pandemic, pneumonia was frequently reported in patients at onset of, or within 1–2 days of symptoms. In these patients, post-mortem findings were consistent with viral pneumonia with no lung consolidation and histological evidence of tracheitis, bronchitis, bronchiolitis, and intra-alveolar haemorrhage.
- During the 1957 Asian H2N2 pandemic, the onset of illness in fatal cases was also typically abrupt, often with rapid deterioration in younger patients. Influenza could be cultured from post-mortem lung tissue in 75% cases.
- Respiratory virus outbreaks among bone marrow transplant recipients are associated with extremely high mortality. Histological changes in bronchial biopsies at post-mortem are consistent with viral pneumonia in

patients where RSV, PIV, rhinovirus, and adenovirus have been detected.

Secondary bacterial pneumonia
- Some influenza patients in 1918 seemed to develop pulmonary bacterial complications after apparent resolution of the influenza illness. In these 'delayed' cases of pneumonia, a marked exudative broncho-pneumonia is the prominent post-mortem feature.
- Studies during pandemics indicate that one or more bacterial pathogens including pneumococci, haemolytic streptococci, *Haemophilus influenzae*, and staphylococci are recovered from blood or respiratory secretions. Overall, *Staphylococcus aureus* has been identified in the majority of bacterial pneumonias complicating proven influenza infections.
- *Staphyloccocus aureus*, *Streptococcus pneumoniae* and *Haemophilus influenzae* have been frequently cultured in blood or sputum from hospitalised elderly patients with influenza and rhinovirus infection.
- Nursing home outbreaks of parainfluenza 1 have been associated with pneumococcal pneumonia and bacteraemia in up to 20% patients.
- A review of influenza-related paediatric deaths in the US during 2003/04 identified 153 fatal cases. The median age was 3 years and the majority of children were previously healthy. Around 30% deaths occurred within 3 days of onset of symptoms. Methicillin-susceptible and resistant *Staphylococcus aureus* were identified in 24% of the cases.

Control of respiratory viruses
Specific vaccination
The diversity of respiratory viruses and frequency of antigenic drift makes vaccine preparation for respiratory viruses challenging.

- Inactivated influenza vaccines contain haemagglutinin from two A (H1N1 and H3N2) subtypes and one B strain. Protective efficacy of 70–95% in healthy adults is obtained when there is a good match between the vaccine and circulating strains. Vaccine efficacy is reduced in the elderly, but is still associated with 19–63% reductions in hospitalisation for pneumonia and influenza, and 17–39% reductions for all respiratory conditions
- As outbreaks of influenza occur in well immunised elderly subjects, enhanced vaccine effectiveness by adjuvantation, improved formulation or alternative routes of delivery are under evaluation.
- Several inactivated RSV vaccine candidates containing subunit proteins or peptide fragments, and chimeric proteins are in stages of clinical development.
- Live attenuated virus vaccines delivered intransally may offer potential advantages over injectable preparations. Mucosal IgA may give broader immunological protection at the site of entry and reduce the peak and duration of virus shedding. However, as individuals acquire partial immunity throughout life by frequent exposure to respiratory viruses, replication of live attenuated virus vaccines in adults may be limited reducing induction of desired local and humoral immune responses.
- Live attenuated parainfluenza virus vaccines are immunogenic in seronegative children, but induce limited responses among seropositive recipients.
- Highly efficacious live attenuated adenovirus vaccines used in military camps virtually eliminated outbreaks; however withdrawal of vaccine due to commercial

reasons resulted in re-emergence of the virus in this high-risk population.

Specific antiviral therapy

- Two classes of drug are available for influenza: M2 inhibitors (amantadine) and neuraminidase inhibitors, (zanamivir and oseltamivir).
- Amantadine use is limited by inactivity against influenza B, adverse effects and rapid emergence of drug resistance.
- In acute influenza in children and adults, treatment with neuraminidase inhibitors shortens the duration of symptoms and the time to return to normal daily activities by 1.5 days (30%) and reduces antibiotic use when compared with placebo.
- Meta-analysis of placebo-controlled trials of oseltamivir for acute community-acquired influenza in adults shows significant reductions in lower respiratory tract complications and hospitalisations including among those aged >65 years (Fig. 8.6.2).
- Ribavirin inhibits RSV replication by blocking transcription. Prompt therapy with inhaled ribavirin in RSV-infected bone marrow transplant recipients may reduce progression to pneumonia and improve outcome, however, its efficacy in established RSV disease is questionable.
- Passive immunisation against RSV can be achieved with polyclonal or monoclonal antibodies.
- Palivizumab is a humanised mouse monoclonal IgG, directed against the virus F surface protein, that blocks virus-induced cell fusion and has neutralising activity against RSV A and B. Monthly palivizumab infusions during the winter seasons are effective in the prevention of severe RSV disease in high-risk children.
- RSV fusion and replication inhibitors are under development to reduce progression to lower respiratory disease in children
- Picornavirus capsid binders have broad *in vitro* antirhinoviral activity by blocking virus attachment and uncoating. However clinical trials produced only modest improvements in symptom relief.

AUTHOR'S TIP

Antibiotic therapy

Bacterial complications of influenza and respiratory viruses include bronchopneumonia, bacteraemia and sepsis. Antibiotic selection should include anti-staphylococcal and pneumococcal activity

---

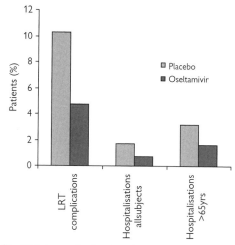

Fig. 8.6.2 Impact of oseltamivir on lower respiratory tract (LRT) complications and hospitalisations in influenza

Further reading

Bhat N et al. Influenza-associated deaths among children in the United States, 2003–2004. NEJM 2005; **353**: 2559–2567.

Falsey AR et al. The 'common cold' in frail older persons: impact of rhinovirus and coronavirus in a senior daycare centre. J Am Ger Soc 1997; **45**: 706–711.

Human Influenza. In: *Textbook of Influenza* KG Nicholson (ed.), Oxford: Blackwell, 1998.

Johnston SL, Papadopoulos NG (eds) *Respiratory Infections in Allergy and Asthma*, Marcel Dekker, 2003.

Kaiser L et al. Impact of oseltamivir treatment on influenza-related lower respiratory tract complications and hospitalizations *Arch Intern Med* 2003: **163**: 1667–1674.

Nicholson KG et al. Acute viral infections of upper respiratory tract in elderly people living in the community. *BMJ* 1997; **315**: 1060–1064.

8.7 Respiratory tuberculosis

Epidemiology

World-wide there are approximately 9 million new clinical cases of tuberculosis (TB), with1.8 million deaths each year, and 32% of the world population is infected with TB as judged by a positive tuberculin test. HIV co-infection is increasingly linked to TB, particularly in sub-Saharan Africa but now also with rising frequency in South Asia and China. In developed countries TB increasingly is a disease of the overseas born. In England and Wales in 2007, of the 8417 cases seen, less than 22% were in the white ethnic group, whereas over 72% were in persons born abroad, with the majority of cases being in those of South-Asian, Black-African, or Chinese ethnic origins. The rate for those UK-born (including ethnic minority groups) was 4.4/100000pa, for those born abroad 103.3/100000pa. The rate in the Black-African population born abroad at 309/100000pa, was ten times higher that that for the UK-born Black-African, and the rates is the South-Asian group were 6 times higher in the non-UK born. Only a minority of cases occur within 1–2 years of initial entry, when the highest rates are found. Second and third generation immigrants still have higher rates than native born white persons. In the white population, over half the cases are in the over 55s representing reactivation of disease acquired earlier in life. Rates range from 1/100,000pa at age 0–15 to >15/100,000 in the over 80's with males having higher rates in the white population. In older white persons it is thought that the substant ial majority of cases are due to reactivation of disease acquired in childhood or adolescence when TB was much commoner in the UK.

Clinical approach

Suspicion of respiratory TB is a synthesis of 3 elements: a) the clinical setting (for which a knowledge of the above epidemiology is important), b) symptoms, and c) CXR appearances (see later). Of the common respiratory symptoms, cough, weight loss, fever, night sweats, breathlessness and haemoptysis, only fever and night sweats are statistically more associated with TB than other respiratory conditions.

Examination

- Unless there is extensive lung involvement, or a significant pleural effusion there are seldom signs in the lung.
- General examination may show evidence of TB at other sites, particularly cervical lymphadenopathy.

Investigation

- CXR defines extent and the clinical pattern raises suspicion (see later).
- Bacteriology is crucial both to confirm the diagnosis and to obtain drug susceptibility testing. Three early morning sputums should be sent for TB microscopy and culture if the patient is expectorating.
- If no spontaneous sputum is produced consider induced sputum, or preferably bronchoscopy with washings targeted to the areas of X-ray abnormality (with appropriate infection control measures).
- Blood tests may be normal and only give non-specific abnormalities.
- Tuberculin testing is usually unhelpful in pulmonary TB as it does not differentiate between disease and infection, and may be falsely negative due to illness or co-morbidities e.g. HIV co-infection.
- Tuberculin testing should be performed for suspected TB pleural effusion and isolated mediastinal lymphadenopathy.

Chest radiography

No X-ray pattern is absolutely diagnostic of TB, but some patterns are very suggestive, but still can be mimicked by other diseases. There is a strong predilection for the upper zones, particularly the posterior segments. Disease in the lower lobes is usually in the apical segments. The shadowing initially is an infiltrate, which can then become confluent with cavitation and loss of volume developing. In association with HIV-infection the pattern becomes increasing less typical as immunosuppression progresses.

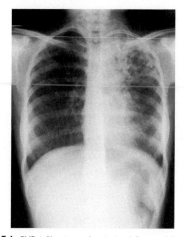

Fig. 8.7.1 CXR: infiltration and cavitation left upper lobe 5–8% of respiratory TB presents as a pleural effusion.

This is associated with a strongly positive tuberculin test and the fluid is a lymphocyte rich exudate. It is usually within 3–12 months of primary infection. Pleural biopsy gives granulomas in 50–60% of cases and 50–60% are culture positive.

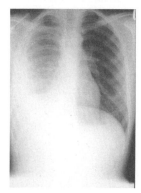

Fig. 8.7.2 CXR: right pleural effusion.

5–8% of respiratory TB presents as isolated mediastinal lymphadenopathy, associated with a strongly positive tuberculin test. CT scan may show lymphadenopathy with central hypodensity (caseation). Mediastinoscopy is only needed if either the tuberculin test is weak or negative (to exclude lymphoma or sarcoidosis) or if there is not some reduction in gland size after 2 months standard treatment.

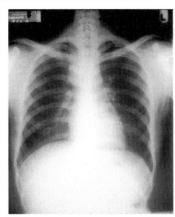

Fig. 8.7.3 CXR: right paratracheal lymphadenopathy.

Classical miliary TB occurs in a few % of cases. The full X-ray picture is easy to spot, with homogenous micro-nodules of 1–2mm spread throughout all lung zones. The early stages are more subtle and are best seen on HRCT scans. The diagnosis is usually easily confirmed with positive cultures, and often scanty-positive microscopy positive bronchial washings
- A lumbar puncture and CT scan should be carried out in classical miliary TB even in the absence of symptoms.
- 30% of such cases will have either LP or CT abnormalities, showing CNS involvement.
- Such CNS involvement then needs a 12-month regimen and corticosteroid treatment (see Chapter 8.8).

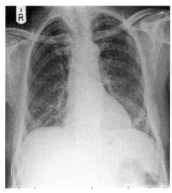

Fig. 8.7.4 CXR: classical miliary TB.

AUTHOR'S TIPS
- In ethnic minority groups, pleural effusion or isolated mediastinal glands with a positive tuberculin test, should be treated as TB until proved otherwise.
- Cavititation is active TB is highly (>0.00001) correlated with sputum microscopy positivity for AFB. If 3 spontaneous sputum tests are negative for AFB, the diagnosis of TB should be reconsidered.

Commencing treatment
- If sputum or respiratory secretions are microscopy positive, or the probablility of TB is high after samples have been sent, TB treatment should be commenced.
- Treatment should be with rifampicin, isoniazid, pyrazinamide and ethambutol as Rifater® plus ethambutol 15mg/kg (to the nearest 100mg), unless there is significant renal impairment.
- Pyridoxine (10mg) is not routinely required unless there are risk factors for peripheral neuropathy – e.g. diabetes, alcoholism, malnutrition or HIV-positivity.
- U&Es and LFTs should be checked pre-treatment, to confirm normal renal function and give a base-line for LFTs
- Visual acuity using Snellen chart should be checked, full ophthalmolgical assessment is not necessary.
- Patients starting on TB treatment should be notified to the Consultant in Communicable Disease Control.
- Consideration should be given to named HIV-testing to find/exclude co-existent HIV infection.
- Material sent to the lab should be screened by auramine stain and cultured using rapid liquid culture.
- An assessment of likely adherence with treatment should be made before starting treatment and consideration given to Directly Observed Treatment (DOT) with a three times weekly regimen.
- Isoniazid 15mg/kg, rifampicin 600–900mg, pyrazinamide 2.0–2.5gm, and ethambutol 30mg/kg should be given thrice weekly, most conveniently Monday, Wednesday and Friday under direct observation if this is used.
- A risk assessment for drug resistance should be made, particularly if there is any prior treatment history, and a rifampicin resistance probe requested on any microscopy or culture-positive material if concern exists.
- Adherence to medication should be monitored at least monthly with pill counts and random urine tests for rifampicin.
- If a large contact tracing exercise is likely e.g. in a school or a hospital or care facility confirm that the organisms seen/isolated is *M.tuberculosis* by appropriate gene probe before embarking on the contact tracing (with attendant publicity).

Treatment in special situations
- Diabetes – standard treatment plus pyridoxine.
- Pregnancy – standard treatment, only streptomycin and prothionamide to be avoided.
- Liver disease – standard treatment but regular LFTs – weekly first 2 weeks, then 2-weekly.
- Renal disease – rifampicin, isoniazid and pyrazinamide in standard dosages. Reduced dosages of ethambutol or streptomycin. Moxifloxacin 400mg od is an acceptable alternative.
- HIV-positive. TB takes precedence. Standard treatment, adjust HAART if necessary to avoid rifampicin interactions.

Infection control
- Suspected respiratory TB if admitted should be to a single side ward until results of 3 sputums known.
- Sputum microscopy cases remain infectious until 2 weeks standard treatment.
- Masks are only needed for suspected or proven MDR-TB cases.

- Suspected or proven MDR-TB should be in a negative pressure room if in hospital.
- NICE Guidelines and JTC 2000 guidance give criteria for cessation of respiratory isolation.

During treatment

- Regular LFT monitoring is not needed unless these are abnormal pre treatment or unless the patient has pre-existing liver disease or is Hep B or Hep C positive.
- Modest elevations of the transaminases are not uncommon in the pre-treatment LFTs of TB patients and usually improve rapidly with treatment.
- 3% of individuals will develop hepatitis/jaundice due to the drugs, with a raised bilirubin or a rise in transaminases to >5x normal.
- If this happens treatment with rifampicin/isoniazid and pyrazinamide should be stopped.. If the patient is not unwell and the form of TB is non-infectious, no treatment needs to be given until liver function returns to normal.
- If the patient is unwell, or the sputum microscopy positive within 2 weeks of starting treatment, some form of treatment needs to be given until the LFTs improve. Streptomycin and ethambutol with appropriate checks should be used unless clinically contraindicated or drug resistance is known or suspected.
- Pyrazinamide is the most likely drug, followed by rifampicin and then least likely isoniazid. Treatment re-introduction, if cessation of treatment is needed, follows the reverse order of probability.

Schedule for re-introduction of anti-TB drugs

A detailed schedule for drug re-introduction is given in the 1998 Joint TB Committee Guidelines (see Further reading).

At 2 months

- If a positive culture is obtained, if the organism is fully sensitive then pyrazinamide and ethambutol can be stopped. If the organism is resistant then treatment should be modified as per NICE Guidelines.
- If cultures are negative, stop pyrazinamide and ethambutol.
- If a culture is positive but susceptibilities are outstanding, continue all 4 drugs until they are known. Only stop pyrazinamide and ethambutol once full susuceptibility is confirmed, total duration of treatment however does not need extending beyond 6 months.
- Continuation treatment with rifampicin/isoniazid as Rifinah® should continue for 4 months (unless drug resistant).

Management of drug resistance

The management of drug resistance depends on the drug resistance pattern, which must be followed (unlike in opportunist mycobacteria (see later)).

Monoresistance

- Streptomycin: this does not alter the effectiveness of standard treatment and no modification is needed.
- Isoniazid: Isoniazid should be stopped and treatment should be with 2 months initial rifampicin, pyrazinamide and ethambutol. The continuation phase should then be with 7–10 months of rifampicin and ethambutol.
- Pyrazinamide: The usual cause of isolated pyrazinamide

resistance is *M.bovis*. Pyrazinamide should stopped and treatment should be with 2 months rifampicin, isoniazid and ethmabutol, followed by a continuation phase of rifampicin and isoniazisd for 7 months.

- Ethambutol: ethambutol mono-resistance is very uncommon. It does not affect the efficacy of standard 6-months short course chemotherapy which should be continued.
- Rifampicin: Isolated rifampicin resistance is uncommon, accounting for only 5–10% of rifampicin resistance. The finding of rifampicin resistance, particularly on a gene-probe, SHOULD BE TREATED AS MDR-TB, with the patient isolated as for, and treated for MDR-TB until proved otherwise.
- If rifampicin monoresistance is confirmed on full susceptibility tests then a regimen of 18 months isoniazid and ethambutol, supplemented by an initial 2 months pyrazinamide should be used.

Multiple resistance

- The commonest multiple resistance is combined isoniazid and streptomycin resistance. This should be treated as per isolated isoniazid resistance, but the use of a 3 times weekly DOT regimen (with appropriate dosage adjustments) should be considered.
- Other combined (non-MDR) resistances are uncommon and need to be discussed on a case by case basis with an expert in TB management.

MDR-TB

- MDR-TB is defined as high level resistance to rifampicin (the main sterilising drug) and isoniazid (the main killing drug) ± other TB drugs.
- Fortunately this occurs in only 50–60 new cases/year in the UK. Most of these have a history of prior treatment abroad, with prior treatment increasing the risk 15-fold.
- Lithuania, Latvia, Estonia, Cote D'Ivoire and the Dominican Republic all have MDR-TB rates of over 5% of cases.
- MDR-TB can now be subdivided into:
  (a) Basic MDR-TB with only rifampicin and isoniazid resistance.
  (b) MDR-TB with rifampicin and isoniazid resistance, plus some other drugs including pyrazinamide and ethambutol.
  (c) XDR-TB – extremely resistant TB, with resistance to rifampicin, isoniazid,pyrazinamide, ethambutol, and at least aquinolone and one rejectable amikaar, capreomycin kanamycin.
- The finding of rifampicin resistance should lead to appropriate isolation and treatment.
- Proven or suspected MDR-TB SHOULD NOT BE TREATED without the input of a physician experienced in such cases.
- The principles of treatment are:
  (a) Use at least 5 drugs to which the organism is, or is thought likely to be, susceptible, including 1 injectable if available until culture negative. At least 3 drugs to be continued, for at least 9 months after becomes culture negative.
  (b) Transfer the patient to another hospital/physician unless both expertise AND a negative pressure room co-exist at the same location.
  (c) Close liaison with the Mycobacterium Reference Centres and Unit of the HPA is essential.

During the continuation phase

- Check sputum, if still being produced, or if clinical progress is unsatisfactory at 4 months. A positive TB culture at 4 months is regarded as treatment failure, and should lead to repeat drug susceptibility tests and a molecular probe for rifampicin resistance.
- NEVER ADD A SINGLE DRUG TO A FAILING REGIMEN.

At end of treatment

- End of treatment CXR as baseline for future comparison.
- If no drug resistance, adherence good and no residual complications, discharge with advice to patient and GP to refer back if symptoms recur (unlikely relapse rate 0–3% for standard TB). Only follow up if continuing clinical problem or doubt about adherence.
- If isoniazid resistance follow up at 6 and 12 months. If MDR-TB long term follow-up.

Contact tracing/new entrant screening

NICE guidelines (2006) set out who to screen and how to screen, including the use of interferon-gamma assays (IGRAs). The main aims of such screening is to (a) detect those with disease, particularly pulmonary; (b) identify those with latent TB infection who may benefit from treatment; and (c) those without immunity who may benefit from BCG vaccination. Between 1–10% of new TB cases, are found through screening of household contacts, with the majority of cases being in the non-BCG'd contacts of sputum smear-positive disease on the first attendance. Only 1 in 200 of new entrants are found to have active TB on entry to the UK.

Treatment of latent TB infection (LTBI)

- Such individuals are tuberculin positive, preferably confirmed by a positive IGRA test, aged up to 35 years and identified through new entrant or contact screening.
- It is important to confirm that there is no evidence of disease – lack of symptoms, normal CXR, and examination, as the regimens below are only suitable for treatment of LTBI.
- Treatment with either rifampicin and isoniazid (3RH) or isoniazid for 6 months (6H) is recommended.

Further reading

Citron KM, Thomas GO. Ocular Toxicity and ethambutol. *Thorax* 1986; **41**: 737–739.

Dye C, Scheele S, Dolin P, *et al.* Global burden of tuberculosis. Estimated incidence, prevalence and mortality by country. *JAMA* 1999; **282**: 677–686.

Health Protection Agency. Focus on TB. Annual Surveillance Report 2006. England, Wales and Northern Ireland. London: HPA Centre for Infections.

Joint Tuberculosis Committee of the British Thoracic Society. Chemotherapy and management of tuberculosis in the United Kingdom: recommendations 1998. *Thorax* 1998; **53**: 536–548.

Joint Tuberculosis Committee of the British Thoracic Society. Control and prevention of tuberculosis in the United Kingdom: recommendations *Thorax* 2000; **55**: 887–901.

National Collaborating Centre for Chronic Conditions (for NICE). *Tuberculosis: clinical diagnosis and management of tuberculosis and measures for its prevention and control.* London: Royal College of Physicians 2006. ISBN 1 86016 227 0.

Ormerod LP, Skinner C, Wales JM. Hepatotoxicity of antituberculosis drugs. *Thorax* 1996; **51**: 111–113.

Ormerod LP, Green RM, Horsfield N. Outcome of treatment of culture negative tuberculosis (respiratory and nonrespiratory) Blackburn 1996-2000. *J Infection* 2002; **45**: 88–89.

8.8 Non-respiratory tuberculosis

Epidemiology

The overall epidemiology follows that of TB in general (see Chapter 8.7). However non-respiratory TB occurs with increased frequency in all non-white ethnic groups. Non-respiratory sites account for only 20% of cases in the white population, but nearly 50% in minority groups. Lymph node TB, 90% in the cervical glands, accounts for nearly half of all non-respiratory TB. Some patients will have both respiratory and non-respiratory TB.

Treatment

All forms of non-respiratory TB should be treated with 6 month's rifampicin and isoniazid, supplemented by 2 months' initial pyrazinamide and ethambutol, with the sole exception of CNS disease (see sub-section), unless there is drug intolerance or drug resistance. Modification of treatment for drug resistance or intolerance is as for respiratory TB (see Chapter 8.7). The drug treatment of all cases of TB should be under the management of either a respiratory or infectious disease physician, or if a child in conjunction with a paediatrician.

Lymph node TB

Clinical

- 90% of cases involve the cervical nodes.
- 10% of those with cervical nodes also have mediastinal lymphadenopathy with no visible lung lesion on CXR.
- Are usually 'cold' without the warmth and erythema of pyogenic infection.
- Usually painless and of gradual onset but can be painful if enlargement is more rapid.
- Central caseation leads to fluctuance, which can then lead to discharge and then sinus formation.
- Constitutional symptoms, weight loss, fever, malaise, night sweats, are seen only in a small minority of patients.
- Peristent lymphadenopathy for over 4 weeks in an ethnic minority patient should be regarded as TB until proved otherwise, and investigated accordingly.

Investigations

- CXR may show other disease.

FNA is useful for cytology but does **not** give enough material for TB culture.

- If there is any hint of fluctuance aspirate the node with a wide-bore (white needle) after a little local anaesthetic in the overlying skin. Obtaining even a small amount of pus from a 'cold' node is sufficient to start treatment.
- If no pus can be obtained, node biopsy for histology *and* culture should be performed.
- The finding of granulomatous histology supported by a positive Mantoux allows treatment to start pending culture results. Only 60–70% of cases are culture confirmed.

During treatment

- Enlargement of current nodes, or the development of new nodes, occur in 20% of cases, and do not imply treatment failure, but are usually immunologically mediated.
- 5–15% of cases have a degree of persistent lymphadenopathy at the end of treatment.

After treatment

- 5–10% may develop new glands or enlargement of glands after cessation of treatment. These are almost invariably sterile if aspirated or biopsied. They are immunologically mediated, due to reaction to tuberculo-proteins from disrupted macrophages.
- Short courses of steroids may be needed to suppress these phenomena.
- TB drug treatment should only be restarted if there is a positive culture for *M. tuberculosis*.

Bone and joint TB

Clinical

- 50% of all cases are spinal, largely thoraco-lumbar.
- Back pain may be present for weeks or months before the diagnosis, with some local tenderness.
- The disease begins as a discitis involving inferior and superior borders of adjacent vertebrae, leading to loss of disc space.
- Kyphosis and angulation are later features.
- Paraspinal and extradural abscesses can form, the former sometimes presenting as a para-spinal mass, or a psoas abscess pointing in the groin.
- 50% of bone and joint TB is non-spinal and can involve virtually any bone or joint.
- Any subacute mono-arthritis in an ethnic minority patient should have TB high in the differential, particularly if pus can be aspirated or there is sinus formation.

Neurological signs or symptoms in the legs, or sphincter disturbance suggest spinal cord compression.

Investigation

- Plain radiology can initially be normal.
- CT or MRI are the investigations of choice for suspected spinal TB.
- Needle or open biopsy may be needed to make the diagnosis.
- Surgeons need to be reminded not to place all material in formalin but send TB cultures.

Treatment

- Surgical intervention in spinal disease is only indicated if there are neurological signs or symptoms.
- Management should be jointly with an orthopaedic surgeon who manages the mechanical aspects of disease, but not drug treatment.

Gastrointestinal TB

Clinical

- Approx 1/3 present as an acute abdomen mimicking appendicitis or with acute intestinal obstruction.
- The other 2/3 are more gradual usually with abdominal pain if there is a degree of intraluminal disease, or distension if there is ascites due to peritoneal disease.
- Only 25–30% have any CXR evidence of respiratory TB.
- Systemic symptoms of weight loss, fever, and malaise are found in over 50%.

Investigations

- Ultrasound may show ascites or bowel masses.
- Small bowel studies may show strictures, fistulae and skip

lesions. They *cannot* distinguish between Crohn's disease and TB.
- Caecal and colonic lesions can simulate carcinoma: colonoscopy is useful.
- Ascitic fluid is a lymphocyte-rich exudate.
- Laparoscopy is the investigation of choice in asctic/peritoneal presentations.

Treatment
- Bowel resection is only required if there is mechanical obstruction.
- 10% of female cases will have secondary infertility.
- In an ethnic minority patient with granulomatous changes in the bowel on biopsy, it is much safer to first treat for TB than Crohn's disease, than vice versa.

TB meningitis
Although making up only 1–2% of cases of TB, the diagnosis is very important because of the morbidity and mortality, particularly if the diagnosis is delayed or missed.

Clinical
- Onset is insidious usually over a few weeks with headache and malaise.
- Focal neurological signs or confusion follow (Stage 2 disease), and later coma (Stage 3).
- Prognosis crucially depends on the clinical stage at start of treatment, so suspicion and early diagnosis are important.

Investigation
- CXR is normal in over 70% of cases but may show acute miliary disease.
- LP shows a lymphocytosis (rarely above 500/ml), with a raised protein and reduced glucose.
- Microscopy for AFB is rarely positive.
- PCR tests for AFB are misleading and give false negative results in 20-40%, do *not* use.
- Baseline CT or MRI may show initial increased meningeal uptake, tuberculomas, or hydrocephalus.

Treatment
- Treatment is for a minimum of 12 months with rifampicin and isonaizid, supplemented by 2 months' initial pyrazinamide and a fourth drug. Ethambutol, streptomycin (not intrathecal) or prothionamide can be used.
- Steroids, starting at prednisolone 40–60mg/day, tailing over several weeks are now recommended for all cases of TBM.
- Tuberculomas can develop during treatment.
- Repeat CT scanning is needed if there is clinical deterioration.
- Shunting may be needed if hydrocephalus develops.

Miliary TB
- Acute classical miliary TB (see respiratory).
- Cryptic miliary TB presents as a PUO, with weight loss and high ESR.
- Biopsies from liver and bone marrow may show granulomata. EMU, liver, and bone marrow are the best sites for culture.

- Fever should respond within 2 weeks if a trial of treatment is given.

Urological TB
- Sterile pyuria should lead to EMU x 3 for AFB.
- Urine microscopy for AFB is unreliable for diagnosis because of genital mycobacteria (*M. smegmatis*), and the use of intravesical BCG for bladder cancer.
- IVP shows chronic clubbing of calyces, there may also be intra-renal calcification.
- Steroids for 2 months might be of benefit if there is ureteric stenosis, but this may need temporary stenting.
- Chronic TB cystitis leads to severe frequency due to marked bladder capacity reduction. An ileal loop may be needed after TB treatment is completed to increase bladder capacity.
- Chronic prostatitis or epididymitis or testicular masses in ethnic minority patients have TB in the differential diagnosis.

Gynaecological TB
- Salpingitis or endometritis are usually found during investigation of infertility.
- Granulomatous histology on D&C or fallopian tubes are very suggestive and bacteriology should be sought.

Skin TB
- Half is due to underlying lymph node, bone or renal disease (scrofuloderma).
- Chronic skin lesions in ethnic minority individuals, particularly if granulomatous, should be considered suspicious (remember leprosy).

Pericardial TB
- Apparent cardiomegaly is seen on CXR, echo confirms the degree of pericardial fluid.
- Pericardial fluid is a lymphocyte rich exudates.
- Prednisolone beginning at 60mg/daily tailing over 3 months is given as well at standard TB treatment.
- Steroids significantly reduce death, the need for pericardiocentesis and pericardectomy.

Other sites
Chronic abscesses or sinuses in ethnic minority patients should have TB actively considered with histology and cultures sent.

Further reading
British Thoracic Society Research Committee. Six-months versus nine-months chemotherapy for tuberculosis of lymph nodes: final results. *Respir Med* 1993; **87**: 621–623.

National Collaborating Centre for Chronic Conditions (for NICE) *Tuberculosis: clinical diagnosis and man agement of tuberculosis and measures for its prevention and control.* London: Royal College of Physicians 2006. ISBN 1 86016 227 0.

Non-Respiratory TB. In Davies PD *et al. Clinical Tuberculosis*, 4th edn. London: Hodder Arnold, 2008.

8.9 Opportunist (non-tuberculous) mycobacteria

Epidemiology

Opportunist mycobacteria, also called non-tuberculous mycobacteria, atypical mycobacteria and mycobacteria other than tuberculosis (MOTT) can be found throughout the environment. They can be isolated from water (including tap water), soil, milk, dust and from various animals and birds. They are very low grade pathogens in humans and person to person spread is vanishingly rare. Because of this it is not necessary to isolate patients (having proved it is **not** TB) or to contact trace. Because of their ubiquitous distribution, which can include hospital water supplies and even bronchoscope cleaning systems, it is very important to determine whether an isolate or isolates is/are significant and differentiate them from contamination. Because they are acid-fast bacilli they cannot be differentiated from *M. tuberculosis* microscopically, but require PCR tests for speciation to differentiate them from the *M. tb* complex, which requires either microscopy-positive or culture positive material. There are some regional variations in the commonest organisms. *M. kansasii* is overall the commonest, *M. xenopi* is the commoner in South East England, and *M. malmoense* in Scotland and Northern England.

Who may get them?

Essentially to get true disease there has to be either reduced immunity and/or tissue damage to allow these very low grade pathogens to cause disease. Three scenarios are the main settings:-

1. Cervical lymphadenopathy usually in the under 5's due to their immature immune system, due to *M. malmoense* or *M. avium intracellulare* (MAC). Histology shows granulomata, and often AFB on microscopy (which is uncommon in true lymph node TB), and the tuberculin test is often weak or negative. (treatment is by excision of the affected node(s) and not by drug treatment.

2. In HIV-positive individuals with CD4 counts of under100/ ml, particularly MAC can cause a disseminated infection with positive blood cultures for AFB from the buffy coat layer of blood. Lung infiltrates, lymphadenopathy and colonic disease can also occur. These problems are now less much less with the introduction of HAART, and prophylaxis against MAC with macrolides in such individuals.

3. In persons with lung damage due to COPD, or other lung conditions causing scarring, including previous TB, and cystic fibrosis, these organisms can cause disease which is indistinguishable from respiratory TB, with similar symptoms and lung CXR appearances. Pleural effusion and isolated mediastinal lymphadenopathy are rarely X-ray features with these organisms. The great majority of cases are in middle-aged to older smokers with a mild male predominance.

Is it true infection or contamination?

The significance of an isolate can only be derived by considering the type of specimen from which the *Mycobacterium* has been isolated, the number of isolates, the degree of growth and the identity of the organism. Usually a positive culture from a sterile site, particularly if there is granulomatous histology is sufficient, but for other sites particularly the lung there should be multiple isolates, preferably separated by at least 7 days, and a consistent clinical and X-ray picture. Single isolates of fast growing organisms such as *M. chelonae* or *M. gordonae* without much clinical or X-ray abnormality are usually environmental contamination.

Drug susceptibility results

Unlike in true TB where the drug susceptibility results have to be scrupulously adhered to, drug susceptibility results in the opportunist mycobacteria are not often helpful and are often misleading and can cause confusion and even panic. All the opportunist mycobacteria are genetically resistant to pyrazinamide. They are often reported resistant to many other drugs on single agent testing, which bears no correlation to response to clinical combinations. This is because drugs which are reported as resistant as single agents, work synergistically when used together, and are effective. Rifampicin and ethambutol are the key drugs. Drug susceptibility results are only of utility in *M. kansasii* infection, and possibly to predict macrolide susceptibility.

Clinical patterns (HIV negative)

Pulmonary disease

- This accounts for 90–95% of all the disease with *M. kansasii*, *M. malmoense*, *M. xenopi* and *M. avium intracellulare* (MAC).
- One cannot differentiate beween these species or from *M. tuberculosis* radiologically.
- Cavitation is seen in 50–70%.
- More chronic presentations and colonisation followed by disease are seen in cystic fibrosis and other forms of bronchiectasis.

Lymph node disease

- Largely confined to ages 1–5 years.

Other sites

- *M. fortuitum* or *M. chelonae* tend to infect skin or soft tissues after surgery or penetrating trauma, with recurrent abscess or fistula formation.
- *M. marinum* occurs following skin tauma in swimming pools or aquaria so-called 'fish tank granuloma'.
- *M. ulcerans* may cause chronic indolent necrotic skin ulcers 'Buruli ulcer' which may be seen in immigrants or asylum seekers from Equatorial Africa.
- Infection of bone, joints and the genitourinary tract are rarely seen.

Clinical patterns (HIV positive)

Pulmonary disease

- Disease only involving the lung accounts for only 5% of opportunist mycobacterial infection in these patients.
- Symptoms are similar to HIV-negative patients but haemoptysis is less common.
- As with standard TB in HIV-positive individuals cavitation is not common. Diffuse interstitial, reticulonodular, or alveolar infiltrates are seen.

Lymph node disease

- Can sometimes seen and can be associated with skin lesions. Safer to treat as standard TB until culture results available.
- Can be part of the immune reconstitution (IRIS) syndrome, in severely immunocompromised patients starting on HAART.

Other extrapulmonary sites
Intrabdominal lymphadenopathy, skin lesions and other sites can also be a manifestation of the IRIS syndrome. Corticosteroids may be needed to reduce the immune response in the short term.

Treatment
Recommendations for some organisms is based on some controlled clinical trials, but the evidence base is not as robust are for the treatment of *M. tuberculosis*.

HIV negative individuals
M. kansasii: pulmonary disease
- A regimen of rifampicin and ethambutol for 9 months gives a >95% cure rate in HIV-negative individuals.
- If there is obvious immuno compromise including HIV-positivity, then treatment for 15–24 months, or until cultures have been negative for at least 12 months would be advised.

M. kansasii: extrapulmonary disease
- Lymph node disease in young children should be treated by excision.
- In HIV-negative treat for a minimum of 9 months with rifampicin and ethambutol. Addition of a macrrolide, prothionamide or streptomycin may need consideration, if the response is poor.
- In HIV positive individuals if disseminated disease (bacteraemia) then give rifampicin, ethambutol and clarithromycin. Improvement of the immune system on HAART may allow cessation of these drugs after some months.

MAC, M. malmoense, M. xenopi: pulmonary disease
- Trials by the BTS have shown that up to 15% of such individuals do not respond to 24 months' treatment.
- Individuals with these infections have a high 5-year mortality from cardio-respiratory failure, of between 25-40%, with *M. xenopi* having the worst prognosis.
- In those who are fit enough, and the disease is unilateral, surgical excision and continuation of drug treatment is an option.
- Treatment is with rifampicin and ethambutol for 24 months, plus a third drug, either isoniazid, clarithromycin or ciprofloxacin is best.
- The results of the most recent study of rifampicin and ethambutol with either clarithromycin or ciprofloxacin show no greater efficacy but mild species differences.
- For *M. avium* 2 years' treatment with rifampicin ethambutol and ciprofloxacin is best, with isoniazid being

an alternative if ciprofloxacin is not tolerated; for *M. malmoense* and *M. xenopi*, 2 years rifampicin, ethambutol and clarithromycin is best.

MAC, M. malmoense, M. xenopii: extrapulmonary disease
- Lymph node excision in children.
- As for respiratory disease.

Fast growing organisms e.g: M. chelonae, M. gordonae, M. fortuitum, M. abscessus. pulmonary disease
- Surgical excision if possible.
- Rifampicin, ethambutol and clarithromycin in the first instance.
- Cure may not attainable.
- Consult JTC Guidance for more detail if needed.

Extra-pulmonary disease
Consult JTC Guidance.

HIV-positive individuals
Improving the immune system with HAART is probably more important than active mycobacterial drug treatment.

M. kansasii: pulmonary or disseminated
Rifampicin and ethambutol for 24 months +/- clarithromycin.

MAC or M. xenopii: pulmonary or disseminated disease
- Rifampicin, ethambutol and clarithromycin for 24 months.
- HAART may need to be modified because ofrifampicin interactions.

Fast growing organisms
As for HIV negative

Further reading
Banks J, Jenkins PA. Combined versus single antituberculosis drugs on the in vitro sensitivity patterns of non-tuberculous mycobacteria. *Thorax* 1987; **42**:838–842.

British Thoracic Society. *Mycobacterium kansasii* pulmonary infection: a prospective study of the results of nine months of treatment with rifampicin and ethambutol. *Thorax* 1994; **49**: 442–445.

Joint Tuberculosis Committee of the British Thoracic Society. Management of opportunist mycobacterial infections: Joint Tuberculosis Committee guidelines 1999. *Thorax* 2000; **55**: 210–218.

Research Committee of the British Thoracic Society. First randomised trial of treatments for pulmonary disease caused by *M. avium intracellulare*, *M. malmoense*, and *M. xenopi* in HIV negative patients: rifampicin, isoniazid and ethambutol versus rifampicin and ethambutol. *Thorax* 2001; **56**: 167–172.

8.10 Fungal and parasitic lung disease

Fungal lung disease occurs primarily in those with a background of immune compromise or underlying pulmonary disease. Fungal lung infections have increased in incidence over recent decades as the number of patients at risk has increased. This is due to a combination of iatrogenic causes (e.g. increased organ transplantation and prescription of immunosuppressant medications) and the emergence and increasing prevalence of HIV. Worldwide travel has increased, leading to exposure to a greater range of fungal infections. There has fortunately been a corresponding increase in the range of available treatments. However, untreated pulmonary fungal infections still result in appreciable morbidity and mortality. It is critical that physicians have a high index of clinical suspicion, allowing early diagnosis and appropriate treatment of these conditions.

Aspergillus

This filamentous fungus is capable of causing a variety of patterns of pulmonary disease. When spores are inhaled into the healthy lung they rarely cause morbidity. However, they can cause a variety of disease manifestations in those who are immunocompromised or those with asthma or chronic lung disease. These syndromes are distinct clinical entities and more than one may occur in the same patient. Traditionally three types of pulmonary disease due to the inhalation of *Aspergillus* species were described. This categorisation is still valid but sub-categories have been included as further manifestations of this disease are recognised:

1 Immune-mediated *Aspergillus* disease:
   (a) Atopy.
   (b) Allergic bronchopulmonary aspergillosis (ABPA).
   (c) Hypersensivity pneumonitis (HP).
2 Aspergilloma.
3 Aspergillosis.
   (a) Chronic pulmonary aspergillosis.
   (b) Invasive aspergillosis.

1 Immune-mediated Aspergillus disease

(a) Atopy

IgE-mediated atopy (type I hypersensitivity) to fungal spores. Atopy to *Aspergillus* species leads to a positive skin-prick test in 10–25% of patients with asthma when exposed to *Aspergillus* spores. Other features of ABPA are not detected in this condition.

(b) ABPA

A type I plus type III hypersensitivity reaction to the inhalation of *Aspergillus fumigatus* spores. This can be divided into ABPA with seropositivity (ABPA-S) alone or ABPA with central bronchiectasis (ABPA-CB).

Essential criteria for diagnosis of ABPA:
- Asthma (long history).
- Immediate skin-prick positivity.
- Total IgE >1000ng/ml (unless taking steroids).
- ± Eosinophilia (blood) >1000mm^3.

Additional diagnostic criteria for ABPA-S:
- Current or previous pulmonary infiltrates.
- Increased serum IgG (precipitins) and IgE (RAST) to A. fumigatus.

Additional essential criterion for ABPA-CB:
- Central bronchiectasis.

Clinical features (not all of these need be present):
- Wheeze.
- Long history of asthma which has recently worsened (often requiring recurrent courses of oral steroids).
- Fever.
- Pleuritic chest pain.
- Cough with expectoration of brown mucus plugs which may contain airway casts.
- Haemoptysis.
- Late presentation may be with features of end-stage lung disease such as dyspnoea, cyanosis, cor pulmonale and clubbing.

Investigations:
- Cytological examination of sputum may reveal fungal hyphae or eosinophilia.
- CXR may demonstrate fleeting pulmonary infiltrates (tending to involve the upper lobe), bronchiectasis and mucoid impaction.
- CT appearances in ABPA-CB are of proximal bronchiectasis, predominantly in the upper lobes.

Treatment:
- Prednisolone, initially at high doses (40mg/day) for 1–2 weeks but then gradually reduced to maintenance doses (5–10mg/day). Monitor total IgE as a marker of response.
- Anti-fungal medication. Oral itraconazole 200mg BD for 4 months is of benefit in cases of steroid dependant ABPA. LFTs and aspergillus precipitins should be monitored regularly. Voriconazole is emerging as an alternative anti-fungal agent.
- Symptoms of wheeze should be treated with bronchodilators.
- If mucus plugging is severe, bronchial aspiration may be required.

(c) HP (Previously known as extrinsic allergic alveolitis (EAA))

See Chapter 7.8, p. 148

Examples include Malt worker's lung (*Aspergillus clavatus or fumigatus*) and Farmer's lung (*Aspergillus umbrosus*).

2 Aspergilloma (Mycetoma)

- Growth of a fungal ball of *Aspergillus fumigatus/flavus/ niger* in a pre-existing cavity in the lung.
- Commonly follows tuberculosis but may occur in the setting of any cavitary lung disease.
- Often asymptomatic and detected on CXR.
- May present with haemoptysis.
- Rarely presents with systemic symptoms or cough.
- Diagnosis is usually radiological.
- Sputum may contain fungal hyphae.
- Aspergillus precipitins may be present.
- Treatment only indicated if symptoms are present. Treat haemoptysis with drugs (tranexamic acid), surgery (resection) or arterial embolisation. Itraconazole may reduce size of fungal cavity but does not act rapidly enough to be of use in life threatening haemoptysis.

3 Aspergillosis

(a) Chronic pulmonary aspergillosis

This rare disease usually occurs in those with mildly impaired host defences and older patients with chronic lung disease. It is a slowly progressive disease with local invasion (but *not* dissemination) occurring over weeks or months. There may be an aspergilloma present prior to disease onset. Patients complain of a prolonged (>3 month) history of chronic productive cough and systemic symptoms such as malaise, fever and weight loss. Haemoptysis is common. CXR changes include new or expanding cavitation, pleural thickening and consolidation, primarily in the upper lobes. Blood tests reveal high inflammatory markers. Serum aspergillus precipitins (IgG) may be positive. The organism may be isolated from sputum, BAL or pleural fluid or biopsy samples. Treatment is with anti-fungal therapy such as voriconazole 200mg BD for 1–6 months. Alternative anti-fungal agents include itraconazole or amphotericin B. Interferon gamma is emerging as a possible future adjunctive therapy. Surgery is occasionally required.

(b) Invasive pulmonary aspergillosis

Invasive pulmonary aspergillosis is a severe disease, responsible for significant mortality amongst those with immune system compromise. *Aspergillus fumigatus* is the commonest cause of this condition but the contribution of other *Aspergillus* species is increasing.

Major risk factors include:

- Neutropenia (especially <500cells/mm^3 for >10 days or persistent dysfunction).
- Transplantation.
- Prolonged high dose corticosteroids (>3 weeks).
- Haematological malignancy.
- Cytotoxic therapy.
- Advanced AIDS (usual CD4 <100cells/mm^3).
- Admission to ICU.

Clinical features:

- Symptoms of a pneumonia that fails to respond to standard antibiotic therapy.
- Pleuritic pain, haemoptysis or unexplained fever in a patient with major risk factors.
- Rarely, presents as a tracheobronchitis with airway inflammation and ulceration.
- Dissemination may occur, leading to involvement of other organs such as the CNS.

Investigations:

- **CXR** may demonstrate cavitation, wedge opacities and/or nodules(s).
- **CT** may show small nodules ± surrounding haemorrhage (halo sign) or central necrosis (air-crescent), consolidation or ground-glass opacification. CT should be performed early in order to look for this disease in patients who are immunocompromised and have unexplained fever.
- **Histological** examination of thoracic biopsy specimens may reveal fungal hyphae.
- **Culture** (e.g. of sputum or BAL fluid) may demonstrate growth of *Aspergillus* spp. This is diagnostic alone if the patient has major risk factors and the organism is cultured from a normally sterile site.
- **Galactomannan** is a polysaccharide component of the fungal cell wall that is released by *Aspergillus* spp.

during growth. The galactomannan test is an ELISA which tests for the presence of this antigen and is highly specific (89%) but less sensitive (71%) for invasive disease. Testing of sera should be performed twice a week in a high risk patient who is unwell to enable early diagnosis of invasive aspergillosis. False positive results may occur within 5 days of taking beta-lactam antibiotics.

- **PCR** for *Aspergillus* antigen may become a useful diagnostic test in the future

Treatment:

Prompt treatment is essential and reduces mortality in this condition.

- Anti-fungal medications: the treatment of choice is oral voriconazole (e.g. 6mg/kg BD on day 1 then 4mg/kg BD until day 7 then oral 200mg BD). Limited studies of combination therapy suggest a possible role for combining the use of capsofungin with voriconazole or amphotericin.
- Adjuvant therapies directed at treating the underlying immunocompromise include GM-CSF, granulocyte transfusions and IFNγ
- Reduce immunosupressants where possible.

Further information & patient support:

http://www.aspergillus.org.uk

Endemic mycoses

These dimorphic fungi cause disease in endemic areas. They are easily missed if the patient presents in a non-endemic area and the travel history is not taken carefully. The disease is usually self-limiting if host immunity is intact. However, when T-cell mediated immunity is impaired or exposure is great, severe or disseminated disease may occur.

PCP

Pneumocytis jeroveci causes a fungal pneumonia in those with impaired T-cell immunity such as malignancy or HIV. This condition is described further in the Chapter 9.2 (p. 210).

Yeast infections

Candida

Although *Candida* spp. often colonise the respiratory tract, primary *Candida* infection of the lungs is rare. Fungal pneumonia due to *Candida* occurs when heavy colonisation of the oral cavity occurs or in the setting of disseminated disease (candidaemia). This is most often seen in the ITU or in those with neutropenia. Diagnosis relies on the culture of *Candida* spp. from a normally sterile site. This condition is described further in Chapter 9.1 (p. 202).

Cryptococcus neoformans

Inhalation of *Cryptococcus* spp. in those with impaired immunity (e.g. due to HIV) can lead to pulmonary infection. There may be no pulmonary symptoms or symptoms may be those of cough, dyspnoea and chest pain. Rarely acute respiratory failure may occur. In HIV the organism commonly disseminates or spreads to the CNS, leading to severe disease with a high mortality. This disease has fallen in incidence as a result of the widespread use of anti-fungal prophylaxis in high risk patients.

Moulds

Rare fungal mould infections affecting the lungs include **mucormycoses**, **zygomycoses** and **fusariosis**. Mucormycosis is an opportunistic fungal infection with a very high mortality and should be treated by early surgical

Endemic mycosis (causative organism)	Endemic regions	Clinical features	Diagnosis	Treatment
Histoplasmosis (*Histoplasma capsulatum*)	Mid-west (along river valleys) and southeast USA Parts of Central America and the Caribbean (especially Puerto Rico and the Dominican Republic) Africa (especially Nigeria+ Niger) Asia	• Asymptomatic: *nodules or calcified lymph nodes on CXR in a healthy individual* • Acute: *systemic flu-like illness ± multilobar infiltrate on CXR following high level exposure to histoplasma* • Chronic: *Progressive lung disease and cavitation on CXR in those with prior underlying lung disease* • Disseminated: *Multi-organ disease and organ failure with reticulonodular CXR infiltrates in immunocompromised individuals* • Rarities: *Broncholithiasis, granulomatous mediastinitis, fibrosing mediastinitis*	• Antigen detection test on blood or urine (up to 95% sensitive) • Smear or culture of sputum/ BAL fluid/ blood/ urine/ bone marrow aspirate (may take 4 days or more to become positive) • Serology (takes weeks to become positive)	Treat if: • Immunocompromised host • Symptoms > 1 month • Disseminated disease • Respiratory failure Treat with: • Oral itraconazole 200mg BD for 2–4 months • If chronic disease fails to respond after 12 weeks or the patient requires parenteral therapy then commence amphotericin B • Corticoteroids may be used to reduce the inflammatory response
Blastomycosis (*Blastomyces dermatitides*)	Mid-west and southeast USA Canadian great lakes	• Progressive pneumonia • Respiratory failure • Rarely disseminated disease involving the meninges	• 10%KOH digest test of respiratory secretions • Rapid staining of BAL fluid • Open lung biopsy may be required • Serological tests have poor sensitivity	• Treat severe disease with amphotericin B • Once stable this can be switched to oral itracona- zole 200mg BD for at least 6 months
Coccidioido- mycosis (*Coccidioides immitis*)	Parts of southwest USA Mexico and areas of South America	• Pneumonia (sometimes with effusions) • Erythema nodosum or multi- forme • Life-threatening meningitis • Severe pulmonary disease and ventilatory failure may occur in immunocompromised patients • Cavitating nodules may occur	The organism is difficult to culture and diagnosis usually relies on an accurate travel history in combination with a characteristic lymphocytic CSF (or neutrophilic or eosinophilic) or positive serology.	Usually self-limiting but if severe disease or meningitis treat with: • Fluconazole (or itracona- zole or posaconazole) for life • Or amphotericin B if the onset is acute and severe
Paracoccidioido- mycosis (*Paracoccidioides basiliensis*)	Parts of Central & South America (especially Brazil)	• Typically presents as a chronic pulmonary disease • May be acute and disseminated in an immunocompromised host	• Culture sputum/BAL • Stain lung biopsy sam- ples	• Treat with oral itracona- zole for 6 months

Fig. 8.10.1 Table of endemic mycoses

resection combined with amphotericin B. Zygomycosis and fusariosis have clinical presentations that are similar to aspergillosis. Zygomycosis fails to respond to voriconazole. These organisms especially cause fungal infection in those with haematological malignancy.

Anti-fungal therapy

Antifungal prophylaxis is recommended for those at high risk of fungal infection (e.g. cotrimoxazole in those with HIV and low CD4 counts to prevent PCP).

Treatment of fungal infections is often empirical with oral azoles or intravenous amphotericin B. If the specific organism is identified targeted antifungal therapy, taking drug sensitivities into account, should be prescribed. Echinocandins are of use in treating azole-resistant *Candida* infections.

Parasitic lung disease

Tapeworms

Hydatid disease
Echinococcus granulosus causes cystic pulmonary disease in sheep rearing areas. Oral ingestion of food contaminated with eggs from dog or sheep faeces leads to infection of the liver. Spread to the lungs may then occur across the diaphragm or via blood or lymph. Intact cysts cause symptoms due to compression of surrounding tissues and presentation may be with cough, chest pain or dyspnoea. Cyst rupture leads to pneumonia, hypersensitivity reactions or haemoptysis. Diagnosis is by serology and radiology. Surgery should be performed to excise an intact cyst if possible, even if no symptoms are present. Anti-helminth medications (albendazole or mebendazole) can be used to prevent recurrence or secondary bacterial infection.

Echinococcus multilocularis is a rare infection occuring in the Arctic, Northern Europe and Asia. It presents with a lung mass on CXR.

Flatworms

Lung flukes (Paragonamiasis)
Paragonimus spp. (esp. *westermani*) cause a pulmonary syndrome in SE Asia, S America or Africa. Parasitic larvae are ingested in undercooked crabs or crayfish. These penetrate the intestinal wall and migrate through the peritoneum,

diaphragm and pleura to the lung, where they mature into adult flukes. Presentation may be with fever, cough, haemoptysis, chest pain, lung abscess or pleural effusion. CXR may reveal pleural or parenchymal lesions or both. Diagnosis is on the basis of detection of eggs (in bronchial tissue or secretions) or serology. Eosinophilia is usual. Treatment is with praziquantel (75mg/kg/day for 3 days) or bithionol.

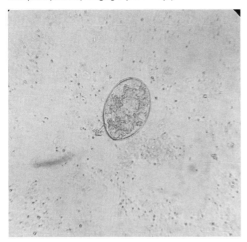

Fig. 8.10.2 Paragoniamasis (See Plate 6).

Blood flukes (Schistosomiasis)
Schistostoma japonicum causes disease in the Far East. *Schistostoma mansoni* and *haematobium* cause disease in sub-Saharan Africa and South America. Larvae from water snails penetrate human skin (when washing or swimming) and pass through the blood to the lungs and/or liver and into the circulation. Patients may present with 'Katayama fever' (dry cough, fever, SOB, wheeze, malaise) or more chronic symptoms due to pulmonary hypertension. CT may reveal small nodules, reticulonodular shadowing or areas of ground-glass. Diagnosis is made by detection of eggs in stool or urine, or by serology. Eosinophilia may be present. Treatment is with praziquantel. Steroids can be used in addition to reduce the immune response in Katayama fever. Artemether may be used as adjunctive therapy in acute disease as this has been found to be active against immature forms of the parasite.

Roundworms
Roundworm infection follows the oral ingestion of eggs or skin penetration by larval stages. These eggs or larvae may then cause an eosinophilic pneumonia (Löffler's syndrome) as they pass through the lungs. Alternatively, adult worms may cause obstruction in the bronchial tree (e.g. tracheal obstruction secondary to *Ascaris lumbricoides*) or, in an immunocompromised host, dissemination may occur (e.g. hyperinfection syndrome due to *Strongyloides stercoralis* in patients with HIV or HTLV-1).

Parasitic causes of Löffler's syndrome include:
- *Ascaris lumbricoides*.
- *Strongyloides stercoralis*.
- *Ancylostoma duodenale*.
- *Necator americanus*.
- *Trichinella spiralis*.
- *Toxocara canis/catis* (visceral larva migrans).

Clinical features of Löffler's syndrome include:
- Symptoms of paroxysmal cough, wheeze, dyspnoea and haemoptysis (pneumonitis).
- Blood (and sputum) eosinophilia.
- Raised total IgE.
- Hepatosplenomegaly.
- Transient migratory patchy infiltrates on CXR.

Diagnosis is by recognition of these clinical features. The exact organism can be determined by serology or detection of larval stages in bronchial secretions or of larval stages in stool or duodenal aspirates. *Trichinella spiralis* may be diagnosed on muscle biopsy.

Treatment is with thiobendazole, albendazole or mebendazole. In some cases (e.g. visceral larva migrans) adjunctive steroids may be indicated.

Tropical pulmonary eosinophilia
This is an asthma-like syndrome occurring due to infection with *Wucheria bancrofti* or *Brugia malayi*. Following a mosquito bite, larvae enter the body, producing microfilaria that become trapped in the lungs. Patients complain of cough, dyspnoea and nocturnal wheeze, and systemic symptoms such as fever, weight loss and malaise. Symptoms fail to respond to asthma medications. Blood tests reveal eosinophilia (>3000 cells/mm^3), raised total IgE, leucocytosis and raised inflammatory markers. Firm diagnosis relies on detection of anti-filarial antibodies (IgG and/or IgE) in the blood or, rarely, on detection of microfilaria on a nocturnal blood smear. Radiographic changes are of diffuse reticulonodular shadowing, miliary mottling or prominent hila. Treatment is with diethylcarbamazine (6mg/kg/day for 3 weeks). Untreated, pulmonary fibrosis may result.

Dog heartworm
Dirofilaria immitis (or *repens*) is transmitted from dogs to man via a mosquito bite. A solitary nodule on CXR, which is positive on PET scan, may result. This diagnosis therefore needs to be considered in tropical or subtropical areas in the differential diagnosis of lung cancer. It is usually a benign condition not requiring treatment.

Protozoa
Malaria
Plasmodium falciparum or *Plasmodium vivax* can cause pulmonary complications by sequestration of parasitised red blood cells in the lungs. This may result in cough, dypnoea and pulmonary oedema. Occasionally respiratory failure may result due to ARDS. The diagnosis of malaria is made on the basis of a blood smear. Treatment varies from region to region and is constantly changing due to patterns of drug resistance. Up to date advice can be found at: http://www.elsevier.com/framework_products/promis_misc/malaria_guidelines.pdf

Amoebiasis
Entamoeba histolytica usually infects the liver but may spread to the lung by direct invasion or via blood or lymphatic drainage. Pulmonary involvement may result in amoebic lung abscesses, pleural effusions, empyema or RLL consolidation. Pus resulting from this infection is characteristically similar in appearance to anchovy sauce. Diagnosis is made on the basis of active trophozoites in sputum or pleural pus, serology or sometimes by culture. Cysts or trophozoites may be detected on stool microscopy but these may be due to other *Entamoeba* spp. so microscopy should be combined with a PCR assay. Treatment is with metronidazole but resistance may occur. Diloxanide

furoate should be co-administered in order to eliminate the cysts.

Pulmonary leishmaniasis

Leishmania donovani infection is transmitted by the sandfly and causes leishmaniasis. Pulmonary involvement may occur in the presence of immunocompromise for example due to HIV or lung transplantation. A pneumonitis, pleural effusion or mediastinal lymphadenopathy may result. Diagnosis is by detection of leishmania amastigotes in bronchial secretions or tissues. Treatment is with amphotericin B (liposomal) and pentamidine. Oral miltefosine is beneficial in visceral leishmaniasis but its exact role on infections with pulmonary involvement is yet to be established.

Further reading

Bateman ED. A new look at the natural history of *aspergillus* hypersensitivity in asthmatics. *Resp Med* 1994; **88**(5): 325–327.

Herbrecht R, Denning DW, Patterson TF, *et al.* Voriconazole versus amphotencin B for primary therapy of invasive aspergillosis *N Engl J Med* 2002; **347**: 408–415.

Hinson KF, Moon AJ, Plummer NS. Bronchopulmonary aspergillosis. A review and a report of eight new cases. *Thorax* 1952; **7**: 317.

Kuzucu A. Parasitic diseases of the respiratory tract. *Curr Opin Pulm Med* 2006; **12**(3): 212–221.

Li YS, Chen G, He HB, *et al.* A double-blind field trial on the effects of artemether on Schistosoma japonicum infection in a highly endemic focus in southern China. *Acta Trop* 2005; **96**: 184–190.

Pfeiffer CD, Fine JP, Safdar N. Diagnosis of invasive aspergillosis using a galactomannan assay: a meta-analysis. *CID* 2006; **42**:1417–27.

Pound MW, Drew RH, Perfect JR. Recent advances in the epidemiology, prevention, diagnosis and treatment of fungal pneumonia. *Curr Opin Inf Dis* 2002 **15**:183–194.

Ross AG, Vickers D, Olds ER, *et al.* Katayama syndrome. *Lancet Infect Dis.* 2007; **7**(3): 218–24.

Sambatakou H, Dupont B, Lode H, *et al.* Voriconazole treatment for subacute invasive and chronic pulmonary aspergillosis. *Am J Med.* 2006; **119** (6): 527.

Stevens DA, Schwartz HJ, Lee JY, *et al.* A randomized trial of itraconazole in allergic bronchopulmonary aspergillosis. *N Engl J Med* 2000; 16; **342**(11): 756–62.

Soubani AO and Chandrasekar PH. The clinical spectrum of pulmonary aspergillosis. *Chest* 2002; **121**: 1988–1999.

Vijayan VK. How to diagnose and manage common parasitic pneumonias *Curr Op Pulm Med* **13**: 218–224.

Yao Z and Liao W. Fungal respiratory disease. *Curr Opin Pulm Med* 2006; **12**: 222–227.

Zmeili OS and Soubani AO. Pulmonary aspergillosis: a clinical update. *Q J Med* 2007; **100**: 317–334.

The immunocompromised host

Chapter contents

9.1 Pneumonia in the non-HIV immunocompromised patient

This chapter addresses the complex problem of 'pneumonia' (abnormal pulmonary infiltrates) in immunocompromised patients without HIV infection. It is structured as follows:

- The approach to the immune compromised patient with pulmonary infiltrates.
- The patterns of lung disease seen in some common clinical scenarios of immunosuppression.
- The major organisms causing opportunistic infection.

Approach to the immune compromised patient with pulmonary infiltrates

The lung is the organ most commonly affected by complications of immunosuppression. The term 'pulmonary infiltrates' can refer to many different disease processes (Table 9.1.1): although infections are the commonest cause, not all infiltrates are infections, and infection may co-exist with non-infectious processes in this population.

When managing an immune compromised patient with lung infiltrates, consider the whole picture, including risk factors and routes of infection. Many factors contribute to the 'net state of immune suppression':

- The immune defect (due to underlying malignancy, drugs, radiotherapy, autoimmune disease, functional defects). Different defects are associated with different complications and infections (see Table 9.1.2). Functional defects may not be apparent on simple blood tests.
- Recent antimicrobial prophylaxis or treatment. Prophylaxis may defer rather than prevent the development of infection.
- The patient's past history: pre-existing lung disease increases the risk of infection, and previous complications of immunosuppression may recur.
- Damage to other host defences: disruption of skin or mucosal barriers by tumour, mucositis, surgery, intravascular devices, catheters, drains.
- The risk of aspiration, increased by sedation, mucositis, debility and myopathy.
- Co-infection with immunomodulating viruses (CMV, EBV, HHV 6–7, HBV, HCV).
- Comorbidity (e.g. renal failure, malnutrition, ischaemic heart disease, alcoholism, cirrhosis, diabetes).
- Environmental exposure: consider the geographical prevalence of mycobacteria and endemic fungi (e.g. histoplasma), other occupational exposures such as aspergillus, zygomycetes and nocardia in gardeners and farmers, cryptococcus in pigeon breeders.
- Reactivation of existing infection (CMV, herpes viruses, tuberculosis, aspergillus).
- Infection from donated transplant organs or blood.

Clinical features

Pneumonia in the immune compromised patient often presents with non-specific symptoms of fever and malaise. Absence of fever does not exclude infection, and fever may be due to malignancy or drugs. Sputum is often not purulent, and may be absent.

Rate of onset of symptoms may help diagnosis, e.g. acute onset (<24 hours) raises suspicion of oedema, haemorrhage or embolism.

Thorough *physical examination* is essential. There may be few specific respiratory findings, but look for clues such as the absence of crackles despite marked infiltrates and hypoxia in PCP, or squeaks and wheezes in obliterative

bronchiolitis. Systemic examination may reveal extrapulmonary infection (e.g. meningitis with cryptococcal pneumonia, or endocarditis with staphylococcal lung abscess).

Investigations

Radiology: a 'clear' CXR does not exclude pulmonary pathology in this population, and CXR appearances are nonspecific. HRCT is more sensitive than CXR (detected abnormality in 50% of febrile neutropenic patients with normal CXR), and may become abnormal several days before CXR. Some CT appearances are diagnostic, (e.g. thromboembolism, obliterative bronchiolitis) and CT can localise a target for bronchoscopic lavage or biopsy, but infections and non-infectious processes can have similar appearances.

Serology is generally unhelpful in this group due to inability to raise antibodies acutely in response to infection. It may demonstrate past infection and hence risk of reactivation.

Any *sputum* should be analysed for fungi, mycobacteria, PCP and viruses as well as routine microbiology. It is relatively insensitive, and organisms may represent upper airway colonisation rather than lung infection. Sputum induction with hypertonic nebulised saline has a lower diagnostic success rate in this population compared to HIV-positive patients, but should be considered if bronchoscopy is not feasible. Nasopharyngeal washing and tracheal suction aspiration are alternative routes for obtaining respiratory secretions, with a similar risk of contamination.

Bronchoscopy with BAL is diagnostic of infection in approximately two-thirds of cases, and should be considered early if infiltrates are detected. Sensitivity is higher for diffuse alveolar infection (e.g. PCP) than for localised invasive disease (e.g. fungal nodules). Lavage site should be guided by CT findings. Send lavage fluid (BALF) for bacteria, fungi, mycobacteria, PCP and viruses, plus differential cell count and cytology. Other tests (cryptococcal antigen testing, CMV PCR) may be available. Negative findings on BAL are regarded as sufficient to exclude infection in contexts such as suspected idiopathic pneumonia syndrome, but if CT suggests focal infection such as fungal disease, negative BAL does not exclude this. Some authorities recommend additional sampling techniques such as protected specimen brushing, but this has not been proven to add sensitivity to BAL and (where feasible) transbronchial biopsy.

Table 9.1.1 Some causes of pulmonary infiltrates in the immune compromised patient

---

- Infection (opportunistic or non-opportunistic)
- Drug-induced lung disease
- Radiation pneumonitis
- Pulmonary oedema
- Pulmonary embolism
- Pulmonary haemorrhage
- ARDS
- Bronchiolitis obliterans organising pneumonia
- Transfusion-associated lung injury
- Diffuse alveolar damage
- Alveolar proteinosis
- Post-transplant lymphoproliferative disorder
- Recurrence of underlying disease in lungs (e.g. metastatic carcinoma, leukaemia, lymphoma)

Transbronchial biopsy (guided by recent CT) may detect malignancy, organising pneumonia or drug-induced lung disease, and is more sensitive than BAL for invasive infections (e.g. mycobacteria, aspergillus). It should be considered in all cases when BAL is performed, weighing the potential benefit against the risk of pneumothorax and bleeding.

Percutaneous lung biopsy under radiological guidance is useful in diagnosis of peripheral nodules, and *surgical lung biopsy* remains the definitive method to sample the lungs for diffuse or focal processes when the patient's condition permits. Specimens should be sent for microbiological analysis as well as histopathology.

Overall approach

In all patients the aim should be to obtain a definitive diagnosis of infective/non-infective disease as soon as possible, with low thresholds for CT scanning, bronchoscopy and biopsy. Exclusion of infection with BAL allows treatment with corticosteroids for many non-infective pathologies. Delay in diagnosis is associated with markedly worse outcome. However, if the patient is unwell or profoundly immunosuppressed, broad-spectrum empirical therapy should be started without waiting for the results of special investigations.

Critical care and non-invasive ventilation

The mortality rate in immunosuppressed patients who require invasive ventilation for respiratory failure is very high, approaching 100% in many series. The management of these patients requires honest and careful assessment of the ceiling of treatment, involving discussion with the patient, their family, and intensivists. Non-invasive face-mask ventilation has been shown to reduce the rate of intubation and hence mortality when applied early, before the onset of hypercapnic respiratory failure.

Clinical scenarios

Neutropenia

Neutropenia is the most important risk factor for pulmonary infection in immune compromised patients. It is a major dose-limiting side effect of cytotoxic chemotherapy, which both decreases neutrophil numbers and causes chemotactic and phagocytic defects, but it is seen in many other conditions that decrease production or increase consumption of neutrophils. It is defined as an absolute neutrophil count (ANC) <1.5×10⁹/l. The risk of infection increases with:

- Degree of neutropenia – increased risk if ANC <1.0, severe infection probable if ANC <0.1.
- Duration – relatively low risk of infection if neutropenia lasts <7–10 days (e.g. chemotherapy for solid tumours), high risk after 10 days with risk of multiple and recurrent new infections.
- Rate of onset – risk of infection lower in chronic neutropenias (e.g. severe aplastic anaemia/idiopathic neutropenia) than in patients with rapidly declining counts due to chemotherapy.

Neutropenic fever is defined by a single oral temperature >38.3°C (or 38°C over at least 1 hour). Bacteraemia is documented in 20% of cases of febrile neutropenia. Although no originating site of infection can be determined in 20–50% of febrile neutropenic cancer patients, 90% of such patients are likely to have infections, fever in the remainder being due to transfusions, drugs or tumour. Sputum production and pulmonary infiltrates may be absent in neutropenic patients with pneumonia.

Pathogens

The most common infectious complications of neutropenia due to chemotherapy are bacterial infections, including gram-positive bacteria (*S. aureus*, *S. epidermidis*, streptococci) and Gram-negative bacteria (enterobacter spp., *E. coli*, *Klebsiella*, *Pseudomonas*).

Invasive fungal infection with aspergillus, candida or mucor becomes more likely in profound, prolonged neutropenia (ANC <0.1).

Solid organ transplantation (SOT)

Pulmonary complications of lung transplantation are considered elsewhere.

Timing of pulmonary infections after transplantation

First month: the risk of infection is due more to surgery and intensive care than to immunosuppressive therapy. Prolonged ventilation increases the risk of nosocomial pneumonia. Surgery, sedation and pain impair cough and increase risk of aspiration pneumonia. Nosocomial bacterial infections predominate, e.g. gram negative pathogens (inc. *Legionella*, *Pseudomonas*), *S. aureus* and MRSA.

2nd to 6th months: sustained immunosuppression favours the emergence of opportunistic pathogens (aspergillus, nocardia, MTB, PCP, listeria), and viruses (most commonly CMV, also EBV and respiratory viruses).

After 6 months, if graft function is stable enough to allow reduced immunosuppression, community acquired organisms cause the majority of respiratory infections (pneumococcus, *Haemophilus*, *Legionella*, respiratory viruses). Patients who require augmented immunosuppression for graft rejection remain vulnerable to opportunistic pathogens, particularly *Aspergillus*, PCP, *Cryptococcus* and *Listeria*.

Liver transplantation

Liver transplantation involves lengthy surgery in physiologically vulnerable patients. Prolonged ventilatory support is often required. Most lung problems occur within 2 months of transplantation; around half are non-infective.

ARDS has an incidence of 5–15% with 80% mortality after liver transplantation. Risk factors: sepsis, transfusion, aspiration, use of OKT3.

Transudative pleural effusions (usually right sided, sometimes bilateral) due to lymphatic disruption are common – look for an alternative cause if not resolved by third week post transplant, or unilateral and left sided. *Right-sided diaphragmatic weakness* is common, due to phrenic nerve damage, and usually resolves spontaneously by 9 months.

Hepatopulmonary syndrome (hypoxaemia due to intrapulmonary vascular dilatation in chronic liver disease) and *portopulmonary hypertension* (pulmonary hypertension in advanced liver disease with portal hypertension) are normally diagnosed preoperatively, but are not immediately reversed by transplantation and are associated with reduced survival.

Pulmonary metastatic calcification: Development of calcified pulmonary nodules after liver and renal transplantation, possibly due to secondary hyperparathyroidism.

CXR usually shows single or multiple nodules or airspace opacification; calcification is not always apparent on plain films. CT scanning or technetium bone scanning (demonstrating tracer uptake in lungs) can confirm diagnosis, and exclude differential diagnoses. Rarely leads to a restrictive ventilatory impairment; no specific treatment is available.

Post transplantation lymphoproliferative disorder (PTLD): see Box 9.1.1.

Renal transplantation
Around one-third of pulmonary complications after renal transplantation have a non-infectious aetiology.

Pulmonary oedema is seen most often in the first few weeks post transplant, due to sodium/water retention with graft dysfunction and over hydration.

Venous thromboembolism is relatively common, accounting for two thirds of non-infectious pulmonary complications.

Pulmonary metastatic calcification (as in liver transplantation, above) may become apparent or progress after renal transplantation, rather than resolving as might be expected.

PTLD: see Box 9.1.1.

Haematopoietic stem cell transplantation (HSCT; bone marrow transplantation)
The spectrum of lung disease following HSCT is very dependent on the time following transplantation: see the 'timeline' in Fig. 9.1.1.

Pre-transplant conditioning: myeloablative conditioning includes high doses of chemotherapy ± total body irradiation (TBI) to ablate bone marrow and destroy tumour cells. *Non-myeloablative conditioning* uses less toxic regimens and is associated with fewer pulmonary complications.

Box 9.1.1 PTLD
Lymphoproliferative disorders (usually B cell lines) following HSCT or SOT range from benign lymphoid hyperplasia to frank malignant lymphoma. They typically occur within 6 months of transplantation (but can be years later), in 4% kidney, 2% liver, and 1–24% allogenic HSCT (highest with HLA mismatched donors, T-cell depleted donor stem cells, and ATG/monoclonal anti C-cell antibodies used for treatment of GVHD). Pre-transplant EBV seronegativity is a strong risk factor. PTLD may be asymptomatic or present with fever and weight loss, and may cause pulmonary nodules or hilar/mediastinal lymphadenopathy. HRCT may show ground glass 'halo' around nodules, interlobular septal thickening and airspace consolidation, mimicking many infections. Lesions are usually basilar, subpleural and peribronchial. Diagnosis is by percutaneous needle or surgical biopsy, occasionally by BAL cytology. PTLD is treated by reducing immunosuppression and giving anti-B cell monoclocal antibodies, and also (in HSCT) with EBV-specific cytotoxic T cells. Prognosis is variable, but poor in HSCT with underlying haematological malignancy.

Pre-engraftment phase (first 30 days after HSCT): neutropenia, mucositis, IV lines and impaired mucociliary clearance are the main risk factors for infection. Bacteria (Gram-negative or Gram-positive organisms) and fungi are the commonest causes of pulmonary infections in this phase.

Early post-engraftment phase (days 30–100 after HSCT): persistently impaired cell mediated and humoural immunity. Allogenic HSCT recipients at greater risk of infection than autologous due to the effects of graft versus host disease (GVHD) and the immunosuppressive drugs used to treat it. The most important pulmonary pathogens are fungi

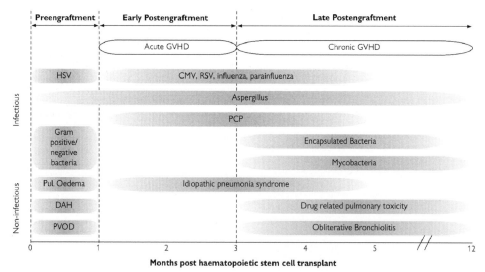

Fig. 9.1.1 Timeline of pulmonary complications post haematopoietic stem cell transplant. GVHD: graft versus host disease; HSV: herpes simplex virus; CMV: cytomegalovirus; RSV: respiratory syncytial virus; PCP: *Pneumocystis jirovecii* pneumonia; DAH: diffuse alveolar haemorrhage; PVOD: pulmonary veno-occlusive disease

(aspergillus, and in those unable to tolerate prophylaxis, PCP) and viruses (notably CMV, which may present much later if prophylaxis used, as well as other respiratory viruses).

By the *late postengraftment phase* (>100 days after HSCT), reconstitution of the immune system is nearly complete in autologous transplants, but allogenic recipients who develop chronic GVHD have persistent defects of cell mediated and humoural immunity and reticuloendothelial function. In these patients, encapsulated bacteria (e.g. *H. influenzae*, pneumococcus) and mycobacterial infections are the most important pathogens, in addition to opportunistic pathogens seen in early postengraftment phase.

Non-infectious complications of HSCT
Pulmonary oedema (cardiogenic or non-cardiogenic) is an early complication of HSCT. Cardiac function may be impaired by chemotherapy (e.g. daunorubicin). Chemotherapy, TBI or sepsis may increase permeability of the alveolar-capillary membrane causing non-cardiogenic oedema as seen in ARDS. Treatment is supportive with diuretic therapy and treatment of underlying infections.

Engraftment syndrome: fever, erythematous rash and non-cardiogenic pulmonary oedema coinciding with neutrophil recovery after HSCT, which may be more common with use of colony stimulating factors. May respond to steroids, but mortality is high in those who progress to respiratory failure.

Diffuse alveolar haemorrhage is a complication of the pre-engraftment phase with dyspnoea, non-productive cough, fever and hypoxaemia. Haemoptysis is surprisingly rare. CXR shows diffuse infiltrates particularly of the mid/lower zones, sometimes preceding symptoms by several days. BAL shows the classic finding of progressively bloodier aliquots of BALF (without organisms). High dose methyl-prednisolone 0.5–1g/day for several days followed by tapering prednisolone over 2 weeks dramatically reduces mortality rates of 50–80%.

Idiopathic pneumonia syndrome: diffuse lung injury occurring after HSCT for which an infectious aetiology is not identified. Median onset is at 40 days, but it can occur in the pre-engraftment period or months later. Risk factors include TBI, intensive conditioning regimes, and acute GVHD. Criteria for diagnosis are multilobar infiltrates on CXR or CT, signs and symptoms of pneumonia, and abnormal pulmonary physiology (increased A–a gradient, restrictive pulmonary function tests), plus exclusion of infection with BAL or transbronchial biopsy. On histology, diffuse mononuclear infiltrate with diffuse alveolar damage is seen. IPS may progress rapidly to respiratory failure requiring ventilation, with high mortality (70%). No specific

treatments are available, although some respond to methylprednisolone 1–2mg/kg/day; etanercept has been proposed as a possible treatment.

Obliterative bronchiolitis is a common late complication of allogenic HSCT, associated with chronic GVHD; it is rare after autologous transplants. Risk factors include low FEV_1/FVC pre-HSCT, increasing age, and viral chest infection in first 100 days. The onset is insidious, with dry cough, dyspnoea and wheezing. Auscultation may find crackles, wheezes, inspiratory squawks or all three. Fever is rare. CXR is usually normal or hyperinflated; HRCT shows mosaic pattern of hyperinflated lobules with reduced vascular marking alternating with normal areas, most obvious on expiratory films. Spirometry shows airflow obstruction without bronchodilator reversibility. Formal diagnosis requires exclusion of infection by BAL.

Delayed pulmonary toxicity/restrictive syndrome is late pulmonary injury in autologous HSCT (originally described after high-dose breast cancer chemotherapy) with restrictive spirometry, impaired diffusing capacity, and ground glass pattern on HRCT. Generally responds to steroids.

Pulmonary veno-occlusive disease occurs rarely after HSCT; it may be due to chemotherapy. Patients have dyspnoea, normal lung function, and no infection. Right heart catheterisation shows pulmonary hypertension with no emboli. Lung biopsy confirms the diagnosis. Treatment with immunosuppression and vasodilators is of questionable efficacy.

Post transplant lymphoproliferative disorder: See Box 9.1.1. Pulmonary lesions may also be due to relapse of underlying malignancy, e.g. lymphoma.

Bronchiolitis obliterans organising pneumonia (BOOP) may follow successful treatment of CMV pneumonitis, be related to chronic GVHD, or be idiopathic.

Organisms

Different forms of immune defect are associated with different spectra of pathogens, as summarised in Table 9.1.2.

Conventional bacterial infections
Common things being common, immunocompromised patients are at risk from non-opportunistic bacteria. Organisms are frequently nosocomial and multiresistant.

Nocardia
Nocardia is predominantly an infection of immunocompromised subjects, associated with cell-mediated immune defects due to steroid use, haematological malignancy or transplantation. Presentation is subacute with fever, dry cough, and weight loss; less commonly dyspnoea, pleuritic pain or haemoptysis. CXR/CT typically shows nodules or

Table 9.1.2 Infections associated with different types of immune defect

Immune defect	Predominant pathogenic organisms
Neutropenia or phagocyte defect	Bacteria: staphylococci, streptococci, Gram-negative bacilli (enteric and non-enteric), *Nocardia*
	Fungi: *Candida*, *Aspergillus*, mucormycosis
T-lymphocyte deficiency	Viruses: CMV, HSV, VZV, EBV, respiratory viruses
	Intracellular bacteria: *Legionella*, mycobacteria, *Listeria*, *Nocardia*
	Fungi: *Pneumocystis jiroveci*, *Histoplasma capsulatum*, *Cryptococcus neoformans*
	Parasites: *Toxoplasma gondii*, *Strongyloides stercoralis*
B-lymphocyte deficiency, hypogammaglobulinaemia, hyposplenism	Encapsulated bacteria: *Streptococcus pneumoniae*, *Haemophilus influenzae*, *Neisseria meningitides*

masses that may cavitate, but may show parenchymal infiltrates, subpleural plaques or effusions. It can be complicated by empyema (25%), mediastinitis, pericarditis, and superior vena cava syndrome. The incidence is reduced by septrin as PCP prophylaxis, but may occur after prophylaxis has ceased.

Nocardia are not usually found in the respiratory tract, so isolation of the filamentous branching gram-positive rods from sputum or BAL is diagnostic. The diagnosis can also be made by aspirating extrapulmonary disease such as skin abscesses. The laboratory should be warned that nocardia is a possibility, to allow appropriate processing. Tissue biopsies show a mixed cellular infiltrate, rarely with granulomata. Treat with sulphonamides for 6–12 months.

Tuberculosis and other mycobacteria
The incidence of TB is increased in all types of immune compromise. The risk is higher in endemic areas, e.g. 0.5–2% post-SOT in USA/Europe but up to 15% in India. Most infections are due to reactivation of latent disease. It is a late complication of transplantation; fever is the most common symptom. CXR may show focal infiltrates, a miliary pattern, effusions, or more rarely (<5%) diffuse interstitial infiltrates or cavitating lesions. Diagnosis is usually made from sputum or bronchial washings. Tuberculin skin testing has a high false negative rate in immune suppression; a newly positive skin test suggests active disease, but this is rarely seen. There is little data regarding interferon γ assays in immune compromised patients.

Combination treatment regimes should be used. Isoniazid hepatotoxicity can be problematic in liver transplants. Rifampicin increases clearance of tacrolimus and cyclosporine, increasing risk of rejection, so monitor drug levels closely. Mortality is high (25–40%) in those who cannot complete the course of treatment.

Non-tuberculous mycobacteria (NTM) cause more frequent and severe infections in the immune compromised. There are many NTM species: refer to current guidelines for management. Prolonged treatment is required and mortality is high; control rather than eradication of infection may be the best achievable outcome.

Fungi
Pneumocystis pneumonia (PCP, Pneumocystis jirovecii)
Risk factors for PCP include prolonged glucocorticoid use, malignancy (esp. haematological, and with use of purine analogues e.g. fludarabine) and transplant. Defective cell-mediated immunity probably leads to reactivation of latent disease. It presents with dry cough, dyspnoea and usually fever; the onset is often more rapid in non-HIV than in HIV. Clinical examination is often normal, with no crackles. There is marked arterial oxygen desaturation on exertion. CXR (and HRCT) may show bilateral perihilar alveolar infiltrates (less commonly isolated nodules, lobar consolidation, cavities/cysts, pneumothorax); CXR is normal in up to 30%. WCC is usually normal, LDH may be raised.

Diagnosis is usually by identification of the organism (e.g. direct immunofluorescence) in induced sputum or BAL fluid: sensitivity is lower than in HIV (60%) as the burden of infection is usually lower. If clinical suspicion is high and sputum/BAL is negative, consider transbronchial or open lung biopsy. If the patient is unwell, begin empirical treatment: BAL remains positive for at least a week. Treat with high-dose septrin for 14–21 days, or iv pentamidine, dapsone+trimethoprim, clindamycin+primaquine or atovaquone if intolerant. If unwell, add high dose steroids

for five days, tapering over two weeks. Expect a response within five days.

The risk of PCP reduces with use of septrin prophylaxis (from 16% in allogenic HSCT to <0.5%), but bone marrow suppression limits tolerability in up to a third; dapsone and nebulised pentamidine are less effective (7% and 3% incidence PCP).

Invasive pulmonary aspergillosis
Aspergillus infection (most commonly *A. fumigatus*, also *flavus, niger* and >20 other species) is a major cause of disease in the immune compromised, associated with prolonged neutropenia, glucocorticoid therapy, HSCT, SOT, HIV, anti-TNFα therapy and chronic granulomatous disease. It is the leading infective cause of death in allogenic HSCT.

The symptoms are non-specific: non-productive cough, fever (may be absent in HSCT), dyspnoea, pleuritic chest pain, haemoptysis (due to angioinvasion & pulmonary infarction), pneumothorax. Disease may progress rapidly over days.

CXR may be normal or show peripheral nodules which may coalesce. CT is more sensitive: look for the 'halo sign' of a ground-glass rim around pulmonary nodules, due to haemorrhage. This is distinct from the 'air crescent sign', which may appear in later stages of invasive aspergillosis with resorption of necrotic tissue by neutrophils (Fig. 9.1.2).

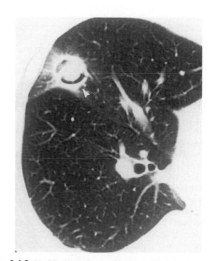

Fig. 9.1.2 Nodule (arrow) caused by *Aspergillus* infection, illustrating both the halo and air crescent signs.

The diagnostic gold standard is isolation of the organism on culture of tissue from lung biopsy. Culture is required to distinguish *Aspergillus* from other fungi. Aspergillus in sputum or BAL fluid can represent colonisation or contamination rather than invasive infection, and BAL sensitivity is low (30–50%). However, if aspergillus is isolated it is usually treated, if the clinical scenario suggests a high risk of infection.

ELISA for serum galactomannan (a fungal wall component released in invasive aspergillosis, often before radiographic change) is sensitive and specific in HSCT and haematological malignancy, less so in SOT. Beta-lactam antibiotics can cause false positives; antifungal treatment reduces sensitivity.

Treatment: reduce immunosuppression if possible. Voriconazole shows a higher response, lower mortality and fewer adverse reactions than liposomal amphotericin B; caspofungin is an alternative if other drugs are not tolerated. Treatment should continue for at least 2 weeks after clinical/radiological appearances have resolved, which may take months. The condition may relapse if neutropenia recurs.

Cryptococcus neoformans (cryptococcal pneumonia)
Risk factors: impaired cellular immunity including HIV, malignancy (esp. lymphoma), transplantation, corticosteroids, cirrhosis, renal failure, diabetes, chronic lung disease, TNFα antagonists. It presents acutely or insidiously with cough, dyspnoea, fever and other non-specific symptoms. CXR/CT commonly shows peripheral nodules, sometimes cavitating, less commonly lobar infiltrates, adenopathy, effusions.

Diagnosis: identification of the organism (Indian ink stain) in sputum or BALF is specific, as it is a rare contaminant. Serum cryptococcal antigen is positive in ~70% non-HIV patients with cryptococcal pneumonia and suggests aggressive disease; it can be used to monitor disease. Pleural fluid and BAL cryptococcal antigen may be helpful. Most patients with pneumonia also have extrapulmonary disease: consider CT head/LP to exclude cryptococcal meningoencephalitis. Treat with amphotericin and flucytosine for 14–21 days followed by fluconazole PO for 6–12 months.

Candida pneumonia
The significance of *Candida* isolated from the respiratory tract is often debated because of the frequency of oral contamination, but true *Candida* pneumonia is a severe complication of immunosuppression or critical illness, with a poor prognosis. It may follow aspiration or candidaemia, and often causes high fever. Radiological findings include nodules and consolidation; *Candida* may also cause empyema. Because of the risk of contamination of sputum/BALF, definitive diagnosis requires lung biopsy. Treat with amphotericin or fluconazole.

Pulmonary zygomycosis (including mucormycosis)
The zygomycetes are ubiquitous fungi in soil or decaying vegetation; *Mucor* spp. are most familiar, but *Rhizopus* spp. are commoner pathogens. Lung infection is due to inhalation; risk factors include neutropenia, diabetes, IVDU, malnutrition, trauma/burns, steroids, haematological malignancy, transplant, and iron overload treated with desferrioxamine.

Infection causes rapid onset of fever, cough, dyspnoea and haemoptysis (may be massive, due to angioinvasion). The pneumonia is diffuse with infarction and necrosis; CXR/CT may show cavitation with air crescent sign, nodules, or effusions. BAL sensitivity is low, the gold standard is lung biopsy tissue culture. Treat with amphotericin; consider surgical resection if planning HSCT as the risk of recurrence is high.

Viruses

Cytomegalovirus (CMV) pneumonia
Clinical CMV infection may be due to reactivation or to transmission from seropositive transplant or blood donors. The main risk factor is defective cell-mediated immunity, especially in allogeneic HSCT. The risk depends on the infection history of donor and recipient, so is lowest when both are seronegative. Ganciclovir prophylaxis is effective, but its tolerability is limited by neutropenia; disease may occur 1–4 months after stopping prophylaxis. CMV infection

is itself immunomodulatory and predisposes to PCP, *Aspergillus* infection and graft rejection.

CMV pneumonia commonly presents with flu-like symptoms, low grade fever, dyspnoea, dry cough and hypoxia, progressing to respiratory failure. Blood tests may show leucopenia, thrombocytopenia, hepatitic liver function. CXR appearances are variable, classically bilateral subtle diffuse infiltrates, sometimes lobar consolidation or small nodules. HRCT shows ground glass opacities or small centrilobular nodules.

The gold standard for diagnosis is demonstration of 'owl's eye' viral inclusion bodies on lung biopsy, but this is frequently impractical. Serology is useful to determine past infection status but not as a test for acute infection unless seroconversion is demonstrated in a suggestive clinical context. CMV antigenaemia and quantitative blood PCR testing are rapid and specific; a rise in values may prompt pre-emptive treatment before disease is apparent.

BAL cytology (visualisation of nuclear/cytoplasmic inclusion bodies) is specific but insensitive. Conventional culture takes weeks, replaced by shell-vial assay (early antigen detection using immunofluorescence with monoclonal antibodies to CMV) which takes 2–3 days and is more sensitive, but not specific. Culture of CMV in BAL fluid defines systemic infection but not necessarily pneumonia. CMV PCR on BALF is being evaluated.

Treatment of may be started pragmatically on basis of compatible clinical/radiological features, preferably with detection of CMV on BAL. Treat with IV ganciclovir for 2–4 weeks, plus CMV-specific immune globulin in severe cases. Mortality is high, up to 85%, with relapse in up to a third.

Other respiratory viruses
RSV and influenza are epidemic in winter/spring, adenovirus and parainfluenza occur throughout year. In SOT recipients, LRTI from these viruses is more common than in the general population, manifest as fever, dyspnoea, cough and wheezing normally in 2nd–6th months post-transplant.

RSV pneumonia after HSCT causes bilateral interstitial infiltrates and high mortality. RSV also causes otitis media and sinusitis. Ribavirin may help if given early enough.

Adenovirus infection may cause fatal pneumonia 2–3 months post-HSCT, as well as pharyngitis, tracheitis, bronchitis, enteritis, cystitis, or disseminated disease. It can be cultured from pharynx, respiratory secretions or urine. There is no proven effective prophylaxis or treatment.

HSV, since aciclovir prophylaxis, is now a rare cause of pneumonitis in preengraftment phase of HSCT. It is due to reactivation, so only seropositive patients are at risk.

HHV-6 has been reported to cause pulmonary infiltrates after HSCT, and may account for some cases diagnosed as IPS.

Parainfluenza is a cause of URTI, laryngotracheitis, bronchiolitis, and pneumonia after HSCT. URTI precedes LRTI: nasopharyngeal lavage may allow diagnosis before pneumonia (cultures positive 9 days after symptoms). Fatal once respiratory failure occurs; there are reports of benefit from ribavirin.

Human metapneumovirus is a recently described and sometimes fatal cause of lung disease after HSCT.

Further reading

Abramson S. The Air Crescent Sign. *Radiology* 2001; **218**: 230–232.

Kothe H, Dalhoff K. Pneumonia in the immunocompromised patient. *Eur Respir Mon* 2006; **36**: 200–213.

Kotloff RM, Ahya VN, Crawford SW. Pulmonary Complications of Solid Organ and Hematopoietic Stem Cell Transplantation. *Am J Resp Crit Care Med* 2004; **170**: 22–48.

Pizzo PA. Fever in Immunocompromised Patients. *New Engl J Med* 1999; **336**: 309–316.

Rañóa A, Agustía C, Jimeneza P, *et al.* Pulmonary infiltrates in non-HIV immunocompromised patients: a diagnostic approach using non-invasive and bronchoscopic procedures. *Thorax* 2001; **56**: 379–387.

Shellito J. Symposium: The Compromised Host. *Proc Am Thoracic Soc* 2005; **2**: 397–460.

9.2 Infection in the HIV compromised host

Since the first, consistent reports of HIV infection in the early 1980s, the speed at which advances in our understanding of this condition have taken place is unparalleled in medicine. The introduction of HAART in 1995, plus effective chemoprophylaxis against opportunistic infections, has transformed the natural history of HIV infection from one with a uniformly gloomy outlook to a condition with an associated life-span perhaps not much less than that of the general population in the developed world. Despite this it remains a huge global health problem. For respiratory physicians this is important as the lungs are the site most commonly affected by opportunistic infections (OI).

The UNAIDS estimated that in 2007, 33.7 million individuals were living with HIV infection. Two-thirds of these are within sub-Saharan Africa. Approximately 21.5 million people have died since 1990 as a result of HIV infection. Possibly up to 50% of these have been due to TB. In the US there are about 1 million infected individuals; whilst the UK has around 72,000. Survey data suggest that almost one third of these people do not know they are infected. Thus it is depressingly common to see patients presenting *in extremis* with undiagnosed HIV infection and opportunistic disease. The major groups of affected individuals within the UK are men who have sex with other men (MSM) (40% of cases), heterosexual women (30%), heterosexual men (20%) and injecting drug users (<5%). New cases are more frequently heterosexual than MSM; and are four times more likely to be black-African than any other ethnic group.

This chapter describes respiratory infections in individuals with known or suspected HIV infection. It provides a general approach to assessment, and then covers specific, important pulmonary infections relevant to UK practice.

General approach to the HIV patient with pulmonary infection

The immune dysregulation associated with HIV means that a wide spectrum of organisms may be responsible for pulmonary infection (Table 9.2.1). However, it is important to remember that *Pneumocystis jirovecii* pneumonia (PCP) and bacterial pneumonia are the commonest causes of acute, life-threatening HIV-related respiratory disease. Mycobacteria (and in particular TB) should not be forgotten; nor that more than one pathogen can be demonstrated in up to 20% of cases. Although there may be helpful pointers in the history, examination and initial simple investigations, often the decision needs to be taken to start empiric therapy prior to obtaining a definitive diagnosis. This is discussed in more detail later in this chapter.

Important points in assessment

The degree of immunosuppression

It is possible to map specific respiratory conditions to the level of an individual's immuno-suppression. This is most easily assessed using blood CD4 T-lymphocyte counts, which generally are inversely related to the degree of immune dysfunction. In an HIV-uninfected individual the normal absolute CD4 count is between 500–1500 cells/µl. During the course of untreated HIV infection this will almost certainly fall to near undetectable levels after several years. Different organisms should be considered depending on the blood CD4 count. When the CD4 count

Table 9.2.1 Causes of pulmonary infection in the HIV compromised

Bacterial
Streptococcus pneumoniae
Haemophilus influenzae
Staphylococcus aureus
Pseudomonas aeruginosa
Escherichia coli

Mycobacteria
Mycobacterium tuberculosis
Mycobacterium avium-intracellulare complex
Mycobacterium kansasii
Other non-tuberculous mycobacteria

Fungi
Pneumocystis jirovecii
Cryptococcus neoformans
Histoplasma capsulatum
Penicillium marneffei
Aspergillus spp.
Coccidioides immitis
Blastomycetes dermatitidis

Parasites
Toxoplasma gondii
Strongyloides stercoralis

Viruses
Cytomegalovirus
Adenovirus
Herpes simplex

is >200 cells/µl, bacterial pneumonia and TB are most likely. At lower CD4 counts, PCP, fungal and non-tuberculous mycobacterial infections are additional possibilities. It should be remembered that PCP can occur at higher CD4 counts (especially in people with physical indicators of immune suppression such as oral thrush; or very high HIV plasma loads). It may also be seen occasionally during acute (primary) HIV infection when there is a profound, transient fall in systemic immunity. Blood CD4 counts may fluctuate on a day to day basis; and it can be helpful to also know either the CD4:CD8 ratio or CD4 percentage (of all T and B lymphocytes), which are rather more stable measures. The latter can be related to blood CD4 absolute counts if one remembers that a CD4 of 200 cells/µl is usually 14%, and CD4 of 400 cells/µl is roughly double that at 27%.

Patient medication history

Patients who are using effective HAART (sustained suppression or near-suppression of plasma HIV load for at least 3 months) have a greatly reduced (50–80%) risk of severe respiratory illness. This is particularly the case for PCP and TB; though rather less so with bacterial pneumonia. The use of specific OI prophylaxis (such as PCP prophylaxis with co-trimoxazole taken at an effective dose for at least 2 weeks) is also relevant; as this may suggest alternative diagnoses (than in this example, PCP) or raise the possibility of the development of resistance to the prophylactic agents. Medication (e.g. the antiretroviral, zidovudine or prolonged use of antibiotics such as rifabutin) can lead to neutropenia and a subsequent increased risk of systemic bacterial infections and invasive fungal infections

Mode of infection

Injecting drug users are at greater risk of bacterial pneumonia and TB.

Travel, residence and ethnic origin

PCP is found more frequently in European and US studies than those from the developing world, where TB and bacterial pneumonia predominate. However patients who have previously lived in TB-endemic areas are inevitably at a much greater risk of active TB when resident in the West than the native populations. Reactivation of certain other conditions should also be considered in individuals who have lived or travelled to certain parts of the world. These include fungi such as *Histoplasma capsulatum* (the Americas, Africa and many parts of Asia), *Coccidioides immitis* and *Blastomyces dermatitidis* (predominantly the Americas and Africa), *Penicillium marneffei* (South-East Asia) and worm infections including *Strongyloides stercoralis* (same distribution as *Histoplasma*).

A history of previous PCP or TB increases the likelihood of recurrent infection. Recurrent bacterial infection may lead to bronchiectasis; which in turn will promote further acute respiratory disease with the types of organisms usually associated with this condition.

Non-infectious diagnoses should also be considered. These will be discussed in Chapter 9.3.

Clinical features

Systemic symptoms such as fever, weight loss, and fatigue are present to a variable extent in many respiratory infections. In themselves, therefore, they may provide little additional diagnostic information.

Progressive breathlessness (usually worsening over the space of several days to weeks) is regarded as characteristic of PCP. A pattern of sudden deterioration on a gradual background may result from pneumothorax (which again is typically associated with PCP).

Cough with sputum is suggestive of bacterial pneumonia or mycobacterial disease. Dry cough of gradual onset is more indicative of PCP in a patient with a CD4 count <200 cells/μl. Although community acquired viral pneumonias (e.g. influenza A) do not appear to be any more common in HIV infected subjects, they will be missed if not actively sought. In presentation they often mimic PCP.

Haemoptysis is suggestive of mycobacterial or fungal causes. Pleuritic chest pain can occur in all infections but is more commonly noted with bacterial pneumonia.

Pleural effusions may be found in any patient with pneumonia but are more commonly associated with bacterial (small to medium size), mycobacterial (any size) infections; malnutrition, renal impairment, fluid overload (small and bilateral) or malignancy (including lung cancer, primary effusion lymphoma and Kaposi sarcoma). They are rare in PCP.

Hepatosplenomegaly can be found in disseminated mycobacterial or fungal disease, lymphoma or multicentric Castleman disease (angio-follicular hyperplasia).

Lymphadenopathy is suggestive of similar diseases, though smooth, non-tender and symmetrical nodes in the neck, axillae and groin are present in many asymptomatic HIV-infected individuals who are not receiving HAART.

Investigations

Serology. Pneumococcal urinary antigen is helpful in suspected bacterial pneumonia. It has a similar sensitivity (approaching 80%) and specificity (approximately 95%) in HIV infected and uninfected individuals. Urine testing for *Legionella* antigen may also be of value; whilst in appropriate cases, urine and blood *Histoplasma* polysaccharide antigen tests have good sensitivity; although false positives can occur in *Blastomyces* and *Coccidioides* spp. infected individuals. Serum cryptococcal antigen has excellent specificity; though is less sensitive in local (e.g. pulmonary) cryptococcal infection than in disseminated disease, where cryptococcaemia is more likely to be present (e.g. >90% positive in cryptococcal meningitis). Serology (acute and convalescent) can be sent for atypical organisms such as *Legionella pneumophila*, *Mycoplasma pneumonia* and *Chlamydia* spp.

Lactate dehydrogenase (LDH) is elevated in up to 90% of patients with PCP; however it is also increased in several other infections (in particular mycobacterial disease and histoplasmosis) as well as lymphoma and lymphocytic interstitial pneumonitis (LIP). As such it lacks diagnostic specificity.

Blood cultures

The increased rates of bacteraemia and septicaemia in HIV-related bacterial pneumonia mean that blood cultures are reported to be positive 40 times more frequently than found in HIV-negative controls. It is important that good-quality blood cultures for both bacteria and mycobacteria (where appropriate) are obtained.

Exercise oxygen saturation. Transcutaneous oximetry may be used in HIV-infected patients to assess for exercise-induced oxygen desaturation. This is of most value in discriminating subjects with a first episode of PCP and normal or near normal chest radiographs, from other causes of this clinical picture. It is generally regarded as a fall to less than 90% from a baseline of ≥95%, following exercise which increases heart rate towards 80% of predicted maximum.

Arterial blood gas analysis provides more information than oxygen saturations. For a given severity of clinical disease a wider arterial oxygen gradient (A–aO$_2$) is found in those with PCP or other causes of alveolitis compared to bacterial pneumonia. Fewer than 10% of patients with PCP have a normal PaO$_2$ and a normal A–aO$_2$.

Lung function testing may confirm decreases in gas transfer, DLCO, which mirror exercise desaturation in those with PCP. However it is not a test which can distinguish between the different underlying aetiologies of a given clinical picture – and is therefore of little diagnostic value.

CXR may show focal areas of consolidation, diffuse infiltrates, nodules or pneumothorax. The radiological pattern may be helpful as shown in Table 9.2.2.

CT scanning of the chest and mediastinum may be useful when the CXR is normal or equivocal. HRCT may reveal the typical ground-glass appearance of an alveolitis that is often found in PCP. However the features lack specificity for this condition. It may also aid in the diagnosis of non-infectious causes such as pulmonary embolism, idiopathic pneumonitis and lymphocytic interstitial pneumonitis. HRCT can also aid in guiding a more directed BAL. Mediastinal imaging may reveal unsuspected lymphadenopathy. Central necrosis of these nodes is usually regarded as indicating either mycobacterial or, less commonly, fungal disease or IRIS (immune reconstitution inflammatory syndrome).

Table 9.2.2 Common chest radiograph findings in the HIV-infected individual

Chest radiological finding	Diagnosis
Normal	Pneumocystis pneumonia (PCP)
	Viruses
	TB
Focal infiltrate	Bacteria (S.pneumoniae, H. influenzae)
	Mycobacteria
	Fungi (Cryptococcus, Histoplasma, Aspergillus, Coccidioides)
	Complex bacteria e.g. Nocardia
	Pulmonary Kaposi's sarcoma or lymphoma
	PCP (an apical infiltrate if on prophylactic nebulised pentamidine)
Diffuse infiltrate	PCP (classical presentation)
	Mycobacteria
	Respiratory viruses
	CMV
	Bacteria
	Fungi
	Toxoplasma
	Lymphocytic interstitial pneumonia
	Non-specific interstitial pneumonia
Diffuse nodules	Mycobacteria
	Fungi (small nodules)
	Kaposi's sarcoma, lymphoma (large nodules)
Cavities	Bacteria (S. aureus, S.pneumoniae Klebsiella)
	TB, M. kansasii
	Fungi
	PCP may appear to cavitate if pneumatoceles present
Pleural effusion	Bacterial
	TB
	Primary effusion lymphoma
	Lung cancer
Pneumothorax	PCP
	Mycobacteria
Mediastinal adenopathy	Tuberculosis
	Other mycobacteria
	Fungi
	Kaposi's sarcoma
	Lymphoma
	Castleman's disease

Microbiology. All patients who are expectorating sputum spontaneously should have samples sent for Gram stain, culture and sensitivity together with samples for staining for acid-fast bacilli and mycobacterial culture. Ideally early morning (or overnight) specimens should be sent on 3 separate occasions to maximise diagnostic sensitivity for mycobacteria.

Induced sputum (IS) may be more helpful, as spontaneous sputum samples are inadequate for the routine diagnosis of PCP. Here, samples are obtained by inhaling hypertonic saline via an ultrasonic nebuliser. Given the possible risk of nosocomial aerosol transmission of e.g. TB, IS should be performed in a well-ventilated setting or a negative-pressure environment, away from other patients. The sensitivity of induced sputum for PCP varies markedly (between 50–95%). This probably reflects the degree of local experience in both sputum sample production and interpretation. Thus, a negative test result from IS should prompt further investigations – typically bronchoscopy and BAL. Once the sample is in the laboratory, immunoflouresence staining enhances yield when compared to standard Grocott silver staining. IS is also helpful in patients with suspected TB who are either spontaneous sputum smear negative or not producing sputum. In such patients IS has a similar yield to bronchoscopy and BAL.

Bronchoscopy allows airway and alveolar sampling, as well as direct visualization of the proximal airways. In the latter case it is of more assistance in the diagnosis of non-infective complications discussed in the next chapter in known or suspected HIV infected. A good quality BAL (composed of mainly alveolar cells with few bronchial epithelial cells) should be obtained and analysed for bacteria, mycobacteria, viruses, fungi and protozoa. *Pneumocystis jirovecii* cannot be cultured. Therefore histochemical examination for this organism is important (see earlier in chapter). BAL has a sensitivity of around 90% for *Pneumocystis jirovecii*. BAL is also helpful in suspected fungal pneumonia; where the organism may be detected with antigen testing e.g. *Cryptococcus* antigen.

Transbronchial biopsy (TBB) is usually reserved for patients in whom other investigations have failed to provide a diagnosis. The sensitivity of TBB for PCP is up to 90% when used as the sole diagnostic test. It is greater than 95% when combined with BAL. However there is a relatively high complication rate with an increased risk of pneumothorax or pulmonary haemorrhage.

Overall management approach

A balance needs to be sought between obtaining a definitive diagnosis and treating empirically for the likeliest pathogens (which may be multiple). If the patient is sick, treatment should be instituted for what is often bacterial pneumonia, PCP or mycobacterial disease. In this situation, investigations need to be tailored to what is practicable, though without specific pulmonary samples it may be difficult to obtain a final diagnosis.

Non-invasive ventilation and intensive care

Respiratory support with e.g. CPAP can be initiated in those with evidence of hypoxia and no hypercapnia. Patients who require ICU admission for pulmonary infections are often those who are presenting with a first severe HIV-related illness. With the improvement in treatment of OI and the benefits of HAART, HIV-infected individuals should not be excluded from full ventilatory assistance if deemed appropriate. Recent studies suggest that overall survival from ICU is similar to that of a non-infected population at greater than 65%. In general unless a patient has a clear cut-terminal illness (e.g. lymphoma unresponsive to therapy), they should be offered admission and comprehensive ICU care. One also needs to consider other co-morbidities, as well as the wishes of the patient when reaching a decision about this. Prognostic factors that appear to carry a worse outcome for HIV positive patients admitted to ICU include lower haemoglobin, lower blood CD4 count, higher APACHE II score and need for mechanical ventilation. The largest single group of patients who require ICU admission will have PCP. Here further factors associated with mortality include increasing age, the presence of pneumothorax and mechanical ventilation with a strategy which does not use low tidal volumes. The latter is especially interesting as unlike the majority of other prognostic factors, this can be influenced favorably during the ICU admission itself.

Immune reconstitution inflammatory syndrome (IRIS)

This intriguing condition was originally noted in the context of treatment for HIV negative mycobacterial disease several years ago, where subjects on effective therapy would have a paradoxical deterioration in their symptoms following an early initial improvement. It is thought to be the clinical manifestation of a returning immune response directed against specific antigen. IRIS will be discussed in more detail in the chapter on non-infectious respiratory complications of HIV infection, though is most commonly reported (in up to one-third) of HIV patients with systemic mycobacterial or fungal infections who start HAART. There is no diagnostic test for IRIS; and it should only be accepted as the cause of symptoms when other possibilities such as drug failure (due to resistance, non-adherence or adverse effects) or new opportunistic diseases have been excluded.

Specific infections

Bacterial pneumonia

Bacterial pneumonia occurs two to four times more frequently in HIV-infected individuals than the general population. Risk factors include previous pneumonia, injecting drug use, cigarette smoking and declining CD4 count. The clinical presentation, assessment and treatment are broadly similar to that of non-HIV infected individuals, as discussed in Chapter 9.1. The most common pathogens in the general population are also largely those encountered in HIV infected subjects. The key differences and special considerations in the HIV-infected patient are outlined.

- Bacteraemia is up to 100 times more common with a diagnostic rate of blood culture being 40-times that of HIV-uninfected patients.
- CXR may be atypical with diffuse infiltrates present in up to 50%.
- Lobar or segmental consolidation may result from a wide variety of bacterial, mycobacterial, fungal and viral pathogens.
- Pleural effusions occur twice as often and empyema and pleural abscess are also seen more frequently.
- As the CD4 count falls to <200 cells/µl more unusual organisms are implicated. These include *Staphylococcus aureus* and *Pseudomonas aeruginosa*.
- *Nocardia asteroides* infection can occur at low CD4 counts although the use of trimethoprim/sulfamethoxazole (TMP-SMX, co-trimoxazole) as PCP prophylaxis may have decreased its overall incidence. Diagnosis is made by identification of the organism in sputum or BAL.
- *Rhodococcus equi* can occur in subjects with very low CD4 counts who have a history of exposure to farms and farm animals. Identification of the organism by culture of sputum, BAL or blood is diagnostic.

- Treatment for the presumed or confirmed causative organisms should be based on local guidelines and resistance patterns. In practice it is often sensible to treat with a broad spectrum antibiotic such as co-amoxiclav or a 'second' or 'third' generation cephalosporin in the first instance, even if PCP is suspected.

Pneumocystis jirovecii pneumonia

P. jirovecii (formerly called *P. carinii*) is a fungus that causes infection specific to humans. To avoid confusion, the term PCP remains to describe PneumoCystis Pneumonia. Serology shows that most people have been exposed to *Pneumocystis* in childhood. However latest evidence suggests that re-infection is the main source of clinical disease. Evidence for nosocomial transmission exists but is limited. Before the advent of prophylactic therapy and HAART, PCP occurred in up to 80% of HIV-infected individuals with AIDS and was the first OI described in this context. PCP is now much less common and is seen mainly in individuals of unknown or undisclosed HIV status; or HIV-infected individuals not using adequate PCP prophylaxis or HAART (see later). PCP has been reported from all parts of the world.

Clinical presentation

Almost 90% of cases occur in HIV-infected persons with blood CD4 T-cell counts <200 cells/µl (or a CD4 T-cell percentage <14%). Other risk factors for disease in subjects not receiving effective HAART include oral candidiasis, oral hairy leukoplakia, unintentional weight loss, recurrent bacterial pneumonia, previous PCP and high plasma HIV load. The most common presentation is with gradually progressive exertional dyspnoea, malaise and a dry cough. However, there may be a wide variety of respiratory symptoms. There is often little to find on examination, although there may be some fine inspiratory crackles audible at the lung bases. Radiological findings are described in Table 9.2.2.

Diagnosis

The use of transcutaneous oximetry to assess for exercise induced desaturation has been validated in the case of PCP with normal or near normal CXR. Patients with a given severity of disease have a wider arterial oxygen gradient (A–aO2) than other causes of pulmonary infection. Radiological findings (Table 9.2.2) may be of assistance. Definitive diagnosis requires identification of the organism either by silver or immunoflourescence staining from pulmonary secretions or tissue. Molecular amplification methods of detection are not routinely used, though early studies using upper and lower respiratory tract specimens suggest they may be helpful.

Empiric treatment vs bronchoscopy – debate exists regarding whether or not a definitive diagnosis is required. The controversy arises from the high frequency of PCP found in the pre HAART era – and hence the good positive predictive value of compatible symptoms in patients with a CD4 count of <200 cells/µl. However as PCP has become less common, so symptoms are less predictive of PCP; and it is advisable that diagnosis should now be actively sought. This is further supported by the following: (1) 20% of HIV-infected patients presenting with respiratory symptoms who are thought to have PCP do not have this diagnosis; (2) response to treatment of PCP typically takes 4–7 days. Thus, if the diagnosis is incorrect the patient may have had increased time on potentially toxic drugs; (3) if empiric treatment fails, one may need to consider bronchoscopy at a point when the patient is more unwell and therefore at greater risk of complications including post-bronchsocopy deterioration; (4) there is frequently more than one pathogen present – and BAL specimens may provide information about this.

Management

On the basis of clinical findings and prior to commencing treatment, the severity of PCP can be stratified into mild, moderate and severe disease (Table 9.2.3). This categorization can assist clinicians in their choice of appropriate drugs with proven efficacy. These are outlined in Tables 9.2.3 and 9.2.4. On the basis of an NIH Consensus Statement concurrent adjuvant glucocorticoid therapy is advocated in those with moderate or severe pneumonia (Table 9.2.3). The benefit has been demonstrated if glucocorticoids are started within 72 hours of specific anti-PCP therapy. It should be noted that co-trimoxazole, dapsone, and primaquine must not be given in glucose-6-phosphate dehydrogenase deficient patients as they are at risk of haemolysis. Thus, levels should be checked prior to commencing treatment.

Co-trimoxazole for 21 days is first-line treatment for HIV-patients with PCP regardless of severity provided there are no contraindications. This regimen is effective in up to 90% of patients with mild disease and in 70% of those with severe pneumonia. Adverse reactions to co-trimoxazole are common and usually become apparent between days 6 and 14 of treatment. Neutropenia and anemia, rash (which may be severe), fever and abnormal liver function tests occur most frequently. Patients receiving co-trimoxazole should be monitored with full blood count, liver function, and urea and electrolytes at least twice weekly. HIV-infected individuals have higher rates of adverse reactions on cotrimoxazole; the reason for this is unclear. If minor, rash can often be managed with the use of systemic antihistamines and careful monitoring to ensure no deterioration occurs.

Individuals with moderate to severe disease (Table 9.2.3) should be given 120mg/kg/day intravenously in three to four divided doses for three days, followed by 90mg/kg/day intravenously for the remaining 18 days. This strategy appears to be equally efficacious as giving the higher dose for 21 days, but has a lower incidence of bone marrow disturbance. The difficulties of giving prolonged intravenous therapy means that many clinicians will switch patients who demonstrate a good and sustained response to oral from intravenous therapy after approximately a week. in mild-moderate disease either co-trimoxazole 1920mg orally three times daily for 21 days or the IV regimen can be given.

Second-line agents. Current evidence suggests little difference in efficacy for the recommended second-line agents and the choice of regimen is often determined by patient tolerance and the ability to take oral or IV medication. There should be a treatment crossover period of 48 hours unless toxicity to the first-line agent has developed. Expert advice should be sought in patients who are failing to respond.

Clindamycin and primaquine in combination has a better toxicity profile than IV pentamidine. This makes it a preferable second-line agent, where it is effective in approximately 70% of patients. Methaemoglobinemia due to primaquine occurs in up to 40% of patients. However this can be reduced if primaquine 15mg once daily is used in place of 30mg once daily. Diarrhoea is common on clindamycin and if it develops stool samples should be sent for Clostridium difficile toxin.

Trimethoprim – dapsone is an appropriate option for mild-moderate PCP. Asymptomatic methaemoglobinemia occurs in the majority of patients (secondary to dapsone). Approximately 50% will develop mild hyperkalaemia secondary to trimethoprim. This drug combination is tolerated in approximately one-third of patients who have developed late, non-severe but persistent rash with co-trimoxazole.

Intravenous pentamidine is mainly reserved for those with severe disease in whom there has been therapeutic failure on co-trimoxazole. Nephrotoxicity, hypotension, leucopenia,

Table 9.2.3 Stratification of disease severity in PCP

	Mild	Moderate	Severe
Symptoms and signs	Dyspnoea on exertion with or without cough and sweats	Dyspnoea on minimal exertion and occasionally at rest; cough and fever	Dyspnoea and tachypnoea at rest; persistent fever and cough
Oxygenation PaO$_2$ room air, at rest in kPa (mmHg)	>11.0 (>83)	8.1–11.0 (61–83)	≤8.0 (≤60)
SaO$_2$, at rest on air	>96	91–96	<91
PAO$_2$-PaO$_2$* in kPa (mmHg)	<4.7 (<35)	4.7–6.0 (35–45)	>6.0 (>45)
CXR	Normal or minor peri-hilar shadowing	Diffuse interstitial shadowing	Extensive interstitial shadowing with or without diffuse alveolar shadowing
First-choice treatment	Trimethoprim-sulfamethoxazole	Trimethoprim-sulfamethoxazole	Trimethoprim-sulfamethoxazole
Second-choice treatment	Clindamycin-primaquine	Clindamycin-primaquine	Clindamycin-Primaquine or intravenous pentamidine
Trimethoprim-dapsone		Trimethoprim-dapsone	
Third-choice treatment	Atovaquone	Intravenous pentamidine	
Fourth choice	Intravenous	Atovaquone	

pancreatitis and hypo- or hyper-glycemia are relatively common. The long half-life of pentamidine means that adverse effects may arise at any time (even several days or weeks after the drug has been discontinued).

Further support. CPAP can be helpful in hypoxic patients and may avoid the need for mechanical ventilation. This is especially helpful in the first few days of therapy; or if the patient deteriorates post-bronchoscopy. Failure to respond to apparently 'appropriate' treatment may result from a number of factors; which should be carefully sought and excluded. These are summarised in Table 9.2.4.

Mycobacterium tuberculosis
As a genuine and global pathogen, TB can present in all HIV infected individuals at any stage of HIV infection. The T cell defects associated with HIV mean that the chance of an individual who has latent TB infection progressing to active clinical disease is 50–100 times greater than background rates in HIV negative subjects. This translates roughly as a reactivation rate of 5% per year compared to a *lifetime* risk of 5% in HIV-negative individuals.

Clinical presentation
Patients with higher CD4 counts (>350 cells/μl) present in a similar manner to HIV-negative patients with TB. The immune dysregulation associated with falling blood CD4 counts means that as the CD4 count drops to below 200 cells/μl, patients are more likely to have non-pulmonary, disseminated and multi-organ disease. Pulmonary manifestations are also often different at low blood CD4 counts. 'Typical' chest radiographic cavitation is replaced by pulmonary infiltration, pleural effusions and mediastinal lymphadenopathy,

Diagnosis
TB diagnosis relies on a similar approach to that used in HIV- uninfected subjects. Samples for AFB smear and culture should always be obtained. If a patient is producing sputum then this should be examined for acid fast bacilli. Although this is less likely to be positive than in HIV-negative subjects, blood, urine and bone marrow cultures are more frequently diagnostic. The tuberculin skin test (which relies on good cell-mediated immunity) is of fairly limited value in co-infected patients, especially in those with a blood CD4 count below 200 cells/μl.

Treatment
Drugs. Standard 'four drug' treatment with a rifamycin (usually either rifampicin or rifabutin), plus isoniazid, pyrazinamide and ethambutol for two months followed by consolidation with rifamycin and isoniazid is the treatment of choice for drug sensitive disease. Vitamin B6 (10–25mg once daily) is usually also given to protect against isoniazid-induced peripheral neuropathy. Six months' treatment is advocated for most patients; though should be prolonged to nine months in those with cavitary pulmonary disease, or positive cultures after two months' treatment where the organism is known to be drug sensitive and patient adherence is very good. The prolonged duration of therapy is designed to reduce the higher risk of relapse that has been reported in these sub-groups. Treatment adverse events are common. Moderate to severe rash, hepatotoxicity or gastro-intestinal disturbance occurs in up to 40% of co-infected subjects. This is in part due to the overlapping toxicities with HAART. The best example of this is the peripheral neuropathy that will almost certainly result if isoniazid is given together with the nucleoside reverse transcriptase inhibitor stavudine.

Table 9.2.4 Treatment schedules for *Pneumocystis jirovecii* pneumonia

Drug	Dosage	Notes
Trimethoprim-sulfamethoxazole	Trimethoprim 20mg/kg IV q24h and sulfamethoxazole 100mg/kg IV q24h in 2–3 divided doses for 3 days then reduced to trimethoprim 15mg/kg IV q24h and sulfamethoxazole 75mg/kg IV q24h in 2–3 divided doses for 18 further days	Use in moderate to severe PCP Dilute 1:25 in 0.9% saline infused over 90–120 minutes
	Same daily doses of trimethoprim-sulphamethoazole PO q24h, in 3 divided doses for 21 days	Use in mild to moderate PCP
	1920mg (2 trimethoprim-sulphamethoxazole double strength tablets) PO q8h for 21 days	
Clindamycin-primaquine	Clindamycin 600–900mg IV q6h or q8h IV and primaquine 15–30mg PO q24h for 21 days	Methaemoglobinemia Less likely if dose of 15mg PO q24h of primaquine is used
	Clindamycin 300–450mg PO q6h to q8h and primaquine 15–30mg PO q24h for 21 days	
Pentamidine	4mg/kg IV q24h for 21 days	Dilute in 250mL 5% dextrose in water and infuse over 60 minutes
Trimethoprim-dapsone	Trimethoprim 20mg/kg PO q24h in 3 divided doses and dapsone 100mg PO q24h for 21 days	
Atovaquone	750mg PO q12h for 21 days	Give with food to increase absorption
Prednisolone	40mg PO q12h, days 1–5 40mg PO q24h, days 6–10 20mg PO q24h, days 11–21	Start corticosteroid as soon as possible and within 72 hrs of commencing specific anti-PCP treatment, if PaO$_2$ <9.3 kPa (<70 mmHg)
Methylprednisolone	IV at 75% of dose given above for prednisolone	

Drug-drug interactions are common in HIV patients with TB. One of the main pharmacokinetic areas of concern is that between rifamycins and antiretroviral drugs. Rifampicin is a potent inducer of the cytochrome P-450 system. Non-nucleoside reverse transcriptase inhibitors (NNRTIs) and protease inhibitors (PI) are metabolised using cytochrome P-450. Thus reduced concentrations of the NNRTIs and PIs and the development of resistance to HIV can occur if used in combination with rifampicin. Rifabutin is a less potent inducer of the cytochrome P-450 system, but is also a substrate of the same enzyme. Hence drugs such as PIs which inhibit the cytochrome P-450 system will lead to increased serum concentrations of rifabutin. Although there are limited clinical trial data with this drug, most clinicians feel that it is as effective as rifampicin when treating TB.

Timing of commencing HAART. The first priority for the TB/HIV co-infected patient is to treat TB. The optimal time to start remains unclear. A suggested approach is (1) in those with a CD4 count of >200 cells/μl to withhold HAART for the duration of TB treatment; (2) in those with a CD4 count <200 cells/μl but >100 cells/μl to delay HAART until the patient is established on anti-TB therapy (usually up to two months); (3) to start HAART as soon as possible in those with a CD4 count of <100 cells/μl (usually after about two weeks, based on physician assessment).

Drug resistance is twice as common in HIV co-infected individuals. Multi drug resistance and XDR (extremely drug resistant) TB is an increasing global problem. This is likely to be due to rapid progression from latent to active infection combined with delayed diagnosis of disease through atypical presentation.

IRIS is commonly associated with TB. Its diagnosis and management is discussed in more detail in the next chapter.

Other mycobacterial infections

These are generally seen in subjects with blood CD4 <100 cells/μl. Isolated pulmonary disease is less common than disseminated infection. It can occur most frequently with *Mycobacterium avium-intracellulare complex* (MAC), *Mycobacterium kansasii*, and *Mycobacterium xenopi*. Diagnosis is based on a positive culture from a usually sterile site (e.g. blood or bone marrow), or multiple positive respiratory samples with consistent symptoms. Treatment usually consists of a macrolide and ethambutol with or without a rifamycin.

Fungal infections

Cryptococcus neoformans

Clinical presentation
In the lungs infection can present as either primary pulmonary cryptococcosis or often as part of a disseminated infection complicating cryptococcal meningitis. The former presents in a similar manner to other respiratory infections.

Diagnosis
Can be made by direct staining for the organism in sputum, BAL or CSF. Cryptococcal antigen (CrAg) in high titres in the blood suggest dissemination but are often negative with primary pulmonary disease, in which case BAL fluid CrAg is a reliable test.

Treatment
Treat with either IV liposomal amphotericin and flucytosine in meningitis and disseminated disease; or high dose fluconazole if there is more limited pulmonary disease. Generally, HAART should be commenced as soon as possible, though IRIS may be more likely if HAART is started early.

Aspergillosis

Aspergillosis is relatively rare in HIV-infected individuals compared to those with severe immunocompromise from other causes. It is usually seen in the context of profound immunosuppression (blood CD4 counts <50 cells/μl). This may also be associated with neutropenia from drugs such as co-trimoxazole or zidovudine; or the use of systemic glucocorticoids. Diagnosis rests on the clinical picture plus radiology with or without identification of aspergillus from lung specimens. The diagnostic utility of measuring galactomannan in blood or lung has not yet been defined in the HIV-infected patients. Treatment is similar to that used in other patients, with either voriconazole or liposomal amphotericin B being first choice therapies.

Candida

Candidal infection of the trachea, bronchi and lungs is rare in HIV-infected individuals. Although isolation of candida in the sputum is common it usually represents colonization of the oropharynx.

Endemic fungi

Histoplasma, *Coccidioides*, *Blastomycoses*, *Paracoccidioides*, and *Penicillium* infection are rare in the UK; though should be considered in patients with significant immunosuppression who have spent time in parts of the world where these fungi are endemic (see earlier in chapter). The typical presentation is with disseminated disease rather than isolated pulmonary infection. Just as with cryptococcal infection, patients may have a variety of skin lesions present. These will often be culture positive if biopsied. Treatment should be undertaken with specialist input, though in an emergency, IV amphotericin B will be effective.

Viral infections

Community-based viral infections including Influenza A and B occur with equal frequency in HIV-infected and non-infected patients.

Cytomegalovirus (CMV)

Clinical presentation
Symptoms are generally quite non-specific but may mimic PCP.

Diagnosis
CMV can be isolated in the BAL fluid of up to 50% of patients presenting with low CD4 counts but less than 5% of those patients will have a genuine CMV pneumonia. A definitive diagnosis of CMV pneumonia requires identifiable or characteristic intranuclear and intracytoplasmic inclusions in a lung fluid specimen. A high plasma CMV DNA plasma copy (>5000 copies/ml) within the blood increases the risk of future end-organ disease.

Treatment
Treatment, if required, is with IV ganciclovir or oral valganciclovir.

Further reading

Breen RA, Swaden L, Ballinger J, et al. Tuberculosis and HIV co-infection: a practical therapeutic approach. *Drugs* 2006; **66**(18): 2299–2308.

Lipman MCI, Baker RW, Johnson MA (2004). *An Atlas of Differential Diagnosis in HIV Disease*, 2nd ed. New York: The Parthenon Publishing Group.

Lipman M, Breen R. Immune reconstitution inflammatory syndrome in HIV. *Curr Opin Infect Dis* 2006;**19**(1): 20–25.

Miller R, Lipman M. Acquired Immunodeficiency Syndrome and the Lung: Pulmonary Infections. *Clin Resp Med* 2008 433.

Mofenson LM, Oleske J, Serchuck L, et al. Treating opportunistic infections among HIV-exposed and infected children: recommendations from CDC, the National Institutes of Health, and the Infectious Diseases Society of America. *MMWR Recomm Rep* 2004; **53**(RR-14): 1–92.

Pozniak AL, Miller RF, Lipman MC, Freedman AR, Ormerod LP, Johnson MA, et al. BHIVA treatment guidelines for tuberculosis (TB)/HIV infection 2005. *HIV Med* 2005; **6**(Suppl 2): 62–83.

The Health Protection Agency. Testing Times - HIV and other Sexually Transmitted Infections in the United Kingdom: 2007. 2007 Nov 23.

UNAIDS/WHO. 2007 AIDS epidemic update. `http://www.unaids org/en/KnowledgeCentre/HIVData/EpiUpdate/EpiUpdArchive/2007` 2007 [cited 2008 Jun 15]; Available from: URL: `http://www.unaids.org/en/KnowledgeCentre/HIVData/EpiUpdate/EpiUpdArchive/2007`

9.3 Non-infectious HIV-related lung disease

Before the widespread introduction of HAART, reduced patient survival plus the inevitability of acute opportunistic infection meant that chronic, usually non-infectious lung disease was less relevant to HIV and respiratory physicians. This has now changed; and such conditions are often encountered in clinical practice. Just as with HIV-related infectious diseases, an individual's level of immunosuppression (measured by blood CD4 T-cell count and HIV plasma load) provides a useful guide to those illnesses that are likely to occur in a given clinical setting. For example, pulmonary Kaposi sarcoma (KS) is seen mainly in subjects with very low blood CD4 counts, and is now much less common, therefore, in populations using HAART. Conversely, as patients live longer, COPD and lung cancer are more frequently encountered, irrespective of CD4 count.

Natural history studies pre-HAART reveal a progressive loss of pulmonary CD4 T cells and an associated CD8 T-cell alveolitis in the HIV-infected lung. The immune dysregulation also involves macrophage activation and widespread changes in local cytokine production.

> **AUTHOR'S TIP**
> Several of the conditions that will be discussed in this chapter are thought to arise from these particular effects; or, in the case of immune reconstitution inflammatory syndrome (IRIS), when this is reversed by HAART.

General approach

The clinical approach to the patient is similar to that outlined in the Chapter 9.2. In those with severe immunocompromise (essentially a blood CD4 count of <200 cells/µL), opportunistic infections must be considered in the common clinical presentations of e.g. breathlessness, sputum production and systemic illness.

> **AUTHOR'S TIP**
> The importance of obtaining tissue or lung fluid samples, again, cannot be over-emphasised; and diagnostic procedures often required with suspected non-infectious diseases include CT-guided biopsy, VATS or open lung biopsy, and mediastinoscopy/mediastinotomy and biopsy. Transbronchial needle aspiration and endoscopy/bronchoscopic biopsy techniques are also more frequently used as part of the diagnostic work-up

Non-infectious pulmonary conditions can be broadly classified as neoplastic, inflammatory (both alveolar and airway) and vascular.

Malignancy and HIV

Kaposi sarcoma was the first malignancy clearly associated with the HIV pandemic. Other important tumours and tumour-like conditions include lymphomas, lung cancer and Castleman disease.

KS

KS is the most common malignancy seen in HIV-infected individuals. Co-infection with Human Herpes Virus 8 (HHV-8, also known as KS Herpes Virus, KSHV) is a pre-requisite for its development; though HIV drives the neoplastic process such that it is approximately 1000 times more frequent in this setting than in HIV-uninfected populations. It occurs at a considerably greater rate in men who have sex with men, and black Africans, than in other HIV positive individuals. It primarily involves muco-cutaneous tissues but is also found at other sites including the lung, lymph nodes and gastro-intestinal tract. Pulmonary KS can involve any of the intra-thoracic structures. Up to one-third of patients with known extra-pulmonary KS will have clinically evident lung involvement. This rises to 50% at autopsy.

Clinical features

The symptoms and signs associated with pulmonary KS are often non-specific but gradual-onset breathlessness and cough (with or without haemoptysis) are the most common presenting features. Careful examination of skin and mucous membranes, in particular, should be undertaken, as often KS involvement will be present at these sites in affected individuals.

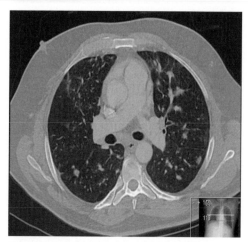

Fig. 9.3.1 CT Thorax of Pulmonary Kaposi Sarcoma demonstrating the bronchovascular distribution of nodules.

Diagnosis

Chest radiographic and CT features are variable. These include parenchymal nodules (often bronchovascular in distribution), consolidation, pleural effusions (which are often haemorrhagic) and intra-thoracic lymphadenopathy. KS lesions are quite distinctive on bronchoscopy. They are flat or raised red or purple plaques. Endobronchial biopsies are usually not performed as there is a risk of bleeding from these vascular tumours. However an experienced bronchoscopist may wish to confirm this diagnosis if there is no evidence elsewhere for KS. Unexplained pleural disease is probably best assessed using VATS.

Treatment

- This depends on the degree of cutaneous and visceral involvement; though will always be offered to patients with pulmonary disease.

- HAART should be given if it is not already prescribed. This will reduce KS lesions in 50–80% of individuals over a several month period. However IRIS-related worsening of KS has been reported. It is not particularly common, though needs to be considered if the patient has apparently worsening disease on HAART.
- Systemic chemotherapy is usually warranted with lung involvement, especially if the patient is symptomatic, or has rapidly progressive disease. Liposomal anthracyclines are most commonly used – with good results. As in other malignancies, a patient's performance status and co-morbidities need to be taken into consideration; though single agent chemotherapy is usually well-tolerated.
- Current treatments have improved median survival with pulmonary KS from less than six months to greater than five years. A worse overall prognosis is associated with hypoxia, pleural disease and low blood CD4 counts at presentation.

Lymphoma and lymphomatous conditions
Just as with KS, oncogenic viruses are important in the pathogenesis of a number of lymphomas. Most non-Hodgkin lymphoma (NHL) is associated with Epstein–Barr virus; whilst primary effusion lymphoma (PEL) and multi-centric Castleman disease (MCD) are linked to HHV-8. The latter two conditions are rare in non HIV-infected subjects. PEL (also known as body cavity-associated lymphoma) presents as an effusion with no identifiable tumour mass. Castleman disease (mult-centric angio-follicular hyperplasia) mimics the features of disseminated mycobacterial disease or lymphom. In both MCD and PEL, the outlook is poor as they are often not considered at an early stage of a patient's diagnostic pathway. Hodgkin disease also occurs at a greatly increased incidence in HIV-infected populations. Investigation is similar to that for NHL. It is recommended that all individuals who are diagnosed with a lymphomatous condition are offered an HIV test, if this has not been performed recently.

NHL
NHL is several hundred times more common in HIV-infected subjects. Although its incidence has decreased by half following the introduction of HAART, it remains a leading cause of mortality; and can occur at any blood CD4 count (though is more common with declining immunity). There is a preponderance of high grade, aggressive B cell lymphomas (mainly Burkitt type, centroblastic or immunoblastic). Pulmonary involvement is either with parenchymal nodules, pleural effusions or intra-thoracic lymphadenopathy. B type symptoms are more frequently seen than in pulmonary KS; and the differential diagnosis often rests between lymphoma and mycobacterial disease. Clinical features that might suggest lymphoma include elevated lactate dehydrogenase (>1000 IU/L) and lack of lymph node central necrosis on CT scanning. It should be stressed that these are very insensitive markers, and diagnosis relies upon good quality tissue biopsy.

Treatment is with similar regimens to those used in HIV negative populations. It is clear that the addition of HAART greatly improves outcome (through a reduction in chemotherapy – and HIV-related opportunistic infections). However drug-drug interactions are common and need to managed expectantly. Overall median survival has risen from less than six months to several years.

Lung cancer
Although not regarded typically as an HIV-associated malignancy, recent data suggest that lung cancer is approximately three to four times more common in HIV-infected individuals than in the general population. The vast majority are cigarette smokers; though they are, on average, younger than other lung cancer patients, with a higher than expected frequency of non-small cell adenocarcinoma tumours. Injecting drug users appear to be particularly at risk – though this may be confounded by higher smoking rates in this population. Unlike the other malignancies described, there appears to be little association with CD4 counts; and only a modest decrease, if any, in incidence with the use of HAART. This may reflect the different oncogenic process involved in lung cancer development compared to that in KS and lymphomas.

Clinical presentation
Although symptoms and signs are similar to those in HIV-negative individuals, systemic symptoms including fever are more frequently encountered. Patients also tend to have more advanced disease at diagnosis.

Diagnosis
Chest radiographs and CT scans are as expected for lung cancer, although the differential diagnosis is inevitably more broad in the context of HIV infection and immuno-suppression. The primary tumour site is often peripheral, and pleural effusions are present in 25% of cases. Assessment and staging is similar to that undertaken in the general population.

Treatment
There is evidence to suggest that the diagnosis may not be considered at an early enough stage of a patient's illness. Inevitably investigation may have focused upon infectious causes of the reported symptoms. As a result, lung cancer can appear to be more rapid and less amenable to surgical cure in this population. However, if surgery can be performed, the outcome is no worse for resectable lesions than that seen in HIV negative subjects. The majority of individuals, however, are incurable and receive best supportive care with symptom control. Median survival is approximately four weeks from diagnosis with nearly 100% mortality at two years in most reported series.

IRIS
Paradoxical symptomatic deterioration following the start of appropriate treatment has been reported by TB physicians for over 50 years. The use of HAART, with resultant profound and rapid changes in immunity, has led to similar clinical events in HIV infected individuals, and been termed IRIS. They are thought to arise from an over-vigorous interaction between antigen and the host immune response. This typically occurs within a few weeks of starting HAART, though can be up to months later in certain cases. It has been associated with a wide variety of organisms as well some apparently non-infectious antigens. However it is most commonly seen in individuals with TB, cryptococcosis and non-tuberculous mycobacterial infection. Here it has been reported in 15–35% of HIV-infected patients using HAART.

Clinical presentation
IRIS has two common presentations. Using TB as an example these are:
- Paradoxical IRIS – where the patient is on treatment for active TB, is getting better and then starts HAART with a subsequent clinical deterioration.
- Post-HAART TB-IRIS, where an asymptomatic individual starts HAART and develops a rapid-onset and very

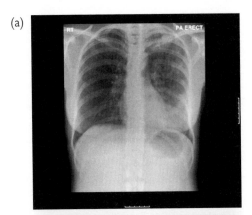

(a)

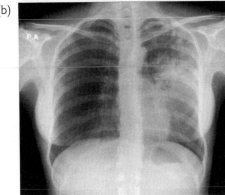

(b)

Fig. 9.3.2 Chest radiography before and after commencing TB treatment 35-year-old woman with TB-IRIS. The first chest radiograph (a) was before the initiation off HAART and anti-tuberculosis treatment. The second chest radiograph (b) was taken during the onset of immune reconstitution and demonstrates increased infiltrates in the left mid-zone.

inflammatory episode of TB. This is often termed 'unmasking' of a previously unknown and untreated infection. In either case, symptoms and signs are variable, though there is usually a degree of systemic upset. Expansion of intra-cerebral or mediastinal masses, or increases in pericardial fluid volume may be life-threatening, though this is relatively rare.

Diagnosis

There is no laboratory test that helps to distinguish IRIS from other causes of clinical deterioration, such as alternative undiagnosed infection or malignancy; non-adherence to treatment; drug resistance, malabsorption, hypersensitivity or drug-drug interaction. Hence these should always be excluded before IRIS is confidently diagnosed. It is generally accepted patients with IRIS should have a demonstrable effect of HAART – usually a decrease in plasma HIV viral load.

Most studies suggest that individuals at greatest risk of paradoxical IRIS following HAART have low baseline blood CD4 counts (<50 cells/μL) and/or commence antiretrovirals within a few weeks of starting specific opportunistic infection treatment.

Prevention and treatment

- Prior to commencing HAART, patients should be screened thoroughly for active opportunistic infection, to minimise the risk of unmasking IRIS. If clinical disease does occur, the relevant organism should be treated in the usual way. HAART does not normally require discontinuation.

- In cases of mild, paradoxical IRIS, no treatment may be required other than careful observation, as the condition is usually self-limiting. Lymph node disease that is suppurating is often relieved with repeated aspiration. The obtained samples should be cultured, to exclude new or active infection.

- Corticosteroids are beneficial, though have considerable adverse effects and should be reserved for more severe manifestations of IRIS. There is no consensus on dose or duration of treatment. Most clinicians would start with around 30 mg prednisolone equivalent (irrespective of concurrent rifamycin use). In severe cases, expert advice should be sought. In general, HAART is not usually stopped, as there is a risk of rapid decline in systemic immunity and opportunistic disease.

COPD

HIV-infected smokers have an approximately two-fold greater risk of COPD than non-infected smokers. Controlling for degree of tobacco exposure, they also appear to have more anatomical emphysema at presentation. This is further increased in patients who smoke other recreational drugs, in particular crack cocaine. Infection and colonisation with bacteria and fungi (including *Pneumocystis jirovecii*) also predisposes to COPD.

Symptoms are similar to those of COPD and emphysema in the general population. On chest radiography and CT-scanning there is an upper lobe predominance of bullous disease and centrilobular emphysema. Treatment is in line with COPD guidance, though there are some important interactions between HAART and respiratory medications that should be noted. In particular, the protease inhibitor ritonavir increases the effective dose of both inhaled and intranasal budesonide and fluticasone.

Given the increased smoking rates documented in HIV-infected patients, strenuous efforts should be made to encourage smokers to quit. Targeted smoking cessation programmes are not widely available, and to date have not met with much success.

Alveolitis associated with HIV

Patients with HIV-infection can develop a number of sub-acute or chronic alveolar disorders which are often only distinguished on histo-pathology. These are lymphoid interstitial pneumonitis (LIP), non-specific interstitial pneumonitis (NSIP) and organising pneumonia. All present in a non-specific manner, often with dry cough, progressive breathlessness, weight loss and fever. As such they are often mis-diagnosed clinically as opportunistic infection. Diagnosis often requires a combination of clinical, radiology and lung function findings together with tissue biopsy.

LIP

LIP was initially described in children with HIV infection and slowly progressive breathlessness and hypoxia. A milder form has been identified in adults. This is often associated with CD8 T cell infiltration in other tissue sites including the parotid glands – and is known as diffuse infiltrative lymphocytosis syndrome (DILS). Features on HRCT include reticular or nodular opacities, patchy ground-glass attenuation, centri-lobular nodules and soap-bubble like cysts. HAART is a useful treatment of adult LIP. Symptoms and radiological abnormalities will often improve without the need to resort to corticosteroids.

NSIP

Prior to the widespread use of HAART, this disorder was reported relatively frequently in subjects with low CD4 counts presenting with cough, breathlessness and mild fever who were had no evidence for infections such as *Pneumocystis* pneumonia. Diagnosis is based on the characteristic features being present on lung biopsy. These are similar to those of LIP (lymphocytic and plasma cell infiltration) plus also non-specific alveolar septal edema. It is now rarely reported – which probably reflects the much earlier use of effective anti-retrovirals in this population. Treatment, if required, is also with HAART, if this is not already being taken.

Pulmonary hypertension associated with HIV (PAH)

Primary pulmonary arterial hypertension (PAH) is reported to be much more common in HIV infected individuals (six to twelve times that of the general population). Its prevalence in some European cohorts is up to 0.5% of the HIV-positive population. It is diagnosed when an HIV-infected individual develops pulmonary artery hypertension and no secondary cause can be identified. The aetiology is unknown though may be related to associated viral infections such as HHV-8 or HIV itself.

Clinical presentation

Most affected patients are already known to be HIV infected and present with exertional breathlessness. Given its insidious nature, it is often considered, and therefore diagnosed, late in its clinical course. PAH has no apparent association with an individual's level of immunosuppression or clinical stage.

Diagnosis

Diagnosis requires PAH to be confirmed in an HIV infected individual, ideally by right heart catheterisation; together with exclusion of other known causes of PAH. Investigation should include CT chest with pulmonary angiography, as pulmonary embolism is probably also more common in HIV infected subjects, due to protein C, S and anti-thrombin III deficiencies. Tissue biopsies reveal remodelling of the pulmonary arterial tree at various levels as well as plexiform lesions.

Treatment

Treatment is broadly similar to that for HIV negative subjects with idiopathic PAH. One caveat is that calcium channel blockers are generally contra-indicated as they interact with many protease inhibitors, leading to significant hypotension and decreased right heart filling. There is evidence that the use of HAART leads to improvements in symptoms as well as pulmonary haemodynamics. It also reduces the possibility of further respiratory disease, and is therefore given by most clinicians if primary PAH is either suspected or confirmed.

Further reading

Humbert M, Sitbon O, Chaouat A, et al. Pulmonary Arterial Hypertension in France: Results from a National Registry. *Am J Respir Crit Care Med* 2006; **173**(9): 1023–1030.

Lipman M, Breen R. Immune reconstitution inflammatory syndrome in HIV. *Curr Opin Infect Dis* 2006; **19**(1): 20–25.

Lipman MCI, Baker RW, Johnson MA (2004). *An Atlas of Differential Diagnosis in HIV Disease*, 2nd ed. New York: The Parthenon Publishing Group.

Meintjes G, Lawn SD, Scano F, et al. Tuberculosis-associated immune reconstitution inflammatory syndrome: case definitions for use in resource-limited settings. *The Lancet Infectious Diseases* 2008; **8**(8): 516–523.

Ognibene FP, Masur H, Rogers P, et al. Nonspecific interstitial pneumonitis without evidence of Pneumocystis carinii in asymptomatic patients infected with human immunodeficiency virus (HIV). *Ann Intern Med* 1988; **109**(11): 874–879.

Petrache I, Diab K, Knox KS, et al. HIV associated pulmonary emphysema: a review of the literature and inquiry into its mechanism. *Thorax* 2008; **63**(5):463–469.

Spano JP, Costagliola D, Katlama C, et al. AIDS-Related Malignancies: State of the Art and Therapeutic Challenges. *J Clin Oncol* 2008.

Chapter 10

Bronchiectasis

Chapter contents

10.1 Bronchiectasis (aetiology)

Overview

Bronchiectasis is fundamentally an anatomical diagnosis describing abnormal permanent dilatation of airways. It may be suspected clinically in patients with chronic cough and purulent sputum production and confirmed by plain or cross-sectional radiology of the chest. Radiological bronchiectasis without clinical symptoms is an increasingly common finding of uncertain significance.

Epidemiology

No cross-sectional population studies exist but for a DGH population of 250,000 about 100–200 patients could be seen by a respiratory physician with a special interest. The extent of severe disease in developed countries has declined since the advent of vaccination programmes, the decline in tuberculosis, widespread antibiotic use and improvement in living conditions. Balanced against this is an increasing rate of diagnosis of milder disease consequent on the increasing availability of CT scanning in the last 25 years. This has been described as the era of 'modern bronchiectasis'.

Pathophysiology

In the established bronchiectatic airway the key features are those of dilatation with damage to the structural components of the airway wall (elastin, muscle and cartilage). In addition there is fibrosis that may extend into the adjacent lung parenchyma. Chronic inflammation with lymphoid follicles in airway walls and neutrophils in the lumen drives overproduction of abnormally viscid mucus that is poorly cleared, resulting in stagnation and a fertile medium for bacterial colonisation and persistence. This in turn encourages continued inflammation and cytotoxic damage, a continuing 'vicious circle'. The initial factor beginning the process of chronic inflammation may vary, for example an exogenous insult such as toxic gas exposure or foreign body inhalation or an endogenous defect of host defences either congenital or acquired. However, what seems clear is that infection plays a key role both in the development and persistence of the disease.

Aetiology

Although the list of conditions recognised as causing bronchiectasis is long (see Table 10.1.1), in clinical practice the majority of cases are of unknown aetiology. The most commonly identified cause is previous severe pulmonary infection, including tuberculosis. Other relatively frequently identified causes (up to 10% in some series) include ciliary dysfunction, immune deficiency (Stead) and allergic bronchopulmonary aspergillosis (ABPA).

Table 10.1.2 shows causes and associations from 2 recent UK studies in tertiary referral centres (Pasteur, Shoemark). These results are a consequence of quite intensive investigation of a selected patient group; findings in a DGH population are likely to be different.

In practice, investigation into aetiology should be limited to identifying causes that might lead to specific therapeutic interventions over and above conventional treatment of the bronchiectasis and/or provide additional prognostic information for the patient and their family. Clues as to aetiology may come form the history, examination, imaging and microbiological investigations.

Table 10.1.1 Classification of recognised causes and associations of bronchiectasis

Causes of bronchiectasis	
Congenital structural defects	Tracheobronchomegaly (Mounier–Khun syndrome)
	Defective cartilage (Williams–Campbell syndrome)
	Pulmonary sequestration
	Elhers–Danlos syndrome
	Marfan's syndrome
	Tracheomalacia
Obstruction	Tumour
	Foreign body
	External lymph node
Impaired mucociliary clearance	Cystic fibrosis
	Ciliary dyskinesia
	Young's syndrome (bronchiectasis, sinusitis and azoospermia)
Immune deficiency	Common variable immunodeficiency
	Selective immunoglobulin deficiency
	Functional neutrophil defects
	Human immunodeficiency virus
Excessive immune response	Allergic bronchopulmonary aspergillosis
	Lung transplant rejection
	Chronic graft versus host disease
Post-infective	Tuberculosis
	Whooping cough
	Non-tuberculous mycobacteria
	Pneumonia
	Measles
	Adenovirus
	Swyer–James syndrome
Post-inflammatory pneumonitis	Aspiration
	Inhalation of toxic gases
Miscellaneous	Diffuse panbronchiolitis
Associations	Rheumatoid arthritis
	Inflammatory bowel disease
	Systemic lupus erythematosis
	Sjogren's syndrome
	Ankylosing spondylitis
	Relapsing polychondritis
	Yellow nails syndrome (yellow nails, pleural effusions and lymphoedema)

Microbiology

Most published studies of non-CF bronchiectasis in adults show similar microbiological findings. The most commonly isolated organism is *Haemophilus influenzae*. *Pseudomonas aeruginosa* is present in about a quarter of patients in most series and affects patients with more severe disease. *Moraxella catarrha lis* and *Streptococcus pneumoniae* also appear, as do anaerobic organisms. *Staphylococcus aureus* is a less common pathogen whose isolation should prompt consideration of CF as a cause. *Aspergillus* spp. may be cultured from some patients and should prompt consideration

Table 10.1.2 Frequency of causes and/or associations of bronchiectasis from 2 large UK studies (Pasteur, Shoemark)

Cause	Frequency
Ideopathic	26-53%
Post-infective	29-32%
Ciliary dysfunction	1.5-10%
Immune deficiency	7-8%
Allergic bronchopulmonary aspergillosis	7-8%
Aspiration	0-4%
Young's syndrome	3%
Cystic fibrosis	0-3%
Rheumatoid arthritis	2-3%
Inflammatory bowel disease	1-3%
Panbronchiolitis	<1-2%
Congenital	<1-2%
Atypical Mycobacterial	0-2%

of ABPA as a causative factor or aspergilloma as a complication. A proportion of patients will not reveal any pathogenic organisms on some samples. *Burkholderia cepacia* has been reported in patients with non-CF bronchiectasis. Isolation requires special culture media and should be specifically requested in patients with unexplained deterioration. Occasional samples should also be sent for mycobacterial culture, especially in cases with poor response to conventional antibiotics, haemoptysis or fever. Longitudinal studies suggest that, for the majority of patients, sputum isolates show consistent findings over time. This supports the usefulness of knowing a patient's microbiological history in predicting the likely organism causing an exacerbation.

AUTHOR'S TIP

Characterising patients as pseudomonas positive or negative is helpful in clinical management since antibiotic strategies differ between the groups.

The new patient

History, examination and imaging establish a diagnosis of bronchiectasis. Subsequent investigations serve two purposes; to look for an underlying cause (once only) and to guide and monitor ongoing treatment (repeated testing).

History

The symptom complex that should lead to consideration of a diagnosis of bronchiectasis is that of chronic cough with purulent sputum production. There will nearly always be a history of episodic worsening in symptoms often with additional features such as general malaise, joint pains, increasing breathlessness and occasional haemoptysis. Some patients with bronchiectasis may produce little or no sputum between exacerbations. Additional historical features may suggest possible aetiologies.

Important historical features:
- Age at onset of symptoms.
- Associated upper airway features (sinusitis, middle ear infection).
- History of a previous severe infective episode.
- Family history (including infertility).
- Symptoms of gastro-oesophageal reflux disease.
- Asthmatic features in the history (ABPA).

Many patients will have had symptoms for most of their life that they accept as normal; persistence in questioning about sputum frequency, volume, colour and taste (foul taste suggestive of anaerobic infection) are important in establishing a baseline. Equally important is an appreciation of the frequency and nature of exacerbations and their response to specific antibiotics.

Past experience of physiotherapy training and the current practice of the patient are useful to establish at the outset.

Some consideration of the impact of disease on the patient's quality of life is always worthwhile; many patients curtail social activities because of embarrassment about their cough and sputum.

Examination

The majority of patients will have few, if any, physical signs. Crackles and clubbing although classical are rare in modern bronchiectasis. Most commonly a few coarse crackles may be heard over the site of disease. In older patients there may be signs associated with previous surgical interventions for the bronchiectasis itself (lung resection) or for therapy of tuberculosis or other infections.

Radiology (Figs. 10.1.1–10.1.3)

Conventional plain CXR is relatively insensitive; HRCT imaging is the current gold standard. Key CT features include internal airway diameter greater than the adjacent artery (dilatation), failure of airway tapering and thickening of airway walls. In addition mucus plugging of small airways may give rise to a 'tree in bud' pattern. Distribution of disease may give clues as to the aetiology. Proximal or central bronchiectasis suggests ABPA as a possible cause; upper lobe predominance should prompt consideration of cystic fibrosis. Localised disease requires exclusion of an obstructive lesion by fibreoptic bronchoscopy. Most patients

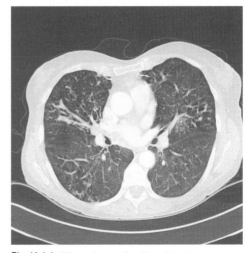

Fig. 10.1.1 CT scan showing dilated branching airways, some filled with sputum, in the right upper lobe together with tree-in-bud appearances in the right lower lobe indicating small airway involvement.

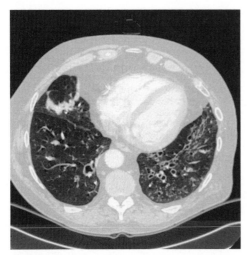

Fig. 10.1.2 CT scan showing patchy consolidation in the right middle lobe, cystic bronchiectasis in the right lower lobe, cylindrical bronchiectasis in the left lower lobe and peripheral nodularity in the left lower lobe indicating small airway involvement.

will have diffuse disease with a lower lobe predominance. A tree in bud pattern in association with nodules and cavitation is suggestive of atypical mycobacterial infection, especially *M. avium* complex. Some patchy consolidative change may also be seen especially if imaging is done in the context of an acute exacerbation.

Comparison with any previous imaging will allow some appreciation of disease progression; it is always worth asking about previous scans, CXR and bronchography (which patients particularly remember). A degree of airway dilatation often occurs in the context of pneumonic consolidation as a temporary phenomenon, this does not constitute

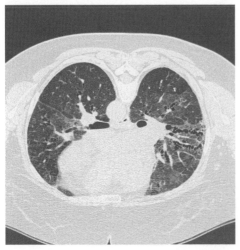

Fig. 10.1.3 Prone HRCT image showing varicose bronchiectasis in the right lung, enhanced in this image by ground glass shadowing in the surrounding lung tissue.

clinical bronchiectasis. Similarly airway dilatation occurring in areas of lung fibrosis, usually termed traction bronchiectasis, rarely gives rise to significant symptoms of its own accord.

Initial investigations

For all patients:

- Blood count for eosinophilia.
- ESR or CRP.
- Serum immunoglobulins.
- IgE RAST to aspergillus.
- Serum IgG precipitins to aspergillus.
- Skin prick sensitivity to aspergillus.
- Sputum culture.

For selected patients with suggestive features:

- Oesophageal studies (aspiration suspected).
- Cilial studies (early onset of lifelong symptoms, middle ear and sinus symptoms).
- CF genotype ± sweat test (upper lobe predominance, infertility, GI symptoms, S. aureus in sputum).
- Seminal analysis (sinusitis and infertility).
- Detailed immunological studies (recurrent infections at multiple sites).
- Fibreoptic bronchoscopy (localised disease on CT).

> **AUTHOR'S TIP**
> IgG subclass testing, auto-immune studies and alpha-1-antitrypsin levels are not clinically helpful.

Lung function

Although diagnostically lung function testing is of no great value, serial monitoring of spirometry helps to identify patients with disease progression that should prompt review of therapy. Reversibility testing helps to identify patients who may benefit from bronchodilator therapy. Most patients will have obstructive spirometry although normal results are not uncommon.

Physiotherapy assessment

An initial assessment by a respiratory physiotherapist with expertise in bronchiectasis is always worthwhile for a new patient. Although many patients with lifelong symptoms will have received physiotherapy instruction in the past this is often remembered by patients as something that is done to them rather than by them. There are a variety of techniques taught by physiotherapists to aid sputum clearance including the active cycle of breathing, postural drainange and autogenic drainage. In addition a number of modern devices are available that are a useful adjunct or replacement for conventional physiotherapy including the Flutter and the Acapella. A detailed assessment will allow the patient and physiotherapist to select the technique(s) that best fits with their lifestyle and abilities. It is always worth encouraging partners to attend these sessions. A second assessment at an interval is useful to assess compliance and deal with problems that may have arisen. Reinforcement of the benefits of physiotherapy by medical staff needs to be frequent. Patients typically settle into a pattern of performing physiotherapy once or twice a day for periods of about 10–15 minutes on each occasion. Those with higher sputum volumes may benefit from more sessions.

Monitoring progress

The above initial assessment will identify a wide range of disease severity amongst patients with bronchiectasis. For those at the milder end of the spectrum with normal lung function, infrequent exacerbations and few if any chronic symptoms, a short period of surveillance in secondary care to ensure stability and educate the patient in the management of exacerbations is probably adequate. Those with lung function abnormality, constant symptoms and more frequent exacerbations will benefit from long term secondary care follow-up. Typically this will include all patients with *Ps. aeruginosa* infection. Patients should have access to a specialist clinic at short notice and be able to get telephone advice easily.

During routine follow-up visits spirometry should be performed and a sputum sample sent. Enquiry into frequency of exacerbations and response to antibiotics together with any change in baseline symptoms will provide an assessment of disease stability.

Further reading

Fowler SJ, French J, Screaton NJ, *et al.* Nontuberculous mycobacteria in bronchiectasis: prevalence and patient characteristics. *Eur Respir J* 2006; **28**: 1204–1210.

Jones AM, Dodd ME, Webb AK, *et al. Burkholderia cepacia*: current clinical issues, environmental controversies and ethical dilemmas. *Eur Respir J* 2001; **17**: 295–301.

King PT, Freezer NJ, Holmes PW, *et al.* Role of CFTR mutations in adult bronchiectasis. *Thorax* 2004; **59**: 357–358.

King PT, Holdsworth SR, Freezer NJ, *et al.* Microbiologic follow-up study in adult bronchiectasis. *Respir Med* 2007; **101**: 1633–1638.

Pasteur MC, Helliwell SM, Houghton SJ, *et al.* An investigation into causative factors in patients with bronchiectasis. *Am J Respir Crit Care Med* 2000; **162**: 1277–1284.

Patterson JE, Bradley JM, Hewitt O, *et al.* Airway clearance in bronchiectasis: a randomised crossover trial of active cycle of breathing techniques versus Acapella. *Respiration* 2005; **72**: 239–242.

Shoemark A, Ozerovitch L, Wilson R, *et al.* Aetiology in adult patients with bronchiectasis. *Respir Med* 2007; **101**: 1163–1170.

Stead A, Douglas JG, Broadfoot CJ, *et al.* Humoral immunity and bronchiectasis. *Clin Exp Immunol* 2002; **130**: 325–330.

Thompson CS, Harrison S, Ashley J, *et al.* A randomised crossover study of the Flutter and the active cycle of breathing technique in non-cystic fibrosis bronchiectasis. *Thorax* 2002; **57**: 446–448.

10.2 Chronic disease management

Bronchiectasis is a chronic airway disorder characterised by bronchial wall thickening and dilatation associated with clinical symptoms of persistent cough productive of sputum and general malaise.

The clinical course is punctuated with acute exacerbations associated with an increase in sputum purulence and volume and worsening malaise.

Aims of treatment

- Survival. The advent of the antibiotic era significantly altered survival in bronchiectasis. There is now debate regarding survival data suggesting that bronchiectasis may not confer reduced survival compared to an age matched population. Thus treatments are not now specifically aimed at improving survival.
- Preserving lung function. Persistent infection in the airways is associated with a vigorous neutrophil dominated inflammatory response with an abundance of proteolytic enzymes which destroy the airway wall. The average loss of lung function has been shown to be of the order of 50ml of FEV_1 per year. By controlling infection we aim to preserve lung function.
- Prevent exacerbations. Exacerbations are unpredictable and result in reduced quality of life. There is clear evidence of a strong correlation between the number of exacerbations per year and reduction in quality of life. An exacerbation in patients with chronic *Pseudomonas aeruginosa* infection may precipitate a hospital admission.
- Reduce symptoms and improve quality of life. There is good evidence that people feel better when they have less sputum and their life is less disturbed by exacerbations.

Principles of treatment

Having ensured that treatment for the underlying cause is established (i.e. immunoglobulin for immunodeficiency), the focus on chronic management is focused on targeting the underlying pathophysiological pathway known as the vicious cycle.

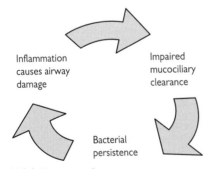

Inflammation causes airway damage

Impaired mucociliary clearance

Bacterial persistence

Fig. 10.2.1 The vicious cycle

Improving airway clearance

People with bronchiectasis should receive instruction from a physiotherapist so that they can perform airway clearance techniques independently at home. The particular technique should be tailored according to information regarding affected lobes from the CT, disease severity, sputum volumes, and patient preference. The most commonly used technique in the UK is the active cycle of breathing, but use of oscillating positive expiratory pressure devices (Acapella or Flutter) is effective and preferred by some patients.

Bronchodilator therapy is helpful for patients with evidence of reversible airflow obstruction.

Mucolytic and hyperosmolar therapies have been proposed as useful adjuncts to physical techniques of airway clearance. Recombinant human DNase (rhDNase) has been studied and found to be of no benefit and indeed increased decline in lung function and exacerbations. Thus rHDNase is not recommended for regular use. Studies of hypertonic saline and inhaled dry powder mannitol are ongoing.

Reducing bacterial load

Patients with bronchiectasis feel better when they have less sputum and less purulent sputum. Mucoid sputum has far less free elastase and myeloperoxidase than purulent sputum and is potentially less harmful to the airways. Antibiotic therapy is aimed at reducing airway bacterial load and improving the amount and colour of the sputum. Bacterial eradication is not always possible because of structural damage and disordered local defences.

Sputum culture is used to characterise the infecting organisms so that an appropriate antibiotic management plan can be put in place for each individual.

The approach to a patient with purulent sputum is shown in Fig. 10.2.2.

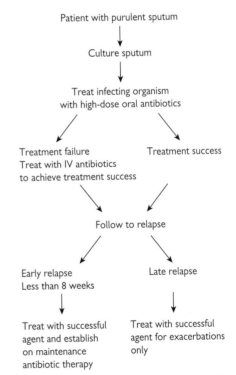

Patient with purulent sputum

Culture sputum

Treat infecting organism with high-dose oral antibiotics

Treatment failure
Treat with IV antibiotics to achieve treatment success

Treatment success

Follow to relapse

Early relapse
Less than 8 weeks

Late relapse

Treat with successful agent and establish on maintenance antibiotic therapy

Treat with successful agent for exacerbations only

Fig. 10.2.2 Approach to antibiotic therapy for a patient with chronic purulent sputum

The principle is to carry out an initial 'clear up' with an antibiotic targeted at the infecting organism and to continue it for a minimum of 2 weeks but longer if necessary to reduce the bacterial load and render the sputum colour as near to mucoid as possible and the sputum volume to the minimum possible.

Treatment success is defined as a reduction in sputum volume and a change in sputum colour to mucoid. The sputum may still culture a potential pathogen but if the patient is well and the sputum is mucoid this is not treatment failure.

Once treatment success is secured the antibiotic therapy is discontinued in order to establish the time to relapse.

Patients can monitor sputum colour and volume at home and are instructed to contact the clinic in the event of a relapse.

If relapse to the original state, (ie: purulent sputum in increasing volumes associated with malaise), occurs early (within 6 or 8 weeks) and there is a history of recurrent frequent exacerbations then after further treatment with the successful agent maintenance antibiotic therapy should be instituted appropriate to the infecting organism. This approach holds whether the infecting organism is *Haemophilus influenzae* or *Pseudomonas aeruginosa* (PA). Patients who have chronic infection with PA are much more likely to require intravenous antibiotics to gain disease control in the first place and maintenance therapy is likely to be nebulised Colomycin.

Sputum culture	Antibiotic therapy
Haemophilus influenzae	Doxycycline 100mg OD Amoxicillin 500mg BD
Streptococcus pneumoniae	Penicillin V 500mg BD Trimethoprim 200mg BD
Staphylococcus aureus	Flucloxacillin 500mg BD
Pseudomonas aeruginosa	Nebulised Colomycin 2 mega units BD

Fig. 10.2.3 Potential therapies for maintenance antibiotic regimen

---

AUTHOR'S TIPS

Maintenance antibiotics in bronchiectasis
Consider if:
- Frequent oral antibiotic courses or greater than four exacerbations per year.
- Rapid relapse (less than 8 weeks) after a course of antibiotics.
- More than two admissions to hospital for IV antibiotics in a year.

Patients who remain well for 3 months or longer without relapse can then simply be given a supply of the successful antibiotic agent to use again in the event of an exacerbation.

It is important for the patient to provide a sputum sample at the beginning of an exacerbation and inform the GP or practice nurse that they are starting antibiotics. Hence the infecting organism is confirmed and in the event of antibiotic failure an appropriate second-line antibiotic can be selected.

Key points
Definition of relapse/exacerbation
- Increase in cough.
- Increase in sputum volume.
- Increase in sputum purulence.
- Increase in malaise.

Treatment of relapse
- Institute antibiotic therapy.
- Send sputum for culture.
- Adjust therapy later based on sputum culture if lack of response.

Anti-inflammatory therapy

There are theoretical reasons why inhaled steroids should be useful in the chronic treatment of bronchiectasis. The host response to chronic bacterial persistence in the airways contributes to airway damage. Clinical studies have been less convincing and inhaled steroids are not recommended outside of routine treatment of any coexistent asthma.

There is one notable exception. Bronchiectasis associated with ulcerative colitis is exquisitely sensitive to oral steroid therapy and control of symptoms is maintained with inhaled steroid therapy.

Immunomodulatory therapy

Azithromycin has been shown to produce benefits in cystic fibrosis in terms of improvement in lung function and reduction in exacerbations.

Azithromycin works through a number of pathways including disruption of bacterial quorum sensing proteins, reduction of production of bacterial virulence factors and reduction of production of host epithelial and phagocytic cell inflammatory cytokines.

Large scale studies in non CF bronchiectasis are lacking but pilot data suggests azithromycin may be useful. Because of absence of long term safety data and randomised clinical trials its use is confined to difficult cases unresponsive to usual maintenance antibiotic therapy in the context of infection with *Pseudomonas aeruginosa*.

Key points
There are important caveats to the use of long-term azithromycin.
- Azithromycin must not be used until infection with non-tuberculous mycobacteria (NTM)is excluded.
- Patients must be warned regarding possible oto-toxicity and to stop therapy immediately if they develop tinnitus.

Patient education

Management of patients with bronchiectasis should become a partnership between the health professionals and the patient. The patient should be involved in defining a management plan having agreed on what they consider to be successful treatment. They can then be involved in decisions regarding the need for long term maintenance therapy and the choice of agent. Furthermore they can be involved in a decision to stop maintenance therapy if they have remained well and exacerbation free for over a year.

It is important that each patient has a clear understanding of the following.

- Individual management plan including a plan for management of an exacerbation.
- Recognition of an exacerbation (symptoms defined earlier).
- Requirement to send sputum for culture in the event of an exacerbation before starting antibiotics.
- How to access advice from health professionals if not responding to management plan.
- Requirement for annual flu vaccine.
- Requirement for follow up and assessment.

Monitoring and follow up

Patients with bronchiectasis require long-term follow-up to ensure that their infections are adequately controlled and their lung function is maintained. Not all patients require long-term follow up in secondary care if they have a satisfactory management plan. The following patients are at risk of more rapid decline or frequent hospital admissions and warrant follow up in secondary care.

- Patients with bronchiectasis in the context of rheumatoid arthritis.
- Patients with *Pseudomonas aeruginosa* infection.
- Patients with immunodeficiency and bronchiectasis.
- Patients with primary ciliary dyskinesia.
- Patients with frequent exacerbations requiring hospital admission.

At follow up the following should be checked

- Current sputum colour and estimation of daily sputum volume.
- Spirometry to assess stability or decline in FEV_1.
- Frequency of exacerbations since last seen.
- Effectiveness of antibiotic therapy in treating exacerbations.
- Effectiveness of maintenance therapy (if applicable) in preventing exacerbations.
- Sputum culture (patient should be encouraged to bring a sample to clinic).
- Patient's concordance with treatment including physiotherapy.
- Patient's understanding of bronchiectasis and the management plan.

A change in frequency or severity of exacerbations should prompt further evaluation of the sputum bacteriology. Furthermore a decline in lung function, general well being and quality of life should prompt reassessment and investigation.

Use of radiology in long term monitoring

The HRCT is used to establish the diagnosis of bronchiectasis. There is no requirement to repeat this on a regular basis if the patient remains well and exacerbation free with stable lung function.

In the event of worsening symptoms and/or decline in lung function it may be helpful to re-evaluate the HRCT appearances as part of a broader strategy of reinvestigation.

The HRCT is useful in the setting of a new growth of NTMa in establishing its significance.

The chest radiograph should be performed during exacerbations requiring hospital admission and other exacerbations associated with chest pain or haemoptysis.

Vaccinations

It is recommended that patients with bronchiectasis have an annual vaccination against influenza.

The pneumococcal vaccine is used as an initial test of functional antibody production. If a bronchiectasis patient who is initially immunocompetent suffers decline with more frequent and severe exacerbations in particular with pneumococcal infection it is worth retesting specific antibody levels.

Other infections in bronchiectasis

NTM are known to cause bronchiectasis and to complicate pre-existing bronchiectasis.

Infection with *Mycobacterium avium intracellulare* is the most common in this setting. There is a characteristic appearance on HRCT of nodular bronchiectasis with florid tree in bud appearance when there is active infection.

Treatment is difficult requiring lengthy courses of multiple drugs often associated with side effects and toxicity. The decision whether or not to treat NTM infection in the context of bronchiectasis depends on whether the same organism is repeatedly isolated, whether there is evidence of clinical deterioration and whether there is evidence of ongoing damage on the HRCT.

It is recommended that treatment is supervised by specialists.

Further reading

Barker AF. Bronchiectasis. *New Eng J Med* 2002; **346**(18): 1383–1393.

Crockett AJ, Cranston JM, Latimer KM *et al.* Mucolytics for bronchiectasis. *Cochrane Database Syst Rev (England)* 2000; **2**: pCD001289.

Davies G, Wells AU, Doffman S, *et al.* The effect of pseudomonas aeruginosa on pulmonary function in patients with bronchiectasis. *Eur Respir J* 2006; **28**: 974–979.

Fowler SJ, French J, Screaton NJ, *et al.* Nontuberculous mycobacteria in bronchiectasis: prevalence and patient characteristics. *Eur Respir J* 2006; **26**: 1204–1210.

Jones AP, Rowe BH. Bronchopulmonary hygiene physical therapy for chronic obstructive pulmonary disease and bronchiectasis. *Cochrane Database Syst Rev (England)* 2000; **2**: pCD00045.

Kolbe J, Wells A, Ram FS. Inhaled steroids in bronchiectasis. *Cochrane Database Syst Rev (England)* 2000; **2**: pCD000996.

Noone PG, Leigh MW, Sannuti A, *et al.* Primary ciliary dyskinesia. *Am J Respir Crit Care Med* 2004; **169**: 459–467.

Vendrell M, deGracia J, Rodrigo MJ, *et al.* Antibody production deficiency with normal IgG levels in bronchiectasis of unknown etiology. *Chest* 2005; **127**(1): 197–204.

Chapter 11

Cystic fibrosis

Chapter contents

11.1 Cystic fibrosis diagnosis

Introduction

CF is caused by mutations in the cystic fibrosis transmembrane conductance regulator (CFTR). Over 1500 abnormalities in this gene have been identified. The gene regulates chloride and sodium transport in secretory epithelial cells. Abnormalities in the gene cause multisystem disease including respiratory disease which is the major cause of morbidity and mortality, and also pancreatic dysfunction leading to malabsorption. Liver disease, diabetes mellitus, osteoporosis, infertility in males, small bowel obstruction, joint disease, vasculitis, sinusitis, and nasal polyps may also occur. There is a high level of sodium and chloride in the sweat which is the basis of the main diagnostic test for this condition. In 1938 70% of patients died within the first year of life but now the median survival is to 36 years in developed countries. In view of the mortality and morbidity associated with this condition it is essential that cases are not missed and appropriate treatment is given. On the other hand a mistaken diagnosis could have a disastrous effect on an individual and their family. Diagnostic procedures therefore must be robust.

Classical cystic fibrosis

The diagnosis is usually made soon after birth due to the development of meconium ileus or recurrent chest infections with, or without, malabsorption and failure to thrive. A positive sweat test and two disease-causing mutations of the CF gene are commonly present.

Atypical cystic fibrosis

There are some atypical cases diagnosed later in life where the diagnosis is difficult. Clinicians must be aware of these atypical presentations. These are patients who usually present late, in adolescence or even adult life, with allergic bronchopulmonary aspergillosis, pancreatitis, sinusitis, nasal polyps, heat exhaustion or infertility. They may have mild pulmonary disease and be pancreatic sufficient with one or no recognised gene mutations.

History

The frequency of presenting features of 20,096 patients in the Cystic Fibrosis Foundation Registry in the USA is as follows: respiratory system 51%; failure to thrive 43%; abnormal stools 35%; meconium ileus and small bowel obstruction 19%; family history 17%; electrolyte imbalance 5%; rectal prolapse 3%; nasal polyps and sinus disease 2%; and biliary disease 1%

Clinical features

Features consistent with a diagnosis are acute or recurrent chest infections often associated with *Staphylococcus aureus*, *Haemophilus influenzae* and/or *Pseudomonas aeruginosa*, together with malabsorption due to pancreatic insufficiency. Older patients may develop diabetes mellitus, osteoporosis, pancreatitis, liver disease, and gallstones. Other features include finger clubbing (which is almost universal), male infertility due to mal-development of the vas deferens, salt depletion in hot climates and chronic metabolic alkalosis.

Screening

More patients are now being diagnosed in the neonatal period due to screening. Some countries in the developed world have extensive screening programmes. Infants with CF have a raised immunoreactive trypsin (IRT) in the blood in the first week of life. This is not specific for CF although sensitive. A second IRT test is carried out at 4 weeks and this is more specific. If this is positive a sweat test is performed. Some screening programmes also include genetic analysis. When screening is carried out it is essential that sweat tests and counselling services are available promptly.

Diagnostic criteria

These were summarised by the Cystic Fibrosis Foundation Consensus Conference:

Clinical features or CF history in a sibling or The screening test	PLUS	Positive sweat test or Positive nasal potential or 2 disease-causing mutations in CFTR

Sweat test

The sweat test is the gold standard for the diagnosis of CF. The test must be performed by accredited laboratories with skill and care especially in collecting the sweat. Sweating is stimulated by iontophoresis of pilocarpine, usually into the skin of the forearm (Fig. 11.1.1). The sweat is collected on a filter paper or by Macroduct test tubing.

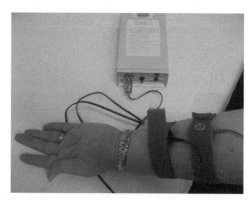

Fig. 11.1.1 A sweat test. Localised sweating is stimulated by iontophoresis of pilocarpine into the skin and then collected on filter paper, gauze or in Macroduct tubing.

The test is reliable after two weeks of age and CF patients have a chloride >60mmol/l and sodium >70mmol/l. Some normal adolescents and adults may have chloride up to 60mmol/l and values of 40–60mmol/l should be regarded as borderline. If a sweat test in an adult is borderline, a repeat sweat test after administration of 9 alpha fludrocortisone for 48hrs (3mg/m2/day) will reduce sodium levels in non-CF but not CF.

Using the conventional method of collection, at least 100mgs of sweat are necessary and 30µL if the Macroduct system is used. As CF is a diagnosis with serious implications for both patients and family, tests should be carried out in duplicate. There are reports of false positive sweat tests. The causes were listed by Wallis (Table 11.1.1).

Table 11.1.1 Some rare causes of false positive sweat tests

Adrenal insufficiency	Glycogen storage disease
Malnutrition	Hypothyroidism and hypoparathyroidism
Eczema	Nephrogenic diabetes insipidus
Fucosidosis	Nephrosis
Glucose-6-phosphate deficiency	HIV infection

Modified from Wallis (2007)

Nasal potential difference (PD)
The PD across the nasal epithelium is more negative in CF patients than controls. The technique requires a co-operative patient and is not useful in the presence of sinusitis or nasal polyps. One electrode is put on the floor of the nose and the reference electrode on the arm (Fig. 11.1.2).

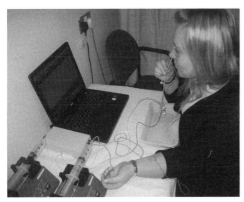

Fig. 11.1.2 Transepithelial nasal potential difference (PD) measurement. An exploring electrode is placed on the floor of the nose and a reference electrode over an area of abraded skin on the forearm. Nasal PD measurements are then taken in the presence of different solutions perfused onto the nasal mucosa.

In CF there is a more negative basal potential difference (due to sodium hyperabsorption), a greater response to amiloride and little response to perfusion with a chloride free solution followed by isoprenaline (Fig. 11.1.3). The technique is not easy and should only be performed by experienced operators. It can in some cases clarify the diagnosis.

Mutation analysis
The identification of two disease-causing mutations in the CF gene confirms the diagnosis. However, over 1500 abnormalities in the gene have been identified and it is not possible to test for them all. A positive test will therefore confirm the diagnosis but if no mutation is identified the diagnosis is not excluded and a sweat test is still required. The commonest mutations are ΔF508 (75%), G551D (3.4%), G542X (1.8%), R117H (1.3%), 621+1G →T (1.3%), Δ1507 (0.5%), and N1303K (0.5%). The presence of two

mutations does not always mean classical CF and the patient may have mild disease presenting with nasal polyps, male infertility or pancreatitis.

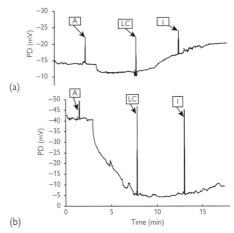

(a)

(b)

Time (min)

Fig. 11.1.3 Transepithelial nasal PD measurements. In a normal subject (a) the amiloride (A) response is small followed by a marked low chloride (LC) and isoprenaline (I) response, in contrast to a CF patient (b) where the amiloride response is large but with very little response to low chloride and isoprenaline.

Imaging the lungs and paranasal sinuses
CT scans of the lung and sinus may indicate bronchial wall thickening and/or parenchymal lung disease. Sinuses are frequently abnormal and polyps are common.

Microbiology
Sputum analysis frequently shows pathogens, the most commonly isolated are *Staphylococcus aureus* and *Pseudomonas aeruginosa*.

Lung function testing
In older children and adults, airflow obstruction may be demonstrated in large or small airways. Patients with severe disease will be hypoxic as measured by blood gases or oximeter.

Semen analysis
98% of males will have azoospermia which is due to maldevelopment of the vas deferens.

Further reading
Alton EW, Currie D, Logan-Sinclair R, *et al.* Nasal potential difference: a clinical diagnostic test for cystic fibrosis. *Eur Respir J* 1990; **3**(8): 922–926.

Andersen DH. Cystic fibrosis of the pancreas and its relation to celiac disease. A clinical and pathological study. *Am J Dis Child* 1938; **56**: 344–399.

Chatfield S, Owen G, Ryley HC, *et al.* Neonatal screening for cystic fibrosis in Wales and the West Midlands: clinical assessment after five years of screening. *Arch Dis Child* 1991; **66**(1:Spec No): Spec-33.

Crossley JR, Elliott RB, Smith PA. Dried-blood spot screening for cystic fibrosis in the newborn. *Lancet* 1979; **1**(8114): 472–474.

Dodge JA, Lewis PA, Stanton M, *et al.* Cystic fibrosis mortality and survival in the UK: 1947-2003. *Eur Respir J* 2007; **29**(3): 522–526.

Farrell PM, Kosorok MR, Laxova A, *et al.* Nutritional benefits of neonatal screening for cystic fibrosis. Wisconsin Cystic Fibrosis Neonatal Screening Study Group. *N Engl J Med* 1997; **337**(14): 963–969.

Hill CM (1998). *Diagnosis. Practical Guidelines for Cystic Fibrosis Care.* Edinburgh: Churchill Livingstone.

Hodson ME. Treatment of cystic fibrosis in the adult. *Respiration* 2000; **67**(6): 595–607.

Kaplan E, Shwachman H, Perlmutter AD, *et al.* Reproductive failure in males with cystic fibrosis. *N Engl J Med* 1968; **279**(2): 65–69.

Knowles MR, Durie PR. What is cystic fibrosis? *N Engl J Med* 2002; **347**(6): 439–442.

Nissim-Rafinia M, Kerem B, Kerem E. Molecular biology of cystic fibrosis: CFTR processing and functions, and classes of mutations. In: Hodson ME, Geddes DM, Bush AB (eds) (2007). *Cystic Fibrosis.* London: Hodder Arnold: 49–58.

Rosenstein BJ, Cutting GR. The diagnosis of cystic fibrosis: a consensus statement. Cystic Fibrosis Foundation Consensus Panel. *J Pediatr* 1998; **132**(4): 589–595.

Southern KW. The challenge of screening newborn infants for cystic fibrosis. In: Hodson ME, Geddes DM, Bush AB (eds) (2007). *Cystic Fibrosis.* London: Hodder Arnold: 109–116.

The diagnosis of cystic fibrosis: consensus statement. 96 Mar; Cystic Fibrosis Consensus Conferences, 1996.

Wallis C. Diagnosis of cystic fibrosis. In: Hodson ME, Geddes DM, Bush AB (eds) (2007). *Cystic Fibrosis.* London: Hodder Arnold: 99–108.

11.2 Managing acute infective exacerbations

Principals of care for acute exacerbations

Patients with CF have better outcomes for nutrition and pulmonary function the two best prognostic predictors for survival when care is delivered by a CF centre.

All adults with CF with an acute exacerbation should be treated by an experienced multidisciplinary team (MDT) based in a CF centre.

There are recognised guidelines for antibiotic management of acute exacerbations in cystic fibrosis.

Epidemiology

There is debate as to what constitutes the precise definition of an acute exacerbation in cystic fibrosis.

Infective exacerbations increase with age.

Repeated infective exacerbations in CF adults are associated with a linear decline in lung function.

Infective exacerbations are a marker of disease severity, a measured variable in studies of survival and an outcome measure in clinical trials.

Pathology and aetiology of acute exacerbations

The basic defect in cystic fibrosis is a mutation in CFTR (the cystic fibrosis transmembrane regulator protein). The resulting basic defect is chloride impermeabilty. The basic defect is expressed in all ductal systems of the body and explains why cystic fibrosis is a multi-organ systemic disease.

The basic defect impairs the local host defences in the airways and sinuses resulting in chronic infection with characteristic bacterial pathogens.

Infective exacerbations are more common during the winter months and can be initiated by the usual respiratory viruses; influenza A and B, RSV and the common cold viruses.

During an acute exacerbation there is an increase in bacterial pathogens, matched by an exuberant self damaging host inflammatory response in the airways consisting of neutrophil elastase, tumour necrosis factor, various interleukins (IL8, IL 6, IL1) and leukotriene B4.

Microbiology of infective exacerbations

Multiple bacterial pathogens can be isolated from a single sputum sample. It is important to decide which is the dominant pathogen causing an acute exacerbation.

CF bacterial pathogens require selective media for culture, grow very slowly and have multiple antibiotic resistance

Culture of bacterial pathogens from CF patients should be undertaken by a specialist CF microbiology laboratory.

Genotyping of Pseudomonas aeruginosa and Burkholderia cepacia from CF patients on at least one occasion is mandatory. This information will decide the outpatient clinic and inpatient segregation for that individual patient.

Bacterial pathogens causing an acute exacerbation

Pseudomonas aeruginosa (PA) is the most common pathogen, infecting 80% of CF adults. PA has a characteristic phenotype producing a protective mucoid exopolysacharide. This mucoid phenotype provides a defence against neutrophil and antibiotic penetration and an explanation as to why infective exacerbations in CF can be controlled but not cured.

Chronic infection with PA is associated with a sharper decline in lung function over time and an increased mortality.

Repeated courses of IV antibiotics result in increased antibiotic resistance. Despite this in vitro antibiotic resistance the patient usually respond in vivo to IV antibiotic combinations.

Bacterial genotyping in CF centres has shown the emergence of transmissible strains of PA within paediatric and adult CF centres in Europe and Australia. Transmissible strains of PA occur more commonly in sicker hospitalised patients and have an increased antibiotic resistance.

CF centres have adopted a policy of segregation for inpatients and outpatients with transmissible strains of PA.

Burkholderia cepacia complex. This bacterial pathogen can be divided into different species by phenotypic and genotypic testing. These different species are commonly called genomovars. Seventeen genomovars are currently recognised. The importance of this division is the association of increased pathogenicity with certain genomovars.

Patients infected with the B cepacia complex have more severe infective exacerbations than those with PA. Some strains of the B cepacia complex are highly transmissible

Chronic infection with the B cepacia complex results in a greater morbidity and mortality than infection with PA. Infection with the B cepacia complex can result in a reduced survival of two decades compared with usual mean survival figures.

The cepacia syndrome is much feared. It is associated with an infective exacerbation which progresses to a necrotising pneumonia (Fig. 11.2.1) and generalised sepsis. At this stage, it becomes untreatable with any antibiotic combination and progresses to death within weeks. It is usually caused by Burkholderia cenocepaca (genomovar 3) but can occur with other strains of the B cepacia complex. This syndrome does not occur with PA.

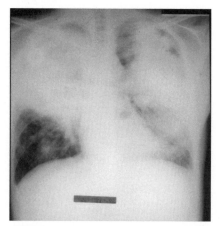

Fig. 11.2.1 Bilateral consolidation typical of necrotising B. cepacia complex pneumonia.

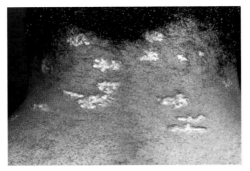

Plate 1 Typical sarcoid cutaneous lesions on nape of neck (see also Fig. 7.9.1).

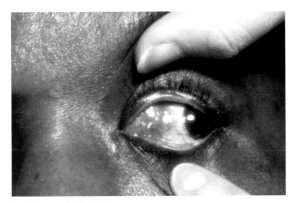

Plate 2 Conjunctival sarcoid nodules (see also Fig. 7.9.2).

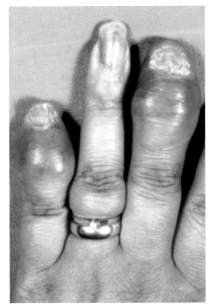

Plate 3 Extensive hand digit distortion with bone cyst formation and associated dactylitis in sarcoidosis (see also Fig. 7.9.3).

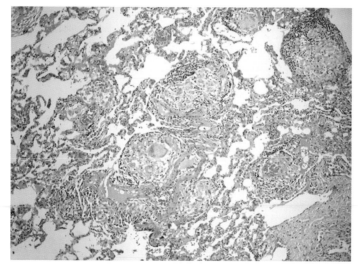

Plate 4 Histological appearances of tightly knit, well formed granulomata formation (see also Fig. 7.9.5).

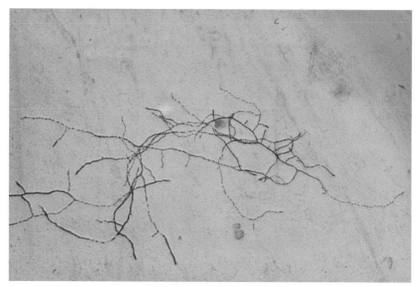

Plate 5 Smear preparation of *Nocardia asteroides* (see also Fig. 8.5.1).

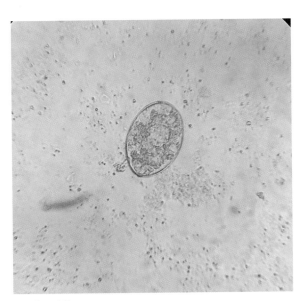

Plate 6 Paragoniamasis (see also Fig. 8.10.2).

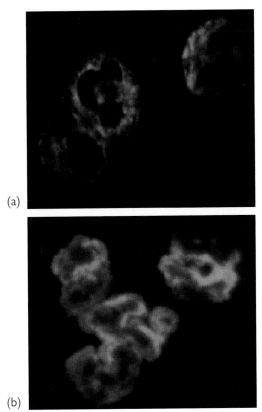

(a)

(b)

Plate 7 ANCA staining by immunefluoresence. (a) C-ANCA with cytoplasmic staining. (b) P-ANCA with peri-nuclear staining (see also Fig. 12.3.3).

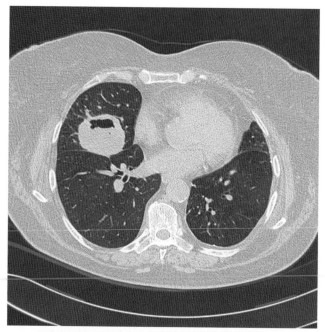

Plate 8 CT scan (lung window) showing cavitating squamous cell tumour right lower lobe (see also Fig. 13.3.1).

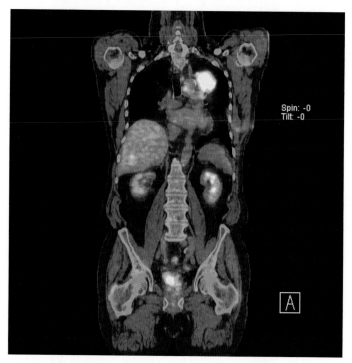

Plate 9 PET CT scan showing increased ^{5}FDG uptake in left upper lobe mass and an unsuspected solitary liver metastasis (see also Fig. 13.3.7).

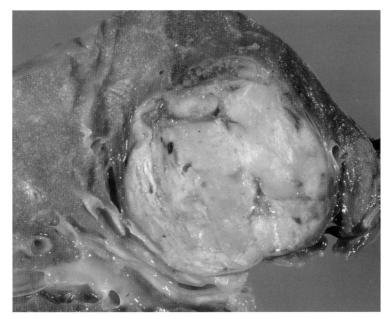

Plate 10 This solitary fibrous tumour is intrapulmonary rather than pleural. The lesion is well circumscribed and, in this region, densely cellular (see also Fig. 13.9.1).

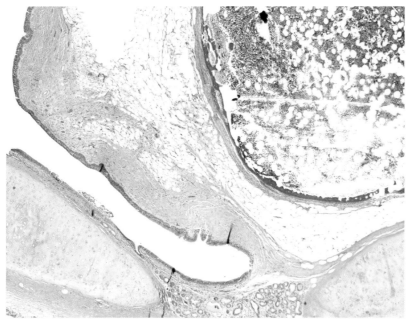

Plate 11 This is an endobronchial chondroid hamartoma. The cartilage plates and seromucous glands of the native bronchus are seen below, the lesion comprising connective and adipose tissue and cartilage, which has ossified and has a substantial component of bone marrow (top right) (see also Fig. 13.9.3).

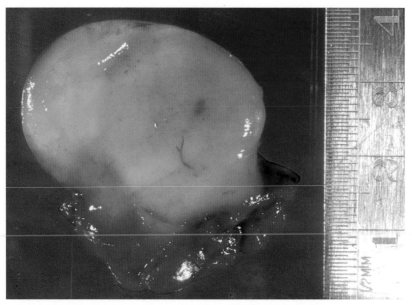

Plate 12 This is a resected pleomorphic adenoma from the main carina. Tracheobronchial wall is present at the base of the lesion, which itself comprises a smooth, rounded mass, which protruded into the trachea and presented as acute onset asthma (see also Fig. 13.9.5).

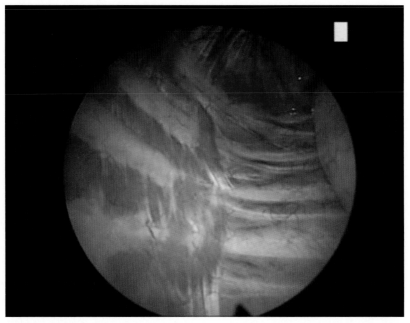

Plate 13 Normal thoracoscopic appearance of parietal pleural surface (see also Fig. 14.2.2).

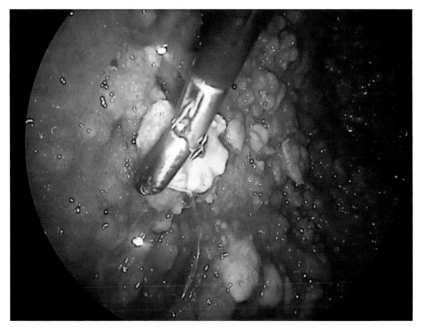

Plate 14 Thoracoscopic biopsy via two-port technique (mesothelioma) (see also Fig. 14.2.3).

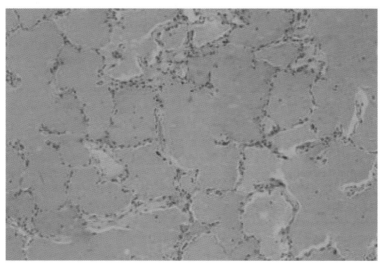

Plate 15 Pathology PAS stain of alveoli filled with lipo-protein in a patient with alveoar proteinosis (see also Fig. 18.1.3).

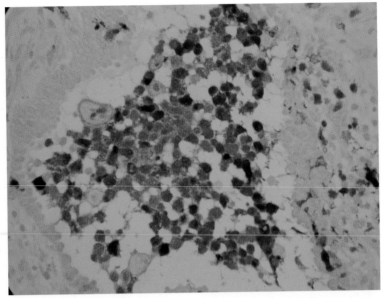

Plate 16 Lung biopsy with Langerhans cells labelled with labelled for S-100 protein (see also Fig. 18.4.2).

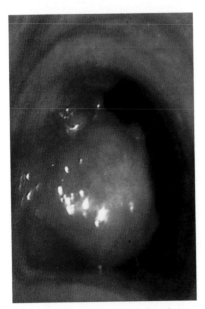

Plate 17 Tracheal tumour visible at flexible bronchoscopy. (see also Fig. 18.6.2).

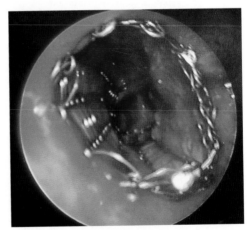

Plate 18 View seen at bronchoscopy following endoscopic resection and stenting (see also Fig. 18.6.3).

CF adults infected with the *B. cepacia* complex have been ruthlessly segregated from other CF patients for many years. This action has resulted in a decline of the incidence (decreased cross infection) and decreased prevalence (increased mortality) of *B. cepacia* complex infection.

Patients infected with *B. cenocepacia* (genomovar 111) are considered unsuitable for transplantation due to poor results after surgery.

Staphylococcus aureus and *Haemophilus influenzae*: these bacterial pathogens previously were responsible for severe infective exacerbations in children. Treatment with long-term prophylactic antibiotics has considerably diminished their pathogenic potential.

S. aureus ((51%) and *H. influenza* (16%) are commonly cultured in sputum without any change in clinical status or need for therapeutic intervention.

Methicillin-resistant *Staphylococcus aureus* (MRSA): MRSA is increasing in patients attending centres and is usually acquired from the hospital environment. There is very little evidence that it causes infective exacerbations

Non-bacterial pathogens and infective exacerbations

Non-tuberculous mycobacteria (NTM): About 4% of CF adults have positive cultures for non-tuberculous mycobacterium (atypical). Positive cultures are often sporadic and therapy is not indicated. Multiple positive cultures and repeated smear positivity may indicate active disease.

Active disease is more often associated with the fast growing NTB (*M. abscessus* and *M. chelonae)*

Active disease due to NTM can be demonstrated on CT scanning.

Infective exacerbations are usually caused by PA and it is difficult to evaluate the exact contribution of NTM to infective exacerbations when isolated repeatedly.

Aspergillus spp.: the fungus *Aspergillus fumigatus* has been found in the sputum of 60–80% of CF patients. Chronically infected CF lung is an ideal environment for this organism

Allergic bronchopulmonary aspergillosis (ABPA) as defined by consensus criteria has a prevalence of about 10–15% in CF patients and is increasing as survival improves. ABPA contributes significantly to infective exacerbations and accelerates decline in lung function. ABPA is probably a significant co-factor with PA in magnifying the severity of an infective exacerbation.

Diagnosing an infective exacerbation

There has been considerable debate as to how an infective exacerbation should be defined and which diagnostic criteria should be employed. However, the physician who reviews the CF patient will have considerable knowledge of the usual clinical status and will easily detect both obvious and subtle decline in health due to an infective exacerbation.

Symptoms of an infective exacerbation

- Increased coughing especially at night.
- Exhaustion/lack of energy.
- Increased sputum quantity or decreased with sputum retention.
- Thicker sputum.
- Bloodstained sputum.
- Dyspnoea and an increased respiratory rate.

- Chest pain (pleuritic or musculoskeletal from coughing).
- Anorexia/weight loss.

Signs
Patient looks unwell with a tachycardia and dyspnoea.

There may be very few signs on auscultation despite a severe infective exacerbation.

CF patients (unlike patients with primary ciliary dyskinesia) rarely wheeze during infective exacerbations.

Increased inspiratory crackles heard usually over the apices of the lungs and at the mouth.

Presence of a pleural rub. These are more common in CF patients than any other respiratory disease (apart from systemic lupus erythematosus).

There is often a difference in intensity of the breath sounds between the two lungs in an individual patient making it very difficult to diagnose a pneumothorax with confidence. A pneumothorax may be difficult to confirm without a chest radiograph but suspicion of a tension pneumothorax may require a lifesaving immediate intercostal drain with no time to do a chest radiograph.

Investigations
Simple spirometry.

If the patient has chest pain do not perform spirometry until a current chest radiograph has been reviewed.

The FEV_1 is remarkably reproducible for an individual patient. A reduction in FEV_1 greater than 10% in the context of the above symptoms and signs denotes an infective exacerbation.

Values for FVC are more variable with infective exacerbations

Blood gases (arterialised capillary blood sample) will decide oxygen requirements (percentage and flow rate) if the patient is hypoxic and the potential need for nasal ventilation if there is an acute rise in carbon dioxide levels.

Chest radiographs usually do not show many new changes with a moderate infective exacerbation.

A chest radiograph should always be done to exclude

- A small pneumothorax: can be difficult to detect on a plain radiograph if the pneumothorax has a posterior location.
- Rib (cough) fractures in the presence of chest wall pain.
- Right upper lobe collapse (more common than left) due to sputum plugs or ABPA.
- Pneumonic consolidation typical of the onset of the cepacia syndrome in a patient chronically infected with the *B. cepacia* complex.

Sputum culture is always repeated at time of a new infective exacerbation to exclude new growth of pathogens such as *B. cepacia* complex and MRSA. Change in antibiotic resistant patterns may indicate acquisition of a transmissible strain of PA.

Haematological investigations
Sequential measurement of C reactive protein (CRP) provides a valuable indication of the severity of the infection and response to treatment.

Blood glucose: 30% of adult CF patients have insulin dependent diabetes. Infective exacerbations are more frequent in diabetic CF patients. Diabetic control is lost during an exacerbation due to infection and treatment (corticosteroids). Continuous blood sugar monitoring is important for management. CF patients can become diabetic for the first time during an infective exacerbation.

Blood cultures should be done if the patient is pyrexial. Persistent temperatures are unusual with an infective exacerbation due to PA in CF. The usual cause of a persistent temperature is an infected permanent IV access device (PORT) or the development of the cepacia syndrome.

Management of an infective exacerbation

The delivery of care for an infective exacerbation should be provided at a CF centre by a multidisciplinary team.

CF patients can become unwell rapidly with an hour infective exacerbation and a CF centre should have a 24-hour open access self admission policy for patients. During the week they should be seen on the same day. At other times they should be able to ring the ward directly for advice and potential admission.

Beds for CF patients should be ring-fenced and used only for CF patients. Usually the adult CF centre will be the only one in the Region and the patients will have nowhere else to go to receive their specialist care.

As the CF adult population increases the CF beds at a centre usually have maximum bed occupancy leading to prioritisation of the sicker patients for admission.

At the start of an infective exacerbation, a clinical decision will need to be made as to whether treatment is undertaken at home or in hospital. Evidence has shown that clinical outcome is better when an infective exacerbation is treated in hospital rather than home.

CF patients often prefer home treatment.

The sickest CF patient can be treated at home receiving IV antibiotics, nasal ventilation, continuous oxygen, and enteral feeding if there is sufficient social support and satisfactory treatment adherence.

Treatment of an infective exacerbation

IV antibiotics

Each patient will have a portfolio of previous sputum cultures facilitating best choice of antibiotic treatment.

There will be records of best responses to IV antibiotics used for previous infective exacerbations.

There should be a low threshold for starting a course of IV antibiotics. A treatment course should be for 10–14 days.

Two antibiotics should be used in combination. Monotherapy is associated with the development of antibiotic resistance.

The 2 antibiotics used should have a different mechanism of action. The usual combination is an aminoglycoside (killing related to peak levels) and a beta lactam (killing related to constant blood level over 24 hours).

Increasingly aminoglycosides are given as a once daily dose to achieve maximum concentration dependent killing and reduce side effects. Beta lactams are given 3–4 times a day.

There is a relatively wide choice of IV antibiotic for combination usage. Large doses of antibiotics are required due to the enhanced metabolism of all drugs in CF patients.

Problem areas

Antibiotic resistance is increasing with repeated courses and with the rising prevalence of transmissible PA. Choice of IV antibiotics is usually made according to the previous best clinical response. Occasionally triple antibiotic therapy is used for multi-resistant PA.

Pan antibiotic resistance occurs with B cenocepacia and makes a suitable antibiotic choice extremely difficult. Triple antibiotic therapy based upon best previous clinical response and prolonged treatment is usually required.

Pregnancy. During pregnanacy there is an increased requirement for IV antibiotics. The penicillins, cephalosporins and monobactms are safe for IV use. Although IV aminoglycosides are safe if blood levels are closely monitored, they are best avoided due to potential oxtotoxicity upon the fetus during the second trimester.

Antibiotic allergy to antibiotics with repeated IV courses is becoming a huge problem. It is severely limiting choice of suitable antibiotics. Serious allergic reactions are common and anaphylactic reactions are not uncommon. It is important to document specific antibiotic allergy. Patients should be provided with an Epipen® (adrenaline) and taught how to self inject. It may be necessary to desensitise patients to useful antibiotics to such as ceftazidime to which they have become allergic. They will need admission to hospital for this procedure.

Physiotherapy and airway clearance

Physiotherapy delivered to a sick patient by an experienced physiotherapist skilled in airway clearance techniques and the intricacies of nebulised drug delivery is crucial for patient recovery.

Clearance of thickened airways secretions can be improved during an infective exacerbation with judicious use of nebulised drugs such as rhDNase and hypertonic saline.

Nebulised bronchodilators prior to physiotherapy have an important role in airway clearance.

The use of overnight IV fluids such as saline or IV aminophylline are useful adjuncts to maintaining airway clearance especially if the patient is sweating, pyrexial or diabetic.

Mobility is crucial. As the patient recovers, mobilisation and gentle exercise under physiotherapy supervision using a saturation monitor and oxygen will also enhance airway clearance.

Oxygen delivery

Repeated blood gases are an essential component of inpatient management of an infective exacerbation.

CF patients have a high inspiratory flow. Correct oxygen delivery with an appropriate high flow rate is important for safety and comfort.

Safe delivery of oxygen is important. Oxygen should be delivered with a fixed concentration mask rather than nasal cannula during an infective exacerbation and especially overnight where uncontrolled oxygen delivery can result in carbon dioxide retention.

Steroids

The beneficial role of oral corticosteroids during an infective exacerbation is uncertain. High doses can cause onset of diabetes and loss of diabetic control in established insulin dependent diabetes

Diabetes control

Infective exacerbations are more common in the 30% of diabetic patients attending a CF clinic. Insulin resistance increases during an infective exacerbation and higher doses of insulin are required or the institution of an insulin pump.

Nutrition

CF patients constitutionally have a high energy expenditure which is elevated further during an infective exacerbation and wasting can occur rapidly and recovery delayed. Commencement of enteral feeding either nasogastric or with the insertion of a feeding gastrostomy will be required.

Complications

Haemoptysis: Small amounts of blood mixed with sputum can be resolved very quickly with IV or oral tranexamic acid (500mg–1g QDS) continued for 5 days.

A large haemoptysis (300–400ml of fresh blood) is an indication for bronchial artery embolisation which is a skilled procedure undertaken by an experience interventional radiologist.

A life-threatening haemoptysis is one of the few indications for endotracheal intubation and ventilation to maintain airway patency. IV vasopressors should be commenced. Terlipressin 2mgm is given as a bolus intravenously and then 2mg 4-hourly until embolisation can be undertaken.

After embolisation the patient should be extubated as quickly as possible and respiratory support provided with non-invasive ventilation (NIV).

Fractured ribs are caused by coughing during an infective exacerbation are a potentially lethal complication. The associated excruciated pain (requiring opiates) inhibits coughing and deep inspiration and optimum airway clearance.

Effective treatment is with intramuscular calcitonin. Dose is 50–100 units per day for 10–14 days. Response is usually within 3–5 days.

Pneumothoraces: these are associated with and cause infective exacerbations. They can be bilateral.

A pneumothorax with an air rim of greater than 2cm will usually require an intercostal drain connected to an underwater drainage system. The tube should be large bore and inserted either in the second intercostal space anteriorly or in the 5–6th intercostal space in the mid-axillary line.

Due to pleural disease or tethering from previous pneumothoraces a further pneumothorax may be both loculated and posterior and a CT scan is required to define the size and location (Fig. 11.2.2.). Intercostal drainage may need to be done with radiological control.

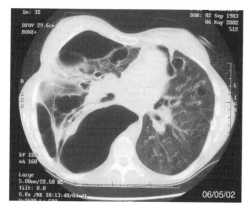

Fig. 11.2.2 Loculated pneumothorax in a patient who had previous pneumothoraces.

Pneumothoraces re-expand slowly in CF patients as the lungs are stiff due to fibrosis and patience is required.

When the lung has re-expanded a pleurodesis should be performed before the tube is removed. Pleurodesis with a 100ml of the patients own blood is common practice. Talc pleurodesis is effective but may compromise the patient as a potential transplant candidate.

Failure of the lung to re-expand requires referral to an experienced thoracic surgeon. The procedure of choice is an apical pleurectomy and surgical pleurodesis performed under videoassisted thoracoscopy (VATS).

Occasionally, the patients may be so compromised that they are unfit for surgical intervention.

Upper lobe collapse is uncommon and usually on the right side. It is due to airways impaction of purulent secretions. ABPA as a cause should be excluded with standard diagnostic tests.

Prompt therapy should be directed at re-expanding the collapsed lobe as chronic collapse will result in permanent loss of lung function.

Therapeutic measures include physiotherapy with intermittent positive pressure breathing to the collapsed upper lobe. Bronchoscopy (fibreoptic) can be used to extract impacted mucous plugs and install rhDNase directly into the lobe.

Antifungal drugs (itraconazole/voriconazole) can be prescribed if ABPA has been diagnosed.

NIV and acute respiratory failure

As a result of an infective exacerbation sick CF patients can fatigue rapidly and develop type 2 respiratory failure.

It is impossible to oxygenate them safely and adequately at night even with controlled oxygen therapy. The acute introduction of NIV can be lifesaving in these circumstances. The benefits are reducing the work of breathing at night, safe oxygenation and increased sputum clearance.

Monitoring treatment responses to an infective exacerbation

An MDT should review twice a week the response to treatment of each patient with an infective exacerbation. Each member should have a significant contribution to the portfolio of each patient's management.

The best objective markers of improvement are reduction in CRP and sputum quantity and an improvement in simple spirometry and body weight towards previous best baseline measurements.

Repeat blood gases and measurements of oxygen saturations.

Qualitative measures of improvement are decline in breathlessness, increased exercise tolerance and patients self expression of improvement in well being.

Failure to improve after first week of an infective exacerbation

Consider changing the patient to a different antibiotic combination after review of most recent sputum culture.

Decline in sputum production with deteriorating lung function indicates retained secretions. Repeat chest radiograph to exclude development of a small pneumothorax or lobar collapse. If no change on chest radiograph introduce or increase pulmozyme to twice a day, add in hypertonic saline.

Review airway clearance techniques.

Monitor blood sugars to exclude the onset of diabetes. If the blood sugars become uncontrolled in an established diabetic put the patient onto an insulin pump.

Monitor overnight oxygen saturations and carbon dioxide levels with a transcutaneous oxygen and carbon dioxide monitor. Have a low threshold for establishing patient on nasal ventilation. Inability to safely oxygenate overnight with a marginally elevated (rather than high) carbon dioxide level.

Infective exacerbations can be prevented or reduced in severity with maximised care.

Further reading

Antibiotic treatment for cystic fibrosis: Report of the UK Cystic Fibrosis Trust Antibiotic Group (2nd edn) (2002). London: UK Cystic fibrosis Trust.

Ashleigh R, Webb AK. Radiological Intervention for haemoptysis in cystic fibrosis. *Roy Soc Med* 2007; **100**(suppl 47): 38–45.

Cystic Fibrosis Foundation. Patient Registry (2005). Annual Report. Bethseda, Maryland.

Ellaffi M, Vinsonneau C, Coste J et al. One year outcome after severe pulmonary exacerbations in adults with cystic fibrosis. *Am J Respir Crit Care Med* 2005; **171**: 158–164.

Goss CH, Burns J. Exacerbations in cystic fibrosis. 1: Epidemiology and pathogenesis. *Thorax* 2007; **62**: 360–367.

Mahadeva R, Webb AK, Westerbeek et al. Management in paediatric and adult cystic fibrosis centres improves clinical outcome *BMJ* 1998; **316**: 1771–1775.

Marshall BC. Pulmonary exacerbations in cystic fibrosis: its time to be explicit! *Am J Respir Crit Care Med* 2004; **169**: 781–782.

Pitt TL, Sparrow M, Warner M, et al. Survey of resis tance of Pseudomonas aeruginosa from UK patients with cystic fibrosis to six commonly prescribed antimicrobial agents. *Thorax* 2003; **58**: 794–796.

Thornton J, Dodd ME, Webb AK, et al. Long term clinical outcome of home and hospital intravenous antibiotic treatment in adults with cystic fibrosis. *Thorax* 2004; **59**: 242–246.

11.3 Chronic disease management

Overview

Cystic fibrosis (CF) is a multi-system condition.

The majority of the morbidity and premature mortality relate to the effects of the chronic suppurative lung disease and exuberant host inflammatory response, and malabsorption due to exocrine pancreatic insufficiency.

Specialist centre care

The management of adults with CF requires a MDT at a specialist CF centre.

The specialist team should comprise physicians, nurses, physiotherapists, dieticians, social workers, psychologists, pharmacists, and administrative support staff.

Survival

There have been significant improvements in quality of life and survival for patients with CF over the past few decades.

Lung function and nutritional status are predictors of patients' survival.

The predicted median age of survival for infants recently born with CF in the UK is over 50 years old.

Pathology of CF lung disease

Pulmonary disease is almost universal in individuals with CF.

The defective CFTR genes causes abnormalities in sodium and chloride permeability in the airway epithelium leading to a decrease in the airway surface liquid and impairment of mucociliary clearance. A combination of airflow obstructive, endobronchial sepsis and an excessive host inflammatory response leads to progressive lung damage. With persistent infection the airways become plugged by thick, mucopurulent material containing bacteria, neutrophils and mucus, the bronchial epithelium become ulcerated, abscesses form and bronchiectasis develops.

The distribution of changes is usually most marked in the upper lobes.

The severe inflammatory changes lead to parenchymal destruction and cyst formation within the lung. Hypertrophy of the pulmonary vasculature and new vessel formation is seen and bronchopulmonary shunting occurs in association with bronchiectasis.

Physiological features of CF lung disease

The early physiological features of CF pulmonary disease are small airway narrowing, air trapping and progressive hyperinflation. In the larger airways damage to the airway wall leads to central airway instability. Later in the disease there is a reduction in lung volume due to the consequence of progressive fibrosis.

The FEV_1 and FVC are reproducible measures of pulmonary function for patients with moderate to severe disease.

The FEV_1 and FVC are used to monitor the progression of CF lung disease and provide an indictor for patients' survival.

Data from specialist CF centres has shown a progressive reduction in the annual rate of lung function decline with each succesive birth cohort of patients over the past few decades.

Management of CF lung disease

Provision for patient review and advice

1 Regular outpatient review is essential. Routine visits should be at least every 3 months or more frequently depending on clinical condition. Ideally, the CF MDT should meet both before and after the clinic to discuss the patients attending that day to plan their long-term management.
2 Patients should have 24-hour access to specialist CF centre care for emergency appointments and telephone advice.
3 Annual assessments should be performed for all patients, including various assessments of CF lung disease (see later in this chapter).

Monitoring of CF lung disease

Spirometry should be measured at each clinic visit and during inpatient admissions unless there is a clear contraindication, such as a current pneumothorax.

Microbiological culture of respiratory secretions is mandatory at each patient visit and during inpatient admissions.

- Sputum samples are more sensitive than cough swabs.
- Use of induced sputum can be considered for those patients who experience difficultly providing sputum samples despite input from a physiotherapist experienced in CF care.
- The samples should be processed by a diagnostic laboratory with expertise in CF microbiology.
- Use of selective culture media for CF pathogens is mandatory.
- Culture for environmental *mycobacteria* should be performed at least once annually.

Postal kits can be used to send samples to the laboratory between clinic visits when more frequent surveillance cultures may be required, such as screening for early *Pseudomonas aeruginosa* infection.

CXR should be performed at least annually, or more frequently if indicated by clinical symptoms/signs or significant fall in spirometry.

Oximetry can be measured at rest and during exercise.

Arterial blood gas, or preferably arterialised capillary blood sample, analysis should be measured at least annually or more frequently if indicated by clinical symptoms/signs or significant fall in spirometry.

Transcutaneous oxygen and carbon dioxide monitoring (TOSCA) can be used to evaluate requirements for overnight oxygen and non-invasive ventilation for patients with moderate-severe respiratory disease at risk of onset of cor pulmonale and/or chronic type II respiratory failure

CT scanning can provide further information of CF lung disease in selected cases, for example, patients who have infection with environmental *mycobacteria*. At present there is insufficient evidence to recommend the use of chest CT-scans on regular intervals to monitor progression of lung disease.

Exercise testing can provide further assessment of pulmonary status and should be considered for patients as part of their annual review assessment.

Physical activity questionnaires and breathlessness scores should be recorded as part of the annual assessment.

Transthoracic echocardiography can provide a non-invasive estimation of pulmonary artery pressure for patients with severe disease at risk of pulmonary hypertension. There are reports of cardiomyopathy in a small number of patients.

Other new techniques, for example measurement of the lung clearance index, are currently research tools and not yet used in routine clinical practice.

Microbiology of CF lung disease

The traditional spectrum of pathogens associated with CF lung disease is surprisingly small, although emerging pathogens such as *Stenotrophomonas maltophilia*, *Achromobacter xylosoxidans*, *Ralstonia* species, and *Pandorea apista* are being more frequently encountered.

Staphylococcus aureus and Haemophilus influenzae

The most common pathogens in early childhood are *Staphylococcus aureus* and *Haemophilus influenzae*.

Meticillin-resistant Staphylococcus aureus (MRSA)

There is no evidence that pulmonary infection with MRSA confers any further disadvantage than with meticillin-sensitive strains of *S. aureus* for patients with CF.

However, infection does limit antibiotic treatment options, may cause problems if infection spreads to other sites, for example if the patient undergoes a surgical procedure, and leads to infection control problems.

The majority of MRSA infections are due to hospital-acquired strains, although whilst the proportion of infections due to community acquired MRSA strains are low in the UK, they are increasing in prevalence in North American CF Centres.

Pseudomonas aeruginosa

The major pathogen in late childhood and adulthood is *Pseudomonas aeruginosa*, with approximately 80% of adults with CF having chronic infection.

Early infection can be eradicated or suppressed by aggressive antibiotic treatment. Left untreated, the organism will adapt to the environment of the CF lung by producing a mucoid exopolysaccharide in a biofilm mode of growth. Once this phenotypic change occurs then eradication becomes impossible.

Chronic *Pseudomonas aeruginosa* infection is associated with an increase in treatment requirements, deterioration in lung function and reduction in life expectancy for patients with CF.

A combination of proactive screening, infection control and aggressive eradication treatment, however, are beginning to reduce the age dependent prevalence of infection.

Burkholderia cepacia complex

Patients with CF are particularly predisposed to infection with a group of organisms known as the *Burkholderia cepacia* complex. Approximately 5–10% of adults patients are infected by these organisms.

Certain strains of these species are highly transmissible between people with CF.

Cross-infection epidemics, with evidence of patient-to-patient transmission, have necessitated the implementation of draconian infection control measures both within and outside hospitals to control spread.

Infection is associated with an increase in morbidity and mortality above that of any other CF pathogen.

Some patients succumb to a necrotising pneumonic illness associated with pyrexia and septicaemia known as the 'cepacia syndrome' (Fig. 11.2.1).

It is probable that certain species within the complex, such as *B. cenocepacia*, are more virulent than others.

There is also a worse outcome following lung transplantation for patients infected with *B. cenocepacia*; patients infected with this pathogen are therefore often excluded from lung transplantation programs.

Environmental mycobacteria

Environmental *mycobacteria* are occasionally isolated from sputum samples of patients with CF.

The diagnosis of active infection and decision to treat the organism in such cases is often difficult. Consistently smear or culture positive cases, or features on a CT-scan suggesting active infection, may help the clinicians' decision.

The fast growing environmental *mycobacterial* species, *M. chelonae* and *M. abscessus*, are more likely to cause clinically significant infection and are particularly difficult to treat.

Some lung transplant centres consider active infection with *M. chelonae* or *M. abscessus* as a contra-indication to transplantation.

Fungi

Although *Candida* and *Aspergillus* species are frequently isolated from sputum of CF patients, in most patients this is not clinically significant and does not require treatment.

Respiratory viruses

Respiratory viruses are responsible for some of the acute exacerbations of pulmonary disease in CF.

Respiratory viral infections, such as adenoviruses, RSV and *Influenza* A and B, can on occasions lead to dramatic falls in lung function, that may take months to recover or can be irreversible.

Treatment

There are a number of treatment options available for CF pulmonary disease.

The management should be tailored to each individual patient, aiming to control infection, preserve lung function, prevent associated complications, and control symptoms whilst minimising the treatment burden.

Nebulisers and compressors

Nebuliser therapy is widely used in treatment of CF lung disease.

It is vital that patients practise cleaning and maintenance of the equipment.

In addition to the traditional nebuliser-compressor systems, new nebulisers are now available that use novel adaptive aerosol delivery, that can reduce treatment time and burden.

Prevention of infection

1. Cross-infection control

There is clear evidence that some CF respiratory pathogens such as strains of *P. aeruginosa* and organisms of the *B. cepacia* complex pose cross-infection risks to others with CF.

All CF Centres should have their own local cross-infection policies for their centre, developed by the CF MDT and hospital infection control team, and guided by Cystic

Fibrosis Trust recommendations. The policy should consider issues of surveillance, hygiene and patient segregation isolation.

Good hygiene should be practised in all outpatient clinics and inpatient facilities to minimise the risk of transmission of pathogens between patients

Mixing of patients should be discouraged both within and outside the hospital environment.

Inpatients should be housed in single en-suite rooms.

Patients infected with organisms of the *B. cepacia* complex should be treated on separate wards from other patients with CF.

Outpatient clinics should be organised according to patients' microbiological status and patients should be prevented from mixing at the clinic visit.

Ongoing microbiological surveillance, including genotyping of *P. aeruginosa* and *B. cepacia* complex strains, is essential.

2. Eradication therapies for CF pathogens
(a) Early P. aeruginosa infection

Early *P. aeruginosa* infection should be treated aggressively to eradicate the organism and prevent progression to chronic infection.

It is important to actively screen respiratory secretions at regular intervals to detect early *P. aeruginosa* infection to allow prompt intervention to eradicate the infection. For patients free of chronic *P. aeruginosa* infection, sputum should be sent for microbiological culture every month. Samples can be collected at outpatient clinic visits or patients given postal specimen kits to send specimens directly to the microbiology laboratory.

The most frequently used regimen used in the UK is nebulised colisitin and oral ciprofloxacin for 3 months. An alternative nebulised antibiotic for use is tobramycin solution for inhalation (TOBI). This may be used either as first line-therapy or second line if a patient is failing to clear early infection with colisitin.

A course of IV antibiotics can be used for any patient unable to tolerate nebulised therapy.

(b) MRSA

Attempts should be made to eradicate MRSA pulmonary infection in patients with CF.

Success is reported with regimens using nebulised vancomycin combined with a course of oral antibiotics.

Nebulised vancomycin is acidic and difficult to tolerate. It is therefore recommended that it be given as a short 5-day course at a dose 200mgs QDS under close medical supervision as an inpatient. A fully supervised test dose and pre-treatment with a bronchodilator is mandatory.

Nebulised vancomycin can be combined with a more prolonged course of two oral antibiotics such as rifampicin and fusidic acid; liver function tests must be monitored during this treatment. Alternative oral antibiotics include clindamycin, trimethoprim or tetracycline if either patient allergy or intolerance, or microbial resistance, preclude use of rifampicin and fusidic acid. Linezolid can be considered as a second-line oral antibiotic, although prolonged courses should be avoided because of potential side-effects.

If first attempts at eradication are unsuccessful, then up to two further courses of eradication treatment should be given.

(c) B. cepacia complex

Although there is no published evidence to support or guide eradication treatment for early infection with organisms of the *B. cepacia* complex, treatment in attempt to eradicate the organism should be considered given the difficult clinical problems associated with infection by this group of pathogens.

Possible treatment options may include nebulised treatment with an antibiotic with good activity against organisms of the *B. cepacia* complex such as meropenem (NB: unlicensed indication) combined with two oral antibiotics with activity against the organism, such as cotrimoxazole, or rifampicim, or chloramphenicol, or ciprofloxacin or minocycline, or a prolonged course of intravenous antibiotics.

3. Vaccination

- *Influenza* vaccination – all adults with CF should be offered an annual influenza vaccination.
- *Pneumococcal* vaccination – pneumococcal vaccination is also recommended for patients with CF
- *Pseudomonal* vaccination – a recent large multicentre phase III clinical trial has shown disappointing results with use of a vaccine to prevent *P. aeruginosa* infection in CF, and at present, there is no clinically effective anti-pseudomonal vaccination available.

Antibiotic therapy for chronic infection
Intermittent IV antibiotic therapy

Some CF centres have adopted an approach of using regular two week courses of IV antibiotics, every three months. The merits of this strategy in comparison with using IV antibiotics courses only for infective exacerbations are unproven, but some individual patients may benefit from this approach.

A combination of an anti-*Pseudomonal* β-lactam with an aminoglycoside should be the first-line IV antibiotic therapy for patients with chronic *P. aeruginosa* infection.

In vitro data and clinical experience suggests a combination of three different antibiotics is most effective for infections with organisms of the *B. cepacia* complex.

Nebulised antibiotics

Nebulised antibiotics are an essential component of the long-term treatment of patients with CF and chronic *P. aeruginosa* infection.

Nebulised antibiotics can cause bronchospasm. They should be administered either preceded by or mixed with a bronchodilator to prevent chest tightness.

The two most commonly used nebulised antibiotics in the UK are colisitin and tobramycin solution for inhalation (TOBI).

Large multicentre clinical studies have demonstrated improvements in pulmonary function and reduction in hospitalisations with use of TOBI in a cycle of 4 weeks on/4 weeks off treatment regimen for patients with chronic *P. aeruginosa* infection and FEV_1 between 25–75% predicted.

Although clinical trial evidence is less robust for the use of nebulised colisitin, there is substantial clinical experience with the use of inhalation or this antibiotic at European CF centres the over many years of that has proved to be a safe and effective therapy for patients with chronic *P. aeruginosa* infection.

Oral antibiotics

Anti-staphylococcal therapy

Although there is some limited evidence of benefit from the use of chronic oral anti-*Staphylococcal* antibiotics in early childhood, there is no evidence that such treatment should be continued in later childhood and adulthood.

Macrolide antibiotics

Long-term treatment with an oral macrolide antibiotic has become an important part of the treatment regimen for most patients with CF.

Studies have demonstrated improvements in lung function, decreased need for hospitalisation and IV antibiotics associated with the use of regular oral macrolide therapy for patients with CF.

The most commonly used macrolide in clinical trials has been azithromycin, although the optimal dose and frequency still remains unclear.

The mechanism of action, whether it is antibacterial, anti-inflammatory, or another property of the drug remains unclear.

Anti-viral drugs

Treatment with oseltamivir, a viral neuraminidase inhibitor, should be commenced immediately if within 48 hours of start of symptoms of suspected influenza infection.

Oseltamivir can also be given as post-exposure prophylaxis for patients in close contact with someone suffering from an influenza illness.

Anti-inflammatory therapy

As the excessive airway inflammatory response in CF plays a major role in the pathogenesis of CF lung disease, anti-inflammatory therapies have been explored as part of the treatment strategies for CF lung disease. However, the most effective anti-inflammatory agent for CF lung disease is an oral macrolide, as outlined in the previous section.

NSAIDs

There are a small number of North American CF Centres that advocate use of NSAIDS as chronic anti-inflammatory therapy for CF lung disease.

Ibuprofen has a narrow therapeutic window, and is associated with potential side effects, in particular gastro-intestinal bleeding and renal problems.

Measurement of serum levels is necessary, but this testing is not widely available.

However, outside of a minority of North America CF Centres there is little enthusiasm for use of NSAIDS in CF lung disease.

Inhaled corticosteroids

Although widely prescribed, the role of inhaled steroids in the management of CF lung disease is unresolved.

Inhaled steroids can help the bronchial hyper-reactivity that accompanies CF.

Some small studies have suggested clinical benefits form inhaled steroids in CF lung disease, however, a recent multi-centre UK study showed no adverse effects from withdrawal of inhaled corticosteroids in adults with CF.

Oral corticosteroids

There is some evidence that oral corticosteroids may slow the rate of progression of CF lung disease. However, for the majority of patients the possible side effects of treatment, such as reduction in bone mineral density, abnormal glucose control, and cataract formation, will usually outweigh the potential benefits.

Other drug treatments

Inhaled bronchodilators

Inhaled and nebulised bronchodilators can give symptomatic relief, and improve airway clearance.

Theophylline

Oral theophyllines can improve sputum clearance through bronchodilation and effects on sputum viscosity.

Recombinant human deoxyribonuclease (DNase) (dornase alpha)

Nebulised recombinant human deoxyribonuclease reduces the viscoelasticity of CF sputum by degradation of extra-cellular DNA within CF mucus.

It can improve lung function and reduce exacerbations.

There is good evidence for benefit in patients with moderate and severe lung disease and some evidence of benefit in mild asymptomatic patients.

Hypertonic saline

There is evidence of reduced respiratory exacerbations, improvement in pulmonary function and increased muco-ciliary clearance with use of 7% hypertonic saline in patients with CF.

Side effects are cough and bronchospasm.

Patients should be pre-treated with a bronchodilator and an initial test dose should be administered under close supervision by an experienced physiotherapist.

N-acetylcysteine

There is no evidence that use of oral or nebulsied N-acetylcysteine is beneficial in patients with CF.

Sodium chromoglycate

There is no evidence that use of inhaled sodium chromo-glycate is beneficial in patients with CF.

Other therapies

Exercise

Regular cardiovascular exercise improves lung function, exercise capacity and well-being and should be actively encouraged as part of the regular therapy for adults with CF.

Exercise programmes should be tailored to the individual patient to take into account patient preference, severity of lung disease, associated comorbidities (such as low bone mineral density and diabetes mellitus), and general level of fitness.

Use of supplemental oxygen may be necessary to maintain exercise capacity.

Airway clearance

Each patient should be taught airway clearance techniques as part of their self-care package by a physiotherapist experienced in CF care.

Various techniques are available, including active cycle of breathing technique, autogenic drainage, high frequency chest wall compression, high frequency oscillation, oscillatory positive expiratory pressure, positive expiratory pressure, postural drainage and percussion. Studies have not demonstrated any technique to be superior to another.

The airway clearance technique regimens used by a patient should be tailored to the individual patient with advice from an experienced physiotherapist.

Non-invasive ventilatory support
Non-invasive ventilatory support was traditionally used in CF lung disease as a bridge for hypercapnic patients to lung transplantation.

However, it can improve symptoms, exercise capacity and respiratory function and should be considered at a much earlier stage for all patients with daytime hypercapnia.

Supplemental oxygen
The oxygen requirements of patients with CF should be assessed on a regular basis.

For many patients with CF, supplemental oxygen will be required to relieve breathlessness and keep the patient ambulatory.

Smoking cessation
Smoking history should be explored for all patients.

Smokers should be counselled and smoking cessation treatment implemented accordingly.

Lung transplantation
Bilateral lung transplantation can further improve the survival and quality of life for patients with end-stage CF lung disease.

Indications for referral include FEV_1 below 30% predicted, a rapid decline in FEV_1, increased need for oxygen therapy and/or non-invasive ventilation, pulmonary hypertension, poor quality of life and increasingly frequent exacerbations despite optimal medical treatment.

A chronic shortage of donor organs means that there is usually a considerable waiting time for patients with CF between listing and receiving a lung transplant, and 30–40% of patients still die whilst awaiting transplantation.

Respiratory complications
Antibiotic allergy
Antibiotic allergies are more common in adults with CF. Antibiotic desensitisation should be considered under hospital supervision when allergies limit treatment options.

Allergic bronchopulmonary aspergillosis (ABPA)
Patients with CF are at increased risk for development of ABPA.

The underlying clinical features of CF lung disease often makes ABPA difficult to diagnose in this group of patients.

Features suggesting ABPA include asthma-like symptoms, new CXR changes, raised eosinophil count, raised total and aspergillus specific IgE, positive aspergillus precipitins, or positive skin test to aspergillus.

Treatment options include oral corticosteriods and/or an anti-fungal agent with activity against *Aspergilllus* species, of which the most commonly used is itraconazole. Itraconazole levels should be measured and liver function tests checked.

Cystic fibrosis related diabetes mellitus (CFRD)
Poor glycaemic control affects sputum viscosity and exacerbates CF lung disease.

There can be an accelerated decline in lung function even for the year or so prior to the advent of clinical CFRD.

An unexplained decline in lung function should trigger close testing for dysregulation of glucose control.

Flying and holidays
Patients deemed to be at respiratory risk from the lower partial pressure of inspired oxygen in flight, should be advised to use supplemental oxygen during the flight.

An in-flight oxygen assessment test using FiO_2 15% should be arranged for patients with moderate or severe lung disease who are planning an aircraft flight.

The inflight risk should be assessed by a clinician experienced in CF taking into consideration the result of the 15% normobaric oxygen challenge together with the patient's FEV_1 and recent clinical status.

Patients should be given course of emergency oral antibiotics to start immediately if they develop an infective exacerbation whilst on holiday and instructions to seek medical attention. They should be provided with a letter detailing their current medial condition and medication, and a treatment protocol if they present to a medical centre with little experience of CF care.

Gastro-intestinal reflux
The contribution of gastro-intestinal reflux should be considered in patients whose respiratory symptoms are not responding to conventional treatment for CF lung disease.

Haemoptysis
Chronic haemoptysis can be a frequent complication in adult patients with CF, often in association with infective exacerbations.

Investigations should include a coagulation screen and a platelet count.

Vitamin K supplementation (phytomenadione 10mg OD) should be given to patients with chronic haemoptysis.

Tranexamic acid (500–1000mgs QDS) can be helpful in limiting haemoptysis.

Consideration should be given to discontinuing DNase until the haemoptysis abates.

A large haemoptysis (>300ml fresh blood) is a medical emergency (see Chapter 11.2).

Intravenous access/totally implantable IV access devices
Totally implantable IV access devices can be a useful aid for patients with difficult venous access or those requiring frequent courses of IV antibiotics.

The use of these devices requires expert care to prevent complications such as infection that invariable necessitates removal of the line, or occlusion. Other complications include line displacement, leakage and venous occlusion.

Nutrition
The nutritional status of a patient with CF influences their lung function and susceptibility to infective exacerbations.

For patients with undernutrition, enteral feeding can improve and stabilise lung function and reduce exacerbations.

Treatment adherence
The CF MDT should monitor adherence with treatment regimens and provide encouragement to the individual patients with their treatment.

The CF MDT should continuously assess the patients' care package, trying to minimise the treatment burden whilst controlling symptoms and preventing disease progression.

Varicella-zoster pneumonia

In cases of chickenpox, patients with CF are at risk of developing varicella pneumonia.

Treatment with acyclovir should be commenced immediately.

Support group

Cystic Fibrosis Trust, 11 London Road, Bromley, Kent BR1 1BY. Tel 020 8464 7211, Fax 020 8313 0472, e-mail enquiries@cftrust.co.uk, website **www.cftrust.co.uk**

Further reading

Antibiotic treatment for cystic fibrosis. Cystic Fibrosis Trust, 2002.

Methicillin-resistant *Staphylococcus arteus* (MRSA). Cystic Fibrosis Trust, 2008.

Clinic guidelines for the physiotherapy management of cystic fibrosis. Cystic Fibrosis Trust, 2002.

Pseudomonas aeruginosa infection in people with cystic fibrosis: suggestions for prevention and infection control. Cystic Fibrosis Trust, 2004.

Standards of clinical care of children and adults with cystic fibrosis in the UK. Cystic Fibrosis Trust, 2001.

The *Burkholderia cepacia* complex: suggestions for prevention and infection control. Cystic Fibrosis Trust, 2004.

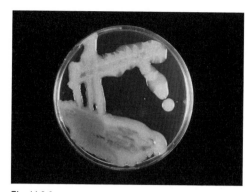

Fig. 11.3.2 Mucoid *Pseudomonas aeruginosa*.

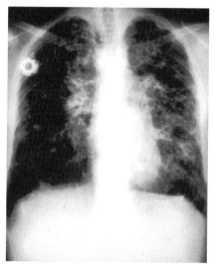

Fig. 11.3.1 Typical CXR features of advanced CF lung disease and the presence of a totally implantable IV access device.

11.4 Cystic fibrosis genetics

CF is the most common life-limiting autosomal recessive (AR) disorder in the white population. Three clinical phenotypes are associated with mutations in the CF transmembrane conductance regulator gene (CFTR) on 7q31–32.

1 Classical CF. Obstructive lung disease, bronchiectasis, exocrine pancreatic insufficiency, elevation of sweat chloride concentration (>60mM), and infertility in males due to congenital bilateral absence of the vas deferens (CBAVD).

2 Non-classical CF. Chronic pulmonary disease 9 pancreatic exocrine disease ± elevated sweat chloride (>60 mM) ± CBAVD.

3 CBAVD.

The incidence of CF in Caucasians of European extraction is 1/2000–1/4000 newborns (1/2500 in the UK). CF is rare in native Africans and Asians. The mutation spectrum and frequency are highly dependent on ethnic background. See Table 11.4.1 for the diagnostic criteria for CF.

More than 1000 mutations in CFTR have been identified (see Table 11.4.2), of which the most common by far is delta F508 (ΔF508). ΔF508 encodes a three-nucleotide deletion resulting in a CFTR protein lacking phenylalanine (F) at postion 508 in the protein. This causes misfolding of the newly synthesised mutant CFTR so that it does not integrate into the cell membrane, but remains in the cytoplasm where it is degraded by the ubiquitin–proteosome pathway. ΔF508 accounts for ~70% of CF alleles, but the exact proportion varies depending on ethnic origin. The next most common mutations are G542X, G551D, delta1507, W1282X, and N1303K, each accounting for only 1–2.5% of known CF alleles. W1282X is common in the Ashkenazi Jewish population. Standard commercial kits for DNA diagnosis usually identify ~29 mutations. In the English population this accounts for ~87% of CF alleles. Thus, using a standard screen, 76% of English patients with CF will have two identifiable CFTR mutations, 22% will have a single identifiable CF mutation, and 2% of patients with CF will have no identifiable mutation. Specialist labs may offer rare mutation screens.

Polythymidine (Poly-T) tracts in intron 8 affect the splicing efficiency of a CFTR allele. The most efficient polymorphism is 9T, 7T has reduced efficiency, and 5T has significantly reduced efficiency. R117H in cis with 5T, with ΔF508 as the other allele, usually results in non-classical CF (pancreatic sufficient), whereas R117H in cis with 9T with

ΔF508 as the other allele typically causes the much milder phenotype of CBAVD without respiratory symptoms. Criteria for the diagnosis of CF (after Rosenstein and Cutting 1998)

Diagnosis requires at least one criterion from each group

Group 1

• One or more characteristic phenotypic features (see below), e.g. chronic sinopulmonary disease, gastrointestinal and nutritional.

• Abnormalities, salt loss syndromes, and male urogenital abnormalities, e.g. CBAVD.

• Sibling with CF.

• Positive neonatal IRT (immunoreactive trypsinogen test).

Group 2

• Sweat chloride >60mM on 2 occasions (≥75mg of sweat is critical to reliability). Some laboratories assay sweat osmolality which is increased in CF (normal range is 62–196mOsm/kg)

• Identification of 2 CF mutations

• Abnormal nasal potential difference (measure of CFTR-mediated ion transport)

Phenotypic features consistent with diagnosis of CF (after Rosenstein and Zeitlin 1998)

• Chronic sinopulmonary disease. Persistent colonisation with typical CF pathogen (*Staphylococcus aureus, Haemophilus influenzae, Pseudomonas aeruginosa, Burkholderia cepacia*), chronic cough and sputum production, persistent CXR abnormalities (bronchiectasis, atelectasis, infiltrates, hyperinflation), airway obstruction (wheezing and air trapping), nasal polyps, X-ray or CT abnormalities of paranasal sinuses, clubbing

• Gastrointestinal and nutritional abnormalities. Meconium ileus (10–20%), rectal prolapse (20%), distal intestinal obstruction, pancreatic insufficiency, recurrent pancreatitis, focal biliary cirrhosis or multilobular cirrhosis, failure to thrive (protein–calorie malnutrition), hypoproteinaemia and oedema, complications secondary to lack of fat-soluble vitamins

• Salt loss syndromes. Acute salt depletion, chronic metabolic acidosis

• Male urogenital abnormalities resulting in obstructive azoospermia. CBAVD.

Table 11.4.1 Functional classification of CFTR alleles (after McKone *et al.* 2003)

Class	Functional effect of mutation	Allele
I	Defective protein production	G542X, R553X, W1282X, R11162X, 621–1G → T, 1717–1G → A, 1078ΔT, 3659ΔC
II	Defective protein processing	ΔF508, Δ1507, N1303K, S549N
III	Defective protein regulation	G551D, R560T
IV*	Defective protein conductance	R117H, R334W, G85E, R347P
V*	Reduced amounts of functioning CFTR protein	3849 +10 kbC → T,2789+5G → A, A455E
Unknown		711+1G → T, 2184DA, 1898+1G → A

*Compared with class II (including ΔF508 homozygotes). classes IV and V have a significantly lower mortality rate and milder clinical phenotype.

See http://www.genet.sickkids.on.ca/cftr for the Cystic Fibrosis Analysis Consortium CF mutation database.

Clinical approach

History: key points
- Three-generation family tree.
- Genotype of affected individual if known.

Examination: key points
Usually not relevant if affected individual is under the care of CF paediatrician/physician or you are seeing another family member.

Investigation
DNA sample for mutation analysis of CFTR.

Genetic advice

Inheritance and recurrence risk
- Autosomal recessive (AR) and so the recurrence risk to parents of an affected child=1/4. The following recurrence risks are based on pedigree analysis and assuming no consanguinity, no family history of CF in a partner, and a CF carrier rate of 1/23 (see below for carrier rates in different ethnic groups). This risk estimate can be substantially modified by CF mutation analysis in the relative and his/her partner (see below).
- Risk to offspring of healthy sib of an affected child is $2/3 \times 1/23 \times 1/4 = 1/138$.
- Risk to offspring of aunt/uncle or half-sib of an affected child is $1/2 \times 1/23 \times 1/4 = 1/184$.
- Risk to offspring of an affected individual is $1 \times 1/23 \times 1/2 = 1/46$.

Variability and penetrance
Homozygosity for ΔF508 and compound heterozygosity or homozygosity for other non-functional alleles are associated with the classical form of CF. Even in classical CF the age of onset and rate and progression of pulmonary disease are very variable (influenced by modifier genes, infection, nutrition, therapy, smoking, etc.). ΔF508 homozygotes vary considerably in their manifestation of gastrointestinal, hepatobiliary, and pulmonary disease. Monozygotic CF twins are more concordant than dizygotic CF twins. The CF phenotype may be modified by loci in the partially imprinted region on 7q 3' of CFTR that determine stature, food intake, and energy homeostasis. All classical cases of CF (ΔF508 homozygotes) have pancreatic insufficiency but there is considerable variability in pulmonary disease. Decline in lung function in CF is associated with colonisation by *Pseudomonas aeruginosa* and *Burkholderia cepacia*.

A partially functional allele in combination with a non-functional allele (e.g. ΔF508) is a typical picture in non-classical CF. However, since the standard screening panel comprises mainly non-functional alleles, many patients with non-classical CF will have only one identifiable CF allele, i.e. those patients in whom clinical diagnosis is most challenging are often those most difficult to diagnose genetically.

In comparison with ΔF508 homozygotes, ΔF508/R117H, ΔF508/A455E, ΔF508/3849+10kb C → T and ΔF508/2789+5G → A are associated with mild clinical manifestations.

Prenatal diagnosis
Possible by chorionic villus sampling (CVS) at 11 weeks gestation if both mutations are known. If a single or neither mutation is known, diagnosis of CF is secure, and paternity is certain, it is possible to offer linkage studies to capture unidentified allele(s) and enable prenatal diagnosis. Pre-implantation genetic diagnosis (PGD) for ΔF508 homozygotes is available in some centres.

Predictive testing
This may be applicable in younger siblings of a child recently diagnosed with CF, in view of the benefits of treatment with prophylactic antibiotics and pancreatic and vitamin supplements.

Other family members
When an individual is diagnosed with CF, and mutation analysis is performed, it is routine practice to offer carrier testing to both parents. Cascade screening of the extended family for the mutation identified in their relative can then be offered. Where an individual is shown to be a CF carrier, population-based screening (see Table 11.4.2) can be offered to his/her partner to determine the risk to their offspring. Carrier testing of children is usually deferred until 16 years when they are of an age to be involved in decision-making and old enough to understand the implications of the result.

Table 11.4.2 Carrier rates and mutation detection rates in different ethnic populations

Population	Carrier frequency	Mutation detection rate with panel appropriate to ethnic group (%)
Ashkenazi Jewish	1 in 23	97
Northern European	1 in 23	90
Hispanic	1 in 46	57
African-American	1 in 65	75
Asian	1 in 90	30

Natural history and management

Potential long-term complications
- Respiratory failure. Pulmonary disease is the main cause of morbidity and mortality in patients with CF. Heart–lung transplantation may be considered for end-stage disease.
- Diabetes. 25–50% have an abnormal glucose tolerance test (GTT) by their 20s and 5% require insulin.
- Liver disease. 5% of adults have cirrhosis and portal hypertension.
- Male infertility. 97% of males with CF have CBAVD with obstructive azoospermia. Pregnancy may be possible with assisted reproductive technology in which case offer mutation analysis to partner.

Surveillance
Evidence is emerging that management of CF in paediatric and adult CF centres results in a better clinical outcome. In the US median survival has reached 31.1 years for men and 28.3 years for women. Survival to the 30s and 40s is no longer rare. Median survival for patients with pancreatic sufficiency (non-classical CF) is 56 years.

Pregnancy in women with CF
Fertility in women with CF is impaired, but successful pregnancy is possible. In a retrospective study from France, of 75 pregnancies, 64 were liveborn (18% premature and 30% low-birthweight), there were 5 miscarriages, 5 therapeutic abortions, and one maternal death. Three women died in the year following a pregnancy, all of whom had a FEV_1

<50% before pregnancy. A retrospective audit of 33 successful pregnancies from Scandinavia found that preterm delivery occurred in 24%. The lung function of women delivering preterm was significantly lower than that of those delivering at term, and they were most likely to have other CF complications including diabetes, asthma, or liver disease. Lung function did not deteriorate during pregnancy, but the need for IV antibiotics was doubled. Women with mild to moderate disease may safely go through pregnancy.

- Offer mutation analysis to partner (offer CVS if partner is a CF carrier).
- Refer to CF physician for assessment of likely impact of pregnancy on respiratory reserve.
- Increased risk of gestational diabetes due to pancreatic insufficiency in women with classical CF.
- Consider the drug regimen of your patient and whether any of the drugs have teratogenic potential.
- Pregnancy should be jointly managed by an obstetrician with special expertise in maternal and fetal medicine and a CF specialist.

Neonatal screening

Most neonatal screening programmes for CF combine assay of immunoreactive trypsinogen (IRT) on a dried blood spot (Guthrie card), with analysis for common CF mutations, e.g. ΔF508. An IRT of 60–70mcg/l is equivocal and >70mcg/l is positive. This approach has been well studied but misses some children with CF and detects more ΔF508 carriers than expected. The excess of ΔF508 heterozygotes is associated with the presence of a second mutation or the 5T allele in some infants. In one study of 57 subjects with positive IRT who were ΔF508 heterozygotes, three had clinical CF at 1 year.

Support group

Cystic Fibrosis Trust <www.cftrust.org.uk>.

Expert advisers

David A. Lomas, Professor, Respiratory Medicine Unit, Department of Medicine, University of Cambridge, Cambridge and Di Bilton, Consultant Respiratory Physician and Director of the Adult CF Unit, Papworth Hospital, Cambridge, England.

Further reading

Dankert-Roelse JE, te Meerman GJ. Screening for cystic fibrosis — time to change our position? [editorial]. *New Engl J Med* 1997; **337**: 997–998.

Durie PR. Pancreatitis and mutations of the cystic fibrosis gene [editorial]. *New Engl J Med* 1998; **339**: 687–8.

Gillet D, de Braekeleer M, Bellis G, et al. Cystic fibrosis and pregnancy. Report from French data (1980–1999). *Br J Obstet Gynaecol* 2002; **109**: 912–918.

Mahadeva R, Webb K, Westerbeek RC, et al. Clinical outcome in relation to care in centres specialising in cystic fibrosis: cross sectional study. *Br Med J* 1998; **316**: 1771–1777.

Massie RJ, Wilcken B, van Asperen P, et al. Pancreatic function and extended mutation analysis in DeltaF508 heterozygous infants with an elevated immunoreactive trypsinogen but normal sweat electrolyte levels. *J Pediatr* 2000; **137**: 214–220.

McKone EF, Emerson SE, Edwards KL, et al. Effect of genotype on phenotype and mortality in cystic fibrosis: a retrospective cohort study. *Lancet* 2003; **361**: 1671–1676.

Mekus F, Laabs U, Veeze H, et al. Genes in the vicinity of CFTR modulate the cystic fibrosis phenotype in highly concordant or discordant F508del homozygous sib pairs. *Hum Genet* 2003; **112**: 1–11.

Neill AM, Nelson-Piercy C. Hazards of assisted conception in women with severe medical disease. *Hum Fertil* 2001; **4**: 239–245.

Ødegaard I, Stray-Pedersen B, Halberg K, et al. Maternal and fetal morbidity in pregnancies of Norwegian and Swedish women with cystic fibrosis. *Acta Obstet Gynecol Scand* 2002; **81**: 689–705.

Rosenstein BJ, Cutting GR. The diagnosis of cystic fibrosis: a consensus statement. *J Pediatr* 1998; **132**: 589–595.

Rosenstein BJ, Zeitlin PL. Cystic fibrosis. *Lancet* 1998; **351**: 277–282.

11.5 Extra-pulmonary manifestations of cystic fibrosis

Introduction
Impairment of the structure of the CFTR is the hallmark of CF. This protein is present in the cell membrane of many organs in addition to the lung; the nose, pancreas, liver, gastro-intestinal track and the reproductive system. This results in CF being a truly multisystem, multi-organ disorder.

The pancreas
Impaired secretory function of the pancreas
Over 85% of all CF people suffer from pancreatic insufficiency (PI). There is a strong correlation between the degree of PI and the genetic profile. Patients carrying class III and IV mutations and who have a relatively preserved CFTR function tend to be pancreatic semi-sufficient or sufficient. In contrast, over 99% of patients who are homozygotes for the Delta F508 mutation have pancreatic insufficiency.

Thickened pancreatic secretions block the pancreatic duct. This is followed by a series of processes starting with duct injury and obstruction and ending with auto-digestion, which start in utero.

Another important function of the CFTR is to mediate the secretion of bicarbonate in the pancreatic duct epithelium. This is an essential component which eases the secretion and solubility of the digestive pancreatic enzymes. The exocrine function particularly of lipase but also of bile reaching the intestine are adversely affected in an acid environment. The failure of sufficient quantities of lipolytic and proteolytic enzymes reaching the intestinal tract leads to steatorhoea and malabsorption.

Clinical manifestations
Symptoms start when lipase and protease levels fall below 5%. The main features in infancy and childhood are combination of hunger and malabsorption. Steatorhoea, with greasy and offensive stool is an early symptom, followed by diarrhoea, abdominal pain and failure to thrive.

Laboratory features reflect malabsorption of fat, proteins and vitamins and include hypoalbuminaemia, anaemia and reduced plasma levels of fat-soluble vitamins.

Diagnosis
Prior to the era of sweat testing, the clinical features outlined earlier made paediatricians suspect CF. In undiagnosed cases, the easiest investigation is measurement of elastase-1 in the stool. Another more cumbersome method is the measurement of fat globules in the stool over a 72-hour collection.

> **AUTHOR'S TIP**
> Even in asymptomatic CF patients, malabsorption may be present. The easiest and most reliable test is the measurement of elastase-1 in a small stool sample.

Treatment
Porcine lipase and protease have revolutionised the management of PI in CF patients. These are now available in different strengths as microspheres in several commercially available preparations.

Pancreatic enzyme supplementations are manufactured in enteric coated preparations. The outer layer is dissolved at a high PH releasing the enzymes.

It is recommended that patients take their enzymes prior to food for ease of compliance. The recommended dose is 500 units of lipase per kg of body weight, but can vary between patients. Younger children are given these preparations as microspheres with a fruit puree or a taste-masking material. The maximum recommended daily dose is 2500 units of lipase per kg per meal or a total of 10,000 units daily.

Adverse effects of pancreatic supplementation include oral and peri-anal irritation. It has been suggested that high doses of lipase might be associated with fibrosing colonopathy.

If symptoms persist despite high doses of enzymes, input from an experienced CF dietitian is needed.

> **AUTHOR'S TIP**
> Common causes of reduced efficacy of pancreatic supplementation include:
> - lack of adherence to treatment;
> - neutralisation of activities by increased acidity in the proximal intestinal tract – try H2-histamine receptor antagonists or proton pump inhibitor;
> - lack of efficacy of that brand for individual – try alternate brand.

Cystic fibrosis-related diabetes mellitus (CFRD)
The role of CFRD in the natural history of CF has increasingly as patients survive longer and hence its prevalence and adverse effects become manifest. The prevalence of CFRD has been estimated to be 5% in all CF patients but ranges between 15–22% in patients over the age of 16.

The impact of pre-diabetic state and diabetes in CF patients:
- accelerated decline in lung function;
- increase rate of pulmonary exacerbations (Fig. 11.5.1);
- premature mortality.

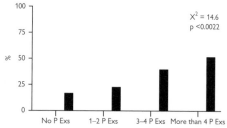

Fig. 11.5.1 Prevalence of CFRD in 499 CF patients in the Southwest region of England according to the frequency of annual pulmonary exacerbations (P Exs).

Pathogenesis of CFRD
Almost all patients with CFRD are pancreatic insufficient. CFRD is probably caused by the insidious physical destruction of Beta cells, leading to decreased insulin levels.

The first biochemical manifestation is delayed secretion of insulin. Post-prandial delay in insulin secretion accounts for impaired oral glucose tolerance test (OGTT) which is one of the main methods of diagnosis of CFRD.

The manifestations of the pre-diabetic state are those of increased numbers of pulmonary exacerbations, accelerated decline in lung function and more pronounced weight loss. Polydipsia and polyurea are occasionally but not often present.

Diagnosis and classifications

There are three methods of diagnosing CFRD:

1. Raised fasting plasma glucose,
2. OGTT results consistent with diabetes as in Table 11.5.1.
3. Raised plasma glucose during continuous glucose monitoring.

CFRD is divided into three categories which might present as different stages:

Category 1: impaired OGTT but normal plasma fasting and random glucose (biochemical diabetes)

Category 2: raised random plasma glucose within the diabetes range but normal fasting glucose

Category 3: raised random and fasting plasma glucose.

Table 11.5.1 The World Health Organization protocol

The UK CF Trust Diabetes Working Group recommends that the WHO classification of diagnosis of diabetes is adapted for CFRD. OGTT must be performed at least 30 days away from acute chest infection.

120 minutes venous blood sample		
Plasma venous sample	< 7.8 mmol/l	Normal
Plasma venous sample	7.9–11.0 mmol/l	Impaired
Plasma venous sample	≥ 11.1 mmol/l	Diabetic

Despite many similarities with type I DM, acute and chronic complications are encountered less frequently and are less severe

Diabetic ketoacidosis has been described but rare. Background diabetic retinopathy is seen in approximately 15% after 5 years and 10% after 10 years of diagnosis of diabetes. More complex proliferative retinopathy with its sight threatening complications is rare.

Microvascular nephropathy has been described, but it is too mild to cause renal failure. Central nervous and cardiac ischaemic events are rare due to a combination of factors including: reduced longevity of patients, absent of other co-morbidity such as hypercholesterolemia and heavy cigarette smoking being unusual.

Screening for diabetes in CF patients

Annual OGGT is recommended as a screening method for CFRD after the age of 12 years. OGTT can be repeated in 12 months if normal or impaired. If the patient has increased symptoms of decline in lung function and weight loss OGTT can be repeated sooner.

Management

A low/reduced calorie diet is not appropriate in CFRD. Adequate nutrition is essential for all CF patients. Patients should not be discouraged from eating high calorie food, but they should not rely on them as the sole source of calories. Rather, patients should be encouraged to adapt a balanced diet. Education is needed to emphasise the difference between usual diabetes and CFRD. Close monitoring of body mass index is important in the management of CFRD.

Insulin replacement is the mainstay of treatment of CFRD. Short acting and long acting preparations are available. Most patients are provided with a combination of both at variable doses according to their eating habits and the results of their glucose monitoring. For patients who require overnight feeding, additional short acting preparations should be prescribed prior to starting the feed.

Oral hypoglycaemic agents are not currently recommended unless patients have a suspected type II features (obesity) or are unable or unwilling to take insulin.

All patients with CFRD should have at least one annual measurement of glycosylated haemoglobin (HB A1C) with the aim of keeping this under 7%.

CFRD is not acontra-indication for either liver or lung transplant. Diabetic CF patients do not have worse transplant outcome, but they are prone to have impaired diabetic control due to surgery and the use of corticosteroids in the early post transplant phase.

Abdominal pain: the gut in CF

Abdominal pain is common in CF patients. In the author's unit 72% of CF patients declared that they had abdominal pain at their an annual assessment questionnaire. Reasons for abdominal pain are illustrated in Table 11.5.2.

Table 11.5.2 Causes of abdominal pain in CF

- Malabsorption due to under-use of pancreatic supplements
- Constipation (Fig. 11.5.2)
- Distal intestinal obstructive syndrome (DIOS)
- Peptic ulceration
- Gall stones and cholecystitis
- Gastro-oesophageal reflux disease (GORD)
- Pancreatitis

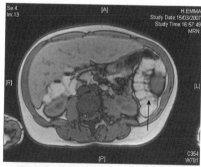

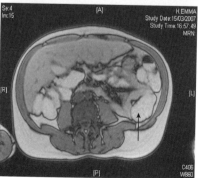

Fig. 11.5.2 MRI of the abdomen showing bowel faecal impaction (white arrows) in a 32 female CF patient with chronic refractory constipation. This patient takes 6 sachets of bulk laxative daily as well as a daily phosphate enema.

Meconium ileus (MI) in infants

The composition of meconium in CF infants differs from that in normal infants. Pancreatic insufficiency plays an important part in the process of formation of MI. It is thought that the mechanisms of MI are: increased level of lactose and other undigested components coupled with dehydrated meconium.

The uncomplicated MI is manifested in the first few days of life with bowel obstruction causing a triad of: constipation, vomiting and distended abdomen with filling in the right lower quadrant of the abdomen. In less than half of cases, complicated MI occurs with features of features of volvulus and bowel perforation with intra-peritoneal infection.

Management of the uncomplicated form is to try to reverse the process by repeated gastrographin enemas. The success rate varies and complications including bowel perforation have been reported.

Management of complicated MI is surgical. This includes resection of the abnormal area and peritoneal toilet. Intestinal anastomosis or temporary stoma may be formed according to the status of the intestinal tract detected intra-operatively.

Distal intestinal obstructive syndrome (DIOS)

The prevalence of DIOS in adult CF patients has been estimated to be 15%. The mechanisms are different from MI. It has been postulated that DIOS occur due to

- sub-optimal management of pancreatic insufficiency;
- dehydrated intestinal content; and
- impaired intestinal motility.

Features of DIOS vary between simple constipation to symptoms of intestinal obstruction including nausea and vomiting. A painful poorly defined mass is often palpable in the right lower quadrant of the abdomen. Normally there are no signs to suggest local or systemic inflammation. If these are present appendicitis or extra-uterine pregnancy in women should be suspected.

Diagnosis is mainly done on clinical grounds. Plain abdominal film may reveal signs of distal intestinal obstruction including dilatation of intestinal loops (Fig. 11.5.3). Abdominal ultrasound, CT scan and MRI may be used to distinguish DIOS from appendicitis.

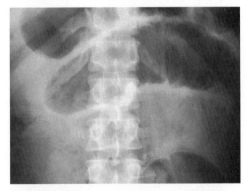

Fig. 11.5.3 Dilatation of the proximal bowel in a 32-year-old patient with repeated episodes of DIOS.

The management of DIOS is now mainly medical. Oral and intravenous fluids for re-hydration are both part of the treatment and prevention. Other measures include:

- Simple laxatives such as lactulose, sodium docusate and Kleen Prep.
- N acetylcysteine (NAC) used in our unit as orange-flavoured sachets (200mg twice daily). NAC is thought to reduce the stool viscosity by breaking the mucoprotein content.
- Gatsrografin is given during acute stages. Gastrografin is a mucosal irritant and an osmotic laxative. The dose is 100ml diluted in 400ml of water daily for three to four days. This could be given orally or through a naso-gastric tube. The same dose could be given as an enema.
- Anti emetics and gastrointestinal lavage can be used in more refractory cases.

Cystic fibrosis liver disease (CFLD)

The bile is more viscous in CF patients than in non CF individuals as with other mucous secretions. Bile plugging at the level of small and medium sized bile ducts results in areas of micro-cirrhosis. This is seen at post-mortem and tends to be asymptomatic.

CFLD is a well recognised feature of cystic fibrosis. Severe decompensated liver disease happens in childhood and adolescent stages. Paradoxically despite the increase in age for CF patients the incidence of liver disease is decreasing.

The incidence of biochemical abnormality and impaired liver architecture is approximately 50%. Liver decompensation,on the other hand, occurs only in less than 5%. There are three stages of CFLD:

1 biochemical: manifested by impaired liver enzymes;
2 structural: in which the images shows fatty infiltration, irregular liver architecture including rough liver edges; and
3 de-compensated liver failure which manifests with portal hypertension, hypoalbuminaemia, ascites and impaired coagulation.

Investigations

All CF patients should undergo measurement of liver function tests at least once a year during their annual assessment. For those with impaired liver function tests, liver ultrasound by experienced radiologist should be done. MRI has an increasing role in identifying the anatomy and complications of liver disease including portal hypertension (Fig. 11.5.4). When clinical or radiological manifestations of complicated liver disease are seen, non-invasive measurement of portal vein pressure and an edonscopy to elucidate and manage oesophageal varices should be implemented.

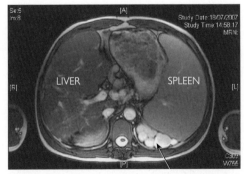

Fig. 11.5.4 An MRI scan of a 22-year-old CF patient with macro nodular liver cirrhosis, splenomegaly and variceal changes in branches of the portal vein (white arrow).

Management

Ursodeoxycholic acid (URSO) is the only medical treatment available. This is a hydrophilic bile salt which is though to increase the 'pourability' of bile salt. It has also been reported that URSO might be protective of both epithelial cells of the bile ducts and of the hepaticocytes.

The benefits of URSO have not been established by randomised controlled trial, but it has been suggested by clinical observation and in one open label study to improve liver biochemistry. It is unlikely that URSO would reverse liver damage.

Liver transplantation (figure 11.5.5) in advanced non-reversible liver disease is advocated in any or a combination of the following circumstances: 1.Portal hypertension with oesophageal varices. 2. Ascitis 3. Biochemical abnormalities of severe hepatic decompensation such as hypo-albuminaemia and impaired clotting factors and 4. Hepatic encepahalopathy.

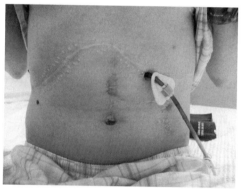

Fig. 11.5.5 A 22-year-old patient who underwent a liver transplant. The patient has percutaneous enterogastric (PEG) feeding with a tube in situ.

Survival rate for liver transplantation is favourable with one year survival reaching 82% and 10 year survival of over 60%. The status of the lungs and microbiology are carefully assessed for liver transplant recipients. Contraindications of liver transplant include:

- Severe ventilatory failure with impaired gas exchange,
- Pulmonary infection with the epidemic strains genomovar III of *Burkhuldria cepacia* (also known as Cenocepacia,) and
- Psychosocial status deemed to influence adherence to life-long administration of cytotoxic agents used to prevent graft rejection and of follow-up in specialist clinic.

Paradoxically the lungs often improve after liver transplant. Possible reasons for this are:

1 reduced intra-pulmonary shunt;
2 probable anti-inflammatory properties of the cytotoxic agents; and
3 improved nutritional status and increased body mass index which tends to occur following liver transplantation.

Reduced bone mineral density BMD (osteomalacia and osteoporosis):

Reduced BMD is now a recognised, preventable and treatable CF complication. Possible reasons are outlined in Table 11.5.3:

Table 11.5.3 Risk factors for reduced BMD in CF patients

- Malabsorption of vitamin D and vitamin K
- Persistent uncontrolled pulmonary infection
- Administration of glucocorticoids
- Reduced body mass index
- Reduced mobility
- Reduced level of sex hormone

Osteoporosis is defined as decreased bone mass which includes loss of bone collagen and bone calcium in a similar proportion. In osteomalacia, the content of calcium in the bones is reduced with a relative preservation of bone collagen. Therefore there is a reduction of the ratio of mineralised/and non-mineralised bone.

Diagnosis is by bone density is measured using dual energy x-ray absorbiometry (DEXA). The frequency of the test should be probably every two years. The significance of the findings are outlined in Table 11.5.4.

Prevention and management

The main aim of management is to treat bone pain and to reduce stress fractures. As reduced BMD is now well recognised early diagnosis and preventive strategies are employed to minimise progressive bone loss.

Prevention and management of reduced BMD is multifaceted. The three main areas are:

1 optimising nutritional intake including vitamin D and calcium;
2 encouraging physical activities; and
3 management of pulmonary exacerbations.

Randomised controlled trials have confirmed that a combination of oral vitamin D, oral calcium and bisphosphonate are effective in the management of reduced bone mineral density. These studies included organ transplant recipients. The effects are similar are for either intravenous pamidronate or oral alendronate.

For patients who are likely to remain on glucocorticoids for a lengthy duration, for example those with allergic broncho-pulmonary aspergillosis, bisphosphonate should start with or shortly after the introduction of glucocorticoids.

Table 11.5.4 outlines the indications for administration of bisphosphonate in CF patients with reduce BMD.

Table 11.5.4 Indications of bisphosphonate treatment

- Reduced Z score on DEXA scan below −2.0 despite optimal treatment
- Reduced Z score below −1.5 in organ transplant candidates or recipients
- Patients likely to have a lengthy course of glucocorticoids
- Patients sustained stress fractures
- Patients with failure to increase weight, body mass index less than 17 and a Z score of less than −1.5

Bisphosphonate is usually a life-long treatment. Musculoskeletal pain is a recognised occasionally associated with the use of bisphosphonate. The mechanism is not established. However, treatment with a short course of prednisolone prior to IV pamidronate suggests an inflammatory mechanism for the pain.

The upper airways in CF patients

It is reasonable to regard the respiratory tract as a passage starts at the nostrils and ends at the alveoli. This fact is true in CF where impaired CFTR in the upper airway is manifested with life long incurable diseases.

Sinusitis and nasal polyps

In the author's unit, over 75% of patients admitted to chronic nasal symptoms and 62% are aware of having chronic sinusitis with acute flare up.

Mucosal inflammation results in narrowing and blockage of the nasal outlets of the maxillofacial and frontal sinuses. This leads to under-developed facial sinuses seen in CF patients. Nasal polyps are probably an exaggerated manifestation of inflamed mucosa. They are histologically different from allergic nasal polyps.

Symptoms of rhino-sinusitis start during childhood with the triad of runny nose, nasal congestion, and post-nasal drip.

Acute on chronic sinusitis often precede symptoms of pulmonary exacerbations. Most patients interpret this as a viral disease (cold) followed by respiratory symptoms

> **AUTHOR'S TIP**
>
> A careful history which rules out viral nasal symptoms in the patients surrounding or when nasal symptoms occur outside the cold season suggest that the patient suffers from acute CF sinusitis.

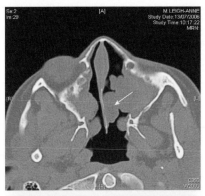

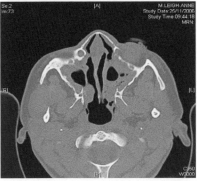

Fig. 11.5.6 MRI of facial sinuses. The right side shows thickened mucosa in both sides with reduced air space in the maxillofacial sinuses. On the left side, there are absent air spaces with obvious bilateral large nasal polyps (white arrow).

Facial X ray should no longer be used to make a diagnosis of sinusitis. Facial CT scan or preferably MRI scan (Fig. 11.5.6) are the investigations of choice. The radiological features are those of thickened mucosa and reduced or absent air spaces.

In chronically infected patients, swabs from sinus secretions often grow *Pseudomonas aeruginosa* and *Haemophillus influenzae* which are implicated in the pathogenesis.

Management

Acute sinusitis responds well to antibiotics provided for pulmonary exacerbations. Oral antibiotics typically with quinolones help with isolated episodes of sinusitis.

Nasal corticosteroids reduce the nasal inflammatory process. Systemic corticosteroids are useful in reducing the size of nasal polyps.

Nasal decongestants are useful symptomatic management during the acute phase, but should be used only for a short period of time to avoid vasomotor disease which is a phenomenon in which the nasal vessels do not constrict after prolong use of decongestant.

Surgical management consists of resection of nasal polyps. Irrigation of the sinuses has also a short symptomatic benefit

The reproductive system and pregnancy

Several surveys showed that CF patients of both genders felt that adequate information about sexual functions and reproduction have not been provided during repeated consultations.

Male CF patients

Almost 97% of male CF patients are infertile due to azoospermia. This is because of bilateral absence of vas deferens and atrophy of the seminal vesicle, ejaculary duct and body and tail of epidydymis. The testicles are normal in architecture and histology and able to produce active sperms. Sexual potency is not affected.

With the increase survival and improved quality of life, male patients are increasingly seeking fertility assistance. Combining sperm harvesting with intra-cytoplasmic sperm injection (ICSI) are the standard methods. The conception rate is variable.

Female CF patients

The fallopian uterine ducts are patent, but the mucous is more viscous and less well hydrated than in normal females. Delayed puberty and abnormal menarche are well recognised in CF female

The reported rate of fertility in female CF patients varies. A conception rate after 2 years of active sexual contact ranged from 20–75%.

We advise that all female CF patients should regard themselves to be fertile and if they do not wish to they should take similar birth control precautions as non CF persons.

> **AUTHOR'S TIP**
>
> Almost all male CF patients are azoospermic. Conversely, all female CF patients should be regarded as fertile and should be given a proper contraception advise if they do not wish to conceive.

CF and pregnancy

Retrospective studies showed no adverse outcome on the mother or the child when FEV_1 was over 50% of predicated values. During a consultation on pregnancy, the discussion should be supportive and sensitively tailored according to the general performance and FEV_1 of the patient.

The following areas need to be discussed.

1 The effect of late stages of pregnancy on lung function especially for those with advanced lung disease.

2 The effect of CF and the CF drugs on pregnancy and the higher rate of miscarriage, extra-uterine pregnancy and pre-term delivery compared to non-CF persons.

3 The higher probability of the child having CF. We advise that the partner seeks counselling and provide blood samples for detection of CF genetic profile.

4 We would seek the views about the patients' ability to care for a toddler.

Further reading

Colombo C, Castellani MR, Balistriri WF et al. Scintigraphic documentation of an improvement in hepatobiliary execretory function after treatment with ursodeoxycholic acid in patients with cystic fibrosis and associated liver disease. *Hepatology* 1992; **15**: 677–777.

Conway SP, Morton AM, Oldroyd B et al. Osteoporosis and osteopenia in adults and adolescents with cystic fibrosis: prevalence and associated factors. *Thorax* 2000; **55**: 798–804.

Edenborough FP, Mackenzie WE, Stableforth DE. The outcome of 72 pregnancies in 55 women with cystic fibrosis in the United Kingdom 1977–1996. *Br J Obstet Gynaecol* 2000; **107**: 254–261.

Elkin SL, Vedi S, Bord S et al. Histomorphometric analysis of bone biopsies from the iliac crest of adults with cystic fibrosis. *Am J Respir Crit Care Med* 2002; **166**: 1470–1474.

Haworth CS, Selby PL, Adams JE et al. Effect of intravenous pamidronate on bone mineral density in adults with cystic fibrosis. *Thorax* 2001; **56**: 314–316.

Jarad NA, Higgs S, Giles K. Factors associated with reduced FEV_1 in adult patients with cystic fibrosis in a relatively affluent area. *Chronic Resp Dis* 2005; **2**: 133–137.

Jarad NA, Giles K. Factors associated with increased rate of pulmonary exacerbations. *Chronic Resp Dis* 2008; **5**: 1–5.

King LJ, Scurr ED, Murugan N et al. Hepato-biliary and pancreatic manifestations of cystic fibrosis: MR imaging appearances. *Radiographics* 2000; **20**: 767–777.

Kopleman H, Corey M, Gaskin K, et al. Impaired chloride secretion, as well as bicarbonate secretion, underlies the fluid secretory defect in the cystic fibrosis pancreas. *Gastroenterology* 1988; **95**: 349–355.

Kotlof RM, FitzSimmons SC, Feil SB. Fertility and pregnancy in patients with cystic fibrosis. *Clin Chest Med* 1992; **13**: 623–635.

Laang S, Thorsteinsson B, Pociot F et al. Diabetes Mellitus in cystic fibrosis: genetic and immunological markers. *Acta Paediatr* 1993; **82**:150–154.

Marshall BC, Butler SM, Stoddard M, et al. Epidemiology of cystic fibrosis-related diabetes. *J Paediatr* 2005; **146**: 681–687.

Raj P, Stableforth D, Morgan DW. A prospective study of nasal disease in adult cystic fibrosis. *J Laryngol Otol* 2000; **114**: 260–263.

Ramsey B, Richardson MA. Impact of sinusitis on cystic fibrosis. *J Allergy and Immunol* 1992; **90**: 547–552.

Rolon MA, Benali K, Munck A et al. Cystic fibrosis-related diabetes mellitus: clinical impact of pre-diabetes and effects of insulin therapy. *Acta Paediatr* 2001; **50**: 1336–1343.

Sawyer SM. Reproductive and sexual health in adolescents with cystic fibrosis. *BMJ* 1996; **313**: 1095–1096.

The Cystic Fibrosis Genotype-Phenotype Consortium. Correlation between genotype and phenotype in patients with cystic fibrosis. *N Engl J Med* 1993; **329**: 1308–1313.

The UK CF Trust bone mineralization document. Cystic Fibrosis Trust Publication 2007. www.cftrust.org.uk.

Van de Meeberg PC, Houwen RH, Sinaasappel M et al. Low-dose versus high-dose ursodeoxycholic acid in cystic fibrosis cholestatic liver disease: results of randomised study with 1 year follow-up. *Scand J Gastroenterol* 1997; **32**: 369–373.

Pulmonary vascular problems/issues

Chapter contents

12.1 Pulmonary embolism

Epidemiology

- The incidence of pulmonary emboli (PE) increases exponentially with age from 5:100,000 in children increasing to 400:100,000 in the over eighties.
- The mortality rate in a clinically stable patient presenting with a PE is 1–2%. Mortality increases with age and co-morbidity. The overall mortality rate which includes patients with significant co-morbid conditions is 12–15%.
- 60–80% of deaths due to PEs are undiagnosed in life, despite post-mortem evidence of earlier 'sentinel' emboli.
- Post-mortem studies consistently show that PEs are responsible for 10% of all hospital deaths, highlighting the importance of thromboprophylaxis in hospital patients.

Aetiology

- Venous thromboembolic disease is a multifactorial condition, resulting from an interaction of genetic factors (known and unknown), external factors and age.
- The major risk factors individually increase the risk of a PE by a factor of 5 or more (Table 12.1.1).
- The minor risk factors increase the risk of a PE by a factor of 2–3 and include the oral contraceptive pill, hormone replacement therapy and long distance travel (travel greater than 8 hours). These factors are more likely to cause disease when combined with genetic or other external factors, and they are not usually considered when assessing the clinical probability of a PE (see later).

Thrombophilias

Thrombophilia is a generic term for conditions in which venous thromboses occur inappropriately. These conditions may be inherited or acquired. Up to 20% of patients with venous thromboembolism will have a recognised genetic clotting abnormality. It is likely that these abnormalities only give rise to problems when combined with one or more additional genetic defects or when interacting with external risk factors.

- For practical purposes it is not worthwhile to routinely test for thrombophilias. Affected patients are no more likely to suffer a repeat event once anticoagulation is stopped than someone not affected, so the result will not alter management.
- Screening patients who might be at risk, such as patients wanting the oral contraceptive pill, is not cost effective.
- Thrombophilia testing is recommended in:
  - a) Patients under the age of 40 with recurrent thromboembolic events and a strong family history of thromboembolic disease in first degree relatives. In such patients combinations of defects or the more serious, but rarer, single defects (Table 12.1.1) are more likely. (However, even a strong family history is a poor indicator of an underlying thrombophilia.)
  - b) Patients who might have disease associated with the acquired anti cardiolipin antibody.

Table 12.1.1 Major risk factors for venous thrombosis

- Major surgery
- Orthopaedic surgery to lower limb/lower limb trauma
- History of venous thrombosis
- Cancer
- Pregnancy/puerperium

Table 12.1.1 Major risk factors for venous thrombosis (Continued)

Reduced mobility – major illness with prolonged bed rest	
Age >70 years	
Thrombophilias:	Antithrombin deficiency
	Protein S deficiecy
	Protein C deficiency
	Antiphospholipid antibodies

Diagnosis

- Pulmonary embolism presents with non-specific symptoms and signs (Table 12.1.2) and is therefore considered in the differential diagnosis of many patients presenting to an acute unit.
- It is important to select only those patients who have a reasonable chance of a PE for further investigation.
- A full history, examination and routine tests, which should include a CXR, an ECG and a full blood count, will help rule out PE in patients with alternative diagnoses such as infection, ischaemic heart disease or chest wall pain.
- The classic ECG findings of right ventricular hypertrophy and strain, or CXR findings of the peripheral wedge shaped infarct or areas of hypoperfusion are rare.

Table 12.1.2 Clinical presentation of pulmonary emboli

Dyspnoea – 73%
Pleuritic chest pain – 66%
Tachypnoea – 70%
Crackles – 51%
Cough – 37%
Tachycardia – 30%
Haemoptysis – 13%
Pleural rub – 3%
Presenting signs and symptoms of patients with a proven PE in the PIOPED study

In a proportion of patients no clear alternative diagnosis can be made and the diagnosis of PE then becomes a reasonable possibility. The patient now enters the clinical algorithm for the diagnosis of PE

Clinical probability

The next step is to assess the clinical probability of the patient having a PE

- The positive and negative predictive value (PPV, NPV) of a test depends on the prevalence of the condition being tested for in the population under investigation.
- The NPV of a test increases when the prevalence is low and decreases when it is high. (To put it another way, you are more able to trust a negative test if the diagnosis was unlikely in the first place!) The reverse applies to the PPV.
- The purpose of the clinical probability is to help the clinician decide on the likely prevalence of a PE in a group of patients presenting with the same clinical features as their patient.

- The clinical probability will determine which test you do next and importantly how you interpret all subsequent tests.
- Several scoring systems, of varying objectivity, have been developed to assess clinical probability. The BTS score is the least well validated but has the benefit of being simple and easy to remember.

Clinical probability scoring systems

Revised Geneva Score	Points
Age > 60 years	1
Previous VTE	3
Surgery/fracture lower limb in last month	2
Active malignancy	2
Unilateral lower limb pain	3
Haemoptysis	2
Heart rate 75–94	3
>95	5
Pain on lower limb deep venous palpation and unilateral oedema	4

Clinical probability	Total points
Low	0–3
Intermediate	4–10
High	>10

Modified Wells score	Points
Symptoms & signs of a DVT	3.0
Alternative diagnosis less likely	3.0
Heart rate > 100	1.5
Immobilisation >3 days or surgery in the previous month	1.5
Previous VTE	1.5
Malignancy	1.0
Haemoptysis	1.0

Score 4 or less: PE unlikely (equivalent to low probability)

This scheme is designed for use with low sensitivity D-dimmer tests eg, SimpliRED, in patients with a low clinical probability.

BTS Score	Points
Is a PE a reasonable diagnosis?	1
Is an alternative diagnosis less likely?	1
Is a major risk factor present?	1

1 point: low clinical probability
2 points: intermediate clinical probability
3 points: high clinical probability

The D-dimer

- The D-dimer test is useful for ruling out a PE.
- Tests have a high sensitivity (a low false negative rate, particularly when the clinical probability is low), but a poor specificity (high false positive rate) which can lead to a lot of unnecessary investigations when the test is used inappropriately.
- Tests with a high sensitivity (>95%) have a very high NPV (few false negatives) in patients with a low or intermediate clinical probability. Most, but not all, of the rapid ELISA kits can be used in these patients.
- Tests with a lower sensitivity can only be used in patients with a low clinical probability, as they have an unacceptably poor NPV (too many false negatives) in other patients. The widely used SimpliRED test falls into this category.

- The D-dimer is not sensitive enough to be used in patients with a high clinical probability.
- A wide range of conditions is associated with increased levels of D-dimer
- D-dimer levels increase with age and this should be considered when dealing with borderline results in the elderly.
- If used appropriately a negative D-dimer can effectively rule out the diagnosis of PE in about 30% of patients.

D-dimer can be raised in

- Venous thromboembolic disease.
- Increasing age.
- Cancer.
- Infection.
- Haematoma.
- Post operative.
- Inflammation.
- Pregnancy.
- Peripheral vascular disease.
- Liver disease.

If the diagnosis of PE cannot be ruled out by the D-dimer, or if the clinical probability is high, then proceed to imaging to confirm the diagnosis.

Imaging

- Multidetector CT pulmonary angiography (CTPA) is the imaging modality of choice for the diagnosis of PE.
- The PIOPED 2 study showed that CTPA has a sensitivity of only 85% (96% when the scan confirmed the clinical probability eg. a positive scan in a high clinical probability patient).
- Large outcome studies show that less than 2% of patients with a negative CTPA suffer a subsequent venous thromboembolic event if left untreated. This would suggest that any missed PEs are not clinically important.
- In the uncommon event of a negative CTPA in a high clinical probability patient, further investigations might be appropriate.
- If the diagnosis is in doubt, investigation of the leg veins is sometimes advocated, since this is where most emboli arise. Thrombi are only found in 35–45% of patients with a known PE (using Doppler ultra sound or CT venography respectively). If thrombi are seen it is reasonable to assume that the patient has had a PE and will need treatment. If negative, this may be because the thrombus has detached completely and gone to the lung, and there is a small risk (less than 5%) of the patient having a further VTE. Further investigations are unlikely to be helpful.
- One large study has shown that there is nothing to be gained from doing routine leg ultrasound with a CTPA.
- It is worth noting that PIOPED 2 also showed a substantial false positive rate in patients with a low clinical probability. In this situation the diagnosis should be reviewed, especially if only a small isolated PE is seen.
- The ventilation perfusion isotope lung scan is only useful if reported as 'normal' or 'high probability', in the former case an alternative diagnosis is sought or in the latter case the patient is treated. Unfortunately these outcomes only occur in 30% of cases, and in the remaining 70% a PE cannot be ruled in or out, and further tests will be required.
- The echocardiogram can detect right heart strain and an increase in pulmonary artery pressure in the case of a large PE, but further objective tests are required to confirm the diagnosis.

Treatment

- Low-molecular-weight heparin (LMWH) should be started as soon as PE is considered a reasonable diagnosis.
- When the diagnosis is confirmed on CTPA warfarin is started and the heparin continued until the INR is in the target range of 2–3, at which point, if clinically stable, the heparin is stopped and the patient is usually discharged home.
- There is a background recurrence rate after an idiopathic PE of about 5% per year (25% at 4 years) once anticoagulation is stopped.
- The risk of a major haemorrhage on long-term warfarin is in the region of 1% per year in patients under 75 years and 5% when older.
- The patient and doctor should consider this risk- benefit profile when discussing how long to anticoagulate.
- Anticoagulation for 3 months is the minimum treatment period, and little is to be gained by continuing beyond this unless opting for lifetime treatment.
- Life long therapy should be considered after a life-threatening idiopathic PE, in patients with severe cardio-respiratory disease, after a second event or in the event of an ongoing major risk factor.

Caval filters

- Filters are considered when a patient suffers recurrent PEs despite adequate anticoagulation or when anticoagulants are contraindicated.
- Filters undoubtedly prevent PEs though there is no evidence that they affect mortality.
- If left in situ they are associated with a significant rise in the incidence of deep vein thrombosis, and thus require ongoing anticoagulation.
- Filters can only be used short term in patients who have contra-indications to anticoagulation and in these patients only removable filters should be used.

Thrombolysis

- Thrombolysis is the treatment of choice for acute massive PE. This is recognised by cardiovascular collapse in a patient with a known or suspected PE or, more commonly, in a patient known to be at risk. Some form of objective test, which in this situation would include an echocardiogram, should be undertaken to confirm the diagnosis. Unfortunately there is often little time for this.
- First-line treatment is thrombolysis with alteplase 50mg IV bolus.
- If thrombolysis fails to restore the circulation various techniques using percutaneous catheters to remove or ablate the embolus have been affective, and in some centres surgical removal might be attempted. Both techniques carry a high mortality rate.
- The role of thrombolysis in less severe PEs remains unclear. In so called sub-massive emboli, characterised by right ventricular strain and an increase in pulmonary artery pressure, thrombolysis may improve recovery time but has no effect on mortality.

Cancer

There is a high recurrence rate of PE in patients with cancer, even when adequately anticoagulated. The rate can be halved using LMWH instead of warfarin and this is now regarded as the treatment of choice in this situation. It would be reasonable to allow for patient choice however, and use warfarin if preferred, converting to long-term LMWH in the event of a recurrence.

Pulmonary embolism and pregnancy

- Diagnosis of PE in pregnancy can present a challenge. Symptoms and signs can be difficult to interpret, the D-dimer is often elevated in the absence of PE and there are concerns regarding fetal exposure to radiation when imaging is required. Given that PE is the second most common cause of death in pregnancy, accurate diagnosis is essential.
- This is one situation where isotope scanning may be appropriate. The CTPA exposes the foetus to less radiation than an isotope scan, but exposes the maternal breasts to significantly more, at a time when they are particularly vulnerable, increasing the risk of breast cancer in the future.
- A half dose perfusion scan, to further minimise the risk to the fetus, in the absence of any active lung disease, has been advocated If the scan is indeterminate then the options are to proceed with a CTPA or rely on further non- invasive tests such as Doppler ultrasound of the leg veins.
- Once confirmed, LMWH is used throughout the pregnancy. Warfarin has adverse effects on fetal development. Warfarin can be started in the post-partum period, if wished.

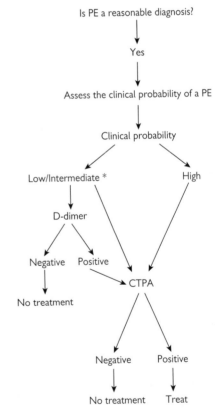

Is PE a reasonable diagnosis?

Yes

Assess the clinical probability of a PE

Clinical probability

Low/Intermediate *   High

D-dimer

Negative   Positive

No treatment

CTPA

Negative   Positive

No treatment   Treat

Fig. 12.1.1 Diagnostic algorithm for suspected pulmonary embolism.

*Low sensitivity D-dimer test are only used in patients with a low clinical probability, high sensitivity tests can be used in patients with both a low and an intermediate clinical probability

---

AUTHOR'S TIPS

- The D-dimer test should not be used as a screening test.
- Only consider testing patients with a reasonable possibility of a PE, after a full history, examination and routine investigations.
- If used appropriately, the D-dimmer can rule out the diagnosis of PE in 30% of suspected cases.

Further reading

British Thoracic Society guidelines for the management of suspected acute pulmonary embolism. *Thorax* 2003; **58**: 470–484.

Baglin T, Luddington R, Brown K, *et al.* Incidence of recurrent venous thromboembolism in relation to clinical and thrombophilic risk factors: prospective cohort study. *Lancet* 2003; **362**: 523–526.

Le Gal G, Righini M, Roy PM, *et al.* Prediction of pulmonary embolism in the emergency department: The revised Geneva score. *Ann Intern Med* 2006; **144**:165–171

Perrier A, Bounameaux H. Accuracy or outcome in suspected pulmonary embolism. *N Eng J Med* 2006; **354**:2383–84.

Scarsbrook AF, Gleeson FV. Investigating suspected pulmonary embolism in pregnancy. *BMJ* 2007; **334**: 418–419.

Wells PS, Anderson DR, Rodger M, *et al.* Derivation of a simple clinical model to categorize patients probability of pulmonary embolism: increasing the model's utility with the SimpliRED D-dimer. *Thromb Haemost* 2000; **83**:416–420.

12.2 Pulmonary hypertension

Definition

The normal pulmonary circulation is a low pressure, high flow system that delivers the output of the right ventricle to the alveolar capillary network during each cardiac cycle for the purposes of gas exchange. Pulmonary hypertension is defined as a sustained elevation of mean pulmonary arterial pressure to greater than 25mmHg at rest, or 30mmHg on exercise. Many diseases can lead to an elevation of pulmonary arterial pressure. Therefore, the term *pulmonary hypertension* is not a final diagnosis, but a starting point for further investigation. In general terms the main causes of pulmonary hypertension are (i) a narrowing or obstruction of the precapillary pulmonary arteries, (ii) an increase in pulmonary venous pressure, or (iii) a persistent elevation of pulmonary blood flow.

Classification

Table 12.2.1 shows the latest World Health Organization (2003) classification of pulmonary hypertension as determined by an international panel of experts. The grouping of causes in this classification takes into account similarities in aetiology, pathology, and haemodynamic assessment at right heart catheterisation. The classification is a useful framework to consider the various causes of pulmonary hypertension, described in more detail below.

Table 12.1.1 Clinical classification of pulmonary hypertension (Venice 2003)

1. Pulmonary arterial hypertension (PAH)
  1.1. Idiopathic (IPAH)
  1.2. Familial (FPAH)
  1.3. Associated with (APAH):
    1.3.1. Collagen vascular disease
    1.3.2. Congenital systemic-to-pulmonary shunts**
    1.3.3. Portal hypertension
    1.3.4. HIV infection
    1.3.5. Drugs and toxins
    1.3.6. Other (thyroid disorders, glycogen storage disease, Gaucher disease, hereditary hemorrhagic telangiectasia, hemoglobinopathies, myeloproliferative disorders, splenectomy)
  1.4. Associated with significant venous or capillary involvement
    1.4.1. Pulmonary veno-occlusive disease (PVOD)
    1.4.2. Pulmonary capillary hemangiomatosis (PCH)
  1.5. Persistent pulmonary hypertension of the newborn

2. Pulmonary hypertension with left heart disease
  2.1. Left-sided atrial or ventricular heart disease
  2.2. Left-sided valvular heart disease

3. Pulmonary hypertension associated with lung diseases and/or hypoxemia
  3.1. Chronic obstructive pulmonary disease
  3.2. Interstitial lung disease
  3.3. Sleep-disordered breathing
  3.4. Alveolar hypoventilation disorders
  3.5. Chronic exposure to high altitude
  3.6. Developmental abnormalities

4. Pulmonary hypertension due to chronic thrombotic and/or embolic disease
  4.1. Thromboembolic obstruction of proximal pulmonary arteries
  4.2. Thromboembolic obstruction of distal pulmonary arteries
  4.3. Non-thrombotic pulmonary embolism (tumor, parasites, foreign material)

Table 12.1.1 (*Continued*) Clinical classification of pulmonary hypertension (Venice 2003)

5. Miscellaneous
Sarcoidosis, histiocytosis X, lymphangiomatosis, compression of pulmonary vessels (adenopathy, tumor, fibrosing mediastinitis)

1. Type
  Simple
  Atrial septal defect (ASD)
  Ventricular septal defect (VSD)
  Patent ductus arteriosus
  Total or partial unobstructed anomalous pulmonary venous return
  Combined
  Describe combination and define prevalent defect if any
  Complex
  Truncus arteriosus
  Single ventricle with unobstructed pulmonary blood flow
  Atrioventricular septal defects

2. Dimensions
  Small (ASD ≤2.0cm and VSD ≤1.0cm)
  Large (ASD >2.0cm and VSD >1.0cm)

3. Associated extracardiac abnormalities

4. Correction status
  Noncorrected
  Partially corrected (age)
  Corrected: spontaneously or surgically (age)

**Guidelines for classification of congenital systemic-to-pulmonary shunts

Epidemiology

Pulmonary arterial hypertension is broadly divided into idiopathic PAH (previously known as primary pulmonary hypertension), and PAH found in association with other conditions. Idiopathic PAH is further divided into familial and sporadic disease. Approximately 10% of patients with idiopathic PAH have an affected relative. Idiopathic PAH is a rare disorder with an estimated incidence of 1–2 per million per year. It is more common in women (F:M sex ratio = 2.3:1). The disease can occur at any age but most commonly between the ages of 20 and 45. Pulmonary arterial hypertension, pathologically indistinguishable from the idiopathic form, can occur in a range of associated conditions (Table 12.2.1). Of the connective tissue diseases, the most common association is with systemic sclerosis, where PAH can complicate the clinical course in 15–20% of patients, in the absence of interstitial lung disease. Other associated conditions include mixed connective tissue disease and systemic lupus erythematosis, and more rarely, rheumatoid arthritis, dermatopolymyositis and primary Sjogrens' sysndrome. There is a well recognised association of PAH with congenital heart disease causing left to right shunts. Overall the prevalence of PAH is 15–30%, but varies depending on the nature of the underlying cardiac defect. Portal hypertension, usually associated with cirrhosis, is associated with PAH in less than 5% of patients. There is an unusually high prevalence of PAH (0.5%) in patients with HIV infection. Epidemiological studies have confirmed the association of PAH with amphetamine-like diet pills. In the 1970s increased numbers of patients with PAH were found to have been exposed to Aminorex. In the 1990s, further studies confirmed an assocation of

PAH with appetetite suppressant drugs of the fenfluramine and dexenfluramine group. An epidemic of PAH also occurred in Spain in 1980s following the ingestion of contaminated rape seed oil. Other more rarely associated conditions are listed in Table 12.2.1. The classification of PAH includes two other rare pulmonary vascular diseases, pulmonary veno-occlusive disease and pulmonary capillary haemangiomatosis. Both are more rare than idiopathic PAH, though the true prevalence is unknown. Persistent pulmonary hypertension of the newborn is a disorder characterised by a failure of vascular transition from fetal to a neonatal circulation and is estimated to affect 0.2% of live-born term infants.

Genetic factors

Familial PAH is a rare autosomal dominant condition with reduced penetrance. It is indistinguishable on clinical or pathological grounds from idiopathic PAH. In 2000, heterozygous germline mutations were identified in the gene encoding the bone morphogenetic protein type II receptor (BMPR-II), located on the long arm of chromosome 2 (2q33). BMPR-II is a receptor for bone morphogenetic proteins (BMPs). BMPs are members of the transforming growth factor-β (TGF-β) superfamily. Mutations in BMPR-II have now been identified in over 70% of cases of familial PAH. Similar mutations are also found in 15–26% of patients thought to have sporadic or idiopathic disease. BMPR-II mutations have been identified in most of the 13 exons of the *BMPR2* gene. The majority (70%) of mutations are nonsense or frameshift mutations. Approximately 30% of the mutations are missense mutations. These cause retention of mutant protein within the endoplasmic reticulum or affect important functional domains of the receptor, such as the ligand binding domain or the kinase domain. Mutations in BMPR-II have also been found in a small proportion (10%) of patients with PAH associated with appetite suppressants and in children with complicated PAH associated with congenital heart disease. Mutations in another TGF-β receptor, ALK-1, have also been reported is association with PAH. ALK-1 mutations are usually found in families with hereditary haemorrhagic telangiectasia, though occasionally some family members develop severe PAH. These findings have highlighted the central role of the TGF-β signalling pathway in the pathogenesis of PAH.

Pathology

Typical morphological appearances include increased muscularisation of small (<200µM diameter) arteries and thickening or fibrosis of the intima, referred to as concentric intimal fibrosis. In severe cases dilatation of small pulmonary arterioles is seen and sometimes fibrinoid necrosis. In the larger elastic arteries, aneurysmal dilatation may occur and atherosclerotic change, the latter being otherwise extremely unusual in the normotensive pulmonary artery. The term plexogenic arteriopathy is used to describe the presence of plexiform lesions (200–400µM), which are tangles of capillary-like channels adjacent to small pulmonary arteries. Plexiform changes are found in some 50% of cases of idiopathic PAH but also in other causes of severe pulmonary hypertension, such as that due to congenital heart disease. Pathologically, in some cases of idiopathic PAH there are changes in the pulmonary venous circulation as well as the arterial. If the venous changes dominate the pathology the diagnosis is pulmonary veno-occlusive disease (PVOD), which has some distinct clinical features (see later in this chapter). Accompanying arterial changes, particularly muscular hypertrophy, often co-exist.

Pulmonary and pleural lymphatics are dilated and long-standing venous hypertension may lead to oedema and fibrosis. A further distinct pathological entity is pulmonary capillary haemangiomatosis (PCH), characterised by the presence of numerous foci of proliferating, congested, thin-walled capillaries, which invade alveolar tissue, as well as pleura, bronchial and vascular tissue.

Clinical features

Symptoms

The three main presenting symptoms are dyspnoea, chest pain and syncope. The severity of symptoms is related to prognosis. Unexplained breathlessness on exertion should always raise the possibility of pulmonary arterial hypertension, particularly in the setting of conditions known to be associated with pulmonary hypertension (Table 12.2.1). The condition may have an insidious onset. Frequently there is a delay of up to three years between the first symptoms and diagnosis. Syncope is an ominous sign, usually reflecting severe right ventricular dysfunction. Other symptoms include lassitude, abdominal swelling from ascites and ankle swelling. Small haemoptysis may occur at later stages.

Clinical signs

Tachypnoea may be present, even at rest. Peripheral cyanosis is common due to a low cardiac output. Central cyanosis occurs later as pulmonary gas exchange deteriorates or right to left shunting occurs through a patent foramen ovale. The jugular venous pulse may be elevated with a prominent 'a' wave, reflecting the increased force of atrial contraction, or, if tricuspid regurgitation is present, there may be a large 'V' wave. There may be a right ventricular heave and a pulsatile liver. On auscultation, forceful closure of the pulmonary valve leads to an accentuated pulmonary arterial component of the second heart sound. There is often a third and fourth right heart sound. The murmurs of tricuspid regurgitation (systolic) or pulmonary regurgitation (diastolic) may be heard. Jaundice, ascites and peripheral oedema may be present at advanced stages of the disease. Cyanosis may be present, though profound cyanosis may indicate the presence of a right to left shunt.

Differential diagnosis

If the symptoms and clinical signs suggest pulmonary hypertension, the differential diagnosis should be considered with reference to the classification in Table 12.2.1. Most importantly the presence of left heart disease, parenchymal lung disease or congenital heart disease should be excluded. Pulmonary hypertension due to chronic thromboembolic disease is important to detect because specific surgical treatment is available. Idiopathic PAH remains a diagnosis of exclusion.

Clinical investigation

The investigation of a patient with suspected pulmonary hypertension involves (i) the exclusion of other underlying causes and (ii) an assessment of severity of pulmonary hypertension and right heart failure for prognosis and treatment.

Blood tests

A thrombophilia screen may reveal clotting abnormalities predisposing to chronic thromboembolic pulmonary hypertension. This should include antithrombin III, protein C and S, factor V Leiden, anti-cardiolipin antibodies, and lupus anticoagulant. Thyroid function should be measured since both hypo- and especially hyperthyroidism are commonly reported associations. An autoantibody screen should be performed to exclude underlying connective tissue disease. Positive antinuclear antibodies can be found in 30–40% of patients with idiopathic PAH. A primary vasculitis is an uncommon cause of pulmonary hypertension, but measurement of antineutrophil cytoplasmic antibodies (ANCA) should be requested. Since there is an increased incidence of unexplained pulmonary hypertension in HIV positive patients, this diagnosis should be considered in all patients.

Imaging

The plain CXR shows enlargement of the proximal pulmonary arteries, which may be dramatic. The proximal right and left main pulmonary arteries are enlarged and peripheral pruning of the pulmonary vascular pattern occurs, giving rise to increased peripheral radiolucency. If heart failure is present the heart may be enlarged and enlargement of the right atrium is seen. The CXR may also give clues to underlying diagnoses such as interstitial lung disease.

A spiral contrast enhanced CT will detect proximal pulmonary arterial obstruction suggestive of acute or chronic thromboembolic disease. A pattern of mosaic perfusion of the lung parenchyma may is also a feature of chronic thromboembolic pulmonary hypertension, and may be the only sign in predominantly distal disease. A high resolution CT scan will pick up unsuspected parenchymal abnormalities, such as fibrosis. CT scanning is also useful to indicate more uncommon forms of PAH, such as PVOD. In PVOD the CT may show a degree of mediastinal lymphadenopathy and septal lines in the lung periphery, presumably indicating lymphatic and venous obstruction.

On the ventilation-perfusion lung scan the pattern of ventilation is usually normal in idiopathic PAH, and uneven ventilation should suggest underlying lung disease. The pattern of perfusion is also virtually normal though small patchy perfusion defects may be present. This is in contrast to the appearance in chronic thromboembolic pulmonary hypertension where segmental or larger perfusion defects persist, often indistinguishable from the pattern of acute pulmonary embolism.

Pulmonary artery angiography is only required if the diagnosis is likely to be chronic thromboembolic pulmonary hypertension. In this situation angiography will provide precise anatomical information regarding the location of vascular obstruction, indicated by abrupt cut-off of vessels or intravascular webs, which may be of great use if surgical endarterectomy is being contemplated.

The main contribution of magnetic resonance imaging (MRI) is in the assessment of patients with suspected intracardiac shunts or with anomalous vascular anatomy; for example, if a shunt is suspected on the basis of right heart catheterisation, but cannot be demonstrated by echocardiography. In addition, MRI can provide further pulmonary angiographic images.

Pulmonary function tests

The typical pattern for standard pulmonary function test for disease confined to the pulmonary circulation is

- Normal lung volumes.
- Normal FEV_1/VC ratio (>0.75), indicating no airflow obstruction.
- Low transfer factor (diffusing capacity, TLco) and low transfer coefficient (Kco).

The low diffusing capacity probably results from a combination of a reduced cardiac output and disease affecting the

small arterioles reducing local perfusion. Additional findings in the pulmonary function tests such as marked airflow obstruction (e.g. severe chronic obstructive pulmonary disease), or a restrictive defect (e.g. pulmonary fibrosis) would indicate the presence of an underlying cause for the pulmonary hypertension. However, subtle changes in lung volumes and mild airflow obstruction have been reported in a proportion of patients with PAH. In some groups of patients at high risk of developing PAH, for example in scleroderma, the Kco can be monitored at intervals. A fall in the Kco, accompanied by breathlessness, may be the first sign of PAH complicating scleroderma.

Exercise testing

Significant PAH is always associated with a reduced exercise capacity. One of the most useful tests of exercise capacity in PAH patients is the 6MWT. A normal distance is greater than 500m. Heart rate and oxygen saturation should be monitored during the test. A low 6MW is predictive of a poor survival. Full cardiopulmonary exercise testing is technically more demanding to perform and is only recommended if the diagnosis is in doubt, for example if there was a need to document cardiovascular limitation on exercise. Peak oxygen uptake on exercise is low and the anaerobic threshold is reduced to about 40% of normal. There is excessive ventilation for a given degree of oxygen consumption or carbon dioxide output, even at rest. There is no ventilatory impairment when underlying lung disease is absent. There is often a pronounced tachycardia at submaximal exercise, and usually arterial oxygen desaturation.

Cardiac function tests

In symptomatic PAH the electrocardiogram (ECG) is abnormal in 80–90% of established cases. However, the ECG has inadequate sensitivity (55%) and specificity (70%) as a screening tool for detecting pulmonary hypertension. The ECG typically shows right axis deviation (more than +120°) in the limb leads. A dominant R wave and T wave inversion in the right precordial leads accompanied by a dominant S wave in the left precordial leads suggests right ventricular hypertrophy. Tall peaked P waves in the right precordial and inferior leads denotes right atrial enlargement. Right bundle branch block is common.

Echocardiography remains the best screening test for significant pulmonary hypertension. It detects the presence and direction of intracardiac shunts. Usually this is possible using conventional transthoracic techniques, but if visualisation is poor or a small shunt is still suspected, then transoesophageal echocardiography may be necessary. In addition, the left ventricle can be reliably assessed to determine whether there is a contribution from left ventricular systolic or diastolic dysfunction to the elevated pulmonary arterial pressure. The function of the right ventricle can also be assessed qualitatively and quantitatively, in terms of atrial and ventricular dimensions and wall thickness. Paradoxical bowing of the intraventricular septum into the left ventricular cavity may be seen during systole, as a consequence of greatly elevated right sided pressures. Newer echocardiography techniques such as 3-D echo and tissue Doppler are being evaluated. Continuous wave Doppler echocardiography is used to measure high flow velocities across cardiac valves. One of the most commonly derived indices in the right heart is the pulmonary artery systolic pressure measured by Doppler echocardiography. The measurement is made from measurement of the velocity of the tricuspid regurgitant jet. About 80% of patients with

PAH and 60% of normal subjects have measurable tricuspid regurgitation. The maximum flow velocity (v) of the regurgitant jet is measured and inserted into the modified Bernouilli equation for convective acceleration pressure change, giving an estimate of right ventricular systolic pressure (RVSP):

$$RVSP = 4.v^2 + RAP$$

Where RAP is right atrial pressure. In the absence of pulmonary valve stenosis, the RVSP is equal to the pulmonary artery systolic pressure (PASP). RAP can be estimated clinically from the height of the jugular venous pressure. There is a reasonable correlation between Doppler estimates of PASP and catheter measurements.

Right heart catheterisation remains the best technique for confirming the diagnosis of pulmonary hypertension and for providing important prognostic information. An elevated mean pulmonary arterial pressure of greater than 25mmHg at rest is the accepted definition, or 30mmHg on exercise. In patients with idiopathic PAH the mean pulmonary arterial pressure may exceed 60mmHg. The pulmonary capillary wedge pressure (PCWP) can also be determined at catheterisation, which is an approximation of left atrial pressure. An elevated PCWP (>15mmHg) generally indicates left heart disease, but can also be elevated in pulmonary veno-occlusive disease. Measurement of the PCWP is often unreliable in the presence of chronic thromboembolic pulmonary hypertension. Sampling of venous blood oxygen saturation as one passes the catheter down from the right atrium to right ventricle may detect a sudden 'step-up' in oxygenation, which would indicate the presence of a left-to-right shunt. Most important is the determination of right ventricular function, which provides important prognostic information. Cardiac output can be determined by thermodilution or the Fick method. Indicators of right heart failure, and hence poorer prognosis, include: i) an elevated right atrial pressure (>10mmHg), ii) an elevated right ventricular end diastolic pressure (>10mmHg), iii) a reduced mixed venous oxygen saturation (SvO_2 <63%) and iv) a reduced cardiac output (<2.5litre/min).

Vasoreactivity studies

A subgroup (10–15%) of patients with idiopathic PAH, and anorexigen-associated PAH, demonstrate a marked reduction in pulmonary vascular resistance following the administration of a vasodilator. These patients are the only group that respond favourably to long-term treatment with vasodilator therapy in the form of calcium channel blockers (see later in this chapter), and are thus an important group to identify. Vasodilator studies are undertaken at the time of right heart catheterisation. The preferred agent is inhaled nitric oxide, or an intravenous infusion of prostacyclin or adenosine. A positive response is defined as a fall in mean pulmonary arterial pressure of at least 10mmHg to below 40mmHg, accompanied by an increase or no change in cardiac output.

Treatment

All patients with suspected severe PAH are best referred to a specialist centre for initial assessment and treatment. A multidisciplinary team approach to planning treatment is preferred with input from respiratory physicians and cardiologists, transplant physicians and cardiothoracic surgeons, radiologists, specialist nurses, and palliative care specialists. Assisting patients to adapt to the uncertainty associated with chronic, life-shortening disease is essential if they are to successfully adjust to the demands of their illness and its treatment. The overall aims are to improve symptoms and quality of life, increase exercise capacity and improve prognosis.

Supportive medical therapy

Patients with right heart failure and fluid retention may require diuretics. Decreasing cardiac preload with diuretics is often enough to alleviate episodes of right heart failure. Caution should be exercised though, because faced with a reduction in vascular filling pressures patients with severe PAH will not be able to increase cardiac output effectively. This may result in systemic hypotension and syncope. Antiarrhythmics may be required for sustained or paroxysmal atrial fibrillation. Patients with severe PAH are prone to this complication because of stretching of the overloaded right atrium. The presence of atrial fibrillation can significantly compromise the already reduced cardiac output in patients with PAH and should be treated aggressively. Rate control with digoxin is possible, but if not contraindicated, pharmacological cardioversion with amiodarone is preferable. Electrophysiological mapping of arrhythmias and ablation of arrhythmogenic pathways may be indicated in selected patients.

Calcium channel blockers

Patients with idiopathic PAH and a documented acute vasodilator response at cardiac catheterisation, as defined above, should be offered long term treatment with a calcium channel blocker. This is associated with very significant improvement in symptoms and prognosis in this subset of patients. Nevertheless, only 50% of those who respond in the cardiac catheterisation laboratory will maintain a long-term response to calcium channel blockers. Calcium channel blockers should be avoided in any patient with significant signs of right ventricular failure, or until this is controlled, because of their negative inotropic effects. For this reason, and the risk of systemic hypotension calcium channel blockers should not be prescribed without confirmation of a vasodilator response at cardiac catheterisation. Indiscriminate prescribing will lead to increased mortality in the PAH population. Treatment should be started in hospital, using diltiazem, amlodipine or nifedipine, and carefully titrated against systemic blood pressure. The aim is to increase the dose to the maximum tolerated.

Anticoagulation

Warfarin therapy to maintain the INR between 2 and 3 is recommended in all patients with idiopathic and familial PAH. Two retrospective and one small prospective study have demonstrated a survival benefit of anticoagulation. Warfarin therapy was shown to almost double survival rate in idiopathic PAH over a 3-year period. The consensus is that patients with PAH associated with connective tissue disease should also receive warfarin, unless contraindicated. The risk-benefit ratio of anticoagulation in other forms of PAH is undetermined.

Oxygen therapy

Oxygen therapy is indicated for symptomatic relief of breathlessness. There are no published trials of the benefit of long-term oxygen therapy in hypoxaemic patients with PAH. Nocturnal oxygen was shown to be of no benefit in Eisenmenger's syndrome. Ambulatory oxygen may be beneficial if there is evidence of correctable desaturation of >4% to less than 90% during a 6MWT. Consideration should be given to in-flight supplemental oxygen for air travel.

Disease-targeted therapies

Over the last 10 years, remarkable advances have been made in the availability of therapeutic agents for PAH. Clinical trails have almost exclusively recruited patients with idiopathic PAH and anorexigen associated PAH, though often include a subset of patients with PAH associated with systemic sclerosis. There are limited published data in other forms of PAH. These agents are used to reduce pulmonary vascular resistance and improve cardiac output. They all improve exercise performance and data support extended survival times for some. Figure. 12.2.1 presents an algorithm summarising the pharmacological approach to treating PAH, based on current recommendations. Disease-targeted therapy is usually only licensed for treatment of patients in NYHA class III and IV.

Prostanoids

Prostacyclin has a half-life in the circulation of less than 2 minutes and thus must be given by continuous intravenous infusion. Although prostacyclin produces acute hemodynamic effects in some patients, most patients experience a fall in pulmonary vascular resistance with long-term use even in the absence of acute improvements. Prostacyclin has been shown to improve haemodynamics, exercise tolerance, quality of life and survival in patients in NYHA class III and IV. Side effects are usually experienced when starting prostacyclin or when escalating the dose. These include jaw pain, cutaneous flushing, nausea and diarrhoea, as well as myalgias. Acute withdrawal of prostacyclin, for example if the infusion pump fails, can cause severe rebound pulmonary hypertension, which can be fatal. Recurrent sepsis due to line infection can also be problematic. Although prostacyclin

remains a proven therapy in PAH, the complexity of its administration, and the availability of newer oral agents, means that this approach tends to be reserved for patients with severe haemodynamic compromise.

Stable analogues of prostacyclin have been developed with longer half lives and improved bioavailability. Iloprost can be given by the intravenous or inhaled route. Treprostinil can be given subcutaneously or intravenously and is approved for use in patients in NYHA class II, III, and IV. Beraprost is an orally available prostacyclin analogue, though the dose may be limited by gastrointestinal side effects. It is presently only available in Japan.

Endothelin receptor antagonists

The orally active, dual selective ET_A/ET_B receptor antagonist, bosentan, has been shown to improve exercise capacity, functional class, haemodynamics, echocardiographic and Doppler variables, and time to clinical worsening in idiopathic PAH. The most significant side effect of bosentan is elevation of the hepatic transaminases, which is usually reversible on stopping the drug. Sitaxsentan and ambrisentan are newer ET_A selective agents with similar efficacy to bosentan in short term studies, and favourable safety profiles. All patients on these agents require monthly monitoring of liver function tests.

Phosphodiesterase inhibitors

Sildenafil is an orally active selective inhibitor of cGMP-phosphodiesterase type 5. It acts by inhibiting the breakdown of cyclic GMP, with vasorelaxant and antiproliferative effects in pulmonary vascular smooth muscle. Sildenafil improves exercise tolerance and pulmonary haemodynamics

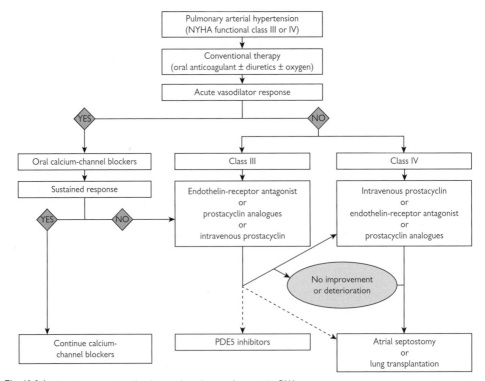

Fig. 12.2.1 Algorithm summarising the pharmacological approach to treating PAH.

in short term studies in PAH. Longer acting PDE5 inhibitors, such as tadalafil, also show promise.

Combination therapy

There is considerable theoretical and experimental evidence to support the use of combinations of the above disease-targeted therapies in PAH. Since PAH is a progressive disease most patients eventually deteriorate on monotherapy. The addition of further agents has been shown to provide clinical benefit, although the evidence for precise recommendations is lacking at present.

Atrial septostomy

Atrial septostomy involves creating a right to left shunt between the atria. The preferred technique is by percutaneous graded balloon dilatation. The rationale for this procedure is that patients with PAH and a patent foramen ovale have improved survival. Creating the shunt reduces right ventricular preload which relieves the failing right ventricle and can increase cardiac output and improve exercise capacity. This increase in cardiac output is at the expense of a reduction in systemic arterial oxygen saturation, but systemic oxygen delivery is usually improved. The procedure is usually reserved for patients who are failing on maximal medical therapy or as a bridge to transplantation.

Transplantation

Transplantation of the lungs or heart and lungs was developed as a treatment for end-stage PAH during the 1980s. The advent of modern targeted therapies has reduced the number of patients referred for transplantation. However, the long-term outcome of patients who remain in NYHA functional class III or IV remains poor. Lung or heart lung transplantation therefore remains an important mode of treatment for patients failing medical therapy. Patients with pulmonary veno-occlusive disease and pulmonary capillary haemangiomatosis have a particularly poor outlook and respond poorly to available medical therapies and should be referred early for transplantation assessment. In general, patients presenting with NHYA class IV symptoms should be referred for transplant assessment at the time of presentation, because their prognosis is poor. Additional indicators of poor prognosis include: i) a six minute walking distance <332 metres, ii) a peak oxygen consumption <10.4 ml/min/kg, iii) a cardiac index <2 l/min/m^2, iv) a right atrial pressure >20mmHg, v) a mean pulmonary arterial pressure >55mmHg, vi) a mixed venous oxygen saturation of <63%. Those with significant improvement after three months medical therapy can be removed or suspended from listing for transplant. The choice of procedure varies between centres but single lung (SLT), bilateral lung (BLT) and heart lung transplantation (HLT) are used in patients with PAH. International Registry figures show that the one-year mortality post-transplantation is highest in patients with idiopathic PAH compared with any other indication. Median survival post-transplantation for idiopathic PAH is between 4 and 5 years.

Prognosis

The prognosis of PAH varies depending on the underlying association or cause. Prognosis is most closely linked to indices of cardiac function, especially cardiac index. Historical data in the period prior to the availability of modern targeted therapies suggest an expected median survival for idiopathic PAH between 2.5 and 4 years, and a 3 year survival of about 60%. The prognosis is worse

for patients with underlying systemic sclerosis, connective tissue disease, HIV disease, and anorexigen-associated PAH. The prognosis for patients surviving to adulthood with PAH associated with a congenital intracardiac defect is substantially better than patients with idiopathic PAH. At least in patients with idiopathic PAH targeted therapies seem to improve survival to some extent, though definitive studies are awaited. Females with severe PAH should be advised that pregnancy carries a very high mortality because of the associated increased burden on the right heart.

Miscellaneous

Pulmonary hypertension is detectable in some 5% of patients with sarcoidosis. This may develop in the context of end stage pulmonary fibrosis due to sarcoid, but also may present as an isolated sarcoid vasculopathy in patients with relatively little parenchymal lung involvement. A falling diffusion co-efficient for carbon monoxide in the face of preserved lung volumes may the first clue to this in a sarcoid patient with worsening dyspnoea. In patients with vasculopathy there may be a marked response to immunosuppression with prednisolone, which is worth trying before embarking on targeted PAH therapy.

The commonest world-wide cause of pulmonary hypertension is said to be schistosomiasis. When one considers how many patients are infected with schistosomiasis this may be true, but true prevalence figures are hard to come by. The clinical picture in schistosomiasis is usually dominated by the effect on the urinary tract (*Schistosoma haematobium*) or liver (*Schistosoma mansoni* and *japonica*). Pulmonary hypertension is thought to be due to granulomata in or adjacent to pulmonary arterioles caused by the reaction to the presence of Schistosome eggs.

One of the commonest causes of pulmonary hypertension is that which occurs as a complication of COPD. The pulmonary hypertension is due to a combination of hypoxic pulmonary vasoconstriction, hypoxia-driven pulmonary vascular remodelling and a reduction in capillary cross sectional area in emphysema. Lung hyperinflation and polycythaemia may also contribute. The prevalence of pulmonary hypertension in patients with severe COPD may be as high as 50%. However, the average mean pulmonary arterial pressure is of the order of 25mmHg and progresses slowly (less than 1mmHg/year). It is likely that ventilatory impairment due to obstructed airways contributes to the majority of the exercise limitation in these patients. Nevertheless, there are relatively unusual cases of COPD in which the pulmonary hypertension dominates. These patients are often profoundly hypoxic, have emphysema on CT scanning and demonstrate a low diffusion coefficient for carbon monoxide. The level of pulmonary hypertension is similar to that seen in idiopathic PAH and these patients warrant targeted therapy for PAH in addition to optimisation of their COPD medication.

Chronic thromboembolic pulmonary hypertension (CTEPH)

Pathogenesis

CTEPH occurs when a clot fails to resolve completely after an acute pulmonary embolic event. The rate of resolution of clots after acute pulmonary embolism varies and is longer in patients with pre-existing cardiopulmonary disease, but normal perfusion should be restored by 4–6 weeks after the acute event. To some extent, the rate of resolution depends on the initial clot burden or the size of the acute pulmonary embolism. If the clot fails to resolve, it becomes organised before it can be completely fibrinolysed. The organised thrombus is incorporated into the wall of the pulmonary artery, becomes covered by endothelial cells and forms a false intima. The organised material occludes the vascular lumen, which increases pulmonary vascular resistance and leads to pulmonary hypertension. The true prevalence of CTEPH is hard to ascertain, because it is not usually sought in patients who are recovering from acute pulmonary embolism (PE), but it almost certainly is underdiagnosed. One well-designed study found that 4% of patients with a history of acute PE had a persistent elevation of pulmonary arterial pressure after two years.

Evidence also shows that those with a higher initial clot burden (massive PE) are more likely to develop CTEPH than those with minor PE. The more widespread use of thrombolysis for acute PE is often assumed to reduce the prevalence of CTEPH, but no data at present support this view. It is of note that some of the classic risk factors for acute deep vein thrombosis (DVT)/PE are not found with increased frequency in the population that develops CTEPH. For example, the factor V Leiden polymorphism, which leads to activated protein C resistance and is found with high prevalence in the population of patients with acute DVT, is not overrepresented in patients with CTEPH.

The prevalence of protein C and S deficiency is increased in patients with CTEPH, although these conditions account for a small minority of patients. In addition, some 10% of patients with CTEPH may have circulating antiphospholipid antibodies. Recent research points to a deficiency in the ability to fibrinolyse established clots as a predisposing factor. Other important predisposing factors include previous splenectomy and inflammatory bowel disease.

Clinical presentation

Clinically, patients often present with persistent symptoms of dyspnoea after an acute embolic event and despite the recommended period of anticoagulation. Up to 60% of patients with CTEPH will have a prior documented episode of previous venous thromboembolism, although some patients may present with gradually worsening dyspnoea in the absence of acute events. A further important finding may be pulmonary flow murmurs, resulting from turbulent flow across partially obstructed large pulmonary arteries, which may be audible on chest auscultation in up to 30% of patients with CTEPH. Otherwise the clinical presentation is similar to that described above for PAH.

Investigation

The work-up of patients referred with a suspected diagnosis of CTEPH requires a multidisciplinary approach involving surgeons, physicians, and radiologists. Imaging plays a key role in determining whether a patient is suitable for the surgical procedure of choice, pulmonary endarterectomy (PEA). Computed tomographic pulmonary angiography with modern multislice scanners is a rapid and non-invasive technique that can provide several important pieces of information in the assessment of patients with suspected CTEPH. CT can assess the presence of any associated lung disease or tumours. Most importantly, a computed tomographic pulmonary angiogram gives an accurate assessment of the extent of proximal organised clots.

Although occlusion of very small arteries cannot be visualised directly in the case of predominantly distal disease, the characteristic appearance of 'mosaic perfusion' suggests the presence of peripheral disease. Ventilation-perfusion lung scans also usually show multiple segmental perfusion defects not matched by defects in ventilation, even in distal disease. Computed tomography can also reveal the extent of right ventricular hypertrophy and dilatation, although this is probably best seen by MRI. Three-dimensional reconstruction of the two-dimensional CT and MR images can help decide whether the distribution of disease is suitable for PEA. The use of a combination of these techniques means that the more invasive traditional pulmonary angiogram can be avoided in most patients. Approximately 60% of cases of CTEPH are potentially suitable for surgery. Of the patients who are not suitable for surgical management, many may be suitable for targeted therapy with the new pharmacological agents described above.

Treatment

Pulmonary endarterectomy (PEA) is a surgical procedure during which organised thrombi are removed from the proximal pulmonary arteries. The procedure is a major operation that usually requires the patient to undergo repeated cycles of cardiopulmonary bypass with cerebral cooling. This ensures a bloodless field of view for the surgeon, who can then enter the left and right main pulmonary arteries via an arteriotomy. The aim is to identify a dissection plane along the base of the false intima and to dissect distally as far as possible. It is often possible to remove organised material as far distally as segmental pulmonary arteries. With successful clearance of proximal clots, the pulmonary vascular resistance can fall dramatically post-operatively, and near normalisation of resistance can be achieved in the long term. Patients are maintained on life-long warfarin and have an inferior vena cava filter sited prior to the operation. Long-term survival is often excellent after a successful procedure with marked improvements in exercise capacity, NYHA functional status and quality of life. The operation itself carries some risk, and perioperative mortality varies between 7–20% depending on the experience of the centre.

There are two main aspects to patient selection for this procedure. Comorbidities are important predictors of perioperative mortality and require careful assessment. A further important consideration is the distribution of the disease, as organised clots need to be anatomically accessible to the surgeon. If the organised material is predominantly of a distal distribution within the pulmonary arteries, that is involves subsegmental vessels, there is a high risk that pulmonary vascular resistance will not decrease after the procedure and that the patient will be left with significant pulmonary hypertension. Patients with persistent PAH following PEA may benefit from the targeted pharmacological therapies detailed above.

Further reading

Abenhaim L, Moride Y, Brenot F, et al. Appetite-Suppressant Drugs and the Risk of Primary Pulmonary Hypertension. N Engl J Med 1996; 335(9):609–616.

Barst RJ, Rubin LJ, Long WA, et al. A comparison of continuous intravenous epoprostenol (prostacyclin) with conventional therapy for primary pulmonary hypertension. New Engl J Med 1996; 334:296–301.

Bonderman D, Skoro-Sajer N, Jakowitsch J, et al. Predictors of Outcome in Chronic Thromboembolic Pulmonary Hypertension. Circulation 2007; 115(16):2153–2158.

D'Alonzo GE, Barst RJ, Ayres SM, et al. Survival in patients with primary pulmonary hypertension. Results from a national prospective registry. Ann Intern Med 1991; 115(5):343–349.

Fedullo PF, Auger WR, Kerr KM, *et al*. Chronic thromboembolic pulmonary hypertension. *N Engl J Med* 2001; **345**(20):1465–1472.

Galie N, Ghofrani HA, Torbicki A, *et al*. Sildenafil Citrate Therapy for Pulmonary Arterial Hypertension. *N Engl J Med* 2005; **353**(20):2148-2157.

Heath D, Edwards JE. The pathology of hypertensive pulmonary vascular disease. *Circulation* 1958; **18**:533–547.

Heath D, Segel N, Bishop J. Pulmonary veno-occlusive disease. Circulation 1966; **34**(2):242–248.

Newman JH, Trembath RC, Morse JA, *et al*. Genetic basis of pulmonary arterial hypertension: Current understanding and future directions. *Journal of the American College of Cardiology* 2004; **43**(12, Supplement 1):S33–S39.

Olschewski H, Simonneau G, Galie N, *et al*. Inhaled Iloprost for Severe Pulmonary Hypertension. *N Engl J Med* 2002; **347**(5):322–329.

Pengo V, Lensing AWA, Prins MH, *et al*. Incidence of Chronic Thromboembolic Pulmonary Hypertension after Pulmonary Embolism. *N Engl J Med* 2004; **350**(22):2257–2264.

Rich S, Kaufmann E, Levy PS. The effect of high doses of calcium-channel blockers on survival in primary pulmomary hypertension. *New Engl J Med* 1992; **327**:76–81.

Rubin LJ, Badesch DB, Barst RJ, *et al*. Bosentan Therapy for Pulmonary Arterial Hypertension. *N Engl J Med* 2002; **346**(12):896-903.

The International PPH Consortium, Lane KB, Machado RD, Pauciulo MW, *et al*. Heterozygous germ-line mutations in BMPR2, encoding a TGF-b receptor, cause familial primary pulmonary hypertension. *Nat Genetics* 2000; **26**:81–84.

Wagenvoort C, Wagenvoort N. Primary pulmonary hypertension: a pathological study of vessels in 156 clinically diagnosed cases. *Circulation* 1970; **42**:1163–1184.

12.3 Pulmonary vasculitis and haemorrhage

Pulmonary vasculitis

The pulmonary vasculitides are a heterogeneous group of rare disorders that result from an inflammatory process damaging the vessel wall and consequent impaired blood flow, ischaemia and tissue necrosis. The clinical manifestation of these vasculitides depends on the site, size, type, and severity of the inflammatory process.

Several classifications of the vasculitides have been described since the original first description of vasculitis by Kussmaul and Maier. Classification based on vessel size is confounded by the fact the vasculitic process does not respect vessel size restrictions. However the classification shown in Table 12.3.1 is frequently applied. The American College of Rheumatologist (ACR) and Chapel Hill classifications allow for standardised comparison of vasculitis but do not help make an early diagnosis in an individual patient since there is an overlap of features between disorders.

Wegener's granulomatosis (WG), Churg–Strauss syndrome (CSS) and microscopic polyangiitis (MPA) are primary small vessel vasculitides linked by an overlapping clinicopathological picture and are frequently called the anti-neutrophil cytoplasmic antibody (ANCA)-associated systemic vasculitides (AASV).

Epidemiology

- The estimated incidence of primary systemic vasculitides is estimated at 11–20/million and the prevalence is 90–278/million.
- There is geographic variation with WG being the most common vasculitis in northern Europe and MPA the most common vasculitis in northern Spain.
- Longitudinal studies have shown an increasing incidence of vasculitis.
- Vasculitis is very rare in childhood and frequently presents from young adulthood onwards.
- There is a seasonal variation in the presentation of WG with an increased rate in winter in Northern Europe.

Aetiology

- The aetiology of vasculitis is unclear.
- Vasculitides have been associated with exposure to silica, quartz, grain, occupational solvents and farming (livestock).
- Drug treatments with propylthiouracil, hydralazine, carbimazole, D-penicillamine, allopurinol and minocycline have been associated with the development of AASV.
- Patients with α_1-antitrypsin ZZ deficiency have a 100-fold increased risk of WG.
- Polymorphisms of genes linked to proteinase 3 overproduction, Fc gamma IIa and III receptors, and adhesion molecules associated with the interaction of neutrophils and endothelial cells have been associated AASV.

Pathogenesis

The pathogenesis of ANCA mediated vasculitis is the best understood. ANCA are auto antibodies, predominantly Ig G antibodies, directed against the cytoplasmic contents of neutrophil granules. The clinically relevant antibodies are directed against the enzymes proteinase 3 (PR3) and myeloperoxidase (MPO). *In vitro* studies have shown that ANCA can activate cytokine primed neutrophils and macrophages with consequent oxygen free radical formation and lysosomal degranulation. *In vivo* murine studies have

shown ANCA vasculitis (alveolar haemorrhage, necrotising pulmonary arteritis and focal segmental glomerulonephritis) can be caused by the transfer of anti-murine MPO Ig G from MPO -/- mice that have been immunised with MPO to mice that lack functioning T and B cells (Rag2 -/-).

Table 12.3.1 Classification of primary and secondary vasculitides.

Primary systemic vasculitis		
Size of vessel affected		
Small	Medium	Large
Wegener's granulomatosis	Polyarteritis nodosa	Giant cell arteritis
Churg–Strauss	Kawasaki's disease	Takayasi's artertis
Microscopic polyangiitis		
Behçet's		
Henoch–Schönlein		
Essential cryoglobinaemia		
Isolated pauci-immune pulmonary capillaritis		
Secondary vasculitides		
Connective tissue disorder	Systemic lupus erythematosus	
	Rheumatoid arthritis	
	Systemic sclerosis	
	Polymyositis	
	Anti-phospholipid syndrome	
	Immune mediated (Goodpasture's)	
Other systemic disorders	Inflammatory bowel disease	
	Autoimmune liver disease	
	Malignancy (haematological and solid organ)	
	Infections (bacterial, fungal and viral)	
	Drugs	
	Sarcoidosis	

These studies are supported by the clinical observation that a pregnant women with active MPO-ANCA positive microscopic polyangiitis gave birth to a newborn with pulmonary haemorrhage and crescentric glomerulonephritis. The newborns blood contained MPO-ANCA Ig G not Ig M. It is presumed that passive transplacental transfer of maternal MPO-ANCA Ig G caused the disease. Corticosteroids and plasma exchange effectively treated the symptoms.

Staphylococcus aureus chronic nasal carriage is associated with WG and relapse of disease. The bacterium contains a protein that mimics the anti-sense sequence of PR-3 incriminating it in the susceptibility for disease.

General principles in the assessment of a patient with vasculitis

Clinical presentation of the vasculitides is variable and careful attention needs to be made to the history taking, clinical examination and investigations. Frequently the investigations may point to a vasculitis in the absence of major symptoms. The principle pulmonary vasculitides are reviewed below and recommended investigations listed in Table 12.3.2.

Table 12.3.2 Investigations for vasculitis. Full blood count (FBC) looking for neutrophilia, eosinophilia, or drop in haemoglobin together with urea and electrolytes (UE) should be routinely done. Mixed cyroglobulinaemia is invariably found with hepatitis C and polyarteritis nodosa with hepatitis B. Vasculitis is found with infections and blood cultures and HIV (human immunedeficiency virus) test should be carried out if indicated. CXR (chest radiograph). ANCA (anti-neutophil cytoplasmic antibody) High resolution computed tomogram (HRCT)

Investigations for vasculitis	
All patients	
Urine dipstick and microscopy	
CXR	
Blood	FBC, CRP, UE
Selected tests depending on presentation	
Blood	ANCA (AASV)
	Blood culture, hepatitis B and C, HIV
	IgE (CSS), Anti-GBM
	Cryoglobulin, Complement
Pulmonary physiology	Dynamic test, flow volume loop
Bronchoscopy	To exclude infection and confirm alveolar haemorrhage. Rarely are mucosal or transbronchial biopsies useful.
Biopsy of relevant tissue	Nasal, lung, kidney
Radiology	HRCT
Neurological	Nerve conduction
Cardiology	Echocardiogram

Specific disorders

WG

WG is the most common pulmonary vasculitis and classically involves the triad of the upper respiratory tract (sinuses, ears, nasopharynx, and oropharynx), lower respiratory tract (trachea, bronchi and lung parenchyma) and kidneys. It is characterised by the histopathological finding of necrotising small vessel vasculitis (arterioles, capillaries and venules) and granulomatous inflammation. Its peak age of onset is 30–50 years. Children and young adolescents are rarely affected.

Upper respiratory features
- Ear, nose and throat symptoms are present in 70% of patients at initial presentation and will develop in 90% of patients throughout their disease history.
- Hearing loss will develop in 15–25% of patients.
- The nasopharynx is involved in 60% of patients and presents with epistaxis, nasal septal perforation, persistent congestion, pain, nasal crusting and mucosal ulcers.
- Saddle nose deformity due vascular necrosis of the cartilage occurs in up to 25 % patients with WG.

Lower respiratory features
Approximately 25% of patients will have limited WG with involvement of the upper and lower respiratory tract only.

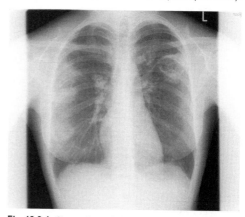

Fig. 12.3.1 Chest radiograph showing bilateral nodular lung changes with cavitation of some of the nodules.

> **AUTHOR'S TIP**
> Frequently overlooked, all patients should have their urine dipsticked for microscopic haematuria and proteinuria if a vasculitis is suspected.

Lung parenchymal
- Lung involvement manifests as symptoms include cough, haemoptysis, dyspnoea or may be silent.
- Abnormalities on the chest radiograph are noted in more than 70% at some point during their disease history.
- Radiological abnormalities include (see Fig. 12.3.1):
  - Single or multiple nodules (20–50%).
  - Cavitation of nodules occur in 66% of cases.
  - Pulmonary infiltrates.
  - Consolidation.
  - Intrathoracic lymphadenopathy (<2%).
  - Rarer findings include pleural effusions, atelectasis and pleural thickening.

Trachea and bronchi
- Granulomatous involvement of the trachea and bronchi will lead to stenosis in 10–30% of patients (see Fig. 12.3.2).
- Symptoms range from non-specific, dyspnoea, 'wheeze', stridor and change in voice.
- Subglottic stenosis invariably occurs in the presence of nasopharyngeal disease.
- Tracheal stenosis is associated with plateauing of both the inspiratory and expiratory limbs of the flow volume loop.
- At the time of bronchoscopy up to 74% of trachea lesion are due to mature scar and only 26% are due to acute inflammation.
- Bronchial stenosis has a female preponderance.

Renal features
- Hypertension.
- Acute renal failure (red cell casts and proteinuria).

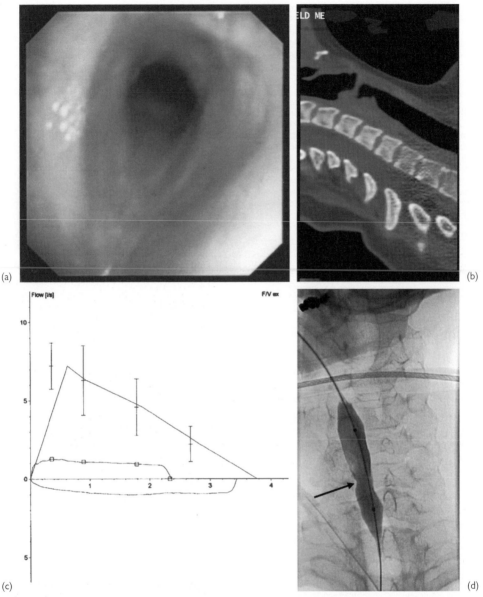

(a)

(b)

(c)

(d)

Fig. 12.3.2 Subglottic stenosis in WG. (a) bronchoscopic finding of fibrous stenosis. (b) CT reconstruction showing stenosis beneath vocal cords; (c) Characteristic plateauing of inspiratory and expiratory limbs of the flow volume loop. (d) Balloon dilation showing waisting of the balloon at the level of the stenosis.

Other organ features:

Occular symptoms of visual disturbance, pain, grittiness and dryness occur in 20–40% of patients with WG. Conjunctivitis, episcleritis and scleritis is found in 15–20% of patients. Prop-tosis occurs in 20% of patients. Posterior uveitis, optic neuritis and retinal haemorrhage are rare but serious complications

Cutaneous manifestations include palpable purpura, ulcerative lesions and haemorrhagic lesions. Neurological presentations include mononeuritis multiplex and cranial nerve palsies. Abdominal and cardiac presentations have been reported.

Intended for research use prior to the advent of ANCA testing two or more of the four ACR diagnostic criteria a listed below have been reported to have an 88% sensitivity and 92% specificity for WG.

- Nasal or oral inflammation (painful or painless oral ulcers or purulent or bloody nasal discharge).
- Abnormal chest radiograph showing nodules, fixed infiltrates, or cavities.
- Abnormal urinary sediment (microscopic hematuria with or without red cell casts).
- Granulomatous inflammation on biopsy of an artery or peri-vascular area.

The ACR criteria were proposed prior to the definition of MPA and poorly differentiate it from WG.

MPA

MPA is a necrotising vasculitis affecting small vessels (capillaries, venules, and arterioles). It is characteristically associated with focal segmental glomerulonephritis. Granulomatous inflammation of the upper respiratory tract, trachea and bronchi are not a feature. It occurs more commonly in men.

Up to 30–60% of patients frequently have a prodromal illness of fever, weight loss, myalgia and arthralgia that precede the diagnosis by up to 2 years.

Pulmonary features

- Diffuse alveolar haemorrhage is the most frequent pulmonary feature occurring in 30% of patients.
- Its presence is associated with a poor prognosis.
- Other features include pleurisy, pleural effusions and pulmonary fibrosis.
- Radiological features are of patchy alveolar changes on CXR without nodules.
- Pulmonary fibrosis develops in up to 11% of patients who have had previous pulmonary haemorrhage and carries a poor prognosis.

Renal features

- Over 90% of patients present with renal involvement.
- Focal segmental glomerulonephritis with fibrinoid necrosis and crescent formation are classically seen.
- Features of microscopic haematuria and proteinuria are found.
- Nephrotic syndrome is uncommon but when present carries a poor prognosis.

Gastrointestinal features

- Gastrointestinal bleeding, abdominal pain, diarrhoea and bowel perforation have been reported in 30–40% of patients.
- Gastrointestinal involvement is more common with MPA than WG.

Neurological features

Mononeuritis multiplex and cerebral vasculitis manifesting as headache, seizures, infarction or haemorrhage has been reported in up to 30% of patients.

Other features

Mild ENT symptoms and ocular symptoms are seen with MPA. However the presence of destructive nasal disease or proptosis would indicate a diagnosis of WG rather than MPA.

Churg–Strauss syndrome (CSS)

CSS is an allergic granulomatous angiitis characterised by small vessel vasculitis, extravascular granuloma and hypereosinophilia. It occurs in patients with a history of asthma and rhinitis. It is named after the two pathologists who described it in 1951. The annual incidence is reported at 2–4/million with a prevalence of 8–11/million. It is discussed in more detail in Chapter 18.2.

Three stages in the natural history of CSS have been described

1 A prodromal stage characterised by asthma and allergy which last for years.
2 A eosinophilic stage characterised by peripheral blood eosinophilia and organ infiltration. This may remit and relapse for several years.
3 A systemic vasculitic phase which may be life threatening.

ANCA patterns in AASV

The AASV are the predominant pulmonary vasculitides and have an overlapping clinical presentation and association with ANCA summarised above and in Table 12.3.3. Two main patterns of ANCA staining are found on indirect immunefluorescence: cytoplasmic (C-ANCA) and perinuclear (P-ANCA).

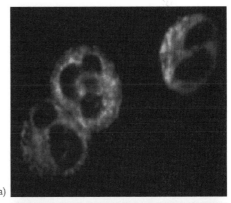

(a)

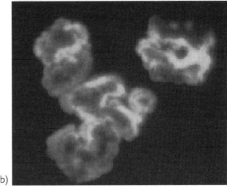

(b)

Fig. 12.3.3 ANCA staining by immunefluoresence. (a) C-ANCA with cytoplasmic staining. (b) P-ANCA with peri-nuclear staining. (See Plate 7.)

Over 90% of C-ANCA is directed against the serine protease PR-3 found in the azurophilic granule. P-ANCA is directed against range of intracellular antigens of which MPO is the most common.

Table 12.3.3 A comparison of the ANCA associated systemic vasculitides Wegener's granulomatosis (WG). Chug-Strauss Syndrome (CSS) and Microscopic polyanglitis (MPA). Diffuse alveolar haemorrhage (DAH). Frequency of organ involvement (*, **, **, ****). High resolution computed tomogram (HRCT). DLCO-diffusing capacity for carbon monoxide. Adapted from Pesci et al, 2007

Clinical features	WG	CSS	MPA
Pulmonary involvement	Nodular lung disease	Asthma	DAH
	Endo bronchial ulceration		
ENT involvement	Nasal destruction	Allergic rhinitis and polyposis	Very rare and mild
Renal involvement	Frequent and severe	Rare and mild	Frequent and severe
Other organ involvement			
Neurological	**	****	**
Cardiovascular	*	***	*
Gastrointestinal	*	***	**
Cutaneous	*	***	**
Investigation			
Radiographic	Nodules with or without cavitations	Transient Infiltrates	Infiltrates
	Infiltrates	Non-cavitatory nodules unusual	Ground glass changes (HRCT)
	Ground glass changes, nodules and stenosis. (HRCT)	Ground glass changes (HRCT)	
Pulmonary physiology	Obstructive/restrictive	Obstructive	Obstructive but can be restrictive in patients who go onto develop fibrosis
	Plateauing of flow volume loop		
	DLCO↑ DAH		DLCO↑ DAH
ANCA prevalence	Up to 90%	Up to 65%	Up to 90%
Immunefluorescence	C-ANCA	P-ANCA	P-ANCA
	PR-3 predominant	MPO predominant	MPO predominant
Pathological biopsy sites	Nasal	Peripheral nerve	Kidney
If clinically indicated	Kidney	Lung	Lung
	Lung		

A positive C-ANCA has up to 90% sensitivity and specificity for active WG. However for CSS and with MPA a positive P-ANCA is only indicative of AASV.

> **AUTHOR'S TIPS**
> - The utility of ANCA depends on its application in high risk populations to maximise its positive predictive value.
> - A negative ANCA does not exclude a vasculitis.

Treatment of AASV

Prior to the advent of immunosuppression with corticosteroids and cyclophosphamide the 1 year mortality for Wegener's was over 90%. It was not until the 1970s with the use of cyclophosphamide was this significantly altered. Cyclophosphamide has remained the mainstay of therapy ever since. However because of its toxicity alternative treatment strategies have been evaluated either to induced remission or maintain treatment. The European Vasculitis Study Group (EUVAS) have proposed a clinical staging system to help guide management, Table 12.3.4.

- Limited disease refers to disease confined to the upper airway.
- Early generalised disease refers to disease without threatened end-organ function. Nodular lung disease falls into this category.

- Active generalised disease refers to disease with threatened end organ function.
- Severe disease refers to critical organ dysfunction, e.g. diffuse alveolar haemorrhage or severe renal failure.
- Refractory disease is any patient who has failed to enter remission despite appropriate therapy. Approximately 10% of patients will fall into this category. Experimental therapy with intravenous immunoglobulin, rituximab, deoxyspergualin and anti-tumour necrosis factor alpha therapy with infliximab have been shown to be effective in small clinical trials or case series.

Treatment for the different stages are summarised in Table 12.3.4.

Once remission has been induced the role of therapy is to maintain disease control on the least level of immunesuppression required. The azathioprine and methotrexate are the best studied however clinical trials are currently underway investigating the role of mycophenolate and leflunomide. The duration of maintenance treatment is unclear.

Co-trimoxazole alone has been shown to cause remission in limited disease and when used in generalised disease with cyclophosphamide and corticosteroids reduced the relapse rate. It is thought co-trimoxazole reduces Staphylococcus aureus nasal carriage. Furthermore co-trimoxazole has a role to prevent Pneumocystis jiroveci infection that carries a significant mortality in the immunesuppressed.

Table 12.3.4 Treatment of AASV based site and severity of disease. Corticosteroid (CS), Azathioprine (AZA), Methotrexate (MTX), Cyclophosphamide (CYC), Plasma exchange (PE), intravenous Ig G (IV IgG), Rituximab (RTX), Deoxyspergualin (DSG), anti-Tumour necrosis factor alpha antagonists (anti-TNFα) and human albumin solution (HAS) Adapted from Pesci *et al,* 2007

Clinical Class	Localised	Early systemic	Generalised systemic	Severe	Refractory
Constitutional	–	+	+	+	+
Renal function	Creatinine < 120 umol/l	Creatinine < 120 umol/l	Creatinine < 500 umol/l	Creatinine > 500 umol/l	Any
Threatened vital organ function	–	–	–	+	+
Induction	Single agent (CS, AZA, MTx)	CYC or MTX +CS	CYC+CS	CYC+CS+PE	Investigational drugs IV IgG, RTX, DSG, anti-TNFα
Dosage	CS (1mg/kg/day) tapered down to 0.25 mg/kg od by 12 weeks				
Recommended	AZA (1mg/kg/day)				
	MTX (20–25 mg/week)				
	Oral CYC (1.5–2mg/kg/day)				
	PE Seven exchanges within first 2 weeks with 60ml/kg plasma exchanged for 5% HAS				
Maintenance	Once remission for is achieved for 3 to 6 months transition to maintenance treatment with AZA (1–2 mg/kg/day) or MTX (20–25mg/week) should be considered				

Monitoring of disease activity and complications

Monitoring disease response to treatment throws up several problems for the physician. Worsening symptoms have attributed to

- Disease relapse:
  - 40–60% of patients with WG will relapse on treatment.
  - 15–25% of patients with CSS will relapse on treatment.
- Infections (10% of infections occur without leucopenia).
- Drug toxicity on cyclophosphamide:
  - 12% of patients will develop cystitis.
  - 8% of patients will develop myelodysplasia.
  - 5% of patients will develop solid organ malignancies.

The role of ANCA in monitoring for disease relapse remains unclear.

Prognosis of AASV

- Even with optimal medical therapy AASV carries a significant 1 and 5 year mortality.
- A 1 year survival figure of 80-85% is reported for AASV as a whole.
- At 5 years a survival figure of 67–78% is reported for WG, 63–69% is reported for CSS and 45–53% for MP.
- Predictors of disease relapse include a diagnosis of WG, ENT or pulmonary or gastrointestinal involvement, PR-3 ANCA and carriage of *Staphylococcus aureus*

Management of airway stenosis in WG

Stenotic airways disease can occur in up to 30% of patients. At the time of bronchoscopy only a minority have active endobronchial disease. Management should be to actively treat WG and avoid interventions. If this is not possible a minimal invasive procedure should be undertaken. These include dilation, corticosteroid injections and conservative laser surgery. Tracheostomy and stenting should be avoided if possible.

Diffuse alveolar haemorrhage

Damage to the alveolar-capillary basement membrane results in filling of the alveolar spaces with blood. Bleeding into the alveolar space subsequently occurs giving rise to diffuse alveolar haemorrhage (DAH). This is a often a finding in AASV. However it needs to differentiated from other causes.

Histologically three patterns are seen:

- Pulmonary capillaritis where there is alveolar wall infiltration with inflammatory cells centred on capillary walls.
- Bland pulmonary haemorrhage where there is bleeding into the alveolar space without inflammatory changes in the vessels or alveoli.
- Diffuse alveolar damage as found in ARSD where the alveoli are oedematous with a hyaline membrane.

Clinical features

- The symptoms of DAH are non-specific.
- Dyspnoea, cough and fever are common.
- Haemoptysis is only present in two-thirds of patients.
- Patients may have clues in their histories to favour one of the diagnoses listed in Tables 12.3.5 and 12.3.6.
- Radiological findings are of diffuse pulmonary infiltrates and ground glass changes on HRCT (Fig. 12.3.4).
- If a baseline value is available for comparison DAH is associated with a drop in haemoglobin.
- If patients are well enough to undertake a diffusing capacity for carbon monoxide (DLCO) test it is elevated.
- Bronchoscopic lavage is characterised by lavage return that fails to clear in contrast to endobronchial bleeding. Lavage should be sent for culture to exclude infection.
- Specific test including urine analysis and serological tests for ANCA, anti-GBM antibodies, anti-nuclear antibodies, anti-phospholipid antibodies and rheumatoid factor as well as complement together with creatinine kinase should be considered.
- Biopsies of the kidneys should be considered if a pulmonary-renal syndrome is suspected.

Treatment

- In severe cases treatment cannot be delayed pending the results of serological or biopsy results.
- If infection and DAH without capillaritis have been excluded immunesuppres and DAH without capillaritis have with corticosteroid (methylprednisolone 1g/day for 3–5 days) with cyclophosphamide (2 mg/kg/day).
- In unstable severe disease due to systemic autoimmune process plasma exchange should be considered.
- Factor VII concentrate have been used achieve haemostasis in severe bleeding.

Prognosis

- Repeated DAH can result in pulmonary fibrosis especially in patients with MP, WG, idiopathic haemosiderosis and mitral stenosis.
- Obstructive features can also develop post DAH.

Anti-glomerular basement antibody disease (Goodpasture's syndrome)

Pathogenesis

The role of anti-GBM antibodies in the pathogenicity of Goodpastures syndrome has been shown *in vivo* studies. Antibodies were passively transferred from humans to monkeys who went on to develop glomerulonephritis. The primary antigen was subsequently identified as component of the α3 chain of type IV collagen of basement membranes.

Table 12.3.5 Causes of diffuse alveolar haemorrhage with pulmonary capillaritis

Primary vasculitis	
ANCA associated vasculitis	
WG	Behçets disease
CSS	Henoch–Schönlein purpura
Microscopic polyangiitis	Pauci-immune pulmonary capillaritis
Secondary vasculitis	
Collagen vascular disease	Mixed connective tissue disease
Rheumatoid arthritis	Polymyositis
Systemic lupus erythematosus	Anti-phospholipid syndrome
Drug-induced vasculitis	
Good pastures syndrome	
Bone marrow transplant	

Table 12.3.6 Causes of diffuse alveolar haemorrhage without pulmonary capillaritis

- Inhalation toxins
- Mitral stenosis
- Severe coagulopathy
- Anti-glomerular basement membrane disease
- Infections
- ARDS
- Idiopathic pulmonary haemosiderosis
- Lymphangioleiomyomatosis
- Tuberous sclerosis
- Pulmonary capillary haemangiomatosis
- Pulmonary veno-occlusive disease
- Neoplasms

Epidemiology

- It is a rare disorder occurring in one in million.
- It is associated with cigarette smoking or exposure to inhaled hydrocarbons.
- Young men are prone to develop pulmonary haemorrhage.
- Pulmonary haemorrhage without renal disease is rare.
- DAH can occur due to bland haemorrhage as well as pulmonary capillaritis.
- An overlap syndrome of AASV and anti-GBM disease exists.

Clinical features

- In 25–30% of patients, a prodromal period of flu like illness occurs.
- Pulmonary manifestations:
  - The insidious onset with symptoms lethargy, dyspnoea upon exertion, and, sometimes, dry cough.
  - Occasionally acute onset with fever, massive haemoptysis and acute respiratory failure.
- Renal manifestations:
  - Usually presents with an abrupt onset of oliguria or anuria.
  - Rarely, the patient's renal involvement is more insidious in onset and he or she remains asymptomatic, progressing slowly until the development of uraemia symptoms

Diagnosis

- Urine analysis.
- Anti-GBM antibodies.
- ANCA, up to 32% of patients testing positive for anti-GBM will test positive for ANCA.
- Renal biopsy. Typical features are a crescentric glomerulonephritis with immunefluorescence microscopy demonstrates a linear deposit along the capillaries.

Treatment

- Plasmapheresis with concomitant use of corticosteroids and cyclophosphamide.
- Patients should be asked to stop smoking.

Prognosis

- Patients who survive the first year with near normal renal function do well.
- Relapses are rare and when they do occur may reflect relapse of the AASV.

Summary

- Pulmonary involvement in primary systemic vasculitis is common especially in the AASV.
- Management relies on early clinical diagnosis and treatment to minimise the morbidity and mortality associated with the disease and its treatment.
- Choice of treatment depends on the clinical severity of disease.
- Advances current medical therapy is unlikely to result in disease free remission and cure the disease in the majority of patients.

Support groups

- http://www.vasculitisfoundation.org
- http://www.vasculitis-uk.org.uk

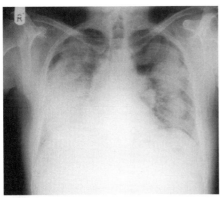

(a)

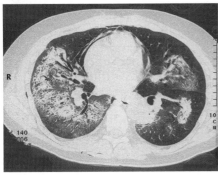

(b)

12.3.4 Radiographic appearance of diffuse alveolar haemorrhage (a) CXR showing bilateral ground infiltrates (b) HRCT showing ground glass changes within which areas of consolidation are seen.

Further reading

Bosch X, Guilabert A, Font J. Antineutrophilic cytoplasmic antibodies. *Lancet* 2006; **368**: 404–414.

Brown K. Pulmonary Vasculitis. *Proc Am Thorac Soc* 2007; **3**:48–57.

Jennette JC, Xiao H, Falk RJ. Pathogenesis of vascular inflammation by anti-neutrophil cytoplasmic antibodies *J Am Soc Nephrol 2006*; **17**: 1235–1242.

Lane SE, Watts RA, Shepstone L, *et al.* Primary systemic vasculitis: clinical features and mortality. *QJM* 2005; **98**: 97–111.

Lee AS, Specks U. Papillary capillaritis. *Semin Respir Crit Care* 2004; **25**:547–555.

Pesci A and Manganelli P. Respiratory system involvement in antineutrophil cytoplasmic-associated systemic vasculitides. *Drugs RD* 2007; **8**:25–42.

Smyth L, Gaskin G, Pusey G. Microscopic polyangitis. *Semin Respir Crit Care Med* 2004; **25**: 523–533.

Watt RA, Lane SE, Bentham G, Scott DG. Epidemiology of systemic vasculitis. A ten year study in the United Kingdom. *Arthritis and Rheumatism* 2000; **43**: 414–419.

Lung cancer

Chapter contents

13.1 Epidemiology of lung cancer

Incidence and mortality

- Lung cancer first emerged as a threat to the public health during the early part of the 20th century and since this time an epidemic of the disease has evolved. Lung cancer is now the leading cause of cancer deaths in the UK and a number of other developed countries.
- In 2004 in England and Wales lung cancer was the second most common cancer diagnosed in the UK (excluding non-melanomatous skin cancer), with more than 30,000 new cases being registered. The most common cancer was breast cancer with 37,000 new cases.
- Lung cancer is predominantly a disease of older people. The commonest age of presentation is between 75–79 years of age and 85% of registrations occur in people over the age of 60 years and 60% of registrations in people over the age of 70 years.
- The male to female lung cancer incidence ratio is approximately 1.5 to 1. The lung cancer epidemic is women is slightly different to that in men in that the peak will occur later and will probably not be as high. At present lung cancer incidence rates continue to increase in older age groups in both men and women, but in younger men the incidence is beginning to fall reflecting a fall in smoking prevalence.
- The incidence of lung cancer rises steeply with increasing levels of social deprivation, and the size of this gradient is higher than that seen for other cancers. In people of working age mortality rates from lung cancer are 4.6 times higher in people who are unskilled manual workers compared to professional people. An analysis of the Health Survey for England found a strong social class gradient in plasma cotinine levels in smokers, even after allowing for number of cigarettes smoked per day. These data suggests that the level of nicotine dependence may well be related to socio-economic status.
- Data from the USA demonstrate that lung cancer incidence rates are higher amongst black people than white people, particularly in the people with more years of education.
- Within Great Britain and Ireland lung cancer mortality rates are highest in people who were born in Scotland, followed by Ireland and then West Africa.
- Lung cancer occurs throughout the world wherever people smoke. Although some of the lowest lung cancer incidence rates are currently found in Africa and other developing countries, as smoking becomes more common the lung cancer epidemic will inevitably follow.

Changes in histological type

In early studies of lung cancer in the 1950s squamous cell carcinoma was by some way the most prominent histological type, followed by small cell lung cancer (SCLC). From the late 1970s a progressive increase in the incidence of adenocarcinoma has occurred, perhaps because the level of some tobacco specific nitrosamines have increase. Recent studies suggest that in women adenocarcinoma is now the most common type of lung cancer, followed by squamous cell, small cell and then large cell, whilst in men adenocarcinoma is now as common as squamous cell lung cancer.

AUTHOR'S TIPS

- A diagnosis of lung cancer carries a poor prognosis and the outlook for people with lung cancer is far worse than that for people with cancers at other sites. Only 25% of people diagnosed with lung cancer are alive at one year and this figure drops to 7% at 5 years. (http://info.cancerresearchuk.org/cancerstats)
- Without treatment SCLC has a median survival or only a few months. With treatment people with extensive disease have a median survival of about 6 months, and those with limited disease have a median survival of 9–12 months. The prognosis of non-small cell lung cancer (NSCLC) is slightly better with one year survival rates of between 25 to 45%.

Aetiology

Cigarette smoking

Cigarette smoking is by some way the most important cause of lung cancer and is believe to be implicated in the aetiology of approximately 90% of lung cancers. The link between smoking and lung cancer was reported in landmark studies by Doll and Hill in the UK and Wynder and Graham in the USA both reported in 1950. These studies were important not only in showing the strength of the association between smoking and lung cancer but also in driving the development of epidemiology. There are earlier studies which reported a link between lung cancer and smoking, notably a case–control study from Germany reported in 1943.

The results of the 50 year follow-up of the British Doctors cohort suggest that in comparison to lifelong non-smokers the incidence of dying from lung cancer is 15 times higher in current smokers and 4 times higher in former smokers. Amongst current smokers the incidence of lung cancer is also strongly related to cigarettes smoked per day (Fig. 13.1.1).

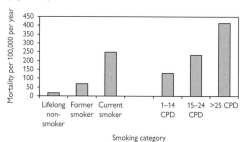

Fig.13.1.1 Lung cancer in the British Doctor cohort.

Cigarette smoking is strongly related to the risk of developing all histological types of lung cancer but overall the associations are strongest with SCLC and squamous cell lung cancer and weaker with adenocarcinoma.

The risk of lung cancer is more strongly related to the duration of smoking that the number of cigarettes smoked per day. In other words amongst people with the same number of pack-years of smoking the risk of developing lung cancer is higher amongst those who have smoked for longer.

The risk of lung cancer falls with time after people stop smoking, but there is still a doubling of lung cancer risk for moderate to heavy smokers compared to never-smokers 30 years after quitting.

The move towards lower tar and nicotine cigarettes has not reduced the risks associated with smoking because smokers rapidly learn to compensate by taking greater puff volumes and blocking ventilation holes and thereby maintain their supply of nicotine.

The association between exposure to environmental tobacco smoke and lung cancer risk is more difficult to study than the association with active smoking, but current estimates suggest a 20 to 30% increase with regular exposure.

Other factors

Diet

There are data from a number of studies which suggest that diets which have higher levels of fruit and vegetables may reduce the risk of developing lung cancer. The main methodological problems with these studies are issue of accurately measuring diet and the problem of not controlling completely for the effect of cigarette smoking.

Occupation

Studies of asbestos textile workers in the UK and insulation workers in the United States suggest that working with asbestos is associated with a 7–10-fold increase in the risk of lung cancer and that this risk peaks 30–35 years after the first exposure to asbestos. Workers who are exposed to tar and soot, arsenic, chromium and nickel may also have an increased risk of lung cancer.

Radiation

Exposure to high levels of radon, for instance in uranium miners, is an established cause of lung cancer. Radon exposure at a much lower level occurs as an indoor pollutant and there are data from a case control study which suggest that this is associated with an increased risk of lung cancer, the risk being approximately double in those people living in houses with the highest level of exposure compared to those with the lowest exposure.

Genetics

There is some evidence that polymorphisms in genes which code for enzymes which may metabolise cigarette carcinogens may have an influence on the risk of developing lung cancer.

Such genes include:

- Enzymes in the cytochrome p450 system (CYP1A1 and CYP2D6).
- Glutathione S-transferase.
- Microsomal epoxide hydrolase.
- NAD(P)H quinine oxidoreductase.
- Myeloperoxidase.

Further reading

Albano JD, Ward E, Jemal A, et al. Cancer mortality in the United States by education level and race. *J Natl Cancer Inst* 2007; **99**(18):1384–1394.

Alberg AJ, Samet JM. Epidemiology of lung cancer. *Chest* 2003; **123**(1 Suppl): 21S–49S.

Doll R, Peto R, Boreham J, et al. Mortality from cancer in relation to smoking: 50 years observations on British doctors. *Br J Cancer* 2005; **92**(3):426–429.

Kiyohara C, Otsu A, Shirakawa T, et al. Genetic polymorphisms and lung cancer susceptibility: a review. *Lung Cancer* 2002; **37**(3):241–256.

Office for National Statistics. Cancer statistics: registrations of cancer diagnosed in 2004, England. MB1 no. 35, 1-88. 2004. London, Office for National Statistics.

Office for National Statistics. Mortality statistics: Cause. Review of the Registrar General on deaths by cause, sex and age, in England and Wales, 2004. DH2 no. 31, i-280. 2005. London, Office for National Statistics.

Pershagen G, Akerblom G, Axelson O, et al. Residential radon exposure and lung cancer in Sweden. *N Engl J Med* 1994; **330**(3):159–164.

Peto R, Darby S, Deo H, et al. Smoking, smoking cessation, and lung cancer in the UK since 1950: combination of national statistics with two case-control studies. *BMJ* 2000; **321**(7257):323–329.

Schairer E, Schoniger E. Lung cancer and tobacco consumption. *Int J Epidemiol* 2001; **30**(1):24–27.

Silvestri GA, Spiro SG. Carcinoma of the bronchus 60 years later. *Thorax* 2006; **61**(12):1023–1028.

The British Thoracic Society. The burden of lung disease: a statistical report from the British Thoracic Society 2006. 2006. London, The British Thoracic Society.

Wild SH, Fischbacher CM, Brock A, et al. Mortality from all cancers and lung, colorectal, breast and prostate cancer by country of birth in England and Wales, 2001-2003. *Br J Cancer* 2006; **94**(7):1079–1085.

Wynder EL, Hoffmann D. Re: Cigarette smoking and the histopathology of lung cancer. *J Natl Cancer Inst* 1998; **90**(19):1486–1488.

Wynder EL. Tobacco as a cause of lung cancer: some reflections. *Am J Epidemiol* 1997; **146**(9):687–694.

13.2 Symptoms and signs (including SVCO)

Lung cancer presents clinically at an advanced stage with 80% of patients having inoperable disease at diagnosis.

- Only 5-10% of newly diagnosed lung cancers present incidentally with asymptomatic lesions on CXRs or CT scans. This proportion is set to increase with the availability of total body screening scans to the asymptomatic general public, and ongoing interval CT scanning following treatment for other malignancies.
- At least 90% of patients with lung cancer are symptomatic at diagnosis and many report having new symptoms for up to a year prior to presentation.
- Patients may present with symptoms relating to the primary tumour, metastatic spread, paraneoplastic phenomena or a combination of these.

Local tumour effects

Cough, dyspnoea, chest pain and haemoptysis are common in patients presenting with lung cancer.

Cough occurs in response to bronchial mucosal ulceration, interruption of bronchial peristalsis, post-obstructive pneumonia and infection; all more common in central airway tumours.

Dyspnoea (new or worsening) is present in up to 60% of patients. It is caused by:

- Persistent infection or atelectasis.
- Central airway obstruction (fixed unilateral inspiratory wheeze or stridor may be audible).
- Pleural and pericardial effusions, thromboemboli, and lymphangitis carcinomatosis (occurring in more advanced disease).

Chest pain is common in localised, operable disease when patients describe an intermittent ache on the side of the tumour. Intractable pain may arise from invasion of chest wall structures in more advanced disease.

Haemoptysis in lung cancer is usually low volume blood streaking of sputum, occurring over a number of days prior to presentation. Massive haemoptysis due to erosion through bronchial or pulmonary vessels occurs infrequently. Lung cancer accounts for around 30% of haemoptysis. In smokers over 40 years of age with haemoptysis, if the CXR is normal, CT thorax followed by bronchoscopy should be pursued as a lung cancer will be diagnosed in 6%.

Effects due to intrathoracic spread

Dysphagia, hoarse voice, pleural effusion, hydropneumothorax, and pericardial effusion or tamponade are usually associated with invasion of intrathoracic structures in this setting.

Pancoast syndrome and superior vena cava obstruction are examples of locally invasive disease, associated with unique symptoms, signs, diagnostic and management challenges.

Pancoast tumours (superior sulcus tumours)

Superior sulcus tumours arise posteriorly in the apex of an upper lobe, in the groove created by the passage of the subclavian artery, near to the brachial plexus. Non-small cell lung cancer (NSCLC) is the most common cause with 5% of NSCLC arising in this area. Other neoplasms, in addition to various inflammatory and infective processes can cause 'Pancoast syndrome' so histological diagnosis is essential.

Clinical features of 'Pancoast syndrome'

- Infiltration of C8, T1, T2 nerve roots causes gnawing pain over the shoulder medial border of the scapula, progressing down the medial aspect of the arm to the little and ring fingers.
- Often delayed diagnosis as a mechanical, musculoskeletal cause is pursued.
- Weakness of the intrinsic hand muscles and loss of the triceps reflex occur.
- Horners syndrome (ptsosis, meiosis, enopthalmos, narrowed palpebral fissure and anhydrosis) may also occur ipsilaterally when C6 and T1 segments of the sympathetic chain are involved.
- There may be associated rib, vertebral body, spinal cord or mediastinal invasion and destruction.

Diagnosis and staging

- CXR may reveal subtle opacity at the lung apex while CT thorax allows visualisation of the tumour and initial staging.
- CT guided biopsy has a diagnostic yield of 90% and is the method of choice for obtaining histology in superior sulcus tumours (fibreoptic bronchoscopy carries a 30–40% success rate)
- MRI scan is essential in potential surgical candidates, to establish the degree of brachial plexus involvement and adds useful information regarding chest wall and vascular invasion.
- A total body PET scan should be performed as in other lung cancer patients considered for radical therapy. Accurate staging is particularly important given the delicate anatomy of the region and high peri-operative mortality.
- Pancoast tumours are typically staged IIB (T3 N0 M0) or greater.

Management and prognosis

Aquequate analgesia should be prescribed, however pain is often resistant to such simple measures.

- Clinical practice is moving towards a tri modality approach to treatment (chemotherapy, radiotherapy and surgery following restaging, to render locally extensive disease operable) which has been associated with 5-year survival rates of up to 46%.
- Vertebral body, rib, subclavian artery or sympathetic chain invasion or N2/3 nodes have a poor prognosis.
- Superior sulcus tumours carry a particularly high risk of brain metastases, however routine pre operative brain scanning and prophylactic cranial irradiation remain controversial areas.

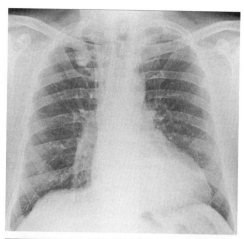

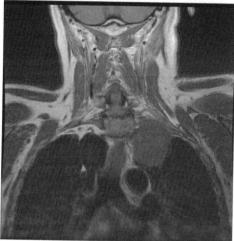

Fig. 13.2.1 Presentation CXR and MRI of a patient with a left Pancoast tumour invading the brachial plexus.

KEY ISSUES

Pancoast tumours

The CXR may be falsely reassuring.

MRI scanning of the brachial plexus is essential in staging potentially resectable tumours.

Superior vena cava obstruction (SVCO)

Lung cancer is the most common cause of SVCO.

It occurs due to invasion or extrinsic compression by tumour or lymph nodes and is frequently accompanied by intravascular thrombosis.

- Present at diagnosis in around 10% of patients with small cell and 2% with NSCLC.
- Its presence at diagnosis is a poor prognostic indicator, particularly in NSCLC where it is a marker of advanced stage.

Clinical features

Reduction of venous return from the upper body is responsible for the distressing symptoms of 'SVC syndrome' (SVCS):

- Oedema, venous distension and plethora of the head, neck, arms and thorax.
- Headache.
- Breathlessness, hypoxia, pulmonary oedema.
- Laryngeal oedema with stridor.
- Symptoms exacerbated by bending forward, lifting arms above the head and lying flat.
- Symptoms and signs of a lung primary or mediastinal mass (cough, hoarse voice, dysphagia).

Severity is determined by the speed and anatomical level (lower is more severe) of vascular occlusion. Chronic obstruction allows the development of collateral venous drainage, in which context patients may be relatively asymptomatic.

In lung cancer, SVCO commonly progresses rapidly over weeks resulting in a florid presentation.

Aetiology

Malignancy accounts for 90% of SVCO with SCLC and NHL being responsible for the majority. Metastatic tumours and primary malignancies arising from the mediastinum are less common causes. Thrombus propagated by central venous lines and pacemaker wires may result in SVCO.

There are many other recognised non-malignant, vascular, infective and inflammatory causes.

Investigation

CTX may demonstrate mediastinal widening, pleural effusion or clear evidence of the primary tumour. Abnormal in 85%.

CT thorax will confirm the presence of a mediastinal mass or other causative process in addition to staging the tumour and confirming the presence of intravascular thrombus and degree and level of venous collaterals.

Tissue diagnosis is obtained by the most minimally invasive approach available and is guided by the radiological appearances.

Management

Immediate. sit the patient up, prescribe oxygen, and analgesia. Treat pulmonary oedema if present. **Definitive** oncological management reflects histological cell type, stage and performance status. Radiotherapy prior to obtaining histology may compromise an accurate tissue diagnosis and the planning of optimal therapy thereafter. Likewise, corticosteroids may alter histology in lymphoma and should be avoided if this diagnosis is a possibility until it can be confirmed. Chemotherapy provides relief of SVCOS in up to 77% of patients with SCLC and radio-therapy in 60–65% of NSCLC. Combined modality approaches may be taken with similar response rates. SVCO relapse rates are 17% and 19% respectively. Symptomatic resolution occurs within 7–21 days of initiating definitive treatment.

Intravascular stenting is performed under radiological guidance and can achieve resolution of headache and facial oedema within 24 hours with improvement of other symptoms within three days.

Stenting does not preclude obtaining histology at a later time or subsequent chemo or radiotherapy and can be performed when the SVC is completely occluded with tumour or thrombus. In lung cancer, symptomatic response rates are 95% with an 11% relapse rate, comparing favourably with chemo and radiotherapy. Stent occlusion can be managed with repeat stenting. Stent migration, vascular trauma and bleeding have been infrequently reported. Current evidence supports a move towards first line use of stenting, particularly in patients with NSCLC.

Anticoagulation is controversial. Some advocate prophylactic anticoagulation in the presence of SVCO and use of low dose warfarin in stented patients to achieve an INR of around 1.6 is common practice. This is not supported by trial data at present and carries a slightly increased risk of intracranial haemorrhage.

Steroids are frequently used in patients with SVCO despite an absence of evidence to support their effectiveness. If prescribed, histology should be obtained first and prolonged, high dose courses avoided.

KEY POINTS

SVCO

Obtain an urgent histological diagnosis and staging before definitive treatment is initiated.

The majority of patients with SVCO do not experience a significant deterioration in the time taken to achieve this.

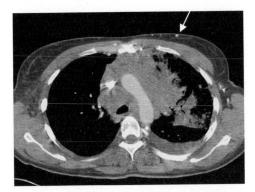

Fig. 13.2.2 SCLC causing SVCO. Multiple chest wall venous collaterals are visable on CT scan.

Effects due to distant metastases

Extrathoracic metastases are present in up to 30% of patients at presentation. Many are asymptomatic.

Common sites are:

Liver which may cause pain, fever, anorexia, weight loss and carries a particularly poor prognosis.

Adrenal glands – clinically silent. Usually detected on CT and or PET scan.

Bone, causing well localised pain, hypercalcaemia and pathological fractures. The vertebrae, ribs, femurs and pelvis are most frequently involved. Extension of vertebral metastases is the most common cause of spinal cord compression in this setting.

Brain, which may present with headache, signs of raised intracranial pressure, seizures, and focal neurological signs.

70% of patients presenting with symptomatic brain metastases have a primary lung malignancy.

Non-specific systemic effects

Cachexia, anorexia, malaise, fever occur in around 20% of patients with metastatic disease and may result in a fall in performance status that precludes palliative chemotherapeutic approaches. Tumour necrosis factor-α is thought to be an important mediator of these symptoms. Although more common in the presence of a heavy tumour load, the syndrome can occur in localised disease.

Paraneoplastic syndromes

These disorders are usually mediated by peptide-proteins with hormonal or immunological activity, produced by the tumour or in response to it, having effects distant from the primary tumour and unrelated to metastases.

- Paraneoplastic syndromes occur in a clinically significant form in 10–20% of patients with lung cancer.
- Importantly, the syndromes may predate diagnosis of malignancy by years when they should stimulate a detailed search for an underlying tumour which may be at a curable stage. They also occur in advanced disease or may herald a recurrence.
- Although specific symptomatic treatment is available for some syndromes, the majority respond to conventional management of the underlying tumour.

Clubbing is the most common paraneoplastic presentation, occurring in up to 30% of patients with lung cancer, most frequently in NSCLC. It is usually asymptomatic. The main diagnostic criteria is a digital profile angle of greater than 180°. Hypertrophic pulmonary osteoarthropathy is the presence of gross digital clubbing with painful peri-articular subperiostial bone deposition, causing swelling of the wrists, ankles and knees. Clubbing may resolve and HPOA improve with treatment of the underlying tumour. Both are recognised in other conditions, particularly chronic suppurative lung disease.

Hypercalcaemia is detected in 1% at presentation and occurs in the course of the disease in 40%. It is most frequently caused by bone metastases but may result from PTHrP production, particularly by NSCLC. Standard management of hypercalcaemia applies. There is little practical value in measuring PTHrP.

Cushing's syndrome occurs in up to 5% of patients with SCLC although detection of high levels of ACTH in serum without related symptoms occurs in more than 50%. The syndrome carries a poor prognosis with an increased risk of opportunistic infections and poor tumour response to chemotherapy. Presentation is tempered by the presence of malignancy and weight loss, psychosis and peripheral oedema are dominant symptoms.

Diagnosis is based on the presence of increased 24-hour urinary free cortisol secretion, increased plasma cortisol and ACTH which does not reduce with a high dose dexamethasone suppression test.

In addition to treatment of the underlying malignancy, symptoms may respond to suppression of ACTH production by octreotide and or steroid synthesis by metyrapone or ketoconazole. Bilateral adrenalectomy has been used in severe resistant cases.

SIADH occurs in 1–5% of patients with SCLC with elevated ADH levels detectable in 70%. Severe hyponatraemia causes changes in mental status, lethargy and seizures.

Diagnosis relies on demonstrating reduced serum osmolality and sodium in the presence of inappropriately high urine osmolality and sodium excretion. Management with fluid restriction is usually adequate but demeclocycline (which blocks the action of ADH in the distal tubules) may be used in highly symptomatic cases.

Neurological paraneoplastic syndromes

- Found almost exclusively in SCLC and are auto-antibody mediated.
- It is useful to test for specific auto-antibodies to make a positive diagnosis which often then leads to a search for an underlying malignancy.
- If specific auto-antibodies are present they can usually be identified in serum, although CSF should also be obtained if the clinical picture is highly suggestive but the serum test is negative or there are any concerns regarding malignant involvement of the central nervous system or co-existent infective diagnoses.

Neurological syndromes and autoantibodies

Syndrome	Auto-antibody
Lambert–Eaton-myasthenic syndrome	P/Q type voltage gated calcium channel auto-ab.
Limbic encephalitis	Anti-Hu (type-1 antineuronal nuclear auto-ab.)
Cerebellar degeneration	Anti-Hu
Autonomic neuropathy	Anti-Hu
Opsiclonus/ myoclonus	Anti-Hu
Retinopathy	Retinal protein auto-ab.
Sensory-motor peripheral neuropathy	Anti CV2 auto-ab.

Lambert–Eaton myasthenic syndrome is the most common of the paraneoplastic neurological phenomena.

- Auto-antibodies to voltage gated calcium channels block acetylcholine release at the neuromuscular junction resulting in proximal muscle weakness, reduced tendon reflexes and autonomic dysfunction.
- Weakness tends be worse in the lower limbs and transiently improves following repeated exertion (in contrast to myasthenia gravis).

- Small cell lung cancer presenting with LEMS has a better prognosis, probably due to its earlier detection.
- Severely disabled patients may require plasma exchange or IV immunoglobulins while oncological treatment is initiated. The other antibody mediated neurological syndromes do not respond to these measures.

Key points

- Paraneoplastic syndromes do not independently preclude curative surgery.
- Most respond to conventional treatment of the underlying neoplasm.

Other recognised paraneoplastic syndromes in lung cancer:

Haematological
- Anaemia
- Leukaemoid reactions
- Thrombocytosis
- Disseminated intravascular coagulation

Renal
- Glomerulonephritis
- Nephrotic syndrome

Cutaneous
- Hypertrichosis languinosa
- Erythema multiforme
- Tylosis
- Acanthosis nigricans
- Pruritus
- Erythroderma

Endocrine and metabolic
- Hypoglycaemia
- Hyperthyroidism
- FSH/LH secretion
- Lactic acidosis
- Hyperuricaemia
- Carcinoid
- Syndrome
- Gynaecomastia

Connective tissue
- Dermatomyositis
- Polymyositis
- Vasculitis
- SLE

Further reading

Anderson NE, Rosenblum MK, Graus F, et al. Autoantibodies in paraneoplastic syndromes associated with small-cell lung cancer. Neurology 1988; **38**: 1391–1398.

Beckles MA. Spiro SG. Colice GL, et al. Initial evaluation of the patient with lung cancer. Symptoms, signs, laboratory tests and paraneoplastic syndromes. Chest 2003; **123**: 1.

Marra A. Eberhardt W. Pottgen C, et al. Induction chemotherapy, concurrent chemoradiation and surgery for Pancoast tumour. Eur Respir J 2007; **29**(1): 117–126.

Rowell, NP. Gleeson, FV. Steroids, radiotherapy, chemotherapy and stents for superior vena caval obstruction in carcinoma of the bronchus: a systematic review. Clinical Oncol 2002; **14**: 338–351.

13.3 Work-up of patients with a suspected diagnosis of lung cancer

Overview

Most patients with lung cancer have advanced disease by the time of diagnosis, limiting the treatment options and prognosis. Early identification and referral of high risk individuals may improve the outlook for a proportion of patients. Treatment options are more varied and complex than in the past and depend on accurate assessment of disease stage and fitness for radical therapies. Multi-Disciplinary Lung Cancer Teams are, for these reasons, now at the core of the management of patients with lung cancer.

Risk factors

The major risk factors for the development of lung cancer are:

- Smoking (current or past).
- Age over 50 years.
- The presence of COPD.
- Previous exposure to asbestos.
- Previous history of head and neck and/or bladder cancer.
- Family history of lung cancer occurring under 50 years of age in a first degree relative.

Symptoms

In its early stages lung cancer usually causes little in the way of symptoms; tumours can grow to a considerable size before patients seek medical advice. Screening of asymptomatic individuals is, as yet, of unproven value and is not likely to become routinely available in the foreseeable future. It is essential, therefore, that clinicians develop a high level of awareness of the early symptoms of the disease, the risk profile of their patients and understand the fact that curative treatment is more likely to be possible the earlier patients are referred to a specialist team. The commonest symptoms are:

- Haemoptysis.
- Cough.
- Breathlessness.
- Chest and/or shoulder pain.
- Weight loss.
- Hoarseness.
- Fatigue.

Many of these symptoms are non-specific and their onset is often gradual. The situation is made more complex because many smokers put down these early symptoms to the effects of smoking itself. It is important to remember that it is not only new symptoms that are of importance, but *changes* in chronic symptoms, such as cough.

Referral and CXR

The factors listed above have been encapsulated into guidelines for the referral of patients with suspected lung cancer by NICE. All patients where there is any suspicion of a diagnosis of lung cancer should have a plain chest X-ray. The vast majority of CXRs are abnormal in patients presenting with symptoms of lung cancer, but around 10% are normal, so it is important to remember that a normal CXR does not exclude the diagnosis. All patients should be referred for their work-up to a rapid access clinic run by a specialist Multi-Disciplinary Lung Cancer Team.

Further investigation

Blood tests

There is currently no reliable tumour marker for lung cancer. Biochemical abnormalities are relatively common and the most important include:

- Hyponatraemia (resulting from inappropriate ADH secretion and seen in both non-small cell and small cell lung cancers).
- Hypercalcaemia (resulting from either bony metastases and the ectopic secretion of parathormone-like substances; more common in squamous cell carcinomas).
- Elevated alkaline phosphatase and lactate dehydrogenase (non-specific but associated with a poorer prognosis).
- Hypokalaemic alkalosis (resulting from ectopic ACTH secretion and strongly associated with small cell lung cancer).

Mild normochromic anaemia and leukocytosis are common and a leuco-erythroblastic anaemia can indicate bone marrow involvement.

CT scanning

A CT scan is the basic imaging modality for the diagnosis of lung cancer after the initial plain CXR and all but moribund patients should have a contrast-enhanced, staging CT scan of the thorax and upper abdomen (see Figs. 13.3.1–13.3.3). CT reports should include an assessment of the stage of disease.

A CT scan should be carried out wherever possible, *prior to any invasive investigation*. This is in order to reduce the number of diagnostic tests by maximising the yield from tests such as bronchoscopy.

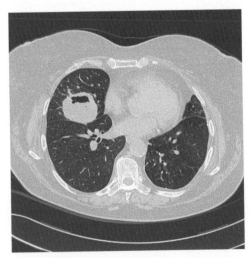

Fig. 13.3.1 CT scan (lung window) showing cavitating squamous cell tumour right lower lobe (see Plate 8).

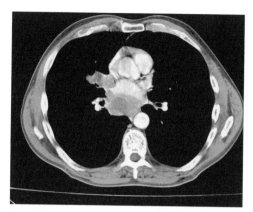

Fig. 13.3.2 CT scan (mediastinal window) showing bulky mediastinal and right hilar lymphadenopathy in a patient with small cell carcinoma.

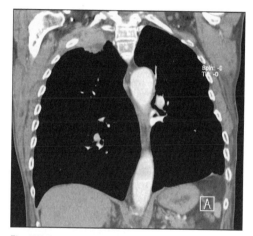

Fig. 13.3.3 CT scan: sagittal reconstruction showing right apical (Pancoast) tumour invading into chest wall.

Tissue diagnosis and staging

Wherever possible the method of biopsy should be chosen to arrive both at a tissue diagnosis of the tumour and the stage of the disease. To achieve this, the site of the most advanced disease that is amenable to biopsy should be targeted. The various biopsy options are listed below in the order of priority broadly in line with this principle:

- Biopsy of a metastasis (e.g. skin, liver).
- Diagnostic pleural tap or image-guided pleural biopsy in patients with a pleural effusion.
- Biopsy of supra-clavicular lymph nodes either by:
  - Needle biopsy of palpable nodes or
  - Ultrasound guided FNA biopsy of impalpable nodes (present in approximately 50% of patients with bulky N2/N3 disease on CT scanning (see Fig. 13.3.4).

- Biopsy of mediastinal lymph nodes. Options include:
  - Transbronchial needle aspiration (TBNA) using a Wang needle via a flexible bronchoscope. *Accessible nodes:* sub-carinal, some pre-tracheal.
  - Endobronchial ultrasound (EBUS) (see Fig. 13.3.5). *Accessible nodes:* sub-carinal, pre-tracheal, hilar.
  - Endoscopic ultrasound (EUS). Accessible nodes: inferior pulmonary ligament, AP window, sub-carinal.
  - Surgical mediastinoscopy or mediastinotomy.
- Bronchoscopy with endobronchial biopsy.
- CT guided needle biopsy of pulmonary mass (Fig. 13.3.6).
- Open surgical biopsy with frozen section (with the option of proceeding to resection).

NB: *sputum cytology is now considered of little value in the diagnosis of lung cancer and should not be used routinely. It may be useful in a small proportion of patients unfit for other, more invasive, investigations.*

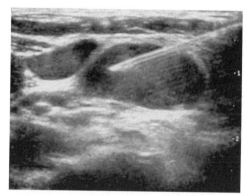

Fig. 13.3.4 US image of FNA in deep cervical lymph.

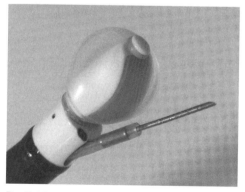

Fig. 13.3.5 Operational tip of an Endobronchial Ultrasound Bronchoscope (EBUS) (Image courtesy of Dr Robert Rintoul).

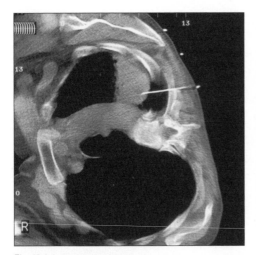

Fig. 13.3.6 CT-guided needle biopsy.

Other imaging modalities

Positron emission tomography (PET) scanning

PET scanning is a form of metabolic imaging which relies on the ability of malignant tissues to take up radiolabelled glucose. The label that is used in lung cancer is ^{5}Fluoro-deoxyglucose (^{5}FDG) which, unlike glucose itself, once phosphorylated, is not further metabolised within the malignant cells. This allows an image to be taken of ^{5}FDG uptake in the cells. PET scanning with ^{5}FDG is non-specific in that many inflammatory disorders will also take up the isotope. In the context of lung cancer this means that differential diagnoses such as tuberculosis, sarcoidosis and other granulomatous diseases can lead to false positive results as can inflammatory causes of mediastinal lymphad-enopathy such as the post-obstructive pneumonias seen in lung cancer. PET scanning is now usually combined with CT scanning to give accurate anatomical correlation of the areas of ^{5}FDG uptake and a typical PET-CT image is shown in Fig. 13.3.7. PET-CT scanning has a greater sensitivity and specificity than CT scanning alone for the assessment of enlarged mediastinal lymph nodes and can also detect unsuspected metastatic disease in around 10% of patients otherwise suitable for radical treatment. Most of the published evidence for the value of PET scanning in lung cancer is in NSCLC and its role in the management of SCLC is not well defined.

The indications for PET scanning in NSCLC include:

- In the final staging of all patients potentially suitable for radical treatment including:
  - surgical resection
  - radical radiotherapy
  - combination chemo-radiotherapy
- In the assessment of some indeterminate pulmonary nodules
- To assess the response after primary chemotherapy or radiotherapy in patients being considered for radical second-line treatments

PET scanning is unreliable for the detection of cerebral metastases.

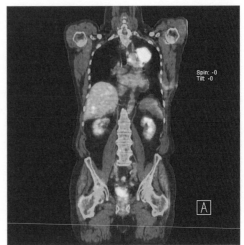

Fig. 13.3.7 PET CT scan showing increased ^{5}FDG uptake in left upper lobe mass and an unsuspected solitary liver metastasis (see Plate 9).

CT and MRI scanning of the brain

Cerebral metastases are common in lung cancer, particularly as the disease progresses. There is no good evidence to recommend routine imaging of the brain in all patients, though some centres carry it out routinely prior to surgery in addition to a PET scan. Certainly a brain scan should be carried out if there is the slightest hint from the history or examination that the patient may have a cerebral metastasis. MRI scanning has a better level of sensitivity and specificity and it the scanning modality of choice if available (see Fig. 13.3.8).

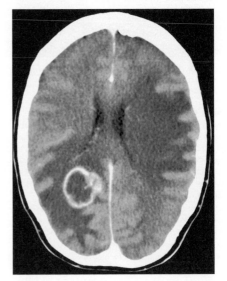

Fig. 13.3.8 CT brain showing ring enhancement of a cerebral metastasis on the right and cerebral oedema adjacent to a left sided metastasis (not itself shown in this image).

Isotope bone scanning

The skeleton is also a common site for metastasis in lung cancer. PET scanning will detect bony metastases of any significant size, but in patients with bone pain who do not require a PET scan for any other reason, an Isotope Bone Scan is useful both for confirming metastatic disease as the source of the pain and for detecting occult bony metastases which may need treatment to prevent pathological fractures.

Staging systems

Small cell lung cancer

CLC is usually staged using the Veteran's Association 1973 classification which divides cases into the following descriptive groups:

- Limited disease: tumour limited to one hemithorax with regional lymph node metastases including hilar, ipsilateral or contralateral mediastinal nodes and/or supraclavicular node involvement.
- Extensive disease: tumour beyond the confines of limited disease.

Assessment of fitness for treatment

Performance status

The functional status or performance status (PS) of a lung cancer patient is central to the assessment their fitness for chemotherapy and radical radiotherapy and is a powerful predictor of survival. It is defined as 'a measure of how well a patient is able to perform ordinary tasks and carry out daily activities'. The commonest scoring system in use in the UK is that proposed by the WHO which is divided into the categories shown in Table 13.3.1:

Table 13.3.1 The WHO PS scoring system

Score	Description
0	Fully active, able to carry on all pre-disease performance without restriction
1	Restricted in physically strenuous activity, but ambulatory and able to carry out work of a light and sedentary nature (e.g. light house work, office work)
2	Ambulatory and capable of all self-care but unable to carry out any work activities. Up and about more than 50% of waking hours.
3	Capable of only limited self-care, confined to bed or chair more than 50% of waking hours.
4	Completely disabled. Cannot carry on any self-care. Totally confined to bed or chair.

Patients with a PS of 0 or 1 are usually considered good candidates for chemotherapy, those with PS 2 as borderline and those with a PS of 3 or 4 unfit for anything but palliative treatments.

Co-morbidities and fitness for surgery

The median age at diagnosis of patients with lung cancer in the UK is 71 years and this, combined with the high prevalence of a history of cigarette smoking means that co-morbidities are common. In particular COPD and ischaemic heart disease commonly make the diagnosis staging and treatment of this patient group more complicated.

The single most important investigation is the FEV_1. In general, the patient may be considered for a pneumonectomy if the FEV_1 is more than 2 litres and for a lobectomy if more than 1.5 litres. At levels lower than these, further assessment of the pulmonary function is usually required and may include one or more of the following:

- Full lung volumes (ideally using helium dilution and body plethysmography).
- Gas diffusion capacity.
- Arterial blood gases.
- An assessment of exercise capacity (which may include formal exercise testing).
- Quantitative perfusion lung scanning.

For the assessment of cardiac fitness there may be the requirement for echocardiography and/or coronary angiography.

Multi-disciplinary team (MDT) working

As stated earlier in the chapter, the complexity of modern diagnosis, staging and treatment means that no one individual specialist has all the skills and experience to properly assess the needs of a lung cancer patient. The MDT is the way that such expertise and complex decision-making is now organised and the management of all lung cancer patients should be decided within that forum.

Patient information and support

Because of the complexity and relative speed of the modern work-up of lung cancer patients, they and their carers require careful verbal and written information and support throughout the care pathway. They usually meet a number of different doctors along the way and the lung cancer Specialist Nurses are in the best position to identify and provide the timely support that is required over this difficult time.

Further reading

British Thoracic Society & Society of Cardiothoracic Surgeons of Great Britain and Ireland. BTS guidelines on the selection of patients with lung cancer for surgery. *Thorax* 2001; **56**(2):89–108.

Kumaran M, Benamore R E, Vaidhyanath R, *et al.* Ultrasound guided cytological aspiration of supraclavicular lymph nodes in patients with suspected lung cancer. *Thorax*, 2005; **60**: 229–233.

National Institute for Clinical Excellence. Diagnosis and treatment of lung cancer. London, 2005. Available at: www.nice.org.uk

National Institute for Healthcare and Clinical Excellence. Referral for suspected cancer. London, 2005. Available at: www.nice.org.uk

13.4 Treatment of non-small cell lung cancer

Introduction

Patients with NSCLC tend to present with advanced disease and it therefore remains a disease with poor prognosis, as shown by Fig. 13.4.1.

Treatment selection is dependent on staging and patient performance status and is best discussed at a multidisciplinary meeting. The staging system for lung cancer has up to now been based on a single centre's experience of around 5000 cases. It has now been completely re-mapped by the International Association for the study of Lung Cancer (IASLC), a worldwide collaboration from 20 countries and 45 different centres to include data from more than 100,000 cases with all stages of presentation of lung cancer. Table 13.4.1 summarizes the new clasification and Table 13.4.2 the new stage groupings.

Table 13.4.1 IASLC staging project: TNM staging

cTNM Clinical Classification	
Primary tumour (T-factor)	
TX	Primary tumour cannot be assessed, or tumour proven by the presence of malignant cells in sputum or bronchial washings but not visualized by imaging or bronchoscopy
T0	No evidence of primary tumour
TIS	Carcinoma in situ
T1	Tumour 3 cm or less in greatest dimension, surrounded by lung or visceral pleura, without bronchoscopic evidence of invasion more proximal than the lobar bronchus (i.e. not in the main bronchus)
T1a	Tumour 2 cm or less in greatest dimension
T1b	Tumour more than 2 cm but not more than 3 cm in greatest dimension
T2	Tumour more than 3 cm but not more than 7 cm; or tumour with any of the following features*: • Involves main bronchus, 2 cm or more distal to the carina • Invades visceral pleura • Associated with atelectasis or obstructive pneumonitis that extends to the hilar region but does not involve the entire lung
T2a	Tumour more than 3 cm but not more than 5 cm in greatest dimension
T2b	Tumour more than 5 cm but not more than 7 cm in greatest dimension
*T2 tumours with these features are classified T2a if 5 cm or less	
T3	Tumour more than 7 cm or one that directly invades any of the following: chest wall (including superior sulcus tumours), diaphragm, phrenic nerve, mediastinal pleura, parietal pericardium; or tumour in the main bronchus less than 2 cm distal to the carina but without involvement of the carina; or associated atelectasis or obstructive pneumonitis of the entire lung or separate tumour nodule(s) in the same lobe
T4	Tumour of any size that invades any of the following: mediastinum, heart, great vessels, trachea, recurrent laryngeal nerve, oesophagus, vertebral body, carina; separate tumour nodule(s) in a different ipsilateral lobe
Regional lymph nodes (N-factor)	
NX	Regional lymph nodes cannot be assessed
N0	No regional lymph node metastasis
N1	Metastasis in ipsilateral peribronchial and/or ipsilateral hilar lymph nodes and intrapulmonary nodes, including involvement by direct extension
N2	Metastasis in ipsilateral mediastinal and/or subcarinal lymph node(s)
N3	Metastasis in contralateral mediastinal, contralateral hilar, ipsilateral or contralateral scalene, or supraclavicular lymph node(s)
Distant metastasis (M-factor)	
MX	Distant metastasis cannot be assessed
M0	No distant metastasis
M1	Distant metastasis
M1a	Separate tumour nodule(s) in a contralateral lobe; tumour with pleural nodules or malignant pleural (or pericardial) effusion
M1b	Distant metastasis

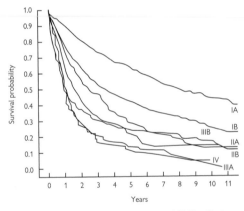

Fig. 13.4.1 Survival curves of NSCLC stages I–IV. Classification from Mountain *et al.* 1997.

Table 13.4.2 IASLC staging project: Stage Grouping

Occult carcinoma	TX N0 M0
Stage 0	Tis N0 M0
Stage IA	T1a, b N0 M0
Stage IB	T2a N0 M0
Stage IIA	T1a, b N1 M0
	T2a N1 M0
	T2b N0 M0
Stage IIB	T2b N1 M0
	T3 N0 M0
Stage IIIA	T1, T2 N2 M0
	T3 N1, N2 M0
	T4 N0, N1 M0
Stage IIIB	T4 N2 M0
	Any T N3 M0
Stage IV	Any T Any N M1

Table 13.4.3 Treatment of NSCLC by stage (from NICE guidelines 2005)

	Stage I	Stage II	Stage IIIA	Stage IIIB	Stage IV WHO 0–1	Stage IV WHO 2	Stage IV WHO >2
Surgery alone							
Radiotherapy followed by surgery							
Surgery followed by radiotherapy							
Preoperative chemotherapy then surgery	a	a	a				
Surgery followed by chemotherapy							
Surgery then chemo- and radiotherapy		a	a				
Radical radiotherapy							
Chemotherapy and radical radiotherapy							
Chemotherapy						a	
Symptomatic treatment/ palliative radiotherapy							
Key							

	First choice for eligible patients
	Suitable for some patients
	Not recommended
a	Unless within a clinical trial

NICE have provided extensive guidelines for the management of lung cancer (February 2005). Their recommendations for treatment according to stage are summarised in Table 13.4.3.

Surgery

Surgery offers the best chance of cure in patients with resectable disease. Typically this is in patients with stage I or II NSCLC but surgery is also sometimes indicated in more locally advanced disease.

Stage I disease (T1a,b,N0,M0) or (T2a,N0,M0)

- Surgery is the primary treatment choice, aiming for clear surgical margins and with curative intent.
- Mortality (death within 30 days of surgery) for all forms of pulmonary resection is 3.5% (systemic review of 16 studies; n = 41105), with a trend for increasing mortality with increasing age.
- Morbidity is 30% (higher for those with more extensive resections.)
- Following successful resection mean five-year survival for stage IA is 69% and for stage IB is 52%.

Choice of operation

- Lobectomy is the procedure of choice (30-day mortality 3%).
- VATs lobectomy appears to be comparable to conventional open lobectomy with potential lower morbidity and mortality.
- More limited resection may be preferable if lung function is very impaired e.g. segmental resection (complete removal of a bronchopulmonary segment) or wedge resection (involving suturing or stapling across non anatomical planes). This can be either via thoracotomy or VATs procedure.
- Further studies comparing limited resection to lobectomy and VATs versus open thoracotomy are required. However local recurrence is commoner with wedge resection than with lobectomy. Distant recurrence can also be commoner if nodal dissection and staging are not done at segmental resection.

Stage II A and B disease (see Table 13.4.2)

- These patients should be considered for surgical resection with curative intent (although no RCTs have compared surgery v other modalities).
- These tumours make up 15–25% of resected cancers.
- Mean five-year survival is 45% for stage IIA and 33% for stage IIB with a survival advantage between 2 and 19% for T1 versus T2, (although larger tumours (T2b) do worse than smaller masses and are now closer in survival outcome to stage III than II A). T3N0 survival is around 44% at 5 years.
- Sleeve lobectomy is an additional approach in centrally located tumours when lung function makes pneumonectomy hazardous. This procedure is especially useful for right upper lobe tumours that encroach onto the main bronchus, as they allow a cross sectional piece of airway plus the right upper lobe to be removed and the upper and lower margins of the main airway are then reanastomosed. Studies have indicated comparable mortality and long-term outcome.

Stage III A disease

- T3 disease or T1, T2 with mediastinal node involvement makes up about 10% of resected patients with NSCLC.
- This stage covers several presentations of lung cancer and making comparisons of results between centres more difficult.
- Completeness of resection and lymph node status influence outcome significantly. Prognosis seems to be worse when mediastinal structures are involved although there have been very few studies considering outcome based on particular structures involved.

Stage III A is a less heterogeneous group now that T3N0 is classified as II B

- Outcome is particularly influenced by nodal status and many with bulky N2 disease will be considered unresectable.
- Surgery alone in those staged at IIIA preoperatively is associated with a relatively poor prognosis and such

patients require careful evaluation by the lung cancer MDT.

- Overall only 25% will be completely resectable and five year survival in those who are macroscopically completely resected is less than 25%.
- Some studies have looked at outcome of complete resection following positive mediastinoscopy versus negative mediastinoscopy with the latter doing better (five year survival 33% compared to 8-31%).
- Patients with negative staging tests but microscopic involvement of the mediastinal lymph nodes found in the pathological specimen after resection may have a five year survival of up to 40%.

Stage IIIB

- This incorporates patients with N2/3 disease and T4 tumours (trachea, carina, SVC, aorta, oesophagus, vertebral bodies) that are generally considered to be inoperable.
- One exception to this is patients with carinal disease in which resections can be performed by resecting the carina and rejoining the main bronchi to the lower trachea. There is little data in this area but one systemic review of 8 series (n = 322) showed mortality of 18%, and 5-year survival of 27%.

Mediastinal lymph node sampling at time of surgery

All patients undergoing surgical resection should have systematic lymph node sampling to provide accurate pathological staging. It is not yet clear whether radical mediastinal lymphadenectomy or lymph node sampling offer any survival advantage over each other. There is little evidence that it does.

Pre-operative assessment

Whilst surgery offers the only realistic chance for cure, some patients are unable to tolerate lung resection. Pre-operative physiological assessment to predict post-operative lung function is therefore vital and is discussed in the section on the work up of lung cancer (Chapter 13.3).

Post-operative complications

- Factors predisposing to postoperative problems include smoking prior to surgery, COPD, diminished health status, poor nutritional status, advanced age and obesity.
- The length of the surgical procedure increases morbidity, with operations lasting more than 3 hours being the critical cut off.
- Surgical complications include: injuries to the recurrent laryngeal and phrenic nerves, broncho-pleural fistula, empyema and wound infection.
- Early complications following thoracotomy are: pulmonary atelectasis, nosocomial infections, respiratory failure and/or persistent hypoxia, pulmonary embolism, aspiration pneumonia, acute lung injury and cardiac arrhythmias.

Post-operative mortality

- Post-operative mortality following thoracotomy is high. In large studies it is ~5% at 30 days and 8% at 60 days, with a higher death rate for men than women.
- Mortality is higher for those over 70 years of age.
- In general mortality increases with disease stage, with a mortality of 1–3% for those undergoing lobectomy for stage 1 disease.
- The major causes of death are pneumonia, respiratory failure and cardiac events.

- In a large series of patients undergoing pneumonectomy at the Mayo Clinic cardiopulmonary complications occurred in 38% of patients. Factors which adversely affected morbidity were age, male sex, associated respiratory or cardiovascular disease, smoking, decreased vital capacity and/or FEV_1, reduced carbon monoxide single breath gas transfer factor, bronchial stump reinforcement, crystalloid infusion and blood transfusion. Mortality was 4.6%, and factors that predisposed to death were cardiovascular disease, haematological disease, pre-operative chemotherapy (not so in other studies), low haemoglobin, low gas transfer and a right-sided pneumonectomy.

Radiotherapy

Radical radiotherapy as sole treatment

Radiotherapy has disappointed as a curative modality. For it to be successful the entire tumour volume (and any known metastatic disease) has to be encompassed within the treatment field. However most of the earlier studies relied on CXRs to establish disease extent. Today, the use of CT and PET scanners allows more precise staging and therefore better patient selection. It also allows more sophisticated targeting of radiotherapy and therefore higher doses to be more safely given

Radical treatments incorporate at least 45 Gray (Gy) in 2 Gy fractions daily to the primary site. Studies using conformal radiotherapy equipment can increase safe delivery to 75 or 80 Gy. This has improved the local control of the cancer but the commonest cause of relapse is the appearance of distant metastatic disease.

Indications

Stage 1 and II

- Radiotherapy is indicated in those who are 'medically inoperable' either because they are unfit for surgery or they decline it.
- There have not yet been studies directly comparing radical radiotherapy to surgery, palliative radiotherapy or no treatment.
- Overall survival post radical radiotherapy from numerous studies has shown a 1-year survival of about 70%, 2-year at 45%, 5-year at 17% (compared to 3-year survival of 0% with no treatment).
- There are very few studies comparing radiotherapy to surgery in comparable patients for obvious ethical reasons but those available show surgery to offer at least double the chances of cure. However it is likely that those in the radiotherapy arms of such studies were less aggressively staged and also tended to be sicker and older than their surgical counterparts.

Stage IIIA and IIIB

- As for Stage I and II disease, radical radiotherapy for stage IIIA and B has been disappointing.
- Two-year survival ranges from 12.5 to 24% (compared to 0–4% for untreated disease) and 5-year survival from 0–17%
- Outcome is more associated with disease bulk than stage. For example a small T4,N0 tumour may have a better prognosis than more bulky early stage disease, which may involve too large a field to be safely irradiated.
- The presence of supraclavicular or contralateral hilar nodal involvement or pleural effusions would make patients ineligible for radical radiotherapy.

Continuous hyperfractionated accelerated radiotherapy (CHART)

This has been a major potential advance for the administration of radiotherapy. In a large randomised trial of CHART versus daily conventional radical radiotherapy showed a significant survival advantage for the experimental arm, especially for squamous cell cancers, both for lung and head and neck tumours. Treatment was given 3 times daily for 3 days at a rate of 1.5Gy every 8 hours to a total of 54Gy. However this study has never been repeated and what might have become a treatment changing moment has been lost because of the difficulty of radiotherapy units getting staff to cover the weekends necessary for treatment and finding sufficient patient numbers to make it more economically viable.

Studies have now assessed CHARTWELL, i.e. CHART with weekend leave, and results may be comparable to the original trial, but it remains a technique in danger of being abandoned.

Combination of radiotherapy with chemotherapy

Given that the main reason for treatment failure is distant relapse, radiotherapy is now being combined with chemotherapy. There have been several trials assessing the ideal timing of the two modalities, either sequential with radiotherapy following chemotherapy, or concurrent, with chemotherapy starting at the commencement of radiotherapy. This timing question has not been adequately answered yet, although concurrent treatment looks more promising.

Neo-adjuvant radiotherapy

There is no evidence that preoperative radiotherapy confers any survival advantage in NSCLC. It in fact may make surgery technically harder due to tissue fibrosis.

Adjuvant radiotherapy

Again, there is no evidence that postoperative radiotherapy has any role. A large meta-analysis has shown that it may infact be harmful. Much of the data considered came from studies between 1960 and 90, and critics raise the problems of inadequate staging, however a more recent meta-analysis produced similar results, in particular suggesting that adjuvant radiotherapy conferred a worse survival than no treatment post resection. For stage IIA disease, the possible role of adjuvant radiotherapy seems less harmful, but confers no survival advantage.

Assessing suitability for radiotherapy

All patients should undergo lung function tests, including lung volumes and gas transfer factor. No minimum values for adequate lung function for the size of planned radiotherapy field have been set and oncologists exercise clinical judgement in this assessment. In patients with FEV_1 <1.0L radical radiotherapy is only suitable if the amount of normal lung irradiated is small. Patients should be strongly encouraged to stop smoking. Patients with poorer performance status do less well and treatment is not usually recommended in those with performance status of WHO classification of 2 or more (see Table 13.4.4). Weight loss prior to treatment is associated with poorer outcome. Increasing age does not appear to affect outcome.

Complications

Early complications include: oesophagitis (if the mediastinum is included in the field), skin reactions, pericarditis and, rarely, acute pneumonitis. Late complications include chronic pulmonary fibrosis and late oesophageal strictures.

There have been few studies documenting treatment related morbidity and quality of life.

Palliative radiotherapy

Radiotherapy remains excellent treatment for many of the manifestations of lung cancer as the natural history progresses:

• Provides relief from haemoptysis in 80% of cases.

• Relieves breathlessness from occlusion of large airways in 60%.

• Effective in treating enlarged lymph nodes, skin and bony metastases.

• For most cases a single fraction of 8Gy has been shown to be as effective as longer higher dose courses, making only a single outpatient visit necessary. The same applies to pain from bony metastases, where one or two fractions a week apart are effective in up to 80% of sufferers.

Brain metastases: most early symptoms are due to cerebral oedema and if these resolve dramatically with steroids, radiotherapy tends to maintain this improvement for a few months. In those who respond poorly to initial steroids, the effects of radiotherapy appear less convincing.

SVCO: radiotherapy may not relieve the symptoms if they have been established for some weeks; stenting the SVC is often more effective. If, however the SVCO is treated early, radiotherapy can provide good control. Usually at least 20Gy in 5 fractions are needed.

Chemotherapy

General indications

The main role of chemotherapy is in patients with advanced disease (stage IIIB and IV). Here chemotherapy can provide symptom relief, improve disease control, better quality of life and increase survival. However, only about a third of patients with this stage of disease are fit enough to receive systemic treatment. NICE have estimated that 1000–5000 patients receive chemotherapy each year yet over 16,000 patients are eligible in terms of disease stage to receive it.

Chemotherapy is generally fairly well tolerated and given on an outpatient basis. A performance status of 0–1 is recommended as these obtain the highest response rates and longer disease-free survival than those with performance status of 2 or worse (see Table 13.5.1, p. 298). Those with poor performance status have a lower response rate, shorter periods of disease control and a higher incidence of Grade 3 or 4 toxicity and risk of treatment related death.

Other poor prognostic factors for patients with NSCLC receiving chemotherapy include male sex, metastases, increased LDH, >5% weight loss and patients >65 years of age.

Second-generation agents

Most important are the platinum based agents such as carboplatin and cisplatin. Their use, in combination with one or two other drugs, has been shown to increase median survival by 1.8 and 4.5 months (Cancer Care Ontario Practice Guideline initiative: four meta-analyses and eight randomised trials). There is significant symptom relief associated with treatment even in the absence of tumour shrinkage, but different trials have shown varying results for quality of life with either no change or an improvement. The platins are associated with side effects of nausea and myelosuppression. Nausea is improved by co administration of antiemetics and intravenous fluids. Carboplatin offers some advantage over cisplatin in that it can be used in patients with poorer renal function and without prehydration. A recent meta-analysis, however, appears to show some survival advantage with cisplatin compared to carboplatin. Survival benefit with cisplatin may be most important in ERCC1 (a DNA repair protein) negative tumours, although more evidence is awaited. Other second line agents include ifosfamide, vinblastine, vindesine, and mitomycin C. Successful regimens have included cisplatin, mitomycin C and a vinca alkaloid.

Third-generation drugs

Gemcitabine, paclitaxel, vinorelbine and docetaxel alone or in a two-drug combination, usually with a platin, have activity against NSCLC. To date trials have not demonstrated any clear advantage of any of these agents over another. NICE guidelines suggest that optimum treatment is a single third-generation drug in combination with a platin. Patients who cannot tolerate platinum based agents should be offered single agent chemotherapy with a third-generation drug. However several studies have compared platinum based regimens to two other second-generation agents and no platin with no significant differences in survival. There is also no evidence that three-drug combinations are any better for survival than two-drug combinations.

The appropriate length of therapy is generally agreed to be 4 cycles, provided there is a response, or at least stable disease after the initial 2. More than 4 courses hardly affects response and increases toxicity.

Second-line chemotherapy

Docetaxel is the recommended agent for second-line treatment. When compared to best supportive care there was a 1-year survival benefit (1-year survival 29% compared to 19%) as well as improved quality of life.

Biological agents

Epidermal growth factor receptor antagonists

EGFR, a receptor tyrosine kinase, is frequently over expressed in NSCLC and plays an important part in tumour cell survival. Two agents have been studied thoroughly in NSCLC, Iressa® (gefitinib); and Tarceva®, (erlotinib). Initial studies with gefitinib showed that when given with initial chemotherapy, there was no benefit for adding the EGFR antagonist. Activity for both agents has only been demonstrated to date if the drug is given after relapse following 1–4 chemotherapy regimens. The most promising study (BR21) from Canada randomised patients with performance status 0–2 at relapse to erlotinib or placebo and showed improved median overall survival from 4.7 to 6.7 months with better quality of life in those given erlotinib. A subsequent trial in a larger group of relapsed patients randomised to gefitinib or placebo only showed trends to a prolonged survival with the active agent. Subgroup analyses in both trials showed significant improvement in survival in Asian patients, especially women, those with adenocarcinomas and in non-smokers.

Separate studies have shown dramatic responses to these agents when patients have somatic mutations in the EGFR gene, also seen most commonly in non-smokers and East Asian patients. However, despite these encouraging responses, patients almost always relapse within a few months. The overall importance of patients EGFR expressions status

and mutation level needs resolving. The potential role of these agents as first-line monotherapy in patients with poor performance status, or as maintenance chemotherapy needs to be explored.

VEGF inhibitor (bevacizumab)

VEGF is important in angiogenesis of tumours. This monoclonal antibody that been shown to increased median survival from 10 to 12.5 months when given in combination with standard chemotherapy for NSCLC. Squamous cell cancers were excluded from the trial due to increased incidence of bleeding complications in this group.

Combination treatment

It is hoped that combination treatment might improve outcome compared to treatment with surgery or radiotherapy alone. There is evidence from other tumour types that combination treatments may be of use. They can take three main forms:

Adjuvant chemotherapy/radiotherapy: cisplatin-based adjuvant chemotherapy can produce a significant survival benefit of 5.3% after curative resection – can we add the stage i.e is Ia and 2 the same benefit? Several studies have reported similar findings and post operative chemotherapy (probably 3 courses of a platinum containing regimen) will become the new standard.

Neoadjuvant chemotherapy: there is some evidence to suggest that preoperative chemotherapy improves survival in early stage NSCLC. There have only been 2 large trials addressing this issue, but a meta-analysis has suggested up to a 5% advantage for neoadjuvant chemotherapy. There is no evidence that chemotherapy increases peri-operative complications, or adds to post-operative mortality. The studies have not contained enough patients to ascertain whether the benefits are greater for early or later stage resectable patients. Three courses of platin based chemotherapy are recommended.

Combined chemoradiotherapy (for patients eligible for radical radiotherapy, with treatments given either sequentially or concurrently). Primary concurrent cisplatin-based chemoradiotherapy for inoperable stage III NSCLC increases survival compared to radiotherapy alone, but can be accompanied by an increase risk of adverse effects. The effects on quality of life are not known. The present standard of care for patients with stage III NSCLC and good performance status (0–1) is sequential chemoradiotherapy. By comparison, in primary chemotherapy, treatment is given in the hope that there will be a tumour response and downstaging of their disease to allow them to proceed to curative surgery or radical radiotherapy.

Lung cancer follow-up

Follow-up depends on the treatment given and disease stage. It is important the follow-up plan is clearly communicated to the patient at each stage.

- Following surgery patients are seen 3-monthly for 2 years and then 6-monthly for up to 5 years. There is no evidence of benefit from follow-up beyond 5 years in those who remain disease-free. Two studies have shown no difference in survival with routine compared to symptom led follow up whilst one has shown better survival in those patients followed up regularly.

- Following radical radiotherapy there should be 9 months of close follow-up with regular CXRs to treat any pneumonitis, identify need for further treatment and assess prognosis. Again there is no evidence of benefit of follow-up beyond five years.

- Follow-up after chemotherapy is determined by anticipated toxicity of treatment, usually of the order of every 1–2 months for the first 6 months.

Those with advanced disease will need to be seen regularly because of the potentially rapid progress of their symptoms and the likely need for palliation. There is evidence that nurse led telephone follow up can be as effective, and preferred by patients on completion of palliative therapy such as chemotherapy.

Further reading

BTS guidelines on the selection of patients with lung cancer for surgery. *Thorax* 2001; **56**: 89-108.

Gilligan D, Nicolson M, Smith I, *et al.* Preoperative chemotherapy in patients with resectable non-small cell lung cancer: results of the MRCLU22/NVALT 2/EORTC 08012 multicentre randomised trial and update of systematic review. *Lancet* 2007; **369**: 1929–37.

Goldstraw P, Crowley J, Chansky K, *et al.* The IASLC lung cancer staging project: proposal for the revision of the TNM staging groupings in the forthcoming (seventh) addition of the TNM classification of malignant tumours. *J Thorac Oncol* 2007; **8** (2): 706–14.

Mountain CF, Dresler CM. Regional lymph node classification for lung cancer staging. *Chest* 1997; **111**: 1718–1723.

NSCLC Collaborative Group. *BMJ* 1995; **311**: 899–909.

NICE guidelines for the diagnosis and treatment of lung cancer 2005.

PORT Meta-analysis Trialists Group. Postoperative radiotherapy in non small cell lung cancer; systematic review and meta-analysis of individual patient data from nine-randomized controlled trials. *Lancet* 1998; **352**: 257–263.

Saunders M, Dische S, Barett A, *et al.* Continuous hyperfractionated accelerated radiotherapy (CHART) versus conventional radiotherapy in non-small-cell lung cancer: a randomised multicentre trial. CHART Steering Committee. *Lancet* 1987; **350**(9072): 161–165.

Scullier JP. The staging of lung cancer. *European Respiratory Monograph on Thoracic Malignancies.* 3rd edn. 2009.

Doroshow JH. Targeting EGFR in non-small-cell lung cancer 2005 *NEJM*, **353**:123–132.

Schiller JH. Comparison of four chemotherapy regimens for advanced non–small-cell lung cancer. *NEJM* 2002; **346**: 92–98.

Van Rens, M. Prognostic assessment of 2,361 patients who underwent pulmonary resection for non-small cell lung cancer, stage I, II, and IIIA. *Chest* 2000; **117**(2): 374–379.

13.5 Treatment of small cell lung cancer

Approximately 20% of all lung cancers are diagnosed as small cell lung cancer (SCLC). Around 60% of these are classified as extensive stage.

Staging
The staging of SCLC has previously been more straightforward than NSCLC, with divisions only into either 'limited' or 'extensive' stage disease. However, the new IASCL staging classification (see Tables 13.4.1 and 13.4.2, p.292), when applied to SCLC does have some prognostic effects (Table 13.5.1), and although most centres are still using limited and extensive stage disease, this may change.
- *Limited stage*: disease confined to one hemithorax (including pleural effusion) plus bilateral hilar or supra-clavicular lymphadenopathy.
- *Extensive stage*: metastatic spread outside the thorax excluding hilar/ supraclavicular nodes.

Given that two-thirds have extensive stage disease on presentation further investigation for distant metastases is always indicated (the most common sites being liver, adrenal glands, brain and bone) as outlined in the following figure:

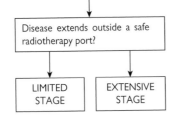

- Clinical evaluation for distant metastases
- CT of chest, liver and adrenals
- FBC/ LFTs/ U&Es /calcium
- Selected imaging of any symptomatic area

Disease extends outside a safe radiotherapy port?

LIMITED STAGE   EXTENSIVE STAGE

Fig. 13.5.1 Staging tests for small cell lung cancer

CT or MRI of the brain is not worthwhile in asymptomatic patients, unless there is weight loss of more than 5 kg.

Table 13.5.1 IASLC staging project : application of the proposed classification to the data basis cases with small cell lung cancer.

Stage	n patients	1-year survival (%)	5-year survival (%)
IA	211	77	38
IB	325	67	21
IIA	55	85	38
IIB	270	70	18
IIIA	1170	59	13
IIIB	1399	50	9
IV	4530	22	1

From Sculier JP. Staging of Lung Cancer. *European Respiratory Monograph on Thoracic Malignancies* 3rd Edition, 2009

Despite the simplicity of the staging system, there are other prognostic indicators for response to treatment and survival. For example, good prognosis is conferred by a high performance status (e.g. ECOG 0-1, see Table 13.5.1 and Chapter 13.3 for the WHO classification) and normal values for sodium, albumin and alkaline phosphatase all of which contribute independently to survival. The combination of performance status and these biochemical values can predict prognosis more closely than just dise-ase extent as determined from clinical and radiological information.

Treatment

Chemotherapy
Chemotherapy remains the mainstay of treatment in SCLC because of the tendency for the tumour to metastasise early. Eligibility for chemotherapy depends more on prognostic features, especially performance status, rather than precise stage of disease. The greatest benefits from treatment are seen in patients with the fewest adverse prognostic features. Those with worse prognostic features can still achieve symptom palliation and survival benefit, but toxicity can be higher and the risks and benefits more finely balanced.

Established poor prognostic factors include performance status ≥2 (ECOG classification), elevated LDH, extensive stage disease, and male sex.

> **KEY FACT**
> If the patient has good prognosis markers at presentation, the 3-year survival following treatment is about 15%.

The natural history of untreated SCLC results in a median survival of only 4–6 months for limited stage disease and 3 months for those with extensive stage disease. This changed with the development of single and then multiple agent chemotherapy in the late 1970s, which extended the survival figures. Initial treatment was with drugs including methotrexate, cyclophosphamide, ifosfamide, adriamycin and vinca alkaloids. By the early 1990s platinum based, two-drug combinations were shown to be as effective as first-line treatment, and easier to give. Most studies have used cisplatin rather than carboplatin and have shown survival benefits at 6 and 12 months in comparison to the older regimens.

Cycle number
Initially chemotherapy was given until a complete response was achieved, or until relapse if the response was only partial. However studies have shown 6 courses to be adequate; fewer courses caused the disease free period of responders to be shorter than after 6 treatments. Maintenance therapy, even at a reduced intensity that initial first-line treatment does not improve overall survival

Dose intensification
This has been the subject of several studies, including bone marrow harvesting followed by very intense chemotherapy. Other forms included late intensification following conventional chemotherapy, weekly treatments, or initial intensification. None of these approaches had any benefit on survival. This suggests that, although one can kill large quantities of the tumour, resistant cells remain which continue to grow and cause relapse.

Second-line chemotherapy

This is usually reserved for those patients who have had a good response to first-line treatment and at least 3 months between the best response achieved and progression. Studies have shown much more modest response rates compared to first-line treatment in SCLC although at least equivalent to first-line chemotherapy in NSCLC. However, response is usually of short duration and there is no outstanding second-line regimen to recommend. Some re-introduce the initial chemotherapy following a period of disease control of at least 1 year, others use drugs such as topotecan or an older regimen to which the patient has not been exposed.

Radiotherapy

SCLC is extremely radiosensitive and radiotherapy therefore also plays an important role in treatment in a number of ways:

Consolidation thoracic irradiation

Review of several studies suggests that this provides a median survival benefit of approximately one month and a 5% improvement in three year survival with the addition of radiotherapy to chemotherapy (19% v 14%). Many studies have shown that thoracic radiation improves control of the primary disease and therefore local symptom control. However its effect on survival is minimised by the disseminated nature of SCLC, with a subsequent high incidence of metastatic relapse. Most studies have reported on a dose range of 40Gy in 15 fractions over 3 weeks, to 50Gy in 25 fractions over 5 weeks.

The timing of the administration of thoracic radiotherapy in relation to chemotherapy has been the subject of debate. Studies have compared early administration (during the first 9 weeks of chemotherapy) to late (after 9 weeks of chemotherapy). They have studied different total doses and also different fractionation regimens including hyperfractionated accelerated radiotherapy. Whilst the latter has been shown to improve survival compared to daily administration, a review of all available studies suggests that the most important factor is getting all the intended chemotherapy to the patient in timely fashion. If this is not achieved, then the timing of the radiotherapy doesn't appear to be important. Studies of radiotherapy timing in which all the chemotherapy was given to more than 80% of the patients had a 6 months better median survival compared to those where the chemotherapy was only fully given to less than 80% of patients.

Prophylactic cranial irradiation (PCI)

This is important given the frequency of cerebral metastases in SCLC and the uncertainty of cytotoxic drugs crossing the blood brain barrier. PCI aims to eradicate microscopic disease before symptoms from brain metastases develop, and is usually most appropriate for those with limited disease who have had a complete response to primary treatment. There is evidence to suggest that this should be given fairly soon after completion of chemotherapy, rather than delayed. Studies show that PCI reduces the incidence of brain metastases, by up to 54% in some studies. A recent meta analysis of more than 900 patients receiving PCI after achieving a complete response with chemotherapy found a reduction in the relative risk of

death of 0.84 (95% CI 0.73–0.97;p = 0.01), which corresponds to a 5.4% increase in the rate of survival at 3 years. Larger doses also reduced the incidence of relapse in the brain, but no improved effect on survival. There is very little evidence pertaining to the effectiveness of PCI in those with extensive disease on survival, although it almost certainly reduces the incidence of brain metastases.

Palliative radiotherapy

As in NSCLC, radiotherapy is an excellent palliative treatment, especially for symptoms caused by relapsing disease. It provides good control of haemoptysis, large airway narrowing, bone pain, superior vena caval obstruction, painful or unsightly lymphadenopathy and skin lesions and sometimes for brain metastases. For most of these, single fractions of 7–8Gy are most effective and convenient.

Surgery

Early data suggested that surgery had no place in the management of SCLC with studies suggesting that patients fared no better than those treated by radical radiotherapy. Since the development of better staging techniques and the understanding that SCLC is often disseminated at presentation the only small cell tumours that are excised are solitary nodules diagnosed post-operatively, and carcinoid tumours in which histology obtained at fibreoptic bronchoscopy was indistinguishable from SCLC. Nevertheless there are several series of resected, genuine SCLC and in general the median survival is better than that of limited stage disease treated by chemotherapy with or without radiotherapy.

AUTHOR'S TIP

Provided optimal staging is performed on a known SCLC which looks operable by lobectomy and that staging includes careful assessment and biopsy of mediastinal nodes, patients can do well and should be considered for surgical resection.

There is less evidence that downstaging with prior chemotherapy effects cure when followed by resection. There is also no study showing any benefit for postoperative chemotherapy, as the numbers undergoing resection are too small for a randomised trial of adjuvant chemotherapy.

Further reading

Auperin A, Aupérin A, Arrigada R, Pignon J-P, et al. Prophylactic cranial irradiation for patients with small-cell lung cancer in complete remission. Prophylactic Cranial Irradiation Overview Collaborative Group. NEJM 1999; **341**(7):524–526.

Goldstraw P, Crowley J, Chansky K, et al. The IASLC lung cancer staging project: proposal for the revision of the TNM stage groupings in the forthcoming (seventh) addition of the TNM classification of malignant tumours. J Thorac Oncol 2007; **8** (2):706–14.

Pignon JP. Role of thoracic radiotherapy in limited-stage small-cell lung cancer: quantitative review based on the literature versus meta-analysis based on individual data. J Clin Oncol 1992; **11**: 1819–1820.

NICE guidelines for the diagnosis and treatment of lung cancer 2005.

Spiro S, Souhami RL, Geddes DM, et al. Duration of chemotherapy in small cell lung cancer: a Cancer Research Campaign trial. Br J Cancer 1989; **4**:578–583.

13.6 PET-CT

Background

Malignant cells are characteristically more glucose avid than non-maligant cells, and it is this that allows their detection using PET-CT scanning. They have up-regulated glucose transport receptors that increase their ability to concentrate glucose compared to normal cells. PET scanning uses this malignancy trait to increase the concentration of trapped radiolabelled deoxygenated glucose to allow detection of malignant tissue. Deoxygenated glucose is radiolabelled with 18 fluorine to make ^{18}FDG. This is injected into fasted patients. Between 40 to 60 minutes is then allowed with the patient resting before scanning, allowing intracellular uptake and concentration of ^{18}FDG and its metabolites to occur. After intracellular uptake, the ^{18}FDG fails to be fully metabolised within the cell and accumulates as ^{18}FDG-6-phosphatase (FDG-6-P). As malignant cells are more glucose and ^{18}FDG avid than nonmalignant cells the concentration of ^{18}FDG-6-P is greater in malignant than benign tissue. Of note, it also greater in other metabolically active tissue such as the heart and brain, as well as in areas of inflammation such as pneumonia, granulomatous reaction and post-radiotherapy. The ^{18}FDG-6-P undergoes decay, producing a positron which immediately collides with an electron producing two photons. These photons are produced at 180° to each other, and are detected by the PET scanner. As more are produced in areas of greater concentration of ^{18}FDG-6-P the scanner detects more photon activity in areas of malignancy and other areas of increased metabolic activity.

Technology

The advent of PET-CT has allowed the anatomic localisation of these areas with far greater precision than when PET was performed without CT. Consequently the diagnostic accuracy of PET-CT is far greater than PET alone. The ability to assess the metabolic activity of lymphadenopathy seen on CT and the increased sensitivity of PET compared to CT in most areas of the body has also resulted in PET-CT having a greater diagnostic accuracy for lung cancer than CT. The use of CT has also reduced the total scan time.

Measurement

It is also possible to quantify the degree of FDG activity seen in areas of uptake. Apart from quantification measures used in research, most reporters use the semiquantitative standardised uptake value (SUV). The SUV is reported from over a region of interest such as a lung cancer, and is calculated using the dose of ^{18}FDG injected, and the patients bodyweight. The time from injection is an important variable that is recorded to allow the measurement to be repeated on follow-up scans if necessary. Various thresholds for reporting a nodule, mass or lymph node have been used, the most common being an SUV of greater than 2.5, although subjective analysis ie whether it looks 'hot' is possibly just as effective in experienced hands.

Clinical utility in thoracic disease

1 Investigating the solitary pulmonary nodule.
2 Staging lung cancer.
3 Assessing treatment response in lung cancer.
4 Staging and assessing treatment response in mesothelioma.

1. The solitary pulmonary nodule (SPN)

SPNs detected on CXR and CT may now be investigated using PET-CT. The decision on whether to assume the SPN is benign, perform a follow-up CXR or CT, perform a biopsy, go straight to resection, or perform a PET-CT scan is dependent on patient preference and the clinical and radiographic parameters. The diagnostic accuracy of PET-CT is dependent upon:

- The size of the nodule, with nodules <1cm in diameter more likely to be false negative.
- The position of the nodule, with smaller nodules less readily characterised within the lower lobes, due to respiratory motion.
- The cell type if malignant, with bronchoalveolar cell carcinoma being a common cause for false negative scans.

A meta-analysis reported a sensitivity and specificity for malignancy of 93.9% and 85.8%. The value of PET-CT is in part dependent on the pretest probability of malignancy. PET-CT may be used to confirm a diagnosis of benign disease in patients with a low pretest probability of malignancy. Generally the value of PET-CT in the management of SPNs is to obviate the need for biopsy. If a nodule is 'PET negative', it is likely to either be benign or of low grade malignancy and may be followed up with a CT scan at one year. If a nodule is 'PET positive', resection is most commonly performed, as biopsy is unlikely to exclude malignancy in these circumstances.

2. Lung cancer staging

PET-CT is used pre-radical therapy in clinically appropriate patients with lung cancer. The PLUS study showed a 50% reduction in futile thoracotomies in patients that underwent PET scanning as part of their work up prior to surgery compared to those that had CT alone.

The degree of primary tumour uptake is in part dependent on both the size of the tumour and the cell type. SCLCs are the most FDG avid.

Its main role pre-radical therapy is in the assessment of the mediastinum and detection of metastatic disease. It has also been shown to be of prognostic importance.

There are a significant number of additional abnormalities demonstrated on PET-CT scans when performed in patients with suspected or biopsy proven lung cancer.

Mediastinal assessment

FDG-PET performance is dependent on node size and the likelihood of other causes of increased uptake such as granulomatous disease. A meta-analysis of node size in FDG-PET has shown a 5% likelihood of maligancy for nodes measuring 10–15mm on CT when PET negative, and a 21% likelihood for nodes measuring >16mm.

False positive scanning is dependent on the underlying prevalence of granulomatous disease. The ranges of reported sensitivity and specificity are 61%–86% and 73% –96%.

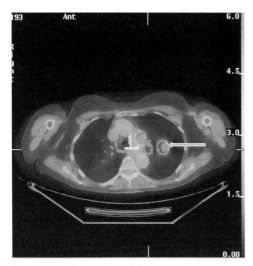

Fig. 13.6.1 FDG avid left upper lobe tumour (long arrow) with FDG avid left hilar (short arrow) and aortopulmonary leymphadenopathy (fat arrow).

Detection of distant metastases:
Several studies have shown that PET-CT detects unsuspected metastases in 10–14% of patients.

Adrenal metastatic disease – PET-CT appears of real value in assessing adrenal disease, with a near 100% sensitivity and very high, 96% specificity.

Bone metastases – this is in part dependent on correlation with the appearance of the area of FDG activity on CT. If the CT appearances are of metastatic disease, PET has a positive predictive value of 98%, if the CT appearance is not of metastatic disease PET has a positive predictive value of 61%. Overall PET has a greater sensitivity than ^{99m}Tc diphosphonate bone scans.

Liver metastases – PET-CT appears more accurate than CT or US, but may not detect sub 1 cm lesions.

Brain metastases are not readily assessed on conventional FDG-PET due to the high metabolic brain activity.

Pleural disease – it appears relatively insensitive, 25%, but of good specificity 90%

Prognosis
PET-CT appears of value in predicting survival. This may be by assessing the SUV of the primary tumour or by assessing the degree of FDG marrow activity.

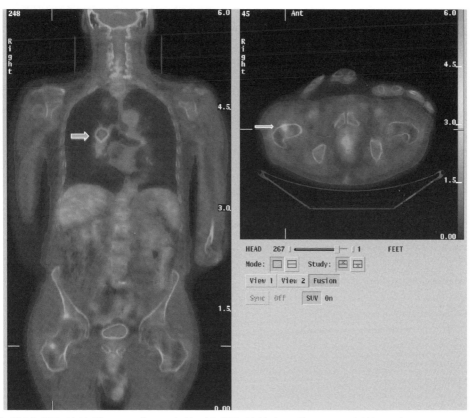

Fig. 13.6.2 FDG avid right hilar tumour (fat arrow) with subtle FDG avid right femoral bone metastasis (thin arrow).

Additional abnormalities
Up to 5–10% of all patients undergoing PET-CT have additional abnormalities such as colonic polyps and thyroid nodules detected.

Its main role may be in the early evaluation of patients undergoing chemotherapy, with a reduction in metabolic activity correlating with continued disease response and survival.

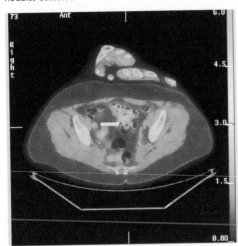

Fig. 13.6.3 Small coincidentally detected FDG rectal polyp (arrowed) detected in a patient with lung cancer.

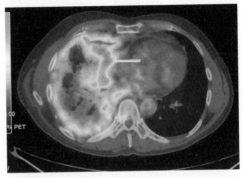

Fig. 13.6.4 Markedly FDG avid mesothelioma (arrowed) in keeping with sarcomatoid histology and a poor prognosis.

Radiation therapy planning
PET-CT has been shown to potentially reduce the volume of non-tumour within the treatment field, reducing toxicity and potentially allowing an increase in dose to the target tissue

3. Assessment of treatment effect in lung cancer
PET has been used post neodadjuvant treatment, as an early assessment during chemotherapy and after completion of therapy. A good response and an early response appear to predict survival.

4. Mesothelioma
FDG-PET has been shown to be of value in detecting areas of disease suitable for biopsy in patients with mesothelioma. It is not sufficiently sensitive to be of value in screening high risk patients, and is not specific, with false positive scans seen post pleurodesis and in patients with other causes of pleural inflammation.

It has been shown to have similar diagnostic accuracy in the detection of mediastinal lymphadenopathy as lung cancer. It detects up to an additional 15% distant metastases compared to CT, and should be performed in all patients being assessed for curative surgery.

Further reading
Ceresoli GL, Chiti A, Zucali PA, *et al.* Early Response Evaluation in Malignant Pleural Mesothelioma by Positron Emission Tomography with [18F]Fluorodeoxyglucose. *J Clin Oncol* 2006; **24**: 4587–4593.

De Geus-Oei L, Oyen WJ. Predictive and Prognostic Value of FDG-PET in Nonsmall-Cell Lung Cancer. *A Systematic Review Cancer* 2007; **119**:1654–1664.

De Langen AJ, Raijmakers P, Riphagen I, *et al.* The size of mediastinal lymph nodes and its relation with metastatic involvement: a meta-analysis. *Eur J Cardiothorac Surg* 2006; **29**: 26–29.

Effectiveness of positron emission tomography in the preoperative assessment of patients with suspected non-small-cell-lung cancer: The PLUS multicentre randomised trial. *Lancet* 2002; **359**:1388–1393.

Erasmus JJ, Macapinlac HA, Swisher SG. Positron Emission Tomography Imaging in Nonsmall-Cell Lung Cancer. *Cancer* 2007; **110**: 2155–2168.

Gould MK, Maclean CC, Kuscher WG, *et al.* Accuracy of Positron Emission Tomography for Diagnosis of Pulmonary Nodules and Mass Lesions: a Meta-analysis. *JAMA* 2001; **285**:914–924.

Hellwig D, Graeter TP, Ukena D, *et al.* 18F-FDG PET for Mediastinal Staging of Lung Cancer: Which SUV Threshold Makes Sense? *J Nucl Med* 2007; **48**:1761–1765.

Truong MT, Marom EM, Erasmus JJ. Preoperative Evaluation of Patients with Malignant Pleural Mesothelioma: Role of Integrated CT-PET Imaging. *J Thorac Imaging* 2006; **21**:146–153.

13.7 Lung cancer screening

Background

Around 80% of lung cancer patients have locally advanced or metastatic disease by the time of diagnosis. Although efforts to improve early diagnosis in symptomatic patients may improve this situation in some patients, it is likely that the bulk of individuals with very limited stage disease will only be detected by some form of population-based screening.

Key elements

For a screening test to be accepted it has to succeed in at least three key areas:
- Provide benefit (usually prolong survival) to the individuals who are found to have the disease.
- Confer no significant danger to the screened population who do not have the disease.
- Should be cost-effective in health economic terms, in other words not impair the capacity of the health service in providing care for others.

CXRs and sputum cytology

Between 1960 and the early 1990s there were five large-scale studies of screening for lung cancer using CXRs, some with and others without the addition of sputum cytology. These were carried out in the UK (as a follow on from the programme of Mass Radiography for TB), the US, and Czechoslovakia. Several of these found a larger number of lung cancers in the screened group and in some a higher proportion of these were surgically resectable. However, in none was an improvement in either lung cancer specific or overall survival demonstrated. All five studies are now recognised to have significant flaws, for example they did not include a proper unscreened 'control' arm, the sample sizes were inadequate and the follow up was not long enough. They are therefore best considered as inconclusive rather than negative.

There is one case–control study from Japan that suggests that CXR screening might still be of value and the current Prostate, Lung, Colo-rectal and Ovarian Trial, funded by the National Cancer Institute, includes randomising the use of plain CXRs in low risk populations.

Low-dose spiral CT scanning

During the 1990s, CT technology advanced significantly, enabling studies using low-dose spiral CT scanning (LDSCT) as a screening tool to be established. The imaging technology has been paralleled by computing power allowing for automated measurements of the dimensions and volume of sub-centimetre nodules to within very low error limits. An example of an image generated in these single-breath hold scans is shown in Fig. 13.7.1.

The current status of research can be summarised as follows:
- The currently published studies of this approach have all been in volunteer groups.
- LDSCT is clearly superior to plain CXRs in detecting early stage disease.
- Over 80% of individuals found to have lung cancer in populations screened using LDSCT have had stage I disease. (This compares with no more than 10% in symptom-detected lung cancer populations.)

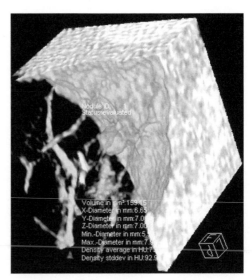

Fig. 13.7.1 Image of 7mm peripheral pulmonary nodule from a low dose CT scan.

- One study (the Early Lung Cancer Action Programme – ELCAP - has estimated an 88% 10-year survival rate in those screen-detected patients with stage I disease.
- No study has yet demonstrated an improvement in mortality outcomes in the screened population, even in high-risk populations.
- The results of the randomised trials that are currently underway will not be available for several years.

Problems of LDSCT screening

Overdiagnosis bias

This is the detection of very slowly growing tumours that are clinically unimportant for the individual patient who is more likely to die of other conditions. There are reports of such clinically undiagnosed lung cancers in post-mortem studies.

Indeterminate nodules and clinical effectiveness

CT can detect very small abnormalities within the lung fields and one of the main issues is how to handle nodules of indeterminate significance. There is morbidity and a small mortality associated with the biopsy and resection of pulmonary nodules. Unfortunately, CT abnormalities are not specific for malignancy and some series report more than 90% of CT nodules to be benign. In a non-randomised Swedish study 78% of the 1520 screened individuals were found to have non-calcified pulmonary nodules but only 68 lung cancers were detected, exposing a very large number of patients to the need for investigation and the associated risks and anxieties. The frequency of benign pulmonary nodules varies widely in different parts of the world, which probably means that each country needs to make its own assessment of the clinical effectiveness and risk of such a programme.

Cost effectiveness

The published estimates of the cost-effectiveness of screening using LDSCT vary hugely and appear to depend as much on the enthusiasm of the authors as the science underlying the analyses. At one extreme, the ELCAP investigators calculated an incremental cost effectiveness ratio of the baseline scan as US$2500 per year of life saved. Others studies have reached very different conclusion with estimates ranging from US$51,001 to US$2,322,700 quality life year adjusted gained. The Health Technology Appraisal panel concluded: 'There are serious shortcomings in the economic data currently available in UK concerning treatment of lung cancer patients. New research is required to provide information needed for a comprehensive economic assessment of lung cancer screening in UK.'

Other potential screening techniques

Several other approaches to the early detection of lung cancer which may, in time lead to technologies useful in population screening are under investigation, though none of them have yet been applied in the context of a randomised trial. They include:

- Identification of genetic profiles that can identify populations at especially high risk.
- Serum proteomics.
- Assessment of methylation biomarkers free circulating plasma DNA.
- Advanced, automated sputum cytology followed by LDSCT and/or autofluorescence bronchoscopy.

- Analysis of the exhaled breath for abnormal patterns of volatile organic substances.

Summary

Currently there is no screening technique that has been demonstrated to alter mortality outcomes even in high-risk populations. Thus screening is currently regarded as a subject of ongoing research by most authorities.

Further reading

Bach PB, Kelley MJ, Tate RC, et al. Screening for lung cancer: A review of the current literature. Chest 2003; **123**: 72S–82S.

Bach PB, Silvestri GA, Hanger M, et al. Screening for lung cancer: ACCP evidence-based clinical practice guidelines (2nd edn). Chest 2007; **132**: 69S–77S.

Gleeson FV. Is screening for lung cancer using low dose spiral CT scanning worthwhile? Thorax 2006; **61**: 5–7.

Henschke CI, Yankelevitz DF, Naidich DP, et al. CT screening for lung cancer: Suspiciousness of nodules according to size on baseline scans. Radiology 2004; **231**(1):164–168.

Okamotoe N, Suzuki T, Hasegawa H, et al. Evaluation of a clinic-based screnning program for lung cancer with a case-control design in Kanagawa, Japan. Lung Cancer 1999; **25**:77–85

Swenson SJ, Jett JR, Sloan JA, et al. Screening for lung cancer with low-dose spiral computed tomography. Am J Respir Crit Care Med 2002; **165**: 433–434.

The International Early Lung Cancer Action Program Investigators. Survival of patients with stage I lung cancer detected on CT screening. N Eng J Med 2006; **355**:1763–1771.

13.8 Carcinoid

Epidemiology

Carcinoid is an uncommon tumour:

- Annual incidence of carcinoid tumours is 1–2 cases per 100,000.
- 1–2% of all primary lung cancers.
- 12% of all carcinoid tumours arise in the lung.

The sex distribution equal overall but the incidence in those aged <50 years for females is almost twice that of males. Peak incidence rates are at 15–25 years and 65–75 years with a mean age of carcinoid diagnosis of approximately 47 years. Atypical carcinoid tumours occur in significantly older patients, usually in the sixth decade.

Pulmonary carcinoid

The most frequent location is the main or lobar bronchi (70%). 30% are peripheral. Regional nodal involvement is found in 10% of cases at the time of diagnosis. Smoking is a risk factor for pulmonary carcinoid and occasionally familial pulmonary carcinoids are found and are associated with the multiple endocrine neoplasia type 1 gene which is situated on chromosome 11 (11Q13).

Pathophysiology

Carcinoid tumours may secrete vaso-active peptides that may be responsible for both clinical presentation and complications. Carcinoids may secrete 5-hydroxytryptamine (5HT) bradykinins, tachykinins, histamine, substance P, adenocorticotrophic hormone, prostaglandins, kallikrein, dopamine, and several other peptides. 5HT production is the most prominent. Carcinoid tumours convert dietary tryptophan into serotonin, and serotonin is then metabolised to 5-hydroxyindoleacetic acid (5HIAA). If there is extensive metabolism of tryptophan in this way as occurs in metastatic carcinoid, then this can lead to a reduction in the synthesis of nicotinamide which can lead to a diagnosis of pellagra (Fig. 13.8.1).

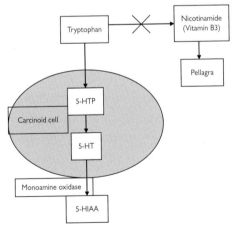

Fig. 13.8.1 5–HT (serotonin) metabolism.

5HT in the systemic circulation causes contraction of smooth muscle leading to bronchoconstriction, increased gastro-intestinal motility, vascular constriction and dilatation as well as platelet aggregation. 5HT and other vaso-active substances are thought to cause carcinoid syndrome and carcinoid heart disease.

Clinical presentations

Pulmonary carcinoid's most frequent symptoms are haemoptysis, cough, recurrent pulmonary infection, fever, chest discomfort, unilateral wheezing (due to endobronchial obstruction) and, if there are metastases (usually liver), then paraneoplastic syndromes can be a presenting feature. However, the frequency of metastatic disease related to pulmonary carcinoid is very low.

Carcinoid syndrome

Carcinoid syndrome occurs in approximately 2% of cases of pulmonary carcinoid. The characteristic symptoms are diarrhoea, flushing, palpitations, and wheezing. Symptoms will be more severe if the tumour drains directly into the systemic circulation (especially liver metastases). Rarely, carcinoid crisis can be precipitated by the release of large volumes of vaso-active substances into the systemic circulation. This can occur after tumour manipulation, induction of anaesthesia, or intubation.

Carcinoid heart disease

This occurs as a late complication of metastatic carcinoid tumours. The heart lesions are characterised by fibrosis of the valve on the right side of the heart due to high exposure to the vaso-active substances. These substances are metabolised in the lung and this is thought to result in a significantly lower exposure to the left side of the heart and hence the fact that only 10% of patients with carcinoid heart disease have lesions on the left side.

Other syndromes

Cushing's syndrome occurs in approximately 2% of patients with pulmonary carcinoid and is characterised by ectopic ACTH production. Although very rare, carcinoid tumours are the most frequent cause of ectopic growth hormone production and can lead to acromegaly.

Diagnosis

The diagnosis of carcinoid syndrome is achieved by obtaining a histological sample either by bronchoscopic biopsy or transthoracic needle biopsy. The tumour tends to be highly vascular and this can result in significant haemorrhage from bronchoscopic or transthoracic biopsies. However, despite some reports of significant haemorrhage, it is usually not a problem. The classic appearances of the tumour at bronchoscopy are either a pink, reddish or yellow smooth-looking tumour.

Imaging

Carcinoid tumours can show on CXR as a solitary pulmonary nodule or lobar consolidation, where endobronchial obstruction has resulted in a post-obstructive pneumonia. Chest CT (Fig. 13.8.2) confirms these findings and, as the liver is usually included in this scan, will show the presence of liver metastases. If that is the case then the primary diagnosis may be obtained from biopsies of the liver metastases. Immunoscintigraphy by somatostatin analogues can be useful in the diagnosis of carcinoid. Carcinoids overexpress somatostatin receptors. [111]Indium-pentetreotide has a sensitivity of 80–90% for the detection of carcinoid tumours and provides information about the localisation of the tumour and is predictive of the response to octeotride therapy (see below). [131]Iodine-metaiodobenzylguanidine ([131]IMIBG) is an analogue of an amine precursor which is taken up by neuroendocrine cells. This analogue has been used for the detection and imaging of neuroendocrine tumours and also as a therapeutic tool. However, the sensitivity is rather lower than the indium analogue at around 70%. FDG PET (Fig. 13.8.3) has limited utility in carcinoid tumours because of a relatively low proliferative activity in these tumours and may have more of an application where there are metastases. Bone scintigraphy shows a high sensitivity for bone metastases than any of the aforementioned analogues.

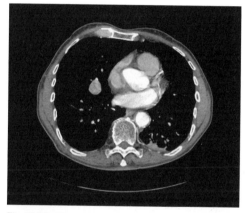

Fig. 13.8.2   CT scan of carcinoid.

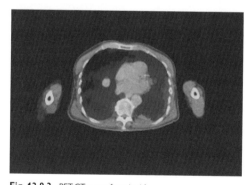

Fig. 13.8.3   PET-CT scan of carcinoid.

Tumour markers

Urinary 5HIAA is the gold standard for the diagnosis and follow-up of carcinoid tumours. It has a specificity of almost 100% but a much lower sensitivity (35%). Urinary 5HIAA levels are influenced by certain foods such as bananas, pineapples and walnuts, and some medications. Platelet 5HT level is a sensitive marker for the detection of small amounts of serotonin production but is not in general usage. Chromogranin A (CgA) is a glycoprotein produced in most neuroendocrine tumours. It is therefore a non-specific detector of such tumours.

Treatment

Surgery

Surgery is the treatment of choice for pulmonary carcinoid and has a high chance of cure. For typical carcinoids, lung-sparing operations are often performed, but in atypical carcinoid, lobectomy is recommended. In small endobronchial carcinoids minimally invasive resection with laser or electrocautery techniques has been successful.

Somatostatin analogues

Somatostatin receptors have five subtypes and are expressed in more than 80% of carcinoid tumours, especially subtypes 2 and 5. Octreotide has a high affinity for these subtypes and can be administered subcutaneously 6–8-hourly. Octreotide improves symptoms in up to 80% of patients and reduces 5HIAA excretion in 72%.

^{131}I-MIBG

This therapy involves higher doses of isotope to deliver a local internal radiation effect to the tumour cells than is used in patients with a positive diagnostic scan. The reported response rates are 60% but the duration of effect is a median of eight months.

Radio-labelled somatostatin analogues

A variety of radio-labelled analogues have been used in patients with [111]indium-pentetreotide scintigraphy. The latter analogue has shown benefits for treatment of small tumours or micro-metastases with improvement in up to 60% of patients. However, side effects include significant renal and haematological toxicity as well as distressing nausea and vomiting.

Interferon alpha

Interferon alpha treatment decreases urinary 5HIAA in around 40% of patients but reduces tumour size in only 15%. Side effects include anorexia and weight loss, fever and fatigue. Interferon alpha therefore has a low therapeutic index and is not usually used.

Systemic chemotherapy

This tends to be used as second-line therapy because of the low therapeutic response of 20-30%. Regimens used include streptozocin and cyclophosphamide or streptozocin and 5-fluorouracil. Third-line therapy using a combination of cisplatin and etoposide may be used in particularly aggressive carcinoid tumour as this regimen tends to help in small cell lung cancer and neuroendocrine carcinomas.

Radiotherapy

Radiotherapy is effective palliation in bone and central nervous system metastases.

Supportive care

Supportive care is particularly important where there are distressing symptoms secondary to the carcinoid syndrome. Flushes may be avoided by not taking food that is known to provoke symptoms, and diarrhoea can be treated with anti-diarrhoea medications. It is also important to consider vitamin supplementation to avoid pellagra.

Hepatic metastases

Surgical resection of liver metastases may benefit patients with limited hepatic disease. However, this is applicable to only a minority of patients. Alternatively, hepatic artery embolisation may be used and is applicable in carefully selected patients to reduce the tumour burden. Median duration of response is 12 months and there are important side effects to consider including renal toxicity and occasional hepatorenal syndrome. The role of liver transplantation in carcinoid syndrome is still under investigation.

KEY FACT

Prognosis

Typical carcinoid has 5- and 10-year survival of 87–100% and 82–87% respectively.

The prognosis for atypical tumours is lower – 5- and 10-year survival 56–75% and 35–56%.

Summary

Pulmonary carcinoid is an uncommon lung tumour that generally has a good prognosis except where the tumour is atypical. Treatment is usually by surgical resection. Metastases may occur and rarely lead to the carcinoid syndrome. Outcomes from chemotherapy and other therapies are improving and new therapies are under investigation.

Further reading

Kosmidis PA Treatment of Carcinoid of the Lung. *Curr Opin Oncol* 2004; **16**(2):146–149.

Kulke MH, Mayer RJ. Carcinoid Tumours. *N Eng J Med* 1999; **340**: 858–868.

13.9 Benign lung tumours

Introduction

Benign lung tumours are relatively rare, accounting for less than 1% of all lung tumours. They comprise a very broad and heterogeneous group of lesions and may be divided or grouped according to their putative cell or tissue of origin. Thus this chapter will consider, amongst others, lesions of bronchial gland, and airway epithelial origin, connective tissue tumours, benign tumours arising from pulmonary lymphoid tissue, vascular tumours and tumours showing neural differentiation. Tumour-like conditions will also be covered. Bronchial carcinoid tumours are low grade malignant lesions and will not be considered in this chapter.

In a clinical sense it is useful to consider whether the tumour is sited predominantly in an airway, or within the lung parenchyma or the pleura, as each location of tumour will have different clinical features. Benign tumours arising in a parenchymal location are often asymptomatic whilst those occurring in a large airway e.g. hamartomas, may have a symptomatic presentation. For each tumour, aetiology (if known or relevant), specific clinical features and pathology will be discussed. Differential diagnosis for each will be considered and treatment, if required, and outcomes will be considered.

Benign pleural tumours

All of these lesions are rare, and some are true neoplasms. The main differential diagnoses for benign pleural tumours include primary or secondary malignancy and organising empyema.

Localised fibrous tumour of the pleura

Although sometimes an incidental radiological finding, patients often complain of chest discomfort, which may be accompanied by cough or breathlessness. This condition is associated with both finger clubbing and hypertrophic pulmonary osteoarthropathy. Some patients can develop spontaneous hypoglycaemia, possibly related to secretion of insulin like growth factors.

These benign tumours usually arise from the visceral pleura but have rarely been described arising from the parietal or mediastinal pleura. Typically they are smooth pedunculated tumours, which can grow to a substantial size (up to 30 cm)

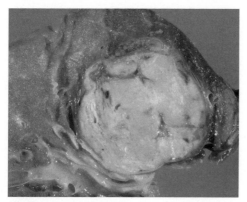

Fig. 13.9.1 This solitary fibrous tumour is intrapulmonary rather than pleural. The lesion is well circumscribed and, in this region, densely cellular. (See Plate 10.)

and may weigh up to 3 kg. Histologically these tumours are low grade spindle cell neoplasms showing a characteristic pattern of variable cellularity, collagen bundles and thick-walled vessels. They have characteristic ultra structural and immunocyto chemical features, the most important diagnostically useful being the frequent expression of CD34 and bcl2. Malignant forms are rare.

Surgical resection is the recommended treatment and is usually curative although rarely local recurrence with a fatal outcome has been described. Thus it is essential to remove the tumour completely to avoid the risk of recurrence, especially since any recurrence may be a higher grade, more aggressive disease.

Solitary fibrous tumours may also occur in the pulmonary parenchyma but these are much rarer than in the pleura.

Calcifying fibrous pseudotumour

This tumour is very rare. They are well circumscribed but not encapsulated and involve the visceral pleura. Surgical resection is the recommended treatment and recurrence is unusual.

Adenomatoid tumour

This is a distinctive mesothelial tumour which is entirely benign and has rarely been reported arising in the pleura.

Blesovsky's Disease (folded lung)

Localised areas of pleural thickening and fibrosis are often identified by chance on a CXR when they may mimic a peripheral lung tumour. They do not usually cause symptoms or functional embarrassment. The contracting pleural fibrosis and scarring causes adjacent lung tissue to fold inwards and collapse and this is particularly seen at the lung bases. Radiologically the characteristic feature is the so-called comet's tail sign and this is particularly well seen on cross sectional imaging. A variety of terms have been used to describe Blesovsky's Disease and include folded lung and rounded atelectasis.

Pleural splenosis

This may occur following trauma, rupture of the spleen and diaphragmatic damage, allowing splenic tissue to be implanted in the pleural cavity. It follows that pleural splenosis almost always occurs on the left side of the chest. Usually patients are asymptomatic and the abnormality is detected as an incidental radiological finding many years after the traumatic episode. Histologically the lesions show normal splenic tissue.

Pleural thymoma and pleural endometriosis are extremely uncommon lesions and are discussed under the section on their pulmonary counterparts.

Benign parenchymal tumours of the lung

These often present as asymptomatic peripheral masses seen on a CXR taken for unrelated reasons. A wide range of tumours are included in this category. These are listed in Table 13.9.1, categorised according to their pathologic classification. Some lesions occur in both peripheral parenchymal and endobronchial locations and will be discussed in the context of the site where they are more frequently encountered. The commonest type of benign parenchymal lung tumour is hamartoma but the list includes a number of extremely uncommon neoplasms of both epithelial and connective tissue differentiation, as well as a number of non-neoplastic tumour-like conditions.

Investigation of benign parenchymal lung tumours

These tumours will often be found incidentally on a CXR when they may mimic a lung cancer. Occasionally, however, they may appear unusually round, smooth and well-circumscribed on chest imaging, suggesting the benign nature of the problem. CT scanning and percutaneous needle core biopsy may give a diagnosis but often the true nature of the lesion is only apparent after resection and full pathologic examination.

As in lung cancer the investigative journey for an individual patient will be predicated by the patient's performance status, comorbidity (especially lung function) and personal wishes.

Specific types of benign parenchymal lung tumour

Soft (connective) tissue tumours

Chondroid hamartoma and related lesions

These tumours, although relatively uncommon, are, in terms of benign lung tumours, the commonest type and account for about 8% of coin lesions seen on CXR. They are commonest in late middle age, show a male preponderance, most are parenchymal and consequently asymptomatic but about 10% are endobronchial and cause endobronchial symptoms. Massive haemoptysis has been described. They comprise a mixture of various connective tissues (fat, cartilage, smooth muscle) and epithelial tissue components, but there is debate as to whether these lesions are truly hamartomas or are true neoplasms. The term mesenchymoma has been proposed and it is now recognised that pulmonary lipomas, chondromas and fibromas may be related neoplasms. These monotypic examples are, however much less common than the heterogeneous 'chondroid hamartoma'. The connective tissue components may calcify, giving the characteristic 'pop-corn' pattern of calcification in some lesions on the chest radiograph.

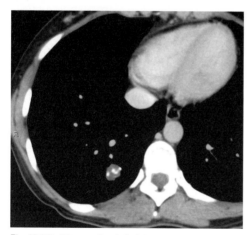

Fig. 13.9.2 CT image of a calcified chondroid hamartoma.

The pathological features of pulmonary hamartomas are the same wherever they arise, be it in the lung parenchyma or as endobronchial growths. They are usually 1–3 cm in size but can grow up to 9 cm. Those arising in a parenchy-

mal location are usually easy to resect, and recurrence or malignant change is exceedingly rare.

Lipomas and chondromas are more likely to be endobronchial. True pulmonary chondromas are extremely unusual, usually multiple and occur more commonly in females. Radiologically calcification is frequent, pathologically bone may be present in some lesions and these lesions occur in the context of Carney's triad (pulmonary chondromas, gastric stromal tumours and paragangliomas). Differential diagnosis of the histology includes chondroid hamartoma and metastatic chondrosarcoma.

Leiomyoma and fibroleiomyoma

These are extremely rare tumours and usually occur in middle aged women. Pulmonary leiomyomas resemble those encountered in other sites. They are well circumscribed.

Angiomyolipoma

These are also extremely rare benign tumours which are hamartomas and composed of a mixture of blood vessels, smooth muscle and fat. Although most commonly found in the kidney they have rarely been reported in the lung.

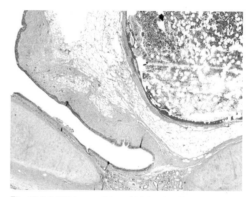

Fig. 13.9.3 This is an endobronchial chondroid hamartoma. The cartilage plates and seromucous glands of the native bronchus are seen below, the lesion comprising connective and adipose tissue and cartilage, which has ossified and has a substantial component of bone marrow (top right). (See Plate 11.)

Inflammatory myofibroblastic tumour

This rare pulmonary lesion is a member of the rare heterogeneous group of so-called inflammatory pseudo-tumours. It has many synonyms and has subsumed a number of previous 'entities' such as plasma cell granuloma and fibrous histiocytoma. It occurs most often in patients aged under 40 years and shows an equal gender distribution.

Most lesions present as localised pulmonary masses which may mimic carcinoma radiologically. Signs and symptoms are dependent on the localisation of the lesion. Rarer endo-bronchial lesions may cause cough, wheeze and haemoptysis. Peripheral lesions give fewer symptoms unless the chest wall is involved.

These lesions show a heterogeneous mixture of spindles cells, macrophages and variable infiltrates of chronic inflammatory cells. Giant cells may be seen. Atypia is rare but the tendency to occasionally invade locally, recur after excision and even rarely metastasise has led some to consider this lesion a low grade malignancy.

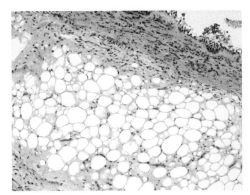

Fig. 13.9.4 Bronchial lipoma showing accumulations of adipose tissue deep to the respiratory mucosa.

Clear cell tumour

This benign lung tumour has also been named the 'sugar tumour'. Less than fifty cases have been reported in the world literature. They tend to occur in middle aged patients who are usually asymptomatic and the tumour is an incidental solitary finding. This is probably a tumour of perivascular epithelioid cells (so-called PEC cells) and the most important differential diagnosis would be with metastatic renal cell carcinoma since the lesion comprises large but banal looking cells with clear cytoplasm containing abundant glycogen. These tumours are quite vascular. The benign pulmonary tumour will not express cytokeratins but will express HMB45. The tumour is usually peripheral and resection is generally curative.

Vascular tumours

Epithilioid haemangioendothelioma

This is a low grade but potentially malignant endothelial tumour, 80% of which occur in women. Age range at presentation is wide (10–60 years),with a median age at 40. Half of the patients are asymptomatic. The remainder complain of cough, and of breathlessness. Typical radiologic findings are the presence of multiple bilateral, sometimes calcified small nodules of 1–2 cm diameter, though solitary masses may occur. Typically this condition is misinterpreted as metastatic disease or old granulomatous inflammation.

Histologically the tumour shows cords and nests of epithelioid endothelial cells set in a rather myxoid stroma. This tumour may also occur in the pleura. The multiple tumours slowly enlarge over a period of years and patients die of respiratory failure.

Other vascular tumours

Haemangioma and lymphangioma are exceedingly rare in the lung. They resemble similar tumours elsewhere in the body and form well circumscribed lesions. They tend to be intrapulmonary but may occur endobronchially. Such a case causing haemoptysis has been described.

Neural tumours

These include nerve sheath tumours, and granular cell tumours. They are all extremely rare occurences in the lung. Nerve sheath tumours comprise both neurofibromas and neurilemmomas which are identical to their counterparts elsewhere. These tumours are sometimes associated with neurofibromatosis. They may be parenchymal but have also been found in the airways and visible on bronchoscopy. Granular cells tumours are more often endobronchial and discussed later.

Parenchymal epithelial tumours

Sclerosing pneumocytoma (sclerosing haemangioma)

Despite the original belief that this was a vascular tumour, hence the term 'haemangioma', it now clear that this is an epithelial tumour showing pneumocyte differentiation.

Table 13.9.1 Benign tumours and tumour-like conditions of the lung

Parenchymal tumours		
Epithelial neoplasms	**Soft tissue and other neoplasms**	**Non-neoplastic conditions**
Alveolar adenoma	Hamartoma	Amyloid tumour
Papillary adenoma	Chondroma	Hyalinising granuloma
Mucinous cystadenoma	Lipoma	Malakoplakia
Sclerosing haemangioma (pneumocytoma)	Fibroma	Endometriosis
Thymoma	Leiomyoma	A-V malformation
Pleomorphic adenoma	Clear cell (sugar) tumour	Lymphoproliferative disorders
	Meningioma	
	Inflammatory myofibroblastic tumour	
	Granular cell tumour	
	Epithelioid haemangioendothelioma	
Endobronchial tumours		
Epithelial neoplasms	**Soft tissue and other neoplasms**	**Non-neoplastic conditions**
Papillomas	Hamartoma	Fibroinflammatory polyps
Squamous papilloma	Chondroma	Amyloid tumour
Glandular papilloma	Lipoma	Foreign body
Mixed papilloma	Granular cell tumour	Bacillary angiomatosis
Bronchial gland adenomas		
Mucous gland adenomas		
Oncocytoma		
Pleomorphic adenoma		

These tumours are commonest in middle age and commoner in women. These lesions are much commoner in East Asia, especially Japan.

The are usually asymptomatic, but cough, pain and haemoptysis may occur.

Pathologically the tumours tend to compress adjacent normal lung parenchyma and most measure under 3cm, though lesions up to 8cm are described. Most are solitary lesions though around 4% are multiple. The two basic histological features of a sclerosing pneumocytoma are the presence of sclerosis and papillary epithelial proliferation but they may show a very wide range of features including alveolar-like spaces and a dual population of larger pale cells and smaller 'stromal' cells. Haemorrage and heamosiderin are commonly present. Immunohistochemistry for cytokeratins and TTF1 are key to the histologic diagnosis.

Mucinous cystadenoma

These are extremely rare tumours, lined by columnar mucin-secreting epithelium, enveloping a uniloculate space filled with mucin. They tend to occur in elderly patients. Cases with borderline malignant histological features have been described. Definitive diagnosis requires surgical excision, which is curative.

Alveolar adenoma

These are well circumscribed tumours. All lobes have been reported to be involved though there is a predilection for the left lower lobe. They comprise micro- and macrocystic spaces, a feature which may be apparent on CT scan, lined by alveolar pneumocytes, all embedded in a variably dense fibrous stroma. These lesions have been described up to 6cm in diameter and are usually asymptomatic incidental findings. Following surgical resection there have been no reports of recurrence.

Papillary adenoma

This is an extremely uncommon parenchymal neoplasm, predominantly found in males of widely ranging age who are asymptomatic. Tumours are well defined encapsulated masses showing a compact growth of true papillae lined by bland epithelial cells which are a mixture of Clara cells, type 2 pneumocytes and even ciliated cells. Surgical excision is curative.

Intrapulmonary thymoma

Primary thymoma has been described both in the lung and pleura and is thought to arise from thymic rests in these tissues. Typically patients with a pulmonary thymoma will present with an asymptomatic peripheral pulmonary nodule. Such ectopic thymomas are identical to those that arise in the thymus but generally are not so obviously surrounded by a capsule. Pulmonary thymomas are usually benign, slowly growing and are cured by complete surgical resection. As with mediastinal lesions, malignant forms do occur. Pleural thymoma has also been described and this presents as an asymptomatic pleural nodule or thickening on chest imaging.

Patients with pleural thymoma may also present with symptoms such as chest pain, fever, cough and weight loss. There is a case report of a patient who presented with an intra pulmonary thymoma who had myasthenia gravis.

Parenchymal tumour-like conditions

There is a wide range of benign lesions which present as masses mimicking neoplasms, yet are non-neoplastic. Many of these lesions, such as rheumatoid nodules, localised

Wegener's granulomatosis, nodular sarcoidosis and infectious granulomatous masses enter the differential diagnosis of benign lung tumours but are discussed elsewhere. Other benign non-neoplastic conditions which may mimic neoplasia include rounded atelectasis (see above), sequestered pulmonary segments and organising pneumonia.

Also included in this category are amyloid tumour, hyalinising granulomas, malakoplakia, thoracic (usually pleural) endometriosis, AV malformations and some unusual lymphoproliferative conditions, which are briefly discussed.

Amyloid tumour

Amyloid tumour in the lung can occur in isolation or as part of systemic amyloidosis. Nodules may be solitary or multiple and can occur endobronchially, when the patient may be symptomatic. Most patients are middle aged.

Localised pulmonary amyloid tumours comprise masses of eosinophilic amorphous material which elicits a foreign-body type giant cell reaction. Calcification or even ossification have been described.

A minority of these patients will have a lymphoproliferative disorder associated with the amyloid and screening for serum paraproteins may be appropriate.

Thoracic endometriosis

This condition is rare and usually affects the pleura or sub pleural lung tissue but occasionally is purely intrapulmonary.

Patients may have an incidental tumour–like abnormality identified on the CXR but catamenial pneumothorax and haemoptysis have been reported.

Arterial venous malformation

Developmental AV fistulae in the lungs have long been recognised and a significant number of cases have been described in the world literature. They represent a vascular hamartoma with abnormal communications between pulmonary arteries and veins. These lesions may be single or multiple and often increase in size with age.

Although the abnormality develops in foetal life, patients usually present in middle age with haemoptysis or features of chronic hypoxia if there is an appreciable arterial venous shunt. These vascular malformations tend to occur in the periphery of the lung and are not infrequently multiple. The treatment of choice is balloon occlusion or embolisation following angiography.

Angiofollicular lymph node hyperplasia (Castleman's Disease)

Although angiofolicular lymph node hyperplasia usually involves mediastinal lymph nodes, it has been reported in the lung and the pleura, and the chest wall. Two specific histological sub types have been described – hyaline-vascular and plasma cell. The hyaline-vascular pattern is much commoner and often presents as a random finding on CXR. However, patients may present with symptoms due to pressure effects. This tends to be a more localised form of disease. The plasma cell pattern is more often multicentric. It is associated with systemic features, lymphadenopathy and hepatosplenomegaly and has an aggressive course. In contrast the solitary form of disease is benign and usually cured by surgery.

Benign endobronchial tumours

Endobronchial tumours usually present with 'bronchial' symptoms such as cough, haemoptysis, breathlessness, wheeze and stridor. Patients may be misdiagnosed as asthma for many years before the endobronchial tumour is identified and treated. Benign papillomatous tumours of the airways include juvenile papillomatosis, solitary squamous cell papilloma, mixed squamous and glandular or pure glandular papillomas and papillary adenoma. All these epithelial neoplasms must be distinguished microscopically from rare soft tissue endobronchial neoplasms and non-neoplastic conditions such as inflammatory polyps, amyloid tumours, inhaled, impacted foreign bodies and endometriosis.

Papillomas

These are usually squamous but glandular papillomas and mixed squamous and glandular papillomas have also been described.

Human papilloma virus has been identified as an aetiological factor in the development of squamous papillomas. Solitary squamous lesions are seen mostly in males (mean age 53). Around a fifth of squamous lesions may show atypia and malignant change, though rare, is reported, emphasising the need for complete excision when possible. Glandular and mixed lesions are extremely unusual, occur equally in both sexes, with a mean age of 65.

Multiple squamous lesions in the form of juvenile papillomatosis of the upper trachea and larynx can rarely affect the lower trachea or large bronchi. These usually occur in young patients and again have been associated with the human papilloma virus.

Bronchial gland tumours

These arise from the sero-mucous glands of the airways. Some, such as muco-epidermoid or adenoid cystic tumours are malignant and beyond the scope of this chapter. Benign bronchial gland tumours usually arise in large airways, protrude endobronchially and thus the characteristic 'bronchial' symptoms of cough and haemoptysis are often seen. Presentation may also be with recurrent episodes of pneumonia due to obstruction by the tumour.

These tumours occur with an equal incidence in males and females. All are rare and can occur at any age.

Histopathologically these lesions are mucous cell, oncocytic and pleomorphic adenomas.

As they do not infiltrate, the overlying bronchial mucosa is usually intact at bronchoscopy.

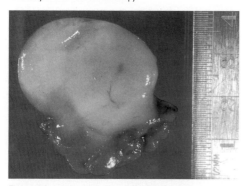

Fig. 13.9.5 This is a resected pleomorphic adenoma from the main carina. Tracheobronchial wall is present at the base of the lesion, which itself comprises a smooth, rounded mass, which protruded into the trachea and presented as acute onset asthma. (See Plate 12.)

Endobronchial non-epithelial tumours

Endobronchial cases of hamartoma and lipoma are well described. Their presentation is typical of obstructive endobronchial tumours and the pathology is as in lesions found in more common sites (see earlier sections).

Granular cell tumour

Bronchopulmonary granular cell tumours are rare and usually develop in middle age. They may be found incidentally or may present with endobronchial symptoms. They may be visible on bronchoscopy and biopsy is often diagnostic. Despite their histologic appearance of infiltrating benign-looking cells with granular cytoplasm, they are of peripheral nerve sheath (Schwann cell) origin and express S100 protein, which is diagnostically useful.

Although these tumours grow only slowly and are almost always benign, resection is the recommended treatment.

Non-neoplastic endobronchial lesions

Bronchial inflammatory polyps

These are polyps consisting of granulation tissue covered by respiratory or a metaplastic squamous epithelium and are related to airway inflammation or trauma. They have been described in conjunction with chronic bronchitis, bronchiectasis and cystic fibrosis and even as a complication of bronchial biopsy. They are generally solitary but multiple polyps have been encountered. They are entirely benign, have no malignant potential and resolve either spontaneously or with antibiotic treatment.

Bacillary angiomatosis

This reactive vascular proliferation usually occurs in the skin and lymph nodes in patients infected with HIV. However it has been described in the respiratory tract where it results in an endobronchial polyp. Chest wall involvement with intra thoracic spread has also been reported.

On microscopy capillaries lined by endothelial cells are admixed with neutrophils, cell debris and often clumps of bacilli. The microscopic appearances differ from Kaposi's sarcoma by the absence of spindle cells and the presence of inflammation.

The treatment for this condition is with macrolide antibiotics.

Conclusion

A large range of benign lung tumours have been described in the literature although they are relatively rare, some extremely so. They often are asymptomatic and detected on routine CXR but may present with endobronchial symptoms if they involve the airway. Benign lung tumours do grow, albeit slowly, and will cause pressure symptoms if not treated.

Definitive diagnosis will almost always require biopsy, though the true nature of the lesion, including its benign nature, often requires full examination of the completely resected lesion.

The treatment of choice is surgical resection if the patient is fit enough.

Acknowledgements

The authors very gratefully acknowledge the help of Jean Elliot (Postgraduate Centre Manager at Stobhill Hospital, Glasgow) with producing the manuscript and Dr Mike Sproule, Consultant Radiologist, Gartnavel General Hospital, Glasgow for supplying some of the images.

Further reading

Travis, WD, Brambilla E, Muller-Hermelink HK, *et al.* (eds.) *World Health Organization Classification of Tumours: Pathology and Genetics of Tumours of the Lung, Pleura, Thymus, and Heart* 2004 Lyon: IARC Press.

13.10 Transbronchial fine needle aspiration

Introduction

Transbronchial fine needle aspiration (TBNA) is a simple bronchoscopic technique which allows sampling of mediastinal lymph nodes, masses adjacent to the airways and sub-mucosal disease. Its main role is in the diagnosis and staging of suspected lung cancer but it also has a role in non-malignant disease such as sarcoidosis. The procedure is extremely safe and the incidence of pneumothorax, pneumo-mediastinum and haemorrhage is low and ranges from 0.05%–0.2%.

Equipment

A variety of needles are available and the key features should include:

1 The needles should be retractable into a protective sheath

2 Insertion length of the needle should be between 13–15mm

3 The needle gauge should be between 18–22 gauge.

Both single-use disposable and partly reusable sheaths are available. The larger gauge needles have a greater chance of yielding some tissue for histological analysis. The choice of needle comes down to individual preference but specific needles may be more suitable for certain circumstances. The Olympus NA-2C-1 needle may be more suitable for an inexperienced user as it consists of a helical metallic outer protective sheath and an inner disposable needle. Hence it is less likely to result in damage to the bronchoscope and the stiffness allows greater precision. An 18 gauge Wang needle may be more appropriate when a patient has suspected sarcoidosis and a histological sample is desirable.

Site selection

A recent CT scan of the thorax should always be reviewed prior to the procedure and the site of the trans-bronchial fine needle aspiration planned. A simple approach is to consider the airway as a clock face and to relate the position of the lymph nodes or mass accordingly. Remember that the CT scan acquires images from the patient's feet upwards, whereas during bronchoscopy we examine the airways from the head downwards. Hence on the CT scan the left side is in the direction of 3 o'clock whereas in the patient at bronchoscopy the left side is towards the 9 o'clock position. This can be corrected by flipping the images of the CT in the vertical axis.

Furthermore, if the patient is being approached from the front at bronchoscopy the anterior aspect is at 6 o'clock whereas the posterior aspect is at 12 o'clock. In contrast on the CT scan the anterior aspect is at 12 o'clock and the posterior aspect at 6 o'clock. Further allowance needs to be made by flipping the image in the horizontal axis. Note this last transposition is not required if the patient is being approached at bronchoscopy from the back of the patient who is lying supine.

The vertical position also needs to be estimated and this can be done by calculating the cartilage rings above or below the carina. For hilar nodes it may be more appropriate to use the origin or relative location of the segmental or lobar bronchi to give the site of aspiration.

Planning and site selection is an important part of TBNA and has an important influence on the yield. With the new multi-slice CT scan reformatting software with virtual bronchoscopy mode and lymph node highlighting will allow the beginner to correctly choose the site of needle aspiration.

Anatomical lymph node site	Position		Vertical position
	Anterior approach	Posterior approach	
Right paratracheal	7–8 o'clock	1–2 o'clock	2–4 interspaces above carina
Left paratracheal	3 o'clock	9 o'clock	Level of carina or one interspace above
Subcarinal	3 o'clock in right main bronchus	9 o'clock in right main bronchus	1 space below carina in right main bronchus
Posterior Carinal	12–12.30 o'clock	5.30–6.0 o'clock	Level of carina
Anterior Carinal	6–6.30 o'clock	12–12.30 o'clock	Level of carina
Right Main bronchial	6 o'clock	12 o'clock	1 space below carina in right main bronchus
Left main bronchial	6 o'clock	12 o'clock	1 space below carina in left main bronchus
Right Hilar	9 o'clock	3 o'clock	Anterior spur of right upper lobe/ proximal portion of bronchus intermedius just below origin of right upper lobe
Left Hilar	3 o'clock	9 o'clock	Origin of left lower lobe bronchus

Fig. 13.10.1 Transbronchial fine needle aspiration (TBNA).

Where anterior approach denotes a bronchoscopy performed on a patient in a semi-recumbent procedure being approached from in front of the patient and posterior approach is where the patient is lying supine and approached from behind. The positions are described as a clockface and the vertical position in terms of cartilage ring spaces.

Technique

The objective is to insert the needle through the airway wall into the underlying lymph node or mass and obtain samples for cytology. The most widely used technique is to appose the hub of the needle onto the airway wall and then advance the needle out. The angle between the airway wall and the needle should be at least 45 degrees and the distal end of the bronchoscope angulated so as to advance the needle as perpendicularly as possible. Once the needle has been inserted fully through the airway an assistant applies suction with a syringe on the distal end and the operator gently manipulates the needle back and forth in the lymph node. This is known as the jabbing method. With the piggy back method the needle is protruding out, and the bronchoscope and TBNA needle is advanced as a single combined unit through the airway wall. In contrast with the cough technique the protruding needle is apposed to the airway wall and the patient is asked to cough gently. The force of the constricting airways pushes the needle through the airway wall into the target area.

Tissue preparation

The samples obtained can be either spread onto slides and then fixed or injected into saline or Cytolite solution for processing. Any tissue specimens that are obtained should be placed in formalin and sent for histopathology. The presence of a cyto-pathologist with rapid staining techniques and appropriate equipment significantly improves the efficacy of TBNA. Once the cytologist is confident that malignant cells are present from a specimen obtained from the highest staged lymph nodes, no further sampling is required. This considerably reduces the time and cost of the procedure. In the absence of rapid on site cytology (ROSE), the author recommends 4 needle passes at each abnormal lymph node site starting from the highest stage lymph node first.

Role in specific diseases

Diagnosis and staging of lung cancer
TBNA has a fundamental role in the diagnosis and staging of lung cancer. In a prospective series of patients with suspected lung cancer, 30% of patients underwent bronchoscopy with TBNA. It was the sole mode of diagnosis in 23% of patients. It provided staging information in 49 % of patients and only 1 in 1.47 procedures were needed to be performed to correctly diagnose or stage one patient. The sensitivity in the literature ranges from 39-78% depending on the prevalence of disease in the study group and methodological variations, but it is a simple procedure that can be performed at the time of initial bronchoscopy. The advantages of TBNA are that it can be established in any bronchoscopy unit with minimal cost. Consequently it can be performed in any individual who is fit for bronchoscopy and can be incorporated into the diagnostic pathway without incurring any delays in the assessment of patients. It also minimises the number of investigations that patients require for both diagnosis and staging.

Role in granulomatous diseases
The yield for TBNA in granulomatous disease is lower than that for malignant disease as predominantly cytological samples are obtained. The diagnosis of sarcoid is based on the presence of granulomas and hence more confidently made when tissue specimens are obtained.

Guided TBNA

EBUS TBNA
Integrated linear array ultrasound bronchoscopes are now available which allow accurate image guided transbronchial needle aspiration. This technique significantly increases the sensitivity of the procedure (over 90%) and allows sampling of lymph nodes as small as 5mm in size.

Superdimension TBNA

This system creates a virtual GPS map of the lung and mediastinum. A virtual bronchoscopy is performed from data obtained from a multi-slice CT and specific landmarks identified. The mediastinal lymph nodes can be marked as specific targets. At bronchoscopy a magnetic locating guide is used to identify the same anatomical points marked on the CT scan and the two pieces of information integrated together. This then allows the operator to navigate the locatable guide to target areas. The catheter is held in position, the locatable guide removed and replaced by a TBNA needle. This technique also significantly improves the sensitivity of TBNA although it is not performed under real time imaging.

AUTHOR'S TIPS

- Perform TBNA prior to any other aspect of the procedure to eliminate the risk of false positive.
- Sample lymph nodes from the highest staging site first e.g. Contra-lateral lymph nodes prior to ipsi-lateral lymph nodes or N2 lymph nodes prior to bronchial hilar lymph nodes.
- Treat all negative results as false negative and consider additional sampling techniques such as endobronchial ultrasound guided TBNA or mediastinoscopy.

Further reading

Harrow EM, Abi-Saleh W, Blum J, et al. The utility of transbronchial needle aspiration in the staging of bronchogenic carcinoma. *Am J Respir Crit Care Med* 2000; **161**(2 Pt 1): 601–607.

Holty JE, Kushner WG, Gould MK. Accuracy of transbronchial needle aspiration of mediastinal staging of non-small cell lung cancer: a met-analysis. *Thorax* 2005; **60**: 949–955.

Patelli M, Lazzari L, Poletti V, et al. Role of fiberoptic transbronchial needle aspiration in the staging of N2 disease due to non-small cell lung cancer. *Ann Thorac Surg* 2002; **73**: 407–411.

Shah PL, Singh S, Bower M, et al. The role of transbronchial fine needle aspiration (TBNA) in an integrated care pathway for the assessment of patients with suspected lung cancer. *J Thoracic Oncol* 2006; **1**; 324–327.

Wang KP, Terry PB. Transbronchial needle aspiration in the diagnosis and staging of bronchogenic carcinoma. *Am Rev Respir Dis* 1983; **127**:344–347.

13.11 Interventional bronchoscopy techniques

Introduction

That portion of a lung tumour which lies within or compresses the bronchial lumen is often the cause of many of its symptoms; examples include cough, haemoptysis, and breathlessness or infection caused by obstructive collapse. There may also be life-threatening large-airway obstruction. The ability to access the large and medium-sized airways with a flexible or rigid bronchoscope enables not only diagnostic and staging procedures to be carried out but also the administration of a number of therapies. The following may be achieved:

- Symptom relief.
- Ablation of large-airway obstructing tumours.
- Stabilisation of life-threatening tracheal obstruction prior to definitive tumour-reducing therapy.
- The eradication of small intra-bronchial tumours.
- The treatment of benign lesions.

Endobronchial treatment techniques fall into three categories.

1 Physical methods of tumour destruction and removal:
   (a) Endobronchial resection and dilatation.
   (b) Thermal laser, diathermy, and argon plasma coagulation.
   (c) Cryotherapy.
2 Biological therapies, with tumour selectivity and a delayed but potentially prolonged effect:
   (a) Brachytherapy.
   (b) Photo-dynamic therapy.
3 Stenting.

Endobronchial resection

Rigid bronchoscopy is normally required for the safe and effective removal or debridement of an endobronchial tumour using suction, forceps, or the bronchoscope tip itself to increase airway calibre. It may be combined with electro-coagulation and other thermal or freezing techniques. It is principally a palliative procedure but can occasionally be curative for benign and low-grade tumours. Endoscopic resection can be life-saving in critical upper-airway obstruction and is also useful to stabilise an airway to allow other treatment (such as brachytherapy) which would otherwise be hazardous. It is often required as a debulking procedure to remove dead tumour after photodynamic therapy.

Thermal destruction/coagulation

There are a number of variants:

NdYAG laser
- Normally used with a rigid bronchoscope to allow good airway control and the management of complications, especially haemorrhage. Small tumours and granulations can be removed using a flexible bronchoscope to deliver laser light.
- Light is transmitted by a coated flexible quartz-fibre, using a non-contact technique.
- F_iO_2 must be less than 30% to prevent fire risk.
- Coagulation occurs at lower powers (30–35watts), vapourization at higher power (40 + watts).
- Complications include bleeding, hypoxia, and bronchial perforation.

Diathermy (electrocautery)
A high-frequency alternating current is used to generate heat, enabling coagulation, cutting or vapourisation of tissue, dependent on the temperature generated
- Uses an insulated probe or snare, in direct or close contact.
- Can be delivered via a flexible bronchoscope, suitably insulated or grounded.
- Used for palliative debulking, the removal of pedunculated lesions, and the eradication of early-stage disease.
- Complications are comparable with thermal laser and include bleeding, airway obstruction, and airway perforation.
- F_iO_2 should be kept below 40% to reduce the danger of endobronchial fire.
- Electrocautery should not be applied to the full circumference of an airway, in order to minimise the risk of bronchial stricture.

Argon plasma coagulation (APC)
This is a non-contact technique using a probe to deliver ionised argon gas to produce coagulative necrosis.
- More superficial than diathermy, causing coagulation to a depth of 2–3mm.
- Effective for haemostasis but not for the debulking of large tumours.
- Minimal risk of airway perforation.
- Can be used with uncovered metal stents.
- Normally requires a power of 40 watts and a gas flow of 2 litres per minute.

Diathermy and APC may be delivered using combined equipment, increasing flexibility of treatment.

Cryotherapy

- Uses freezing to destroy tumour.
- A cryoprobe delivers liquid nitrogen or nitrous oxide, cooling the probe tip to -80°C on expansion (the Joule–Thomson effect).
- Used to treat haemoptysis and to remove obstructing tumour.
- Some of the treatment effect is delayed, and several treatments may be required.
- Can be used with the flexible bronchoscope—don't freeze the videochip!

Brachytherapy

The word derives from the Greek 'βrachis', meaning 'close to'. The technique uses a standard flexible bronchoscopy technique to place a blind-ending catheter or applicator through or alongside an endobronchial obstructing tumour; a radioactive source is then delivered from a safe, attached to its drive-cable. The treatment delivers an intense dose of radiation to a limited volume of tissue, eliminating or minimising radiation damage to surrounding organs. A high dose-rate iridium source is normally used, enabling treatment to be delivered in minutes. Most centres use fractionated regimes.
- Effective for primary and secondary palliation
- Results comparable with external beam radiotherapy
- Potentially curative for small intraluminal tumours

- Offers additional flexibility as an alternative treatment in a number of situations.
- Complications include radiation bronchitis, fibrotic stenosis, and massive fatal haemoptysis variably reported at 3–30%, probably local dose-dependent.

The effect on endobronchial tumours is delayed but progressive and potentially durable. Brachytherapy should be available on a regional or network basis as part of the multidisciplinary management of lung cancer.

Photodynamic therapy (PDT)

The word 'photodynamic' means pertaining or relating to the energy of light, and in a clinical setting implies a tissue-toxic response to light. An intravenous sensitiser is first administered, most frequently the porphyrin derivative, Porfimer sodium. It is selectively taken up by tumour tissue. Exposure of photo-sensitised tissue to laser light of an appropriate wavelength causes the release of highly active singlet-oxygen radicals which cause tumour cell death by thromboxane release, resulting in ischaemic necrosis.

- A flexible or rigid bronchoscope can be used.
- Laser light is delivered by a radial diffuser or a forward-projecting microlens, attached to a flexible light guide.
- Produces a local anti-tumour effect with minimal toxicity to surrounding tissue.
- Porfimer sodium is administered intravenously at a dosage of 2mg per kg.
- Illumination is generated by a Diode laser at 630 nm.
- The recommended dosage using a cylindrical diffuser is 200 Joules/cm, 100 Joules per cm^2 using the microlens.
- A typical treatment, using a 2.5cm diffuser, takes around 8 minutes to deliver.
- Can be used to debulk large obstructing tumours and to eradicate in situ and micro-invasive disease.
- The principal drawback is light sensitisation due to accumulation of the systemic sensitiser in skin. Light protection is required for up to eight weeks.
- Other complications include large-airway obstruction from tumour necrosis, occasional haemorrhage, and late fibrotic stricture.

Both brachytherapy and PDT offer the attractive option of potential cure in early central lung cancer without major loss of lung tissue. Careful post-treatment surveillance is required however, and may be assisted by the use of fluorescence bronchoscopy to identify and delineate recurrent/progressive disease.

Stenting

Tracheobronchial stents are hollow prostheses used to maintain or restore airway patency in malignant (and occasionally non-malignant) airway obstruction.

They are most often placed using a rigid bronchoscope but some can be placed with a flexible bronchoscope, with or without radiological screening.

Most bronchial stents are made either of silicone or metal mesh, especially Nitinol, a Nickel-Titanium alloy which retains its manufactured shape and is extremely biologically inert. Metal stents may be covered or uncovered, the latter only suitable for extrinsic compressive stenosis. They are placed using an applicator passed over a guidewire, then accurately released in the required position within the airway.

- May be life saving in critical tracheal obstruction.
- Useful to stabilise an airway prior to radiotherapy or other treatment which would otherwise be hazardous.
- Should not be regarded as a substitute for definitive tumour-reducing therapy.
- Complications include infection, granulation, and stent migration.
- Uncovered metal stents rapidly embed and epithelialise and therefore cannot be removed; they are to be used with caution in non-malignant disease.
- Late stent fracture has been reported.

Interventional bronchoscopy techniques can be used singly or in combination and should be considered along with standard methods of tumour-reducing therapy. They are best delivered as part of a multidisciplinary airway management service, perhaps involving more than one treatment centre but available on a regional or network basis. Selection of the appropriate technique (or combination of techniques), for a given patient and clinical situation, is of paramount importance.

Further reading

Barber P, Barr H, George J, et al. Photodynamic therapy in the treatment of lung and oesophageal cancers. *Clinical Oncology* 2002; **14**: 110–116.

Barber P, Stout R. High dose rate endobronchial brachytherapy for the treatment of lung cancer: current status and indications. Invited editorial, *Thorax* 1996; **51**: 345–347.

Ernst, Feller-Kopman D, Becker HD, et al. Central airway obstruction. *Am J Crit Care Med* 2004; **169**: 1278–1297.

Herth, Eberhardt R, Ernst A, et al. The future of bronchoscopy in diagnosing, staging and treatment of lung cancer. *Respiration* 2006; **73**: 4.

Saad, Murthy S, Krizmanich G, et al. Self-expandable metallic airway stents and flexible bronchoscopy. *Chest* 2003; **124**: 1993–1999.

Sutedja, Venmans BJ, Smit EF, et al. Fluorescence bronchoscopy for early detection of lung cancer. A clinical perspective. *Lung Cancer* 2001; **34**(2): 157–168.

Pleural disease

Chapter contents

14.1 Normal physiologic fluid volume and cellular contents

In normal conditions, the pleural space contains a small amount of pleural fluid. This small volume of pleural fluid is maintained in the pleural space by a complex interplay of hydrostatic pressures and lymphatic drainage, which allows for steady liquid and protein turnover.

Pathological processes may lead to the development of pleural effusions by causing disequilibrium between the rates of pleural fluid formation, pleural permeability, and pleural fluid absorption. The focus here is on the normal pleural fluid volume, cellular and solute content in normal, physiological circumstances. Normal pleural fluid is a microsvascular filtrate; its volume and composition are tightly controlled. Liquid enters the pleural space through the parietal pleura down a net filtering pressure gradient, and is removed by an absorptive pressure gradient through the visceral pleura, by lymphatic drainage through parietal pleura stomas, and by cellular mechanisms (active transport of solutes by mesothelial cells).

The main function of the normal pleural fluid is thought to be lubrication of the pleural surfaces, enabling transmission of the forces of breathing between the lung and the chest wall. Together with the presence of subatmospheric pressures within the pleural space, this lubrication function enables respiratory movements by a mechanical coupling between lung and chest wall. This lubrication function is supported by the presence of surfactant lipids in normal pleural fluid, which are efficient in terms of boundary lubrication and adherence to biological surfaces, and of hyaluran. Most of what is known about the volume, composition, and dynamics of normal pleural fluid has been obtained from animal studies. Retrieval of the few mililiters of normal pluid fluid in humans indeed is difficult without traumatically disturbing the pleural space: therefore, only a few human studies are available.

Animal studies

Data derived from animal studies are summarised in Table 14.1.1. Although there is a certain degree of concordance as to the total volume and total white blood cell count of normal rabbit and dog pleural fluid, there is a large disparity between the various differential cell counts between the various animal models. The reasons for this disparity include differences in identification of and distinction between macrophages, monocytes and mesothelial cells, and methodological differences in fixation, staining and fluid retrieval techniques (aspiration or lavage), and possible genuine interspecies differences.

Miserocchi and Agostoni collected pleural fluid from the costodiaphragmatic sinuses of rabbits and dogs. In rabbits, 0.46 ml of free fluid could be retrieved from both pleural spaces (0.2 ml.kg-1). In dogs, 0.55 ml or 0.15 ml.kg-1 could be collected. When the volume of fluid adherent to the lung surfaces was assessed and included, volumes of pleural fluid rose to 0.4 ml.kg-1 and 0.26 ml.kg-1 respectively. Total and differential white blood cell counts were performed using a cell counting chamber and May-Gzunwald-Giemsa stained cell smears. In rabbits, 2442±595 cell.µL-1 were present including 31.8% mesothelial cells, 60.8% monocytes, and 7.4% lymphocytes. In dogs, 2208±734 cells.µL-1 were present, including 69.6% mesothelial cells, 28.2% monocytes, and 2.2% lymphocytes. Stauffer et al compared different cytopreparations and different methods of fluid

collection in rabbits: aspiration of the free fluid versus irrigation with 10 ml Hanks solution. The total volume of aspirated pleural fluid volume for both pleural spaces was 0.45 ± 0.12 ml (0.13 ml.kg-1). Total white blood cell count for the original aspirated fluid was 1503± 281 cells.µL-1. Differential cell counts varied with the different methods of fixation (95% alcohol and Papinacolaou stain versus 50% alcohol, 1% polyethylene glycol, and Papinicolaou stain) between 38.6 and 70.1% monocytes, 10 and 10.6% lymphocytes, and 5.5 and 16.6 macrophages. Sahn et al aspirated costodiaphragmatic fluid in rabbits. Total volume of the free pleural fluid in both pleural spaces was 0.45 ± 0.90 ml (0.13 ml.kg-1). Total white blood cell count was 1503 ± 414 cells.µL-1, with 70.1 ± 3.6% monocytes, 10.6 ± 1.8% lymphocytes, 8.9 ± 1.6% mesothelial cells and 7.5 ± 1.5% macrophages. Novakov et al performed aspiration and lavage in rabbits. Volumes and total white blood cell counts were not reported; differential cell counts included 9.25% macrophages, 66.5% monocytes, 8 % mesothelial cells, and 9.75% lymphocytes after aspiration, and 5% macrophages, 60.17% monocytes, 10% mesothelial cells, and 11.08% lymphocytes after lavage. Other measurements of pleural fluid volume have been made by Broaddus, Wang, and Agostoni in rabbits, Mellins in dogs, Wiener-Kronish, and Broaddus in sheep and Miserocchi in various animal models (cats, puppies, dogs, cats, and pigs), as part of studies for other purposes than actual volume measurements. All measurements (except those in puppies) yielded total volumes between 0.04 and 0.28 ml.kg-1.

The solute composition of normal pleural fluid is similar to that of interstitial fluid of other organs and contains 1 to 2 grams of protein 100 ml-1, mainly consisting of albumin (50%), globulins (35%) and fibrinogen. Levels of large molecular weight proteins such as lactate dehydrogenase in the pleural fluid are less than half of that found in serum.

Human studies

Reliable data on the volume and cellular content of pleural fluid in normal humans are scarse, because of the obvious difficulties in retrieving this small amount of fluid without 'disturbing' the pleural environment. The first study addressing this issue was that of Yamada, published in 1933, who punctured the 9th or 10th intercostal space on the dorsal axillary line in a group of healthy Japanese soldiers. In about 30% of cases some fluid was aspirated after a period of rest, whereas in about 70% of cases some fluid was retrieved after exercise. Usually only a few drops of foam was aspirated but in a few cases up to 20 ml could be retrieved. Total white blood cell count was 4500 µL-1 (range 1700 – 6200). Differential cell count showed 53.7% cells similar to monocytes, 10.2% lymphocytes, 3% mesothelial cells, 3.6% granulocytes, and 29.5% 'deteriorated cels of difficult classification'. More recently, a pleural lavage technique was used to retrieve the few millilitres of pleural fluid present in the pleural space of otherwise healthy participants undergoing thoracoscopic sympathectomy for the treatment of essential hyperhidrosis. In analogy with bronchoalveolar lavage (a technique enabling retrieval of small volumes of epithelial lining fluid from the lung), 150 ml of prewarmed saline was injected in, and immediately aspirated from the right pleural space, after induction of a pneumothorax in the setting of a thoracoscopic sympathectomy performed for the treatment of

Table 14.1.1

Species	Mean volume (right & left pleural space) ml.kg-1	Total white blood cell count, µL-1	Macrophages (%)	Monocytes (%)	Mesothelial Cells (%)	Lymphocytes (%)
Rabbits	0.2	2442 ± 595	NR	60.8	31.8	7.4
Dogs	0.15	2208 ± 734	NR	28.2	69.8	8.2
Rabbits	0.13	1503 ± 281	7.6 to 16	38.6 to 70.1	3.7 to 25.4	10 to 10.6
Rabbits	0.13	1503 ± 414	7.5 ± 1.5	70.1 ± 3.6	8.9 ± 1.6	10.6 ± 1.8
Rabbits	NR	NR	9.25	66.5	8	9.75
Rabbits	NR	NR	5	60.17	10	11
Rabbits	0.1	1216 ± 800	NR	NR	NR	NR
Rabbits	0.09	NR	NR	NR	NR	NR
Rabbits	0.22	NR	NR	NR	NR	NR
Dogs	0.1	NR	NR	NR	NR	NR
Sheep	0.12	NR	NR	NR	NR	NR
Sheep	0.04	NR	NR	NR	NR	NR
Rats	0.6	NR	NR	NR	NR	NR
Puppies	1.33	NR	NR	NR	NR	NR
Cats	0.28	NR	NR	NR	NR	NR
Pigs	0.22	NR	NR	NR	NR	NR

essential hyperhidrosis. With urea used as an endogeneous marker of dilution, measured mean right-sided pleural fluid volume was 8.4 ± 4.3 ml. In a subgroup of subjects, right- and leftsided pleural fluid volumes were shown to be similar. Expressed per kg of body mass, total pleural fluid volume in non-smoking, healthy subjects is 0.26 ml.kg-1, which corresponds well with values obtained in animal studies. Total white blood cell count in the pleural fluid of normal non-smoking subjects was 1716 cells µL-1. Differential cell count yielded a predominance of macrophages (median 75%, interquartile range 16%) and lymphocytes (median 23%, interquartile range 18%). Mesothelial cells, neutrophils, and eosinophils were only marginally present. A typical image of a cell smear is shown in Fig. 14.1.1. In a second study using a similar lavage technique, lymphocyte subtyping showed a lower proportion of CD4 positive T cells (30% vs 45.8 %) and a higher proportion of CD8 positive T cells (11.78 vs 9.6 %) and regulatory T cells (CD4+CD25high) in pleural fluid in normal subjects as compared to blood which may suggest that previously described abnormalities in lymphocyte subsets in pleural effusions may not only be a result of the pleural disease itself but also be characteristic of the pleural compartment itself. Interestingly, a small but statistically significant increase in pleural fluid neutrophils was observed in smoking subjects. In addition to revealing the volume and cellular composition of normal pleural fluid (which may be helpful in understanding cellular events occurring in disorders characterised by pleural effusions), this pleural lavage technique allows to study the pathophysiological events in pleural disorders which typically are not associated with pleural effusions, such as pneumothorax and asbestos-related pleurisy.

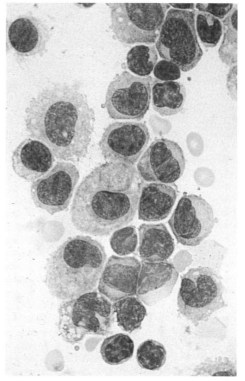

Fig. 14.1.1 A typical cell smear of a pleural lavage sample in a normal, non-smoking subject.

KEY ISSUES

- In normal animals and humans, the pleural space contains a small volume of pleural fluid. In different animal species this volume varies between 0.04 and 0.20 ml.kg-1. In normal humans, the pleural fluid volume is 0.26ml.kg-1.
- This fluid has the solute characteristics of all interstitial fluids, and contains a total of 1000 to 2500 white blood cells per µL. Macrophages/monocytes and lymphocytes are the predominant cell types.
- Pleural lavage is a safe and simple technique allowing the study of normal pleural fluid, and of pleural disease which is not characterised by pleural effusions.

Further reading

Broaddus VC, Araya M, Carlton DP, et al. Developmental changes in pleural liquid protein concentration in sheep. Am Rev Respir Dis 1991; 143: 38–41.

MiserocchiG, Negrini D, Mortola J. Comparative features of Starling-lymphatic interaction at the pleural level in mammals. J Appl Physiol 1984; 56:1151-1156.

Miserocchi G, Agostoni E. Contents of pleural space. J Appl Physiol 1971; 30: 208–213S.

Miserocchi G. Physiology and pathophysiology of pleural fluid turnover. Eur Respir J 1997; 10: 219–225.

Noppen M, De Waele M, Li R, et al. Volume and cellular content of normal pleural fluid in humans examined by pleural lavage. Am J Respir Crit Care Med 2001;7:180–182.

Noppen M, Herregodts P, D'haese J, et al. A simplified thoracoscopic sympathicolysis technique for essential hyperhidrosis: results in 100 consecutive patients. J Laparoendosc Surg 1996; 6:151–159.

Noppen M. Normal volume and cellular contents of pleural fluid. Curr Opin Pulm Med 2001;7:180–182.

14.2 Assessment and investigation of an undiagnosed pleural effusion (including thoracoscopy)

Introduction

Pleural effusions are a common medical problem, affecting over 3000 people per million population annually. They are a manifestation of over 50 underlying diseases, some pleuro-pulmonary and some systemic. The commonest causes of pleural effusion in the USA and UK are heart failure, pneumonia, and malignancy.

The approach to the patient with a pleural effusion requires a structured approach to formulate the likely diagnosis, minimise invasive investigations and guide treatment.

Pathophysiology

The normal pleural cavity contains approximately 0.13–0.06ml/kg body mass of fluid for lubrication during respiration. Pleural effusions arise when the balance between pleural fluid production and its absorption has been disturbed. Transudative effusions occur due to an increase in hydrostatic pressure or reduction in tissue oncotic pressure; whereas exudates accumulate secondary to increased pleural permeability or impaired absorption (e.g. obstructed lymphatic flow). Transdiaphragmatic passage of ascites or peritoneal dialysate from the abdomen, chyle (chylothorax), blood (haemothorax) or rarely urine (urinothorax), bile or CSF may also result in pleural effusion.

History

A thorough history should determine previous asbestos exposure, risk factors for heart failure, tuberculosis exposure, pack-years smoking history, features of malignancy or infection. A drug history is also important as a number of medications have been associated with exudative pleural effusions (Table 14.2.1); http://www.pneumotox.com is a useful resource for further information.

Table 14.2.1

Drugs most commonly associated with pleural effusion
• Amiodarone
• Nitrofurantoin
• Phenytoin
• Methotrexate
• Penicillamine
• Carbamazepine
• Cyclophosphamide
• Cabergoline
• Pergolide

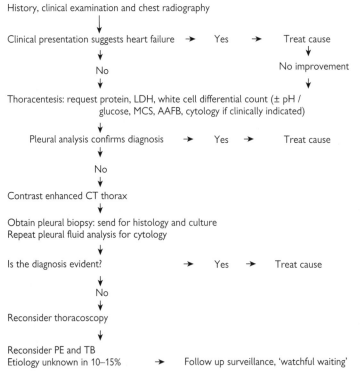

Fig. 14.2.1 Diagnostic algorithm for the patient with an undiagnosed unilateral pleural effusion.

Clinical features

Patients may be asymptomatic but often present with dyspnoea, chest pain or cough. Dyspnoea arises as a consequence of altered diaphragm mechanics (secondary to increased pleural pressure) as well as decreased chest wall compliance and impaired underlying lung function.

Pleuritic chest pain indicates irritation of the parietal pleural surface, ribs or chest wall.

Cough is a non-specific symptom, although expectoration of purulent sputum indicates an infective aetiology.

The presence of constitutional symptoms such as weight loss, night sweats, anorexia, and malaise typically occur with infective causes or malignancy, and joint, skin or eye symptoms may indicate underlying connective tissue disease.

Physical examination reveals a stony dull percussion note with decreased fremitus and absent breath sounds. Clinical detection of less than 250–300ml of pleural fluid is difficult.

Features of heart failure, malignancy and connective tissue disease should be sought.

Investigation

In most cases, the underlying diagnosis is determined by the clinical history and examination supplemented by chest radiography and pleural fluid analysis. A systematic diagnostic approach is outlined in Fig. 14.2.1.

Pleural fluid analysis

Thoracentesis

Thoracentesis (pleural aspiration) is indicated in patients with a newly discovered pleural effusion except where there is a secure diagnosis of heart failure. Diagnostic pleural fluid aspiration using a 21F bore needle is safe and few contraindications exist. Ultrasound guidance should be used if the fluid volume is small or heavily loculated. Therapeutic aspiration of 1-2L of fluid can relieve breathlessness but complete drainage should not be performed prior to CT imaging as superior images are obtained with pleural fluid present.

Table 14.2.2 lists recommended initial pleural fluid tests for effusions of unknown aetiology.

Table 14.2.2

Biochemistry	Protein
	Lactate dehydrogenase (LDH)
	Glucose
	pH (if no blood gas analyser available)
Cytology	Cytological analysis
	Differential white cell count
Microbiology	Grams' stain and culture
	Acid fast bacilli stain and culture

Following diagnostic aspiration note:

Appearance and odour

Pleural fluid may be serous (straw coloured) or blood stained (serosanguineous). Blood stained fluid may occur in malignancy, tuberculosis, pulmonary infarction, trauma, benign asbestos pleural effusion (BAPE) or post cardiac injury surgery (PCIS). A true haemothorax (fluid haematocrit >50% blood haematocrit) is usually related to trauma.

Milky pleural fluid occurs in chylothorax, pseudochylothorax or empyema. Putrid odour suggests anaerobic infection and an ammonia smell is characteristic of urinothorax. The presence of food particles is indicative of oesophageal rupture.

Is the fluid a transudate or exudate?

Differentiation between exudative and transudative effusions aids diagnosis (Table 14.2.3), and all initial pleural fluid samples should be sent for measurement of protein and lactate dehydrogenase (LDH).

In clinical practice, pleural fluid protein levels <27g/l represent a transudate and >35g/l an exudate. In borderline cases, pleural fluid is an exudate if any of Light's criteria apply:

- Pleural fluid to serum protein ratio >0.5.
- Pleural fluid to serum LDH >0.6.
- Pleural fluid LDH >2/3 the upper limit of normal serum LDH.

Light's criteria are very sensitive in determining exudative effusions however misclassification may occur particularly in patients with heart failure taking diuretic therapy or in those with two separate diagnoses such as cancer and heart failure.

Table 14.2.3 Causes of pleural effusions

Transudates	Exudates
Common causes	**Common causes**
Left ventricular failure	Malignancy
Liver cirrhosis 'hepatic hydrothorax'	Parapneumonic effusions
Hypoalbuminaemia	Pulmonary infarction
Peritoneal dialysis	Rheumatoid arthritis
	Mesothelioma
Less common causes	**Less common causes**
Nephrotic syndrome	Empyema
Hypothyroidism	Tuberculosis
Mitral stenosis	SLE
Pulmonary embolism (10–20%)	Other autoimmune diseases
	Benign asbestos pleural effusion
	Pancreatitis
	Post cardiac injury syndrome (Dressler's)
	Post coronary artery bypass grafting
	Hepatic/Splenic/Subphrenic abscess
	Oesophageal rupture
Rare causes	**Rare causes**
Constrictive pericarditis	Yellow nail syndrome
Urinothorax	Chylothorax
Meigs' syndrome	Drugs
Ovarian hyperstimulation syndrome	Sarcoidosis
SVCO	Fungal infections
Malignancy (up to 5% are transudates)	

Differential cell count

The predominant cellular population within a pleural aspirate is determined by the nature of the pleural insult and timing of thoracentesis relative to the injury.

Acute inflammation produces a typically neutrophilic pleural fluid e.g. infection, whereas in chronic pleural effusion, e.g. malignancy or tuberculosis, mononuclear cells prevail. Lymphocytic effusions are common in chronic diseases of insidious onset such as tuberculosis (usually over 80%) or malignancy.

Eosinophilic (>10% of total leukocytes) pleural fluid is often diagnostically unhelpful and occurs in both benign (e.g. air or blood in pleural cavity, drug reactions or Churg–Strauss syndrome) and malignant conditions.

Pleural fluid pH and glucose
Pleural fluid pH should be measured in all cases of suspected pleural infection. All non-purulent samples can be heparinised (in an arterial blood gas syringe) and the pH measured in a standard blood gas analyser. Care must be taken, during pleural aspiration, to avoid contamination with local anaesthetic, e.g. lidocaine, which is acidic and can produce a falsely low pH reading.

Normal pleural fluid pH is around 7.6 (as a result of bicarbonate accumulation in the pleural space). Pleural pH <7.3 reflects a substantial amount of lactic acid production and is seen with intense pleural inflammation. Low pleural fluid glucose (<3.3mmol/l) is seen with a similar spectrum of disease reflecting metabolic activity within the pleural space.

Causes of exudative effusions with low pleural fluid pH and glucose concentration include: complicated parapneumonic effusion and empyema, rheumatoid pleuritis, malignancy, tuberculous pleuritis, oesophageal rupture and lupus pleuritis. Urinothorax is the only transudative effusion to be, rarely, associated with a low pleural fluid pH.

Clinically a pleural fluid pH <7.2 in the context of *pleural infection* indicates a need for urgent pleural drainage. Some data suggest that in malignant pleural effusion, pleural fluid pH <7.3 is associated with a poorer prognosis and lower pleurodesis success rate.

A high pleural fluid pH (>7.6) may be seen with *Proteus*-related pleural infection.

Microbiology
Send samples in a sterile pot and blood culture bottles (may improve the yield of bacterial culture).

Frank pus, turbid pleural fluid, Grams' stain and/or culture positive fluid or a pleural pH <7.2 in the context of clinical infection secure the diagnosis of pleural infection and indicate a need for prompt pleural drainage.

Pleural fluid culture is negative in 40% of those with pleural infection however; amplification of bacterial DNA can provide a diagnosis in a proportion of these cases.

In cases of tuberculous pleuritis direct smears of pleural fluid for acid-fast bacilli (AFB) are positive in <20%, and pleural fluid culture sensitivity <50%. This reflects the low mycobacterial load. Demonstration of granulomata histologically is often required to establish the diagnosis.

Cytology
Pleural fluid cytology has a sensitivity of approximately 60%, dependent on cell type and experience of the cytologist. Yield is increased with detection of a further 27% of cases with analysis of a second, but not third, pleural aspirate.

Immunocytochemistry can improve accuracy of cell type diagnosis and flow cytometry should be requested if lymphoma is a possibility.

Other pleural fluid analysis
Pleural fluid amylase levels higher than the normal range for serum, or a pleural-to-serum ratio >1, are seen in effusions associated with acute pancreatitis, oesophageal rupture, and malignancy (especially adenocarcinoma). Isoenzyme analysis differentiates between amylase of pancreatic or salivary origin.

Pleural fluid cholesterol and triglyceride levels should be requested if chylothorax or pseudochylothorax is suspected. Simple bench centrifugation of turbid/cloudy pleural fluid can aid differentiation from empyema when there is diagnostic doubt. A clear supernatant is seen in empyema as the cell debris sediments whereas a chylous effusion remains milky. The presence of chylomicrons or a triglyceride concentration >1.24mmol/L (110mg/dL) confirms the diagnosis of chylothorax. Whereas the detection of cholesterol crystals at microscopy or a cholesterol level >5.18mmol/l (200mg/dL) is diagnostic of a pseudochylothorax.

Raised adenosine deaminase (ADA) levels are very sensitive for tuberculous pleural effusion however, its specificity is limited. Therefore, measurement is not routinely recommended except in TB endemic areas where low pleural fluid ADA levels effectively exclude tuberculous effusions.

Elevated pleural fluid creatinine (fluid: serum ratio >1) is diagnostic of urinothorax, a condition which arises ipsilateral to an obstructed kidney as a consequence of the passage of urine through retroperitoneal space into the pleural space.

Measurement of pleural fluid rheumatoid factor and antinuclear antibodies is unhelpful diagnostically as levels mirror serum values. The presence of lupus erythematosus ('LE') cells in pleural fluid is diagnostic of systemic lupus erythematosus (SLE) related pleuritis.

Detection of β-transferrin, found in cerebrospinal fluid, confirms the presence of a duro-pleural fistula.

Imaging
CXR
Most pleural effusions are revealed with an erect plain posterior-anterior (PA) ± lateral chest radiograph. Blunting of the costophrenic angle occurs with approximately 200ml of fluid. If the patient is imaged supine (e.g. if ventilated on ICU) hazy opacification of the hemithorax is seen. Subpulmonic effusions can be difficult to diagnose with an erect PA CXR but a lateral view may demonstrate a flattened posterior hemi-diaphragm. Evidence of the underlying cause may become apparent i.e. bilateral effusions with cardiomegaly in heart failure or presence of concomitant lobar collapse or a parenchymal mass in malignant disease.

Ultrasound
Ultrasound is safe and easy to perform. It will confirm the presence of pleural fluid in borderline CXR cases with a sensitivity of almost 100%, and should be used to guide aspiration of small or heavily septated effusions.

CT
Contrast enhanced CT imaging, with pleural fluid in situ and allowing time for contrast medium to enter the tissue phase, allows effective delineation of the pleural surface. Nodular, circumferential or mediastinal pleural thickening and parietal pleural thickening >1cm, all favour malignant disease with sensitivities approaching 100%.

Pleural empyema may be differentiated from lung abscess with thoracic CT. The 'split pleura' sign is often demonstrated in empyema with enhancement of the visceral and parietal pleural surfaces evident. A lenticular shape and compression of surrounding parenchyma is also seen with empyema.

Coincidental endobronchial disease or asbestos related lung pathology may be discovered.

MRI

Although MR imaging is as sensitive as CT for defining pleural disease it is not routinely used for cost and accessibility reasons. However, MR is preferred in patients where minimisation of radiation dose is important e.g. young women with susceptible breast tissue and benign pleural disease.

PET

PET is not routinely indicated in the investigation of pleural effusion however, may aid differentiation of malignant from benign pleural disease.

Pleural biopsy

In cases where pleural fluid analysis is non-diagnostic, pleural biopsy for histological examination should be considered. Tissue can be obtained under direct vision at thoracoscopy or via closed (blind) or imaging-guided percutaneous biopsy.

Thoracoscopic biopsy techniques are most sensitive and should be the method of choice where possible.

Thoracoscopy with pleural biopsy

Thoracoscopy is indicated for patients with undiagnosed cytology negative exudative pleural effusions. It can be performed under local or general anaesthesia, using a single port or two-port technique.

Thoracoscopy allows direct visualization of the pleural surface, biopsy of areas which appear abnormal and therapeutic manoeuvres such as complete fluid drainage ± pleurodesis during the same procedure (Figs. 14.2.2 and 14.2.3). The diagnostic rate is approximately 90% for malignant pleural disease and approaches 100% in tuberculous pleurisy.

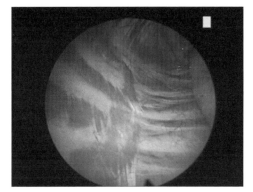

Fig. 14.2.2 Normal thoracoscopic appearance of parietal pleural surface (see Plate 13).

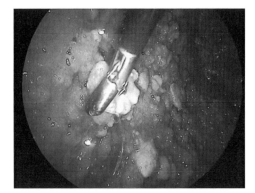

Fig. 14.2.3 Thoracoscopic biopsy via two-port technique (mesothelioma) (see Plate 14).

Contraindications include an obliterated pleural space, significant pleural adhesions, bleeding diathesis, unstable cardiovascular disease or hypoxia (oxygen saturations <92% on room air).

Medical thoracoscopy is conducted under sedation with local anaesthetic and may be carried out as a day-case. A short stay in hospital can be expected if therapeutic talc poudrage has been performed. For details of the procedure see Chapter 69 of the *Oxford Handbook of Respiratory Medicine*.

Thoracoscopy is safe and complications rare. Intra-pleural haemorrhage and air/gas embolism on pneumothorax induction occur in approximately 0.1%. Empyema, local skin infection and port-site pain, which may persist for several weeks, are also recognised. Mortality rates are low (<0.01%).

Closed blind pleural biopsies are performed using an Abrams' biopsy needle. They are indicated in cases of suspected pleural tuberculosis where diffuse granulomatous pleural involvement is seen. Diagnostic sensitivity is around 90% when both pleural histology and culture are analysed. Closed biopsies are less sensitive when pleural involvement is patchy i.e. malignancy.

At least four biopsies are recommended from a single site, and the samples should be placed in sterile saline (for AFB smear and culture) and 10% formaldehyde (for histological examination). Complications are uncommon but include chest pain, pneumothorax (approximately 1% of patients require chest drain insertion) and vasovagal reactions.

Imaging-guided (CT or ultrasound) biopsy is superior to closed biopsies in patients with suspected malignant pleural disease as focal areas of pleural thickening can be targeted (sensitivity 87% for CT-guided biopsy vs 47% for Abrams' biopsy).

Bronchoscopy has no role in the routine investigation of an undiagnosed pleural effusion; however, should be considered if endobronchial pathology is detected during the diagnostic work-up (usually with CT scanning).

The persistent undiagnosed pleural effusion

Despite thorough investigation about 15% of exudative pleural effusions remain undiagnosed. In approximately 15% of these underlying malignancy is eventually proven.

Important diagnoses to reconsider in cases of unexplained pleural effusion include pulmonary embolism and tuberculosis as specific treatment is available to prevent ongoing patient morbidity.

Further reading

Diacon AH, Van de Wal BW, Wyser C, et al. Diagnostic tools in tuberculous pleurisy: a direct comparative study. *Eur Respir J* 2003; **22**: 589–591.

Garcia LW, Ducatman BS, Wang HH. The value of multiple fluid specimens in the cytological diagnosis of malignancy. *Mod Pathol.* 1994; **7**: 665–668.

Hansen M, Faurschou P, Clementsen P. Medical thoracoscopy, results and complications in 146 patients: a retrospective study. *Respir Med* 1998; **92**: 228–232.

Menzies R,.Charbonneau M. Thoracoscopy for the diagnosis of pleural disease. *Ann Intern Med* 1991; **114**: 271–276.

Rodriguez-Panadero F, Lopez MJ. Low glucose and pH levels in malignant pleural effusions. Diagnostic significance and prognostic value in respect to pleurodesis. *Am Rev Respir Dis* 1989; **139**: 663–667.

Sahn SA,.Good JT, Jr. Pleural fluid pH in malignant effusions. Diagnostic, prognostic, and therapeutic implications. *Ann Intern Med* 1988; **108**:345–349.

14.3 Pneumothorax

Definition

- Pneumothorax literally means 'air in the chest'.
- Air becomes trapped between the lung (visceral pleura) and the chest wall (parietal pleura) causing varying degrees of lung collapse.
- Pneumothoraces are divided into **Primary** (the underlying lung is normal) and **Secondary** (associated with lung disease – e.g. COPD and emphysema, interstitial lung disease, cystic fibrosis, infections, etc).
- Pneumothorax may also be **Iatrogenic** (eg transthoracic needle biopsy, central line insertion, acupuncture) or **Traumatic** (e.g. rib fracture, chest trauma, penetrating or blast injury).
- **Tension pneumothorax** occurs when air enters but cannot leave the pleural space, causing a progressive build up of pressure, compromise of the mediastinal structures, impairment of venous return, shock and risk of death

Prevalence

The annual consulting rate for primary and secondary pneumothoraces combined is approximately 24/100,000 (men) and 10/100,000 (women). Hospital admission rates are around 17/100,000 (men) and 6/100,000 (women). Mortality rates are low at 1.3/million (men) and 0.6/million(women).

Epidemiology

Over half of all pneumothoraces are traumatic in origin (trauma or iatrogenic). There is a bimodal age distribution the peaks being attributable to primary (15–34 years) and secondary (over 55 years). Pneumothorax is commoner in men with a ratio of about 3:1 due to a number of possible factors including higher smoking rates, tall thin body habitus and different lung mechanics. Other reported associations of primary pneumothorax include, loud music (`The Pink Floyd Effect'!) type A personality angen, phases of the moon, and falls in humidity and ambient air pressure! Pneumothorax has been reported in families with an autosomal dominance with variable penetrance. Recognised genetic conditions associated with pneumothorax include collagen disorders such as Ehlers–Danlos syndrome, cystic fibrosis, homocystinuria, and alpha 1 antitrypsin deficiency.

Aetiology

Primary

Rupture of pleural blebs and bullae probably plays a role in pathogenesis as they are more frequently seen on CT scans and at thoracoscopy in cases of pneumothorax.

- Subpleural emphysema-like changes are also thought to be important in the aetiology of pneumothorax (Fig. 14.3.2).
- Inflammatory changes typically caused by smoking, in small distal airways cause obstruction and increased pressure in the distal lung parenchyma. This leads to rupture of the visceral pleura and may also cause mediastinal pleural leaks that are also likely to be important aetiologically. Smoking confers a 22-fold increase in relative risk of developing pneumothorax for men and a 9-fold increased risk for women.

Secondary

- Almost any lung disease has been reported as causing secondary pneumothorax. Common causes include:-
  - Airway diseases (e.g. COPD, acute severe asthma, cystic fibrosis).
  - Infections (pneumocystis, tuberculosis, abscess forming organisms, e.g. *Staphylococcus*) (Fig. 14.3.3).
  - Interstitial lung disease (sarcoid, pulmonary fibrosis, histiocytosis X, lymphangioleiomyomatosis).
  - Connective tissue disease (Rheumatoid, Marfans, and Ehlers–Danlos).
  - Tumours (lung cancer, sarcoma).

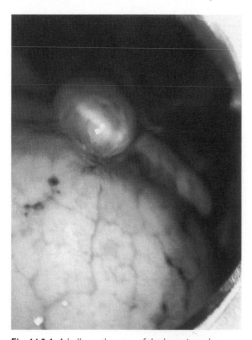

Fig. 14.3.1 A bulla on the apex of the lung viewed thoracoscopically. (Courtesy of Mr T Morgan).

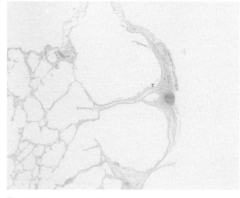

Fig. 14.3.2 Emphysema-like changes just beneath the visceral pleura. (Courtesy of Journal of Bronchology).

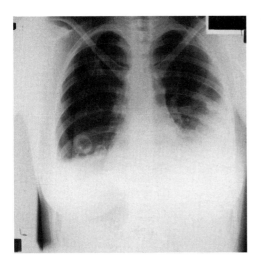

Fig. 14.3.3 This pneumothorax is due to multiple septicaemic staphylococcal abscesses in a young diabetic girl. One of the abscesses has ruptured through the visceral pleura to cause a pyo-pneumothorax. A chest drain is needed.

Clinical features

Symptoms

Primary pneumothorax may not cause any symptoms and may be an incidental radiological finding.

Usually patients will experience a sharp pleuritic pain with or without dyspnoea.

Small pneumothoraces may be overlooked and the symptoms attributed to pleurisy, pneumonia, musculo-skeletal pain, pulmonary embolism or angina.

Dyspnoea is invariably present in secondary pneumothorax and may be severe and associated with respiratory failure even with small pneumothoraces.

Signs

Abnormal signs usually require the presence of a moderate/large pneumothorax.

Hyper-resonance, reduced chest expansion, reduced vocal fremitus and reduced/absent breath sounds may all occur on the affected side.

In a mediastinal air leak a clicking/crunching sound may be heard or palpated, which the patient themselves may also sense.

Subcutaneous emphysema rarely occurs and causes a palpable sub-cutaneous crepitus.

Tension pneumothorax is associated with tachycardia, hypotension, mediastinal shift, and respiratory failure.

Radiology of pneumothorax

A standard PA chest radiograph taken in full inspiration is sufficient.

There is no evidence that routine use of additional expiratory or lateral films increases the diagnostic yield for experienced clinicians.

In cases of bullous lung disease a CT scan may be needed to differentiate pneumothorax from bullae.

CT scanning may be necessary if the plain radiograph is obscured by surgical emphysema.

Estimating the size of a pneumothorax

The clinical status of the patient rather than the estimated size of a pneumothorax should be the main criteria for treatment decisions.

A large primary pneumothorax may not require any intervention whilst a small secondary pneumothorax may require urgent drainage.

The most accurate assessment of the volume of a pneumothorax requires CT scanning. This is not necessary for the majority of patients.

The best method of estimating the size of a pneumothorax is much debated! It is not an exact science, since the lung often collapses leaving an uneven edge.

One reasonable approach classifies pneumothoraces as 'small' or 'large' depending on whether the distance between the lateral chest wall and collapsed lung edge is <2cm or >2cm.

The actual volume of a 2cm pneumothorax is approximately 50%.

Management of pneumothorax

Primary (Fig. 14.3.4 and 14.3.5)

Those with no or minimal symptoms can safely be treated by observation alone and discharged home with review at 2 weeks. They should be provided with verb\al and written instructions to return immediately if they become breathless. Patients with marked dyspnoea and/or a 'large' pneumothorax should undergo simple aspiration (see algorithm).

> **AUTHOR'S TIP**
> If whilst aspirating a primary pneumothorax air is still easily removed after 2.5l have been aspirated, success is unlikely. Give up. Re-X-ray and consider intercostal tube drainage.

If simple aspiration fails and less *than 2.5l of air have been aspirated* a second attempt is worth considering and may succeed in up to one third of cases.

However in most cases if aspiration is unsuccessful, intercostal tube drainage is usually recommended.

Small bore catheters (approx. 14F) may also be used for aspiration and attached to a Heimlich valve or water seal device until the lung re-expands.

New but expensive catheter kits with integral Heimlich type valves may also be equally effective and allow out patient management.

There is likely to be an increasing trend to earlier use of definitive thoracoscopic surgery.

There is no relationship between the risk of a future recurrence and either the size of a primary pneumothorax or the initial method of treatment.

Secondary (Fig. 14.3.5)

The majority of cases will be breathless and require a drainage procedure.

> **AUTHOR'S TIP**
> In COPD and emphysema the symptoms and signs of secondary pneumothorax may be wrongly attributed to the underlying lung disease so that the presence of a pneumothorax is overlooked. Examine the CXR carefully.

If the pneumothorax is 'small' and the symptoms mild, simple aspiration can be tried and the patient admitted for observation.

All 'large' secondary pneumothoraces and all those with significant dyspnoea should be treated with intercostal tube drainage (see algorithm).

Failure of lung expansion or persistent air leak following intercostal tube drainage

- Check tube position on x-ray. Is it kinked or blocked by partially expanded lung?
- If tube is in a good position try high volume/low pressure suction (−10 to −20cm H_2O).
- If the lung fails to expand or air leak persists discuss early (3–5 days) with thoracic surgeons.
- For those patients who are considered too high risk for VATS or thoracic surgery, consider chemical pleurodesis (see Chapter 14.6).

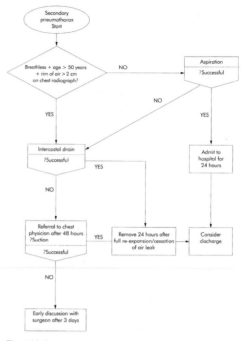

Fig. 14.3.5 Algorithm for the management of secondary pneumothorax. (Courtesy of Thorax/BMJ Publishing Group Ltd.)

Suction

- There is no evidence that routine use of suction is of value.
- Suction may be of use in resolving a persistent air leak, particularly in secondary pneumothoraces. This is debated!
- Early use of suction, especially in large primary pneumothoraces may precipitate re-expansion pulmonary oedema.

Clamping of chest drains

- This is controversial. Some experts favour clamping prior to chest drain removal in order to detect the persistence of an air leak despite radiological evidence of lung re-expansion and therefore prevent unnecessary re-insertion of a chest drain.
- More commonly chest drains are removed *without* clamping once full expansion of the lung for 24 hours has been confirmed radiologically.
- Clamping a chest drain, particularly on non-specialist wards or for patient transfer, may allow the development of a tension pneumothorax.

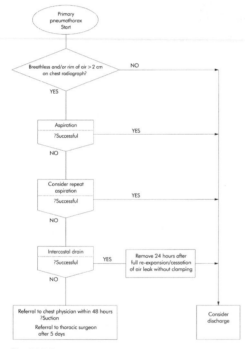

Fig. 14.3.4 Algorithm for the management of primary pneumothorax. (Courtesy of Thorax/BMJ Publishing Group Ltd.)

Size of chest drains

- Size doesn't matter. There is no evidence that large (24–28F) chest drains offer any advantage over smaller ones (14–18F) in the management of pneumothorax.
- Large bore drains may be required in cases of broncho-pleural fistula with a large air leak, typically in secondary pneumothorax and in patients receiving positive pressure ventilation.

Other types of pneumothorax

Tension pneumothorax

This is a medical emergency. A flap of tissue causes a valve effect, allowing air to leak IN but not OUT of the pleural space. A rapid build up of pleural pressure follows, causing shift of the mediastinal structures, impaired venous return, hypotension, shock and dyspnoea. Unless recognised and treated swiftly it may prove fatal.

- Look for reduced/absent breath sounds on the affected side and the trachea pushed *away* from the affected side.
- Remember that a tension pneumothorax can occur in a patient who already has a chest drain in place (that becomes blocked or is inappropriately clamped) and might also be the cause of a sudden, unexplained deterioration in a patient receiving positive pressure ventilation.
- Treat by inserting a large bore cannula into the pleural space through the second intercostal space in the mid-clavicular line. There should be a loud hiss as the air under pressure escapes. A formal intercostal chest drain should then be inserted through the triangle of safety.

Spontaneous haemopneumothorax

Fortunately this is rare, as it can be associated with severe blood loss, which may be life threatening. The bleeding usually comes from torn vessels in adhesions within the parietal pleura (Fig 14.3.6).

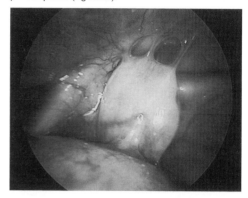

Fig. 14.3.6 Thoracoscopic view of an apical bulla in a young man with recurrent pneumothorax. Note the adhesions from the parietal pleura (rarely these can bleed when torn, causing a haemo-pneumothorax) The subclavian artery can be seen running behind the parietal pleura. (Picture courtesy of Mr. T. Batchelor).

- Early referral to a thoracic surgeon is indicated for repair, which can be undertaken through a thoracoscopic approach.

Catamenial pneumothorax

- Catamenial pneumothorax is a rare form of pneumothorax occurring in association with menstruation.
- Usually recurrent and predominantly right-sided it typically affects 30–40-year-old females.
- The majority of cases have associated pelvic endometriosis with deposits of endometrial tissue on the diaphragmatic and visceral pleural surfaces.
- Defects in the diaphragm that allow air to travel into the pleural space from the abdomen during menstruation may also be important aetiologically.
- Treatment consists of suppression of ovulation or thoracoscopic pleurodesis and patching of any diaphragmatic defects.

Iatrogenic pneumothorax

This is the commonest form of pneumothorax. The usual causes are transthoracic needle biopsy, central venous line insertion, pleural aspiration of fluid, pleural biopsy, transbronchial biopsy, and positive pressure ventilation. Acupuncture and aspiration of breast or thyroid nodules have also been implicated!

- Most cases will resorb without the need for intervention. Simple aspiration with a small bore catheter (8F) will treat most cases. Resorting to intercostal tube drainage should rarely be necessary *except* for patients on positive pressure ventilation who should always have a chest drain inserted.

Complications of pneumothorax

Surgical emphysema

This is caused by air tracking from the pleural space into the subcutaneous tissues. Although unpleasant for the patient this does not usually cause problems and resolves spontaneously within a few days. It may be precipitated by a blocked or kinked drain or a poorly positioned drain with some of the drain holes lying subcutaneously. Rarely, surgical emphysema can compromise ventilation and lead to respiratory failure.

- High flow oxygen (when safe) and subcutaneous drains or incisions are rarely used in troublesome cases (beware infection risk).
- Re-positioning of the chest drain or re-insertion of a large bore chest drain may be necessary. Very rarely tracheostomy may be required.
- Surgical emphysema will be more severe and harder to treat in patients with pneumothoraces who are receiving positive pressure ventilation.

Re-expansion pulmonary oedema

This probably results from alveolar capillaries damaged by the presence of a pneumothorax becoming traumatised as the lung re-expands causing a capillary leak.

Mild forms are quite common after pneumothorax and are more of a radiological phenomenon than a clinical problem.

Re-expansion pulmonary oedema is thought to be common after a large primary pneumothorax in younger patients, particularly in cases where the lung has been collapsed for several days.

Symptoms are usually mild and include cough, breathlessness, and a tight sensation experienced as the lung re-expands.

Rarely, there may be significant pulmonary oedema and respiratory failure, which can even include the other lung such that positive pressure ventilation is required. To minimise the risk of re-expansion pulmonary oedema avoid suction, particularly in the early management of a large pneumothorax, especially if the lung may have been collapsed for several days.

Preventing recurrence of a pneumothorax

Primary

Smoking greatly increases the risk of recurrence and should be discouraged.

Recent developments in VATS have led to some experts recommending VATS pleurodesis for the first episode of primary pneumothorax. This seems extreme since at least half of all cases (more in non-smokers) will never recur.

Individual patient's wishes and lifestyle, however, may sometimes dictate the need for a VATS pleurodesis after the first episode.

In most cases VATS pleurodesis should be recommended following a second pneumothorax (first recurrence) and for a first contra-lateral pneumothorax.

Secondary

As with primary pneumothorax smoking should be discouraged because of the very high association with recurrence as well as the risk of exacerbating the underlying lung disease.

If a patient is fit for surgery, referral for a surgical pleurodesis after the first episode should be considered because of the high recurrence and the increased risk of respiratory failure due to the associated underlying lung disease.

Pleurodesing techniques

Surgical pleurodesis

Whatever technique is used it should involve the 2 principles of:

1 resecting or suturing any visible blebs or bullae usually found on the visceral pleura at the lung apex

2 thoroughly abrading the visceral pleural surface in order to obliterate sub-pleural emphysema-like changes together with varying degrees of resection of the parietal pleura (pleurectomy) in order to seal the two layers of pleura together.

- Both procedures can be achieved through a VATS procedure.
- Mini (transaxillary) thoracotomy and open thoracotomy may result in slightlly fewer recurrences than a VATS procedure and may be the preferred approach in secondary pneumothorax.

Chemical pleurodesis

This is reserved for those who are not fit for thoracic surgery – usually older patients with secondary pneumothoraces.

Talc (2–5g) calibrated to remove small particles should be used as this minimises the chance of systemic absorption and is therefore unlikely to cause ARDS which has been described following the use of uncalibrated talc

Tetracycline (1500mg) has also been used extensively in the past, but is becoming less available and has a higher recurrence rate than talc.

Using 50–100ml of a patient's own blood as a pleurodesing agent has been tried successfully in the management of air leaks following lung resection and may also have a role in pneumothorax.

Talc poudrage at thoracoscopy or the insertion of talc slurry down a chest drain has a success rate of around 90%.

Success is most likely if the lung is re-expanded despite a persistent air leak, as this will encourage apposition of the chemically inflamed pleural surfaces so encouraging pleurodesis.

With continued partial collapse of the lung chemical pleurodesis combined with suction can still be attempted as a last resort in those who are unfit for surgery.

Advice to patients on discharge

- Don't smoke! Smoking greatly increases the risk of recurrence.
- Return to hospital immediately if breathlessness recurs.

Sporting activities

There is no clear evidence on which to base advice. It is probably safe to resume sports immediately, although many physicians advise a 6-week interval between radiographic resolution of a pneumothorax and resumption of sporting activities – particularly contact sports.

Flying

Once again, there is no clear evidence on which to base advice, but most lung specialists and airlines advise an arbitrary 6-week interval between radiographic resolution of a pneumothorax and flying.

Diving
Developing a pneumothorax whilst diving may have seri-ous, even life threatening consequences. After successful treatment for pneumothorax diving should only be consid-ered for those who have undergone the most effective surgical pleurodesing technique, i.e. pleurectomy and pleural abrasion at open/mini thoracotomy. Each case should be reviewed individually and this may involve CT assessment of the lungs and pleural space.

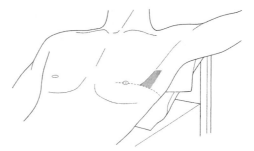

Fig. 14.3.8 The safe triangle. The boundaries are formed by the anterior border of latissimus dorsi, the lateral border of pectoralis major and a line superior to the horizontal level of the nipple. The apex is just below the axilla. (Courtesy of Thorax/BMJ Publishing Group Ltd.)

Further reading

Baumann MH, Strange C, Heffner JE, *et al.* Management of sponta-neous pneumothorax: an American College of Chest Physicians Delphi Consensus Statement. *Chest* 2001; **119**: 590–602.

Coker RK, Boldy DAR, Buchdahl R, *et al.* Managing passengers with respiratory disease planning air travel: British Thoracic Society recommendations. *Thorax* 2002; **57**: 289–304.

Godden D, Currie GP, Denison D, *et al.* British Thoracic Society guidelines on respiratory aspects of fitness for diving. *Thorax* 2003; **58**: 3–11.

Henry M, Arnold T, Harvey J. BTS guidelines for the management of spontaneous pneumothorax. *Thorax* 2003; **58**(suppl ii): 39–52.

Noppen M, Schramel F. Pneumothorax in European Respiratory Monograph. *Pleural diseases* 2002; **22**: 279–296.

Schramel FM, Postmus PE, Vanderschueren RG. Current aspects of pneumothorax. *Eur Resp J* (1997); **10**: 1372–1379.

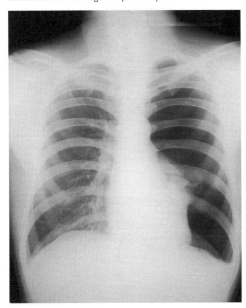

Fig. 14.3.7 This large primary pneumothorax can be successfully treated by a simple aspiration technique or even just observed and be allowed to resolve spontaneously.

14.4 Exudative pleural effusions (excluding malignancy)

Introduction
Pleural effusions are common and have a wide variety of causes. Classification into transudate or exudate assist the clinician in choosing the most appropriate range of tests to secure a diagnosis.

Pathophysiology
Exudates accumulate secondary to factors local to the pleura. There is a disruption in the balance between pleural fluid production and absorption. The mechanism depends on the underlying disease (e.g. obstructed lymphatic flow due to malignant infiltration).

Aetiology
Causes of an exudative pleural effusion are listed in Table 14.4.1. The majority are due to malignancy or infection.

A drug history is also important. Pneumotox.com lists a number of medications that have been associated with exudative pleural effusions. Table 14.4.3 lists the more commonly associated.

Table 14.4.1 Causes of an exudative pleural effusion

Common:
Malignancy
Parapnuemonic effusion
Pulmonary infarction
Rheumatoid arthritis
Mesothelioma
Less common:
Empyema
Tuberculosis
SLE
Other autoimmune conditions
Benign asbestos pleural effusion
Pancreatitis
Post cardiac injury syndrome (Dresslers)
Post coronary artery bypass grafting
Hepatic/splenic/sub-phrenic abscess
Oesophageal rupture
Cardiac failure treated with diuretics
Rare:
Yellow nail syndrome
Chylothorax
Drugs
Sarcoidosis
Fungal infection
Meigs syndrome
Hypothyroidism

Investigations
In clinical practice, pleural fluid protein levels <25g/l represents a transudate and >35g/l an exudate. In borderline cases (protein level 25–35g/l) Light's criteria should be applied (Table 14.4.2).

Table 14.4.2 Light's criteria

Pleural fluid protein/serum protein >0.5
Pleural fluid LDH/serum LDH >0.6
Pleural fluid LDH >2/3 upper limit of normal serum LDH.
The pleural fluid is an *exudate* in the presence of one or more of the above criteria.

These criteria identify more than 99% of exudates correctly but will misclassify approximately 20% of transudates as exudates. If there is concern, then the difference between the serum and pleural fluid protein (the protein gradient) should be measured. If the gradient is >3.1g/dl, then it is a transudate.

Pulmonary infarction
Pulmonary embolism is a common disease and approximately 30% of cases are associated with a pleural effusion. The majority of these are small and unilateral, only causing blunting of the costophrenic angle on the chest radiograph.

The pleural fluid is generally an exudate, but can rarely be a transudate.

Undiagnosed exudative pleural effusions should be investigated for pulmonary embolism. This is best assessed with a high-sensitivity D-dimer assay and a CT pulmonary angiogram.

Drainage may be required to alleviate symptoms, but caution is advised as the patient will require anticoagulation to treat the underlying pulmonary embolism.

Tuberculous pleural effusion
Tuberculous pleuritis results from infection of the pleura with *Mycobacterium tuberculosis*. Pleural TB is one of the most common extra-pulmonary manifestations of tuberculosis and coexists with pulmonary infection in 34–50% of cases.

Since the introduction of public health measures and effective anti-tuberculous agents, the incidence of TB has decreased significantly in the developed world. Unfortunately it continues to be a major health issue globally. According to the World Health Organization (WHO), 8 million new cases of TB and 1.6 million deaths occur each year. Co-infection with HIV contributes to this.

In the UK, tuberculous pleuritis is more likely to be due to reactivation of disease than primary infection.

The clinical presentation is usually acute or sub-acute i.e. < 1 month from onset of symptoms to diagnosis. Symptoms include cough, dyspnoea, fever and chest pain. Co-infection with HIV produces a more insidious onset of symptoms.

Pleural aspiration shows a clear yellow or serosanguineous fluid. This is an exudate and is predominantly lymphocytic. In the very early stages the fluid may be neutrophillic.

Pleural fluid culture for TB is usually only positive in 20–30% of cases.

In areas with a high prevalence of TB, pleural fluid levels of adenosine deaminase (ADA) >35 IU/L in association with a lymphocytic effusion are virtually diagnostic of tuberculous pleuritis.

In areas with a low prevalence of TB, pleural biopsy via thoracoscopy is the gold standard. When microscopy and culture for TB and histological examination for necrotising granulomas are combined there is a high diagnostic sensitivity and specificity.

Therapeutic drainage of the effusion can significantly improve symptoms. In most cases, pleural TB will resolve spontaneously within 2-4 months without treatment. However, 65%

will experience a recurrence of either pulmonary or pleural TB. Treatment is aimed at preventing this.

Standard treatment includes:
- Isoniazid, rifampicin and pyrazinamide for 2 months.
- Isoniazid and rifampicin for a further 4 months.

If a patient comes from an area of isoniazid resistance, then ethambutol should be added until the results of sensitivity testing are known.

Currently, there is insufficient evidence to justify the routine addition of corticosteroids.

Pleural thickening is a common complication in up to 43% of cases. There are no known predictive factors. Empyema is a rare complication that requires pleural drainage.

Drug associated pleural effusion

Although a rare cause of pleural effusion, drugs should always be considered. A detailed medication history is required as patients may not reveal the use of a drug unless specifically asked.

Most cases of drug induced pleural effusion are associated with bilateral pulmonary infiltrates and are predominantly eosinophilic.

Table 14.4.3 Drugs most commonly associated with pleural effusion

Amiodarone	Cyclophosphamide
Nitrofurantoin	L-tryptophan
Phenytoin	Carbergoline
Sodium valproate	Pergolide
Methotrexate	Propranolol
Penicillamine	Clozapine
Carbamazepine	Simvastin

The most common cause of drug-associated pleural effusions is drug-induced lupus pleuritis. While more than 80 drugs have been connected to this syndrome, definite evidence only exists for a handful including:
- Procainamide.
- Hydralazine.
- Isoniazid.
- Methyldopa.
- Chlorpromazine.
- D-penicillamine.
- Quinidine.

Patients with drug-induced lupus pleuritis are symptomatic with fever, pleuritic chest pain, myalgia and arthralgia. The chest radiograph commonly shows bilateral effusions while the pleural fluid is exudative with varying nucleated cell counts. The presence of lupus cells in the fluid, although rare, strongly suggests the diagnosis. Serum antinuclear antibody (ANA) titres are elevated.

The majority of drug-associated pleural effusions resolve upon withdrawal of the drug.

Key points
- Pulmonary embolism should be considered in all cases of undiagnosed exudative pleural effusion.
- A detailed drug history is important.
- Cardiac failure treated with diuretics can produce an exudative effusion and may be unilateral.

Further reading
www.pneumotox.com
www.who.int/mediacentre/factsheets/fs104/en/
Light RW, Lee YCG, *Textbook of Pleural Diseases*. 2nd edn. London: Hodder Arnold 2008

14.5 Transudative pleural effusions

Introduction

Pleural effusions can be classified into transudates or exudates.

This distinction can assist in determining the aetiology of the pleural effusion.

Pathophysiology

A transudative pleural effusion is caused by an imbalance of the hydrostatic or osmotic pressure gradient between the pulmonary capillaries and the pleural space, and the rate of pleural fluid drainage by the lymphatics (Fig. 14.5.1).

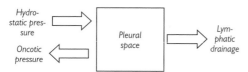

Fig. 14.5.1 Increased hydrostatic pressure or reduced colloid osmotic pressure within the pulmonary vasculature tends to cause leakage of fluid into the pleural space. If the pleural lymphatics are unable to keep up with the fluid influx then a transudative pleural effusion develops.

Aetiology

The causes of a transudative pleural effusion in the UK are shown in Table 14.5.1. Most are secondary to increased hydrostatic pressure, such as in congestive cardiac failure, or to low protein states (decreased oncotic pressure) such as hepatic cirrhosis or nephrotic syndrome. Most, though not all, are bilateral.

Table 14.5.1 Causes of a transudative pleural effusion

Common:
Congestive cardiac failure
Hepatic cirrhosis
Hypoalbuminaemia
Nephrotic syndrome
Less common:
Constrictive pericarditis
Peritoneal dialysis
Myxoedema
Ovarian hyperstimulation syndrome
SVCO
Post-operative basal atelectasis
Sarcoidosis

Although pleural effusions due to pulmonary emboli are usually exudative, they occasionally present as transudates.

Investigation

Unexplained unilateral pleural effusion, or bilateral pleural effusions that are greatly disparate in size, require a diagnostic pleural aspiration.

Pleural aspiration may be deferred in the presence of bilateral pleural effusions in a clinical setting suggestive of congestive cardiac failure, unless there is failure to resolve with appropriate treatment, or atypical features are present.

Atypical features include:

- the absence of cardiomegaly on the chest radiograph;
- unexplained pyrexia;
- clinical suspicion of pulmonary embolism.

Pleural fluid which is watery is very suggestive of a transudate, but most transudates are straw-coloured, and may even be tinged with blood. Additional tests are therefore required to differentiate between a transudate and exudate.

Differentiating between a transudate and exudate

Traditionally a transudate is defined as pleural fluid with a protein level <30g/L, whereas an exudate is defined as pleural fluid with a protein level of >30g/L, in the presence of a normal serum protein.

However in borderline cases (when the protein level is between 25–35g/L) Light's criteria should be used to distinguish between transudates and exudates (Table 14.5.2).

Table 14.5.2 Light's criteria

Pleural fluid protein/serum protein < 0.5
Pleural fluid LDH/serum LDH < 0.6
Pleural fluid LDH < 2/3 upper limit of normal serum LDH.
The pleural fluid is a *transudate* in the presence of one or more of the above criteria.

Treatment

The treatment of a transudative pleural effusion depends on it aetiology.

For example, transudative pleural effusions due to congestive cardiac failure usually resolve within 48 hours after initiation of diuretic therapy. However, one should be aware that a pleural effusion due to congestive cardiac failure partially treated with diuretics may develop the characteristics of an exudate if diagnostic aspiration is subsequently performed.

Transudative pleural effusions due to hepatic cirrhosis should not be treated by serial therapeutic thoracocentesis as they reaccumulate rapidly. Instead diuretic therapy, a low salt diet, and drainage of tense ascites, should be performed in the first instance.

The treatment of a pleural effusion associated with the nephrotic syndrome is to minimise protein loss in the urine so as to increase plasma protein levels. Even if the diagnostic aspiration indicates a transudate, the possibility of pulmonary embolism needs to be considered due to the increased risk of thromboembolism in nephrotic syndrome.

Thus, in most cases, therapeutic drainage of a transudative effusion is not appropriate.

However, in selected patients, large transudative pleural effusions require chest tube drainage for rapid relief of symptoms, followed by pleurodesis to reduce the likelihood of recurrence.

AUTHOR'S TIPS

- Bilateral pleural effusions associated with clinical features of congestive cardiac failure do not require aspiration unless there are atypical features or there is failure to resolve with diuretic therapy.
- Beware of ascribing all bilateral pleural effusions to congestive cardiac failure as up to 25% of cases have an alternative cause.
- When the pleural fluid protein level is borderline (25–35g/L), or in the presence of a low plasma protein level, Light's criteria should be used to accurately classify a pleural effusion into a transudate or exudates.
- Pleural effusions secondary to pulmonary embolism are occasionally transudates.

Further reading

Light RW. *Pleural Diseases* 4th edn. Philadelphia: Lippincott Williams & Wilkins, 2001.

Maskell NA. BTS Guidelines for the investigation of a unilateral pleural effusion in adults. *Thorax* 2003; **58**(suppl. II):8–17.

14.6 Malignant effusions

Epidemiology

Malignant pleural effusion (MPE) is the leading cause of exudative effusions subjected to thoracentesis. Pleural malignancy can occur without the presence of effusion.

Causes

The majority of MPE are the result of metastases to the pleura from other sites:

- Lung (30%).
- Breast (18%).
- Unknown site (10%).
- Lymph nodes (9%).
- Gastrointestinal tract (7%).
- Ovary (6%).

Primary pleural neoplasms (mesothelioma) account for approximately 10% of all MPE.

Pathogenesis

Potential mechanisms of metastatic pleural involvement include one or more of the following:

- Pulmonary artery invasion with microscopic tumour embolization to the visceral pleura and subsequent seeding to the parietal pleura (e.g. lung cancer).
- Pleural invasion from contiguous structures (e.g. diaphragm – ovary carcinoma, lung, mediastinum, breast).
- Hematogenous spread (e.g. breast, ovary).

Once malignant cells nest on pleural surfaces, the main mechanism of pleural fluid accumulation is increased vascular permeability, probably in combination with the obstruction of lymphatic vessels by the parietal pleural metastases.

Patients with cancer may also develop effusions from causes unrelated to direct pleural involvement by tumour ('paramalignant' effusions) such as:

- Post-obstructive pneumonia or atelectasis.
- Pulmonary embolism.
- Lymphatic mediastinal blockade or thoracic duct obstruction (chylothorax).
- SVCO.
- Malignant pericardial effusion and cardiac tamponade.
- Post-radio- or chemotherapy.
- Hypoalbuminemia.

Clinical features

- Dyspnoea (the most common symptom).
- Constitutional symptoms.
- Cough.
- Chest pain (particularly in mesothelioma).

Mean age of patients with MPE is 65 years.

> **AUTHOR'S TIP**
> A pleural effusion in a woman with breast cancer is malignant until proven otherwise.

Imaging

Chest radiographs (see also Chapter 3.8)

Typical radiological appearance of MPE:

- Large unilateral pleural effusion (60%). Malignancy is the most common cause of massive pleural effusions.

- Bilateral effusions with normal heart size (15%).
- The absence of contralateral mediastinal shift in a large MPE indicates:
  - Ipsilateral bronchial obstruction with lung collapse (e.g. lung cancer).
  - Fixation of the mediastinum by malignant lymph nodes.
  - Extensive pleural involvement (e.g. malignant mesothelioma, trapped lung).

CT scan

Features that favour the diagnosis of MPE are:

- Pleural nodularity.
- Parietal pleural thickening greater than 1 cm.
- Mediastinal and circumferential pleural thickening.
- Liver metastases.

More than half of CT scans in MPE do not show any pleural finding other than the pleural effusion.

> **AUTHOR'S TIP**
> Chest CT should be done before the effusion is completely drained to ensure optimal diagnostic utility.

Diagnosis

Pleural fluid analysis

Pleural fluid characteristics in MPE are:

- Exudate according to Light's criteria in 98%.
- Bloody appearance (>10.000 RBC/mm^3) in >40%.
- Lymphocytes predominance in 80%.
- Reduced glucose levels (<3.3 mmol/L) in 10–30%.
- Low pH (<7.3) in 20–35%.
- Adenosine deaminase (ADA) levels <40 U/L in 95%.
- Positive panel of tumour markers (CEA>50 ng/mL or CA15.3>75 U/mL or CA125>2800 U/mL or CYFRA 21–1>175 ng/mL) in about half the cases. Notably, one-third of cytology-negative MPE can be identified by at least one of these markers.
- Positive cytological examination in 50% after a single tap attempt; a repeat aspiration is helpful in an additional 10% of cases. This is the most common way of diagnosing MPE.

Cytological yield depends on:

- Number of submitted specimens.
- Type of tumour (e.g. lower positive results with squamous cell carcinomas, mesotheliomas and sarcomas).
- Tumour burden in the pleural space.
- Expertise of the cytophatologist.

In contrast, the volume of pleural fluid analyzed does not impact the yield of cytologic diagnosis (submission of 5–10 ml may suffice).

> **AUTHOR'S TIP**
> Pleural fluid flow cytometry should be ordered when lymphoma is a consideration.

Closed (blind) pleural biopsy

- 45% sensitivity for MPE.
- Establish the diagnosis of malignancy only in 15% of patients with false-negative cytology.

CT-guided biopsy of the pleura
- High diagnostic yield (85%) in the presence of pleural thickening or nodularity.
- Consider also if only a small effusion is present and pleural fluid cytology is negative.

Medical thoracoscopy
- >95% sensitivity for MPE.
- The recommended procedure when the cytological analysis is negative and a substantial amount of pleural fluid exists in patients who are fit enough.

Thoracoscopy allows:
- Biopsies from the chest wall, diaphragm, lung and mediastinum.
- Staging in lung cancer and mesothelioma.
- Removal of all pleural fluid and talc pleurodesis if macroscopic tumour is obvious.

Prognosis
- Median survival depends upon the site of the primary tumour (5 months, with the shortest in lung and the longest in breast primaries and mesothelioma).
- A pleural fluid pH <7.3 is associated with far advanced disease of the pleural space and a decreased response to pleurodesis.

Treatment

Systemic therapy
- May control effusions in chemo- radio- or hormone-therapy responsive tumours, such as lymphoma, SCLC and breast cancer.
- Some experts favour early pleurodesis in chemo-sensitive tumours. At least, proceed to aspirate symptomatic pleural effusions before chemotherapy.

Observation
- Indicated in asymptomatic patients or when there is no recurrence of symptoms after an initial therapeutic thoracentesis (uncommon).

Therapeutic thoracentesis
- Recommended for the palliation of dyspnoea in patients with a very short live expectancy (Karnofsky performance scale score ≤40).
- Caution should be taken if removing more than 1.5–2 litres on a single occasion.

> **AUTHOR'S TIP**
> Dyspnoea that does not improve after pleural aspiration suggests pulmonary carcinomatous lymphangitis, atelectasis, pulmonary or tumour embolism, or COPD.

Pleurodesis
With pleurodesis, a chemical irritant is injected into the pleural space, creating an intense pleural inflammation, which ultimately leads to the fusion of the visceral and parietal pleura.

Prerequisites for pleurodesis:
- Symptomatic (dyspnoea) MPE.
- Reasonable survival expectancy (>1 month).
- Absence of trapped lung (defined as lung failure to re-expand after drainage of an effusion because of mechanical restriction of the visceral pleura) or mainstem bronchial obstruction.

The most widely used sclerosants are:
- Talc, which is the most effective agent (>90% success rate). Dose: 4g.
- Doxycycline (effectiveness of 75%). Dose: 0.5g.

Pleurodesis can be performed:
- Insufflating dry powder talc (poudrage) through a thoracoscope.
- Instilling, at the bedside, doxycycline or talc (slurry) mixed with saline *via* a chest tube.

The choice of the pleurodesis procedure will depend upon:
- The patient's characteristics (e.g. bedside pleurodesis would be preferred in those with poor performance status or contralateral pleuro-pulmonary involvement).
- The availability of an expert thoracoscopist.

Pleurodesis with doxycycline
Insert a small-bore catheter (10–14F).
- Drain in a controlled fashion.
- Confirm full lung re-expansion with a chest radiograph.
- Inject 500 mg of doxycycline in 100ml of saline into the pleural space.
- Clamp chest tube for 1–2 hours, and then open it for drainage.
- Remove chest tube within 12–24 hours, in the absence of excessive fluid drainage (>250 ml/day); otherwise, a second dose of the sclerosing agent can be administered.
- The entire pleurodesis procedure can be accomplished within <24 to 72 hours.

> **AUTHOR'S TIP**
> A trial of intrapleural fibinolytics may be a useful adjunct therapy for patients with multiloculated MPE who fail to drain adequately, before attempting pleurodesis.

Complications of pleurodesis:
- Pleuritic chest pain and fever (10–30%).
- Rarely, acute respiratory failure (ARDS) following talc administration. Where grade large-particle talc (most particles <10 μm removed) is used, this complication has not been reported. Consider the possibility of an unrecognised air leak if ARDS develops post pleurodesis.

Indwelling pleural catheters
- A chronic indwelling 15.5F pleural catheter is the treatment of choice in patients with trapped lung and is also an effective option if pleurodesis fails.
- Indwelling pleural catheter allows patients to drain pleural fluid regularly or on an 'as required' basis at home.
- A spontaneous pleurodesis will occur in almost 45% of patients.
- The catheter remains in place for a median of 2 months, until death or removal.
- The expensive drainage supplies (suction bottles) counterbalance hospital cost-savings.
- Pleurodesis through the indwelling pleural catheter needs to be explored in future.

Other options
- Reserve pleuroperitoneal shunting or surgery (pleurectomy or decortication) for selected patients with trapped lung or failed pleurodesis. In patients with chylothorax, pleuroperitoneal shunt may preserve nutritional status.
- Bronchoscopic removal of tumour masses in the large airways provoking atelectasis may allow subsequent pleurodesis.

Key points
- Consider the diagnosis of MPE in patients with:
  - A unilaterally large effusion.
  - A known malignancy.
  - A lymphocytic exudate with normal ADA levels.
- Thoracoscopic insufflation of talc may be the optimal technique for pleurodesis in patients with MPE.
- If thoracoscopy is not available or the patient is too frail, bedside pleurodesis with doxycycline or talc slurry is a reliable alternative.
- Consider indwelling pleural catheter in patients with trapped lung or failed pleurodesis.

Further reading
Janssen JP, Collier G, Astoul P, et al. Safety of pleurodesis with talc poudrage in malignant pleural effusions: a prospective cohort study. *Lancet* 2007; **369**: 1535–1539.

Light RW. *Pleural Diseases* 5th edn. Philadelphia: Lippincott Williams & Wilkins, 2007.

Light RW, Gary Lee YC. *Textbook of Pleural Diseases*, 2nd edn. London: Hodder Arnold, 2008.

Rodriguez-Panadero F, Janssen JP, Astoul P. Thoracoscopy: general overview and place in the diagnosis and management of pleural effusion. *Eur Respir J* 2006; **28**: 409–421.

Stather DR, Tremblay A. Use of tunnelled pleural catheters for outpatient treatment of malignant pleural effusions. *Curr Opin Pulm Med* 2007; **13**:328–33.

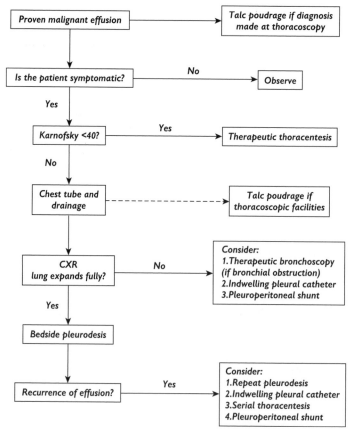

Fig. 14.6.1 Algorithm for treating MPE.

14.7 Malignant mesothelioma

Definition
Malignant mesothelioma is an aggressive, universally fatal, neoplasm arising from the serosal surfaces usually of the pleura (>90%), peritoneum (7%) or rarely the pericardium or tunica vaginalis.

Incidence
There is a global epidemic of mesothelioma. On average one patient dies of mesothelioma every 4 hours in the UK and the incidence is expected to rise until 2015 (Fig. 14.7.1). In Western Europe over 250,000 deaths from mesothelioma are predicted in the next 20–30 years. This reflects the latency period (typically 20–50 years) between prior asbestos exposure and disease onset as use of asbestos was banned in the UK as late as 1999. In the USA, an early ban of asbestos use means the incidence of mesothelioma has peaked, but the disease still kills about 3000 each year. Substantial future increases in cases are predicted in developing countries where asbestos use remains largely unregulated.

Fig. 14.7.1 shows the number of mesothelioma deaths amongst males in Great Britain since 1968 (dots), the inferred past collective dose of asbestos (exposure index) and an estimation of projected male mesothelioma cases to 2050. www.hse.gov.uk/statistics/causdis/proj6801.pdf

Causes
Occupational, and occasionally environmental, exposure to asbestos is the commonest cause. Industries associated with significant asbestos use include shipbuilding, construction and building trades, automotive brake repair and the manufacture of asbestos textiles.

There is no safe threshold of exposure to asbestos although the risk of mesothelioma increases with intensity of exposure and duration since first exposure.

Amphibole asbestos fibres (e.g. crocidolite (blue asbestos), amosite (brown asbestos)) are more carcinogenic than serpentine (chrysotile) fibres (white asbestos).

Other aetiological factors include erionite (a non-asbestos fibre found in Turkey), exposure to ionising radiation, especially thorium dioxide – a radiographic contrast agent used in the 1950s. The role of simian virus 40 (SV40) has been implied, but remains unproven, in the pathogenesis of mesothelioma.

Up to 20% of patients may not have identifiable predisposing factors.

Pathogenesis
Inhaled asbestos fibres can provoke damage (and subsequent carcinogenesis) in pleural mesothelial cells directly, following translocation of fibres from the lung to the pleural surface, or indirectly, through stimulation of oncogenic mediators.

The risk of mesothelioma is related to the biopersistence of the fibres in the lung. Long, slender amphibole fibres are more difficult to eliminate than serpentine fibres, thus accounting for their significantly higher tumorigenic capacity.

Clinical features
The majority of patients are males (reflecting occupational exposure) in their fifth to seventh decades.

Symptoms may include:
- Dyspnoea, particularly exertional.
- Chest pain.
- Constitutional features such as weight loss, sweating and fatigue.
- Ascites is common with primary peritoneal mesothelioma or with peritoneal metastases from pleural mesothelioma.
- Symptoms reflecting involvement of adjacent intrathoracic structures, e.g. oesophagus, spinal cord, superior vena cava.

Paraneoplastic syndromes and distant metastases are uncommon.

Examination commonly reveals a unilateral pleural effusion. Clubbing, if present, often reflects concomitant asbestosis. Subcutaneous masses can occur at the sites of previous pleural intervention, reflecting pleural tract spread.

Diagnosis
Over 95% of patients with mesothelioma develop a pleural effusion and mesothelioma should be considered in all patients with a unilateral exudative pleural effusion or pleural thickening. There are no specific radiological features or blood profiles that allow diagnosis of malignant pleural mesothelioma.

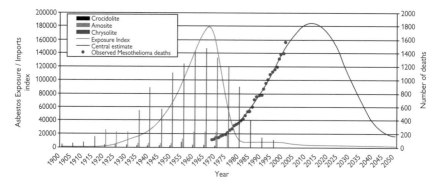

Fig. 14.7.1 Mesothelioma observed and fitted/projected deaths among males aged 20–89, asbestos imports and estimated/projected exposure inde.

Definitive diagnosis can only be made with cytological or histological confirmation.

Histological subtypes

Common histological subtypes include:

- Epithelioid (50–60%).
- Sarcomatoid (10%).
- Mixed (biphasic), a mixture of epithelioid and sarcomatoid components.

These histological subtypes have different gene expression profiles. Differentiating between subtypes is important as they vary in their biological behaviour and prognostic implications.

Staging

There is no universally accepted staging regimen. Staging is more important in research studies than for clinical use.

The Butchart classification and the more recent International Mesothelioma Interest Group (IMIG) staging system (based on the tumour-nodal-metastasis (TNM) classification) are frequently employed in mesothelioma research trials.

Investigations

Imaging

Chest radiography

May demonstrate:

- Unilateral pleural effusion ± mediastinal shift.
- Pleural mass (may be multiple).
- Pleural thickening: focal or diffuse (lung encasement).
- Evidence of previous asbestos exposure: pleural plaques or interstitial fibrosis.
- Local rib invasion.

CT with pleural-phase contrast enhancement

The following features suggest malignant pleural disease but cannot distinguish pleural mesothelioma from metastatic carcinomas (Fig. 14.7.2):

- Pleural effusion with pleural nodularity and enhancement.
- Mediastinal pleural thickening.
- Local invasion e.g. chest wall and diaphragm.

Concomitant features of asbestos exposure e.g. pleural plaques or asbestosis may be present.

MRI

MRI is useful in selected cases to aid definition of localised disease e.g. chest wall or spinal cord invasion.

PET

The clinical role of PET is unclear as it cannot determine malignant pleural disease from inflammatory pleuritis. High pleural standard uptake values (SUV) are associated with a worse prognosis in mesothelioma.

Pleural fluid analysis

Pleural fluid is typically an exudate.

Sensitivity of cytology is low (usually 20-30%) as differentiation between normal, reactive and malignant mesothelial cells is often difficult.

Distinguishing malignant pleural mesothelioma from metastatic pleural carcinoma can be challenging, and usually requires immunostaining with a broad panel of markers e.g. calretinin, epithelial membrane antigen (EMA) etc.

Pleural biopsy

If cytological analysis is inconclusive, pleural biopsy should be performed unless clinically contraindicated.

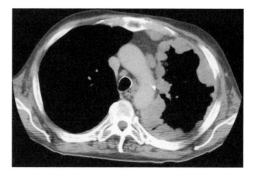

Fig. 14.7.2 CT scan revealing a shrunken left hemithorax with circumferential nodular pleural thickening in a patient with advanced mesothelioma.

Imaging guided biopsies are preferred to blind (e.g. Abrams') biopsies (diagnostic sensitivity 87% v 47% respectively) if pleural abnormality is detected. Thoracoscopy allows simultaneous therapeutic fluid drainage with pleurodesis and diagnostic pleural biopsy (sensitivity 98%)(Fig. 14.7.3).

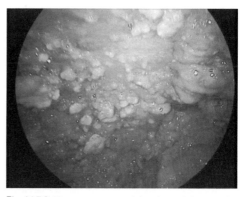

Fig. 14.7.3 Thoracoscopic view of pleural mesothelioma on the parietal pleural surface.

Biomarkers

No specific pleural fluid or serum marker exists to reliably identify mesothelioma.

Pleural fluid and blood levels of soluble mesothelin-related protein (SMRP) are significantly elevated in patients with mesothelioma, particularly epithelioid subtype, but can also be raised in other tumours (e.g. pancreatic and ovarian carcinomas).

The exact role of serum or pleural fluid levels of mesothelin and other potential markers, such as osteopontin and RCAS1 (a type II membrane protein), in malignant mesothelioma is the subject of ongoing evaluation.

Prognosis

The prognosis of mesothelioma is poor with a median survival of approximately 8–14 months although these figures vary dependent on patient selection and how survival was calculated. Long-term survival (>5 years) has occasionally been reported.

Performance status and histological subtype are the most important prognostic indicators. Epithelioid mesothelioma has a better survival compared with biphasic and sarcomatoid subtypes. Staging of mesothelioma at presentation is also related to outcome with a shorter survival seen in those with advanced disease.

Other, weaker, prognostic indicators, associated with an adverse prognosis, have been identified and include age (>75 years), male gender, low haemoglobin, raised lactate dehydrogenase (LDH) and high white blood cell and platelet counts. Clinically the presence of chest pain and >5% weight loss may suggest a worse prognosis.

Treatment

There is no curative treatment for mesothelioma hence management should focus on providing symptom relief and improving patients' quality of life. A multi-disciplinary team approach is recommended to ensure medical, psychological, financial and medicolegal support is provided for the patients and their families.

Psychological support

The psychological aspects of patients with mesothelioma deserve attention, as the issues involved differ from other cancers. Many patients have lived under the anxiety of developing the disease for decades and have witnessed death of previous colleagues from mesothelioma. Amongst some, mesothelioma carries a reputation of horrible death of drowning and suffocation. Anger towards prior employers for lack of provision of occupational protection is common. Medicolegal proceedings often present additional stresses.

Analgesia

Pain is a major issue for many patients. Opiate analgesia is often required and radiotherapy can ease localised pain, e.g. from bone erosion or tract metastases.

In severe and refractory cases percutaneous cervical cordotomy (interrupting the spinothalamic tract at C1– C2), intrathecal analgesia and regional nerve blocks may be considered.

Dyspnoea

Pleural effusions from mesothelioma almost always recur. Early pleurodesis is recommended. In patients with tumour encasing the lung preventing re-expansion ('trapped lung') drainage with an ambulatory indwelling pleural catheter may be useful.

Surgical pleurodesis and, rarely, pleuroperitoneal shunting are alternative options.

Radiotherapy

There is no role for radical radiotherapy alone in mesothelioma. Various fractionation strategies (e.g. intensity modulated radiotherapy (IMRT)) are under investigation.

Palliative radiotherapy can provide good pain relief for localised symptoms.

Prophylactic radiotherapy to sites of pleural intervention can reduce the risk of tract site metastases. However, the value of routine administration to all pleural puncture sites is currently debated.

Chemotherapy

Multi-targeted folate antagonists, e.g. pemetrexed disodium or raltitrexed, in combination with cisplatin have shown a survival advantage of approximately 3 months and may improve quality of life. No other chemotherapy regimens, given intravenously or intrapleurally, have shown proven benefit.

Surgery

As mesothelioma spreads along the serosal surface rather than growing as a defined mass, surgical attempts to eradicate mesothelioma have not been successful. No randomised controlled trials support the use of radical surgery (extrapleural pneumonectomy, EPP) in mesothelioma.

EPP has an operative mortality of approximately 5%, and 25% of patients suffer life-threatening complications. Patients' quality of life is significantly worsened for the first 6 months after EPP. Tumour relapse always occurs if patients survive long enough.

Thoracic debulking with pleurectomy, as a palliative procedure, has not been fully assessed.

Trimodality therapy

As EPP alone does not provide a cure, trimodality therapy, i.e. EPP with adjuvant chemotherapy and radiotherapy, has been tried. Although patients are highly selected, with early stage disease, a good performance status and no significant co-morbidity, no definite survival benefit has been seen and the role of trimodality therapy remains unproven.

Novel approaches

Gene therapy and immunotherapy have both shown promise in preliminary phase trials.

No survival benefit has been seen with photodynamic therapy.

Anti-angiogenic strategies and molecular targeted therapies are being explored.

Compensation (See Chapter 16.3)

Patients with mesothelioma are often eligible for compensation though eligibility and compensation regulations vary among countries.

Prevention and screening in exposed individuals

Anxiety of developing mesothelioma is high among the millions of workers exposed to asbestos worldwide. There is no proven prophylactic therapy, though some evidence suggests that vitamin A may have some protective effect.

No effective screening methods exist. The preliminary data on the use of mesothelin in predicting disease development awaits validation in large studies. Population screening cannot at present be justified as no effective curative treatment exists and no evidence suggests early detection alters outcome.

AUTHOR'S TIPS

- Suspect the diagnosis in all patients with prior asbestos exposure and an exudative pleural effusion regardless of the interval since exposure and exposure intensity. However, absence of exposure does not exclude diagnosis.

- The histological subtype of mesothelioma should be identified wherever possible as the biological behaviour and prognosis differ.

- Focus management on symptom palliation and maintaining quality of life. Psychological support for patients and their families is important but often overlooked by clinicians.

Further reading

Cancer Research UK. `www.cancerresearchuk.org` Jaurand M-C, Fleury-Feith J. Review: Pathogenesis of Malignant Pleural Mesothelioma. *Respirology* 2005; **10**: 2–8.

Musk AW, de Klerk NH, Ambrosini GL, *et al*. Vitamin A and cancer prevention I: observations in workers previously exposed to asbestos at Wittenoom, Western Australia. *Int J Cancer* 1998; **75**:355–61.

Robinson BWS, Musk AW, Lake RA. Seminar: Malignant Mesothelioma. *Lancet* 2005; **366**: 397–408.

Scherpereel A, Lee YCG. Biomarkers for mesothelioma. *Curr Opin Pulm Med* 2007; **13**:339–443.

West SD, Lee YCG. Current Management of Malignant Pleural Mesothelioma. *Clin Chest Med* 2006; **27**: 335–354.

14.8 Pleural effusions in systemic disease

Pleural effusions are associated with a wide variety of systemic diseases with a very broad and wide range of pathophysiology and pleural fluid characteristics. The effusions can be either exudative or transudative depending on the disease process.

Gastrointestinal, obstetric, cardiovascular, and collagen vascular diseases more commonly involve pleural effusions as disease manifestations and often pleural effusions are markers of disease severity.

The highly vascular pleura is sensitive to derangements in capillary permeability from systemic inflammation making the pleural space vulnerable to fluid accumulation. This chapter provides a brief and limited sample of the systemic diseases that are complicated by pleural manifestations.

Gastrointestinal tract

Pancreatitis, intraabdominal abscesses, esophageal perforation, biliary tract disease, and cirrhosis are the more common gastrointestinal diseases associated with pleural effusions (Table 14.8.1). Both exudative and transudative effusions are encountered but exudative effusions are far more common.

Table 14.8.1 Gastrointestinal disease overview

Diagnosis	Pleural effusion characteristics	Pathophysiology
Pancreatitis	Most commonly bilateral; exudative, elevated amylase, elevated levels of phospholipase A2	Transdiaphragmatic transfer of exudative fluid from the pancreas. With pseudocyst get sinus tract from pancreas to pleural space
Subphrenic abscess	Effusions in 60–80% of cases; exudative and neutrophil predominance	Inflammation of the diagphragm increasing its permeability
Oesophageal perforation	Subcutaneous emphysema often present; low pleural fluid pH, often accompanied by pneumothorax. mortality approaches 60%	Acute mediastinitis causing medistinal pleural rupture
Cirrhosis	Transudative; generally should not perform therapeutic thoracentesis as the fluid will reoccur	Many patients with cirrhosis and ascites have small defects in their diaphragms. Low pressure in pleural space sucks ascitic fluid into pleural space

Pancreatitis

Pancreatitis associated pleural effusions are often bilateral, exudative and often bloody. The presence of an effusion in pancreatitis is a negative prognostic indicator. An effusion associated with simple pancreatitis need not require a thoracentesis as long as the patient is not febrile. A pancreatic abscess is a much more serious condition carrying with it a very high mortality rate. In one series, pleural effusions were found in nearly 40% of these patients. The pancreatic abscess must be surgically drained but no specific treatment is required for the pleural effusion.

Chronic pancreatic pleural effusions can develop when a sinus tract forms between a pseudocyst and the thoracic cavity. Men are more likely to develop a pancreaticopleural fistula. These create large effusions often occupying the entire hemithorax. Diagnosis is confirmed by abdominal CT revealing the pancreatic psuedocyst and the sinus tract.

Gynaecologic conditions

Gynaecologic conditions associated most commonly with pleural effusions include ovarian hyperstimulation syndrome (OHSS) and Meigs' syndrome. OHSS results from the overstimulation of the ovaries by hCG and the fertility drug clomiphene. The pathogenesis of OHSS is quite interesting. The leading hypothesis is that elevated levels of IL-6 and VEGF gain access to the systemic circulation and act as capillary permeability factors thus creating the transudative effusions. These effusions are most commonly right sided but bilateral effusions are not uncommon. Withholding the fertility medications is the treatment.

Meigs' syndrome consists of a benign ovarian tumor, ascites, and pleural effusions. Transdiaphragmatic transfer of fluid is the proposed mechanism of the effusion. Treatment is surgical removal of the pelvic tumor.

Cardiovascular system

Post-CABG pleural effusions are very commonly encountered. These are identified in the vast majority of patients but nearly all are small and inconsequential. The large pleural effusions that do occur are divided into early (within 30 days post-op) and late (after 30 days).

More early effusions are associated with internal mammary grafts vs saphenous vein grafts and with the use of topical hypothermia. The effusion is predominately left sided and the characteristic fluid is a bloody exudate with an eosinophil predominance. The most common presenting complaint is dyspnoea.

The late post-op effusions are clear non bloody exudates and lymphocytes dominate. Both early and late effusions will generally resolve without treatment but thoracentesis should be preformed to rule out other causes if the patient is febrile or has chest pain. A therapeutic thoracentesis should be performed if the patient is experiencing dyspnoea. If the pleural effusion continues to reaccumulate a pleurodesis or VATS procedure may be necessary but this is rarely occurs.

Collagen vascular diseases

Collagen vascular diseases are occasionally complicated by pleural effusions that are quite varied in their characteristics Table 14.8.2.

Table 14.8.2 Collagen vascular diseases

Disease	Incidence and patient characteristics	Presentation	Pleural fluid characteristics	Treatment
Rheumatoid arthritis	Between 3–5% of patients with RA More common in men with RA than women Subcutaneous rheumatoid nodules often present	Patients often present with pleuritic chest pain Small to moderate sized effusion Usually unilateral but no predilection for either side	Exudative Low glucose <20mg/dL Low pH <7.20 Often cholesterol crystals and elevated cholesterol level present	Most often the effusions resolve spontaneously No clinical trials available but recommendation is to treat with NSAIDS for 8–12 weeks
Systemic lupus erythematosus	Approximately 16% to 44% of patients More common in women than men	Pleuritic chest pain common Usually small but can be large and occupy >50% hemithorax 50% bilateral	Serosanguinous Exudative Glucose level >80mg/dL pH above 7.20	Very good response to systemic corticosteroids; recommendations: 80mg of prednisone every other day with rapid taper once clinical improvement is demonstrated
Wegener's granulomatosis	22–55% present with small effusions	Patients present with upper and lower respiratory tract involvement and glomerulonephritis; important to consider this disease in patients with parenchymal infiltrates, nodules, and a pleural effusion. Need to measure ANCA	Fluid not well characterised	Cyclophosphamide and high dose steroids treat the underlying disease and the pleural effusion will resolve

Further reading

Abramov Y, Elchalal U, Schenker JG. Pulmonary manifestations of severe ovarian hyperstimulation syndrome: a multicenter study. *Fertil Steril* 1999; **71**: 645–651.

Halla JT, Schronhenloher RE, Volanakis JE. Immune complexes and other laboratory features of pleural effusions. *Ann Intern Med* 1980; **92**: 748–752.

Light RW. Pleural effusions after coronary artery bypass graft surgery. *Curr Opin Pulm Med* 2002; **8**: 308–311.

14.9 Pleural infection

Epidemiology

Pleural effusions occur in up to 40% of patients with pneumonia. Pleural infection affects patients of all ages but is more common in children and the elderly. Men are affected twice as often as women. Its incidence is higher in those with diabetes, alcoholism, substance abuse and chronic lung disease.

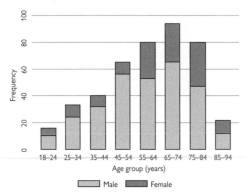

Fig. 14.9.1 Empyema frequency.

Aetiology

The commonest causes of pleural infection are:
- Secondary to a community-acquired pneumonia (70%).
- Secondary to a hospital-acquired pneumonia (12%).
- Primary empyema (5%).
- Post operative (10%).
- Miscellaneous (bacteraemia, oesophageal rupture, IV drug abuse, abdominal infection/collection) (3%).

Pathophysiology

This can be divided into three stages
- *The exudative phase*
The development of the initial effusion is due to increased permeability of the pleural membranes. Fluid moves into the space owing to locally increased capillary vascular permeability. The accumulating pleural fluid has a normal glucose level and pH.
- *The fibropurulent phase*
Secondary bacterial invasion occurs and the high level of fibrinolytic activity in the pleural space is suppressed and tissue plasminogen activator inhibitor 1 and 2 rise. This leads to fibrin deposition over the visceral and parietal pleura and loculations form. Bacterial metabolism lead to increased lactic acid production and fall in pH.
- *The organising stage*
Proliferation of fibroblasts and evolution of pleural scarring. An inelastic peel forms on both pleural surfaces with dense fibroid septations. As solid fibrous peel replaces the soft fibrin lung function is impaired.

Classification

Light's classification of parapneumonic effusions and empyema
- *Class 1* – non significant:

Small <10 mm thick. No thoracentesis required.

- *Class 2* – typical parapneumonic:

>10mm thick, glucose >40 mg/dl, pH > 7.2.
- *Class 3* – borderline complicated:

pH 7.0-7.2 or LDH >1000 Gram stain negative.
- *Class 4* – simple complicated:

pH < 7.0 or Gram stain positive. No loculation or frank pus.
- *Class 5* – complex complicated:

pH < 7.0 Gram stain positive. Loculations.
- *Class 6* – Simple empyema:

Frank pus, single locule or free flowing.
- *Class 7* – Complex empyema:

Frank pus, multiple loculations.

Differential diagnosis

The commonest problem with the differential diagnosis is failure to make the correct positive diagnosis. Often the presentation is indolent (especially in the elderly) with weight loss and anorexia and little fever.

Other possible causes for the effusion include:
- Tuberculosis effusion.
- Malignancy.
- Rheumatoid pleural effusion.
- Pulmonary embolus with associated effusion.

Associated conditions
- Lemierre's syndrome – acute oropharyngeal infection with Fusobacterium species leading to septic thrombophlebitis of the internal jugular vein, septic pulmonary emboli and empyema.

Bacteriology

This differs significantly between pleural infection acquired in the community and those acquire in the hospital setting. In view of this they require different empirical antibiotics. In one large randomised trial throughout the UK the following bacteria were cultured:

Community acquired
- S. Milleri group (32%).
- Streptococcus pneumoniae (13%).
- Other Streptococci (7%).
- Staphylococci (11%).
- Anaerobes (16%).
- Enterobacteriaecea (7%).
- *Proteus* (3%).
- *H. influenzae* (3%).

Hospital acquired
- MRSA (26%).
- Staphylococci (18%).
- Enterobacteriacea (16%).
- Enterococci (13%).
- Pseudomonas (5%).
- Streptococci (10%).

It should be noted that up to 40% of patients with pleural infection do not ever have a positive bacterial culture. This is partly due many having already started antibiotics before hospital presentation.

Investigations

Pleural fluid sampling

Fluid should be sent to the laboratory for glucose, LDH and protein measurements as well as standard cytological and microbiological investigations. A sample of fluid (not frank pus) should also be placed in a heparinised syringe and the pH measured

Imaging

The imaging features of parapneumonic effusion and empyema depend upon the state of evolution of the effusion and the underlying aetiology. The imaging will also often have to be circumstance led, e.g. a ultrasound for ill unstable patients on ITU.

Chest radiology

- In general, a pleural effusion is demonstated often in association with consolidation. The effusion is commonly unilateral. If uncomplicated it behaves like a non-infected sterile effusion with a normal meniscus sign.
- If complicated it may be loculated. It will then have a lentiform, pleural based opacity. If the effusion is within a fissure it may have the appearance of a 'pseudotumour'.

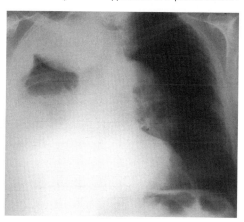

Fig. 14.9.2 CXR of a loculated empyema.

Ultrasound

- The majority of parapneumonic effusions will be septated and may be hyperechoic.
- Whereas septations are readily visualised on ultrasound, pleural thickening is poorly visualised and CT is better.

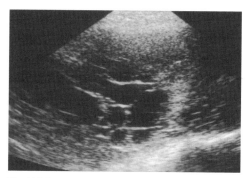

Fig. 14.9.3 Pleural ultrasound showing loculations.

CT

- Useful in trying to distinguish a lung abscess from a pleural collection.
- Also helpful in evaluating the drain position and any residual location in a patient not responding to medical treatment where surgery is being contemplated.
- With a contrast CT, as with other exudative effusions, pleural enhancement is seen.

Differentiating between a lung abscess and empyema on enhanced CT.

The following rules are often useful in distinguishing a lung abscess for an empyema:

Lung abscess

- Often round in shape.
- Vessels passing through or near.
- Indistinct boundary between lung parenchyma and collection.
- Thick and irregular wall, making contact with chest wall at acute angle.

Empyema

- Lenticular in shape.
- No vessels closely associated.
- Compression of surrounding lung.
- Smooth margins creating obtuse angles, following contours of chest.

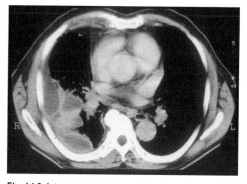

Fig. 14.9.4 Loculated empyema on CT.

Treatment

> **AUTHOR'S TIP**
> - A complicated parapneumonic effusion due to *Proteus* spp. does not result an acidic effusion.
> - The pH of the pleural fluid should be measured (using an arterial blood gas machine and heparinised syringe) in all cases of suggested parapneumonic effusions. This should not be done with frank pus as it will damage the machine. A pH <7.2 is an indication that formal tube drainage will be required.

Antibiotics

As the microbiology is very different between community-acquired and hospital-acquired pleural infection they require different empirical antibiotic regimens at presentation.

Possible empirical antibiotic regimens:

- Community acquired – co-amoxiclav and metronidazole.
- Hospital acquired – meropenem and vancomycin.

Tube drainage

The optimal size of chest tube to use in cases of pleural infection is still a subject of vigorous debate.

However, patients entered into the large UK–MIST 1 trial did just as well if a small-bore drain was inserted initially as a large-bore drain. They also experienced significantly less pain and discomfort. For this reason, the author would always start with a small chest tube (12–14F) and ensure that is was flushed regularly (20ml normal saline 6hrly).

Monitoring response to medical management

The best markers of response to medical management include:
- Falling CRP.
- Settling of a spiking temperature.
- Clinical signs of resolution of sepsis.

In the event that these indices are improving, the author would tend to avoid acting on worrying chest radiology as this often lags significantly behind the patient's improvement.

When patients look as if they have avoided surgery by the narrowest of margins, prolonged oral antibiotics and close follow-up in out-patients with monitoring of the chest radiograph and CRP is advised.

Fibrinolytics

The MIST 1 trial showed no benefit in giving intrapleural streptokinase to patients with pleural infection, in terms of reduced mortality or need for surgery.

The role of other fibrinolytics are still being evaluated and the MIST 2 trial should be reporting shortly.

Nutrition

This is an important cornerstone of management and often overlooked until later in the disease process. Early nutritional assessment and NG feeding if necessary is recommended.

Surgery

Unfortunately 20–30% of patients will fail medical management. If this occurs then prompt referral to thoracic surgery is recommended.

Options include:
- VATS.
- Open thoracotomy with decortication.
- Rib resection with open drainage.

Further reading

BTS guidelines on the management of pleural disease. *Thorax* 2003;**58**(Suppl II):ii1–ii59.

Light RW, Lee YCG (eds). *Textbook of Pleural Disease*. London: Hodder Arnold, 2008.

14.10 Surgery for pleural diseases

Spontaneous pneumothorax

Primary spontaneous pneumothorax

Indications: second episode; persistent air leak (>3–4 days); failure to achieve re-expansion following drainage of a 1st episode, haemopneumothorax, 1st contralateral episode, bilateral pneumothorax. Professions at risk: scuba divers, pilots.

Principles: closure of source of air leak; obtaining pleural adhesions.

Approach: modern literature favours video assisted thoracoscopic surgery (VATS) which usually results in reduced hospitalization, postoperative analgesia and improved cosmesis than thoracotomy with comparable success rate.

Procedure: pleuropulmonary adhesions must be divided to reveal blebs or bullae which should undergo stapled resection. In the absence of visible bullae or blebs blind resection of the apex reduces recurrence. Pleurodesis can be achieved by pleurectomy (either apical or total), pleural abrasion or talc poudrage.

Complications: the risk of recurrence is 2–4%. Pleurectomy and pleural abrasion carry a small risk of postoperative bleeding. The concern regarding the use of talc poudrage in young patients seems unjustified. A long-term survey showed no oncological risk associated with asbestos-free talc. Systemic talc granulomatosis is avoided by the standard use of larger particles (<11% of particles <5 micron). The theoretical risks of adult respiratory distress syndrome and long-term respiratory dysfunction have not been seen in large series reported by Cardillo. Rare complications include: Horner's syndrome and chronic wound pain.

Secondary spontaneous pneumothorax

Indications: It is observed mostly in older people with documented lung disease and because the risks of a second episode are high intervention is recommended after the *first* episode.

> **AUTHOR'S TIP**
> Early referral for surgery is essential if VATS is to be successful. Prolonged pleural drainage increase the risk of pleural sepsis and adhesions which increase the need for thoracotomy.

Principles, approach, procedure: these are largely the same as for primary spontaneous pneumothorax.

Complications: the recurrence rate is higher than for primary spontaneous pneumothorax.

Pleural empyema

Indications: persistent loculated pleural sepsis after tube drainage (intrapleural fibrinolytic therapy, in our opinion, has very little role); chronic pleural thickening causing symptomatic restrictive ventilatory deficit.

Principles: removal of purulent material (*debridement*); removal of inflammatory cortex from visceral and parietal pleural surfaces (*decortication*).

Approach/procedure: the result of treatment must be independent from the surgical approach, either open (standard thoracotomy or minithoracotomy) or VATS. The choice of approach should not compromise the principles

of expeditious removal of parietal and visceral debris without injuring the lung with a low morbidity and mortality rate. The early use of VATS debridement with directed, magnified identification and lysis of pleural adhesions has been shown to have benefits over closed methods. VATS decortication achieving lung re-expansion in more chronic situations is also feasible but is operator dependent. Open decortication remains the standard of care. In those unfit for thoracotomy, rib resection and open drainage via a thoracostomy is an option.

Complications: conversion of VATS to thoracotomy must be accepted at consent, the rate is operator dependent.

> **AUTHOR'S TIP**
> Again, early referral for surgery in the fibrinopurulent phase of the disease increases the success of VATS and redcues the need for open decortication. Initial drainage should be large-bore and image-guided.

Pleural effusion

Indications: undiagnosed, symptomatic or recurrent pleural effusion.

Principles: to obtain a sufficiently large pleural biopsy and to achieve pleural symphysis and in some cases re-expansion of the trapped lung.

Approach/procedure: VATS via one or two 2cm incisions and the insufflation of a sclerosing agent. Among sclerosing agents, asbestos-free talc has proved to be superior to other commonly used agents with a success rate ranging from 81–100%. VATS. VATS pleurodesis has been shown to be more effective than bed-side instillation of a talc slurry. In the 'trapped-lung syndrome' treatment options include: the insertion of a pleuroperitoneal shunt; insertion of a long-term silicone chest drainage tube or attempts to re-expand the lung. Re-expansion can be achieved by visceral decortication which can be performed by VATS. VATS can be effectively performed on a sedated, spontaneously ventilating patient.

> **AUTHOR'S TIPS**
> - Thoracoscopy is indicated after the intial pleural aspiration. Repeated thoracocentesis can be associated with pleural fluid contamination leading to loculation and subsequent empyema.
> - Thoracoscopic talc poudrage represents the treatment of choice for recurrent pleural effusions. Talc slurry represents an alternative in patients not fit for surgery.

Localized (solitary) fibrous tumours of the pleura

Localized (or solitary) fibrous tumour of the pleura (LFTP) (also called subpleural fibroma) is a rare, slow-growing neoplasm.It is thought to be nonmesothelial in origin, not to be associated with asbestos exposure and usually shows a good prognosis, in contrast to diffuse mesothelioma.

The surgical treatment of choice is local removal by VATS with intraoperative assessment of free surgical margins. If the parietal pleura show signs of tumor invasion, a chest wall resection is recommended. Pedunculated lesions can be safely treated with a wedge resection if originating from the visceral pleura or with a local resection with extrapleural dissection if originating from the parietal pleura, provided that the surgical margins are negative.

Mesothelioma

Indications: symptom control, tumour debulking, or radical excision.

Selection criteria: include: fitness for GA, fitness for pneumonectomy and tumour stage.

Preoperative staging should include CT and PET where possible. PET is useful for detecting occult distant disease but not for mediastinal nodes, nor is CT thus mediastinoscopy is mandatory to exclude extrapleural nodal metastases where radical surgery is planned.

Procedures: VATS can be used to perform talc pleurodesis or parietal pleurectomy. VATS decortication can also relieve entrapped lung.

Extrapleural pneumonectomy (EPP) involves the en-bloc excision of the pleura, lung, pericardium and diaphragm. Radical pleurectomy/decortication (P/D) may achieve the same clearance but preserves the lung.

The longest surgical survival has included adjuvant treatment with chemotherapy and radical radiotherapy. In node negative, completely resected epithelial mesothelioma 5-year survival is a goal of treatment. VATS debulking surgery may prolong survival when compared to biopsy alone.

Prospective randomized trials are ongoing in UK to evaluate the respective roles of EPP in the MARS trial and VATS debulking in the MesoVATS trial.

Complications: operative mortality from EPP or P/D is less then 5% in experienced centres. Significant morbidity may occur in up to 50%.

> **AUTHOR'S TIP**
> Mesothelima should be suspected in all males born in the 1940s who present with pleural effusion, thickening or pleuritic pain. Recruitment into clinical trials should encouraged.

Further reading

Baumann MH, Strange C, Heffner JE, *et al.* Management of spontaneous pneumothorax. ACCP Delphi consensus statement. *Chest* 2001; **119**: 590–602.

Halstead JC, Lim E, Venkataswaran R, *et al.* Improved survival with VATS pleurectomy-decortication in advanced malignant mesothelioma. *Eur J Surg Oncol* 2005; **31**: 314–320.

Henry M, Arnold T, and Harvey J, *et al.* BTS guidelines for the management of spontaneous pneumothorax. *Thorax* 2003; **58**: 39–52.

Wait MA, Sharma S, Hohn J, *et al.* A randomized trial of empyema therapy. *Chest* 1997; **111**: 1548–1551.

Waller DA. Malignant Mesothelioma – British surgical strategies *Lung Cancer* 2004; **45S**: S81S84.

Sleep

Chapter contents

15.1 Obstructive sleep apnoea

Definition

Obstructive sleep apnoea/hypopnoea (OSAH) is the term for a sleep disorder characterised by dynamic upper airway obstruction during sleep. It is part of the spectrum of sleep-related breathing disorders, with trivial snoring at one end and repetitive complete upper airway obstruction, causing apnoeas with oxygen desaturations and arousals, at the other.

Apnoeas during sleep can be classified as one of three commonly recognised types: obstructive, central and mixed. An obstructive apnoea is characterised by a respiratory effort during the apnoeic period, while a central apnoea shows neither airflow nor respiratory effort. Mixed apnoeas begin with a central component followed by an obstructive component. Mixed apnoeas are not really a separate entity but sometimes occur in association with both primary obstructive and central aetiologies.

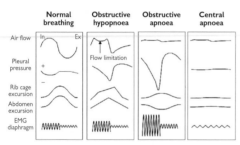

Fig. 15.1.1 Discrimination of apnoea types. Each panel represents one whole breath. Obstructive and central apnoea/hypopnoea are differentiated by the presence or absence of respiratory effort as evidenced by oesophageal pressure, diaphragmatic EMG recordings or other indirect measure of respiratory effort: asynchrony or paradoxical motion of rib cage and abdomen recorded by inductance plethysmography and changes in pulse transit time provide indirect evidence of increased respiratory effort. During partial upper airway obstruction, the contour of the inspiratory flow curve is typically flattened. (Adapted from Kohler M, Bloch KE 2003.)

Historically, an arbitrary definition of an apnoea was made as breathing cessation for longer than 10 seconds; and hypopnoea was a reduction in airflow >50% from the previous stable baseline, lasting >10 seconds, and in some centres, requiring association with a >3% decline in oxyhaemoglobin saturation.

Because >5 apnoeas/hypopnoeas per hour of sleep were found to be uncommon in sleep studies of healthy young adults, the standard definition of OSA became >5 apnoeas per hour of sleep, or >35 per night. The number of apnoea/hypopnoea events increases with age, and therefore many more events per hour of sleep can be normal in the elderly.

Numerical sleep data, which are based on counts of events during a sleep study (e.g. apnoea–hypopnoea index), are commonly used to define OSAH, although they are not very useful in defining overall disease severity and the necessity for treatment. This is partly because there is a poor correlation between symptoms and sleep study findings, and partly due to night-to-night variation in these indices. Because this definition lacks clinical usefulness,

a pragmatic distinction should be made between the sleep study findings of repetitive apnoeas, oxygen desaturations or arousals on their own, and such an abnormal sleep study plus the presence of daytime symptoms (obstructive sleep apnoea syndrome, OSAS). This differentiation is particularly important in patients who are considered to have upper airway resistance syndrome (UARS). It has been shown in clinical studies that certain individuals with UARS show upper airway narrowing leading to sleep fragmentation and excessive daytime sleepiness in the absence of an increased number of apnoeas, hypopnoeas or dips in oxygen saturation.

The definition of OSAS/UARS, which implies clinically significant symptoms and thus requiring consideration of treatment, can be summarised as follows:

> Upper airway narrowing during sleep, causing sufficient sleep fragmentation to result in significant symptoms, usually excessive daytime sleepiness.

Pathophysiology

Although full explanations for OSA still need to be defined, the principal pathophysiologic mechanism of the disorder is dynamic narrowing of the upper airway associated with sleep. The upper airway is defined as the space between the nasal and oral orifices and the epiglottis (Fig. 15.1.2).

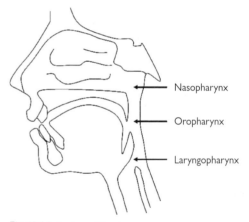

Fig. 15.1.2 Anatomy of the pharynx.

Airway narrowing in patients with OSA can occur at multiple sites of the upper airway, but it happens most commonly in the region of the pharynx, because of its anatomical and functional characteristics. The pharynx consists of a complex muscular tube which serves two major purposes: breathing and swallowing. When the pharynx is being used to breathe, it is held open by dilator muscles. During swallowing it collapses and thereby enables peristaltic movements to propel food. The functional diversity of the pharynx is achieved by the floppy and collapsible muscular tube which also has the capacity of being held open rigidly by dilating muscles. During sleep, the dilator muscles show reduced activity, and consequently some pharyngeal narrowing occurs even in healthy individuals.

The collapsibility of the pharynx can be defined by the critical collapsing pressure (Pcrit) surrounding the oro- and nasopharynx, which has been shown to be abnormally high in patients with OSA. In theory, the upper airway resembles a Starling resistor (Fig. 15.1.3), consisting of a mainly rigid tube (nose), followed by a collapsible part (pharynx), and followed by another rigid tube (laryngeal airway). During inspiration, flow will persist as long as the nasal pressure is greater than the pressure in the collapsible pharynx which will be subatmospheric. In sleeping healthy individuals, airflow continues because inspiratory nasal pressure is approximately 0 cmH_2O and pharyngeal pressure, although subatmospheric, remains above Pcrit (about -10 cmH_2O, subatmospheric). In contrast, it has been shown that the peripharyngeal Pcrit in patients with significant OSA is often about, or even above, 0 cmH_2O during sleep and therefore the pharynx easily collapses and airflow ceases. Simple snorers are somewhere in between.

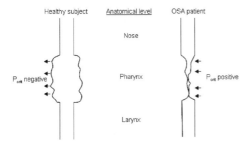

Fig. 15.1.3 Upper airway resembling a Starling resistor. Subatmospheric Pcrit in healthy subjects (left) compared to patients with OSA (right). When external pressure at any point along a collapsible tube (pharynx) is greater than the intraluminal pressure then collapse will occur, but the consequent cessation of airflow will return the intraluminal pressure to atmospheric and may allow the airway to spring open again – this produces snoring. However, if the external Pcrit pressure is greater than that at the nose, collapse occurs at some location along the tube where the transmural pressure equals zero or above, producing an apnoea, rather than just snoring.

As a consequence, clinically significant upper airflow obstruction is determined by factors, such as anatomical abnormalities in the pharynx, or dysfunction of the pharyngeal dilator muscles, which both facilitate the narrowing or collapsibility of the pharynx.

Thus, possible causes of obstructive sleep apnoea can be divided into two major groups:
- Anatomical causes.
- Functional causes.

Anatomical causes of OSA

The most common anatomical factor contributing to the pathogenesis of OSA is neck obesity which compromises upper airway patency by increased loading from the adipose tissue surrounding the pharyngeal lumen, and therefore increases Pcrit. In various observational studies, neck circumference has been shown to correlate with the frequency of apnoeas better than any other index of obesity. Craniofacial abnormalities, like retro- and micrognathia, are also frequently observed in patients with OSA. These conditions are associated with crowding of the pharyngeal space, which decrease the resting cross-sectional area of the upper airway. Studies, using radiological imaging

techniques, have shown that patients with OSA have a smaller pharyngeal cross-sectional area than control subjects (Fig. 15.1.4). It has not been possible to determine a cut-off size for the upper airway that differentiates a patient with OSA from a healthy individual.

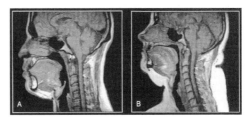

Fig. 15.1.4 MRI images of the upper airway in a healthy control (A) and a subject with OSA (B). Note the crowded airway, with more neck adiposity and a degree of retrognathia. (Adapted from Schwab RJ 1998.)

In children with OSA, the pharynx can commonly be crowded by enlarged tonsils and adenoids; this cause is much less common in adults.

Functional causes of OSA

There is some evidence for a relationship between nasal obstruction and OSA. Data from physiological studies suggest that upper airway narrowing and snoring can be induced by greater subatmospheric pharyngeal pressures, caused by an increased nasal resistance, as would be predicted from the Starling resistor model. The model also predicts that apnoeas would be self terminating as described earlier in this chapter. However, it is unlikely that the pharynx indeed behaves like a simple Starling resistor. This is probably due to surface adhesive forces between the opposed pharynx walls, which will tend to hold the pharynx closed once collapsed, and hysteresis effects. This theory is supported by the observation that the pressure needed to reopen the collapsed pharynx exceeds its closing pressure.

The patency of the pharynx is also influenced by motor output from the CNS to upper airway muscles, which can be differentiated into five striated muscles (m. palatoglossus, m. palatopharyngeus, m. levator palatine, m. tensor palatine, and m. uvulae). In awake subjects, the m. palatoglossus, palatopharyngeus and levator palatini show electromyographic activity during inspiration that keeps the upper airway open during the respiratory cycle. Sleep is generally associated with decreased upper airway muscle activity and tone. In patients with OSA, genioglossus EMG activity is increased during wakefulness compared to healthy controls (probably reflecting increased activity to defend the airway), with a greater proportional decrease at sleep onset. This disproportional reduction of upper airway muscle tone is associated with a higher tendency to upper airway collapse during sleep.

An additional possible pathophysiological explanation for dysfunction of the upper airway in patients with OSA is that there may be a reduced protective reflex mechanism in the pharynx. In healthy subjects, receptors in the pharynx detect pressure falls and provoke an increase of pharyngeal dilator muscle tone which prevents collapse of the pharynx. Repetitive airway narrowing during snoring, smoking and alcohol may injure the mucosa and nerves in the pharynx, interrupting this reflex and thereby facilitating the development of OSA.

Some pharmacologic agents (e.g. alcohol, opiates, benzodiazepines) can promote OSA by inhibition of CNS activity, reflex muscle tone, and thus motor output to upper airway muscles: this decreased muscle tone produces a higher propensity for the pharynx to collapse.

Causes of OSA
Anatomical
- Neck obesity.
- Retrognathia, micrognathia and maxillary underdevelopment.
- Pharyngeal encroachment (e.g. tonsillar and adenoid hypertrophy, acromegaly).
- Chronic nasal obstruction (e.g. polyps, turbinate hypertrophy, rhinitis), possibly plays a minor role in the pathogenesis of OSA.

Functional
- Alcohol.
- Sedative drugs (e.g. opiates, benzodiazepines).
- Sleep deprivation.
- Bulbar palsies.
- Neurological degenerative disorders (e.g.multisystem atrophy).
- Myopathies (e.g. Duchenne muscular dystrophy).
- Hypothyroidism.

Immediate consequences of OSAS
Once significant upper airway obstruction occurs there will be increased inspiratory effort to overcome it. At a specific level of pleural pressure (usually about −15 cmH$_2$O in non-sleep deprived subjects, but down to −80 cmH$_2$O in OSAS) patients tend to arouse from sleep. The recurrent arousals result in two major consequences: sleep fragmentation, which leads to excessive daytime sleepiness, and autonomic changes including elevation of arterial blood pressure.

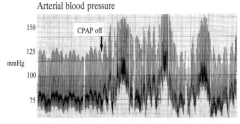

Fig. 15.1.5 Blood pressure swings in OSAS. Arterial tracing during sleep (3½ mins, Finapres device) showing instant return of large systemic BP surges, with each of three apnoea terminations, following removal of affective CPAP in a man with obstructive sleep apnoea.

Long-term consequences of OSAS
OSAS may be associated with various complications, including the following:
- Accidents.
- Arterial hypertension.
- Arrhythmias.
- Myocardial infarction and stroke.
- Cor pulmonale.
- Ventilatory failure.
- Insulin resistance.

- Polycythaemia (in cases with daytime hypoxia).
- Neuropsychological impairment.
- Increased anaesthetic risk.

It must be stressed that a direct causal relationship has not been established for most of these complications. As accidents and cardiovascular complications probably contribute most to the number of premature deaths in patients with OSAS, they will be discussed in detail.

Accidents
The most immediate risk from OSAS relates to falling asleep at the wheel. The risk of causing traffic accidents is elevated 3- to 10-fold in patients with OSAS. Accidents typically occur at night when driving alone on monotonous highways. As the vehicle usually crashes into an obstacle without the driver breaking, the consequences are particularly grave. Therefore, all patients with OSAS should be advised of the following (and recorded in the medical notes!):
- Notify the DVLA at the time of diagnosis, or shortly after. They will send the patient a short questionnaire. If they admit to excessive daytime sleepiness, their driving licence is revoked until they are effectively treated and sleepiness has resolved.
- Do not drive while sleepy.
- Heavy goods or public service vehicle drivers should be advised to stop driving entirely, until the sleepiness has resolved completely. In the case of class 2 licence holders the success of the treatment must be verified by a specialist clinic.

Treatment success is defined as a normal ESS (Epworth Sleepiness Score <10) and evidence of adequate nasal CPAP usage (minimum usage of at least 3 hours per night, every night, verified by downloaded machine data).

Cardiovascular complications
Severe sleep apnoea syndrome (affecting about 1–2% of the male population) is associated with a high cardiovascular risk. Over 10 years, 14% of this group are predicted (by Framingham-index) to experience a stroke and 23% a myocardial infarction – a 37% combined risk.

There are several potential mechanisms of vascular damage operating in sleep apnoea. During each apnoea cycle there are stereotypic rises in blood pressure, usually >30mmHg, and not uncommonly >100mmHg. These rises will induce shear stresses in blood vessel walls – forces that are thought to cause vascular wall damage and initiation of atherosclerosis. Each apnoea is also associated with hypoxaemia and re-oxygenation, which may be disadvantageous through repeated 'ischaemia re-perfusion injury'. Sleep apnoea patients show evidence of increased production of reactive oxygen species, increased systemic catecholamine production, abnormal vascular reactivity, reduced baroreceptor sensitivity and possibly impaired insulin resistance. Furthermore, circulating vascular risk factors (e.g. cholesterol, CRP) have been shown to be elevated in OSA. Thus many features of the sleep apnoea syndrome may potentially contribute to vascular damage. It is difficult to estimate the risk reduction that correcting these factors might produce, because it has not been accurately defined from long-term randomized, controlled clinical trials.

Cor pulmonale can result from severe untreated OSAS which probably constituted the original 'Pickwickian syndrome'. It occurs if a patient has daytime hypoxaemia, most often resulting from co-existing COPD. Chronic hypoxaemia results in pulmonary hypertension and fluid retention, producing the picture of cor pulmonale.

Epidemiology

There are a large number of studies on the prevalence of OSAS in the general population, but the frequency of this disorder is still open to debate, mainly because of controversies concerning clinical diagnostic approaches and the lack of a uniform definition of OSA(S). As a consequence, the reported prevalence of OSA differs considerably between the various population based studies with a range from as low as 0.3% to as high as 26% in middle-aged people. Broadly it is believed that up to approximately 2–4% of the population in Western countries suffer from clinically significant OSAS. The highest frequencies are found in countries with a high prevalence of obesity as there is evidence for a strong correlation between BMI and OSA. The prevalence of OSA has been reported to be >20% in a community sample of middle-aged men with a mean BMI of 30.5kg/m^2.

Ethnic origin seems to influence the prevalence of OSA, since a higher proportion of individuals with African or Oriental origin seem to have OSA compared to whites and Asians.

An inherited basis for OSA is suggested by reports of families with multiple affected members and genetic epidemiologic studies; the genetic basis for upper airway narrowing during sleep has not been defined yet. However, risk of OSA among relatives of patients with the disorder is almost twice that among neighbourhood control subjects. Potential pathogenetic explanations for these findings are provided by familial studies which have demonstrated that craniofacial abnormalities, structural features of the upper airway, and the propensity to develop obesity are at least partially inherited.

There is a strong predominance of OSA in men, 2–3 times more men are affected than pre-menopausal women. Why men are at higher risk for the development of OSA is still unclear, however, hormonal influences on breathing during sleep and fat distribution cannot fully explain this difference. The prevalence in females probably increases after menopause, shifting the male-to-female ratio to 2:1, possibly because body fat is redistributed to the upper body.

OSA occurs in all ages, although the prevalence in children and the elderly has been investigated less thoroughly. Several large population-based studies suggest that the mean age of patients with OSAS at presentation lies between 40 and 50 years. The prevalence of OSA and OSAS seems to rise continually with age and to level off after the age of 65 years. Of note, healthy elderly individuals commonly have a higher frequency of apnoeas/hypopnoeas, which makes the definition of a clinically significant cut-off level of apnoeas even more difficult.

Diagnosis

To date there is no sufficiently precise test in awake patients which diagnoses OSAS. However, there are some typical clinical features that should raise the clinical suspicion of OSAS:

- Sleepiness rather than tiredness.
- Unrefreshing sleep.
- Difficulty concentrating.
- Nocturnal choking.
- Nocturia.
- Witnessed apnoea.

The most common complaint of patients with OSAS is excessive daytime sleepiness. This finding shows a considerable inter-subject variability and the definition of abnormality can be difficult. The most widely used score to assess daytime sleepiness is the Epworth sleepiness scale (ESS) which asks patients to rate their tendency to fall asleep in eight different situations of varying stimulation.

Epworth Sleepiness Scale

How likely are you to doze off or fall asleep in the situations described in the box below, in contrast to feeling just tired?

This refers to your usual way of life in recent times. Even if you haven't done some of these things recently try to work out how they would have affected you.

Use the following scale to choose the <u>most appropriate number</u> for each situation:

| 0 = would <u>never</u> doze | 2 = Moderate chance of dozing |
| 1 = Slight chance of dozing | 3 = <u>High</u> chance of dozing |

Situation	Chance of dozing
Sitting and reading	
Watching TV	
Sitting, inactive in a public place (e.g. a theatre or a meeting)	
As a passenger in a car for an hour without a break	
Lying down to rest in the afternoon when circumstances permit	
Sitting and talking to someone	
Sitting quietly after a lunch without alcohol	
In a car, while stopped for a few minutes in the traffic	

Fig. 15.1.6 Epworth sleepiness scale. An ESS score of ≥10 is generally regarded as abnormally sleepy and requires further investigations to find the underlying cause. Of note, there is no good correlation between ESS and the severity of OSA which might be explained by perception problems of patients with OSA regarding their sleepiness. Furthermore, there are many other possible reasons for excessive daytime sleepiness which are discussed elsewhere in this book.

The bed-partner's account provides important information about what happens during a night, thus a complete medical history includes the patient's partner. The following symptoms are frequently observed by the bed-partner during the night:

- Snoring.
- Apnoeas.
- Restless sleep.
- Choking episodes.

A physical examination of all patients with suspected OSAS is advised as it is important to detect possible causes and complications of OSA. The examination should include assessments of:

- Weight and height (BMI).
- Neck circumference (distribution of fat).
- Craniofacial appearance (e.g. retrognathia, prognathia).
- Oral cavity and pharynx (e.g. size of tongue and tonsils).
- Nasal patency.

- Cardiovascular system (blood pressure, ankle oedema).
- Diabetes mellitus.
- Respiratory system (e.g. lower airway obstruction, chest wall disease, respiratory failure).
- Neurological system (Neuromuscular diseases).
- Signs of predisposing diseases (e.g. hypothyroidism, acromegaly).

The majority of patients with OSAS are male with a tendency to have upper body obesity (neck circumference >17in/>43cm), a retrognathic appearance of the mandible and a history of excessive daytime sleepiness.

Sleep studies

The sleep study is the crucial investigation in the process of making the diagnosis of OSAS. There is a wide choice of equipment available for monitoring sleep, some can be used in an ambulatory setting (home sleep studies) others are only available in specialised hospital centres. Principally, there are three major types of sleep studies:

- Overnight oximetry alone.
- Respiratory polygraphy (RP), which normally includes assessments of snoring, body and leg movement, heart rate, oronasal airflow, excursion of the chest and abdomen in addition to oximetry.
- Full polysomnography (PSG) with EEG, EOG, and EMG, to stage sleep electrophysiologically, in addition to the channels of respiratory polygraphy.

Equipment for oximetry and RP is suitable for home sleep studies, whereas full PSG usually requires a sleep laboratory and a technician to set up and supervise the sleep study during the night.

Overnight sleep studies at home allow patients to sleep in their own environment which may reflect normal conditions better than a sleep laboratory. Furthermore, most of the available equipment can be set up by the patient without any help from technical staff, thus home sleep studies may be cheaper than in-hospital studies.

There may be some limitations in interpretating the results from home sleep studies:

- Home sleep monitoring systems sometimes use sensors which have a different sensitivity and reliability compared to those used in RP or full PSG systems.

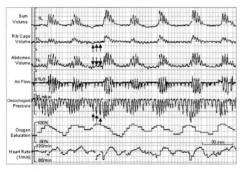

Fig. 15.1.7 Respiratory polygraphy. Recordings obtained from a patient with OSA. Progressive oesophageal pressure swings and paradoxical signals from rib cage and abdominal sensors (arrows) indicate that the apnoeas are obstructive. They are associated with oxygen desaturations, and cyclic alterations in heart rate. (Adapted from Kohler M, Bloch KE 2003).

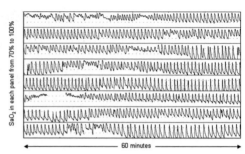

Fig. 15.1.8 Overnight oximetry. Eight hours of overnight oximetry in a patient with severe OSA. Note the many dips >4% in SaO$_2$ with typical saw-tooth appearance.

- It is not possible to tell if the patient is awake or asleep, consequently a home sleep study might be falsely negative, although this is rarely an issue if the patient says he slept.
- Other diagnoses than OSAS might be missed (e.g. periodic limb movements syndrome).

Limited sleep studies (RP) have become the usual routine investigation in most sleep centres as full polysomnography (PSG) is not needed to make the diagnosis of OSA. In fact, there is evidence that most cases that are eligible for CPAP treatment can be identified by oximetry alone. However, false positive oximetry occurs with Cheyne–Stokes breathing (e.g. in heart failure), and when there is a low baseline SaO$_2$ (e.g. COPD) SaO$_2$ oscillates considerably. False negatives can occur in thin young patients who hardly desaturate during apnoeas.

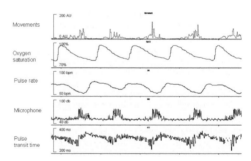

Fig. 15.1.9 Visilab sleep recording (RP device). Recordings obtained from a patient with severe OSA. Oxygen desaturations are associated with cyclic alterations in heart rate, and arousals indicated by movements in the channel. The microphone records periodic snoring, interrupted by apnoeas. Alterations in pulse transit time (similar to oesophageal pressure) shows increases in ventilatory effort during the apnoeas, indicating that the cause of the apnoeas is upper airway obstruction.

In the authors' view, the expertise in interpreting a sleep study is more important than the particular sleep study equipment used. However, any system used should at least allow assessment, directly or inirectly, of the degree of sleep fragmentation and the degree of upper airway narrowing.

Treatment

Patients should not be treated unless the diagnosis of OSA has been established by a sleep study. This is because there are other casues of sleepiness, it is potentially a lifetime diagnosis, and there are driving and DVLA implications. It is also important to state that not all patients need treatment as the current evidence from randomised controlled trials indicates that significant treatment benefits are mainly found in symptomatic patients. Improvement in daytime sleepiness and alertness are the major benefits of treatment, whether it also decreases the risk of cardiovascular events (e.g. myocardial infarction, stroke) or results in improved mortality remains to be proven in appropriately powered randomised controlled studies. However, many experts in the field apply a lower threshold for treatment in patients with additional severe cardiovascular disease, poorly controlled hypertension or heart failure.

There are some key questions which might help in making a treatment decision, these include the following:

- How sleepy is the patient, do the symptoms affect his quality of life?
- Do the symptoms influence the patient's ability to drive or work?
- Is the patient motivated to do anything about it?
- Has the patient underestimated the impact of his sleepiness, or misled the doctor because of concerns over driving issues?
- Is there any underlying cause which can be treated specifically (e.g. hypothyroidism, tonsillar hypertrophy)?
- Is there support from the patients' partner and/or family?

General approaches

The underlying mechanisms and the clinical significance of the disorder should be explained to all patients with OSAS and their partners. It is crucial that they understand why the treatment is important because in most cases it will be a life-long commitment to treatment. Simple approaches to improve OSA severity and symptoms may include the following:

- Weight loss.
- Reduction of alcohol consumption in the evening.
- Avoid sleeping tablets or sedatives.
- Try to sleep in decubitus rather than in supine position.
- Treat underlying conditions such as hypothyroidism, acromegaly, tonsillar or adenoid hypertrophy, chronic nasal obstruction.

Specific approaches

In addition to the above mentioned general measures the appropriate treatment largely depends on the severity and symptoms of OSA.

For snorers and mild OSA
- Mandibular advancement devices.

For significant OSA
- Nasal CPAP.
- Bariatric surgery (e.g. gastroplasty or gastric bypass operations).
- Mandibular/maxillary advancement surgery in highly selected cases.
- Tracheostomy (only if all other treatment options are not effective and the patient is severely compromised by the symptoms).

Nasal CPAP

Nocturnal application of CPAP via a nasal mask is the standard therapy for OSAS. Continuous positive pressure is generated by an airflow turbine pump which maintains a constant supra-atmospheric pressure (about 10 cmH$_2$O) within the tubing, mask and the upper airways. A leak valve built into a tightly fitting nasal mask allows CO$_2$ washout via a continuous leak. The generated positive airflow pressure splints open the pharynx thereby preventing apnoeas, hypopnoeas, snoring and sleep fragmentation.

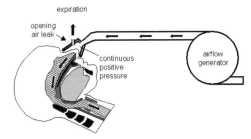

Fig. 15.1.10 The principle of CPAP.

CPAP has been shown in randomised placebo-controlled trials to be an effective therapy in patients with OSAS; it improves excessive daytime sleepiness, quality of life, vigilance, cognitive and driving simulator performance, and daytime blood pressure. Furthermore, blood pressure variations associated with obstructive apnoeas and excessive sympathetic tone are also improved.

Compliance with CPAP therapy is strongly influenced by the severity of the patients' symptoms, the benefit they perceive by the treatment, the support and information given by doctors and other health care workers specialised in sleep medicine. Therefore, most sleep centres in the UK employ a dedicated CPAP nurse or technician, and many centres provide special patient education programmes, including video presentations, informative leaflets and telephone help lines. The compliance with CPAP shows a considerable inter-individual variability which tends to be better in patients with severe OSAS than in mild–moderate OSAS. In addition to the severity of symptoms other factors can predict CPAP use, including whether the patient self-initiated the referral to the sleep centre, the patients' age and co-morbidities. Certain patients refuse to use CPAP because of the initial inconvenience, possible side effects, and for psychological reasons.

Nasal CPAP is a highly effective therapy for moderate to severe OSAS, with complete resolution of sleepiness and large gains in quality of life. To achieve maximal benefits from CPAP a careful induction programme is required.

It is a matter of debate how to derive the required mask pressure, and many different approaches appear to work. Conventionally, after the diagnosis of OSAS has been established by history and a sleep study, the therapeutic pressure is determined during an overnight titration study with a sleep technician present; CPAP pressures are set by manual adjustment in order to abolish apnoeas and minimise arousals. In most cases this is a successful approach but obviously expensive as it requires overnight staffing. Alternatively, 'intelligent', but more expensive, CPAP machines, which automatically adjust the CPAP pressure in response to apnoeas, inspiratory flow limitation, and snoring, can be used to determine what pressure of CPAP is needed, generating similar pressures to manual titrations. As an even less labour intensive alternative, an algorithm (a predictive model which takes into account the dip rate and neck size of a patient) can be used to set an initial CPAP pressure, an approach shown to be as effective as the conventional approach using a titration night, but much less costly.

Patients require subsequent life-long follow-up to maintain their CPAP equipment and solve possible problems. Fortunately, CPAP is a safe therapy and serious side effects are extremely rare. The most common problems encountered include:

- Mouth leakage leads to increased airflow through the nose and out of the mouth, with consequent excessive drying of the mucosa, sore throat, nasal congestion, nasal stuffiness, and rhinitis. This problem is recognised in up to 60% of all patients on CPAP.
- Pain and skin ulceration; most commonly over the nasal bridge.
- Claustrophobia
- Abdominal bloating, usually a minor problem

AUTHOR'S TIPS

- The most effective way to deal with mouth leaks is to either use a chin support to close the mouth or use a full-face mask.
- Initial steps of dealing with nasal congestion are adding humidified air and correcting potential leakage from the nasal mask.
- Nasal congestion can be treated with topical intranasal steroids (e.g. fluticasone) in addition to avoidance of any relevant allergens. Topical decongestant nasal sprays (e.g. oxymetazoline) can also reduce nasal congestion, but treatment duration is limited as therapy lasting more than 5 days can lead to rebound nasal congestion.
- Patients who have obvious nasal polyps, severe turbinate hypertrophy or a distinctive abnormality of the nasal anatomy should be referred to an ENT-specialist for surgical therapy.
- Pain and skin ulceration can be addressed by trying different types of masks (e.g. nasal cushion masks) or patient interfaces (e.g. oracle, an oral CPAP interface).
- Claustrophobia usually settles but it may be worth trying a different patient interface.

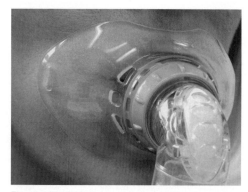

Fig. 15.1.11 Oracle device – delivery of CPAP via the mouth rather than via the nose.

Alternative treatment options

Mandibular advancement devices

For patients with mild–moderate sleep apnoea and patients who cannot tolerate CPAP, fitting a removable mandibular advancement device that is snapped onto the teeth during sleep is a valuable alternative treatment option. Such devices are designed to advance the mandible (usually by 5 to 10mm), thereby enlarging the upper airway calibre. They need to be customised to match the patient's dentition, which usually requires the services of a dentist. Several randomised trials have documented effectiveness of this therapy in improvement of mild to moderate OSA, daytime symptoms and quality of life. However, there are some potential limitations:

- Side effects include tooth and jaw ache, which often lessen with time.
- Effects on teeth and temporo-mandibular joints have to be carefully evaluated as long-term use may be associated with movement of the teeth and alterations to the bite.
- The initial cost (often over £300) is similar to that of a CPAP machine (£250) but mandibular advancement devices usually only last about a year.

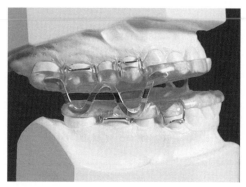

Fig. 15.1.12 Mandibular advancement device. (Adapted from Kohler M, Bloch KE 2003.)

Surgical treatment

With the exception of adeno-tonsillectomy in children and adults with significantly enlarged adenoids and tonsils, surgical treatment is rarely indicated as therapy for OSAS. Although sometimes performed for snoring and OSAS, uvulopalatopharyngoplasty (UPPP), and other surgical techniques such as radiofrequency tissue ablation, and laser-assisted uvulopalatoplasty have not been proven to be effective treatments for OSAS in the few randomised controlled trials performed. Even for snoring the evidence for efficacy is poor.

Pharmacological treatment

To date there is no specific pharmacological treatment available for OSAS. Alerting drugs (such as modafinil) have no place in the routine management of sleepiness in OSAS as it is unclear if these agents help. They are rarely used as an adjunct in selected patients with OSAS in whom excessive sleepiness persists despite optimal adaptation of CPAP therapy.

Further reading

Douglas NJ. *Clinicians' guide to sleep medicine*. London: Arnold 2002.

Jordan A, White D, Fogel R. Recent advances in understanding the pathogenesis of obstructive sleep apnea. *Curr Opin Pulm Med* 2003; **9**: 459–464.

Kohler M, Bloch KE. Sleep-related breathing disorders. *Swiss Arch Neurol Psychiatr* 2003; **154**: 302–309.

Kohler M, Bloch KE, Stradling JR. The role of the nose in the pathogenesis of sleep apnoea and snoring. *Eur Respir J* 2007; **30**: 1205–1215.

Management of obstructive sleep apnoea/hypopnoea syndrome in adults. A national clinical guideline. Scottish Intercollegiate Guidelines Network, 2003, Edinburgh, UK.

Marin JM, Carrizo SJ, Vicente E, *et al.* Long-term cardiovascular outcomes in men with obstructive sleep apnoea-hypopnoea with or without treatment with continuous positive airway pressure: an observational study. *Lancet* 2005; **365**: 1046–1053.

Stradling JR, Davies RJO. Obstructive Sleep Apnoea, definitions, epidemiology and natural history. *Thorax* 2004; **59**: 73–78.

NICE technology appraisal of CPAP for OSA, 2008: `http://www.nice.org/guidance/index.jsp?action=byID&o=11944`

Polotsky VY, O'Donnell CP. Genomics of sleep-disordered breathing. *Proc Am Thorac Soc* 2007; **4**: 121–126.

Pepperell JC, Ramdassingh-Dow S, Crosthwaite N, *et al.* Ambulatory blood pressure after therapeutic and subtherapeutic nasal continuous positive airway pressure for obstructive sleep apnoea: a randomised parallel trial. Lancet 2002; **359**: 204–210.

Schwab RJ. Upper airway imaging. *Clinics in Chest Medicine* 1998; **19**(1).

Smith PL, Wise RA, Gold AR, Schwartz AR, Permutt S. Upper airway pressure-flow relationships in obstructive sleep apnea. *J Appl Physiol* 1988; **64**: 789–795.

Young T, Palta M, Dempsey J, *et al.* The occurrence of sleep disordered breathing among middle aged adults. *N Engl J Med* 1993; **328**: 1230–1235.

Young T, Skatrud J, Peppard P. Risk factors for obstructive sleep apnea in adults. *JAMA* 2004; **291**: 2013–2016.

15.2 Driving

Driving is a task involving a variety of sensory inputs including visual, auditory and spatial awareness which are processed and result in a coordinated motor output. Vigilance and cognitive processing are required to accurately place the vehicle on the road, drive at an appropriate speed and react to external factors.

The ability to drive may be impaired in a range of respiratory and sleep disorders. Examples include confusion caused by hypoxia or carbon dioxide retention, reduced vigilance due to medications causing sedation, or sleepiness resulting from nocturnal dyspnoea or sleep disorders.

Sleepiness

Symptoms of excessive sleepiness that lead to impairment of driving performance can result in accidents. In the UK approximately 25 percent of all motor vehicle accidents (MVAs) are due to sleepiness. There are many causes of sleepiness including lack of sleep, poor quality sleep due to shift work and sleep disorders.

Sleep disorders

There are over 80 sleep disorders recognised in the International Classification of Sleep Disorders. In the UK most patients with sleep and breathing disorders including OSAS are investigated and managed by respiratory consultants. Untreated OSAS patients have an increased risk of being involved in a MVA of up to 6 times that of a normal individual. Patients with other sleep disorders such as narcolepsy are also often referred to specialist respiratory sleep clinics.

Advice regarding the fitness to drive is an important part of the care of any patient with a sleep disorder.

Guidelines

In the UK the body responsible for issuing driving licenses is the Driver and Vehicle Licensing Agency (DVLA). Group 1 licences include drivers of motorcars and motorcycles, Group 2 licences include drivers of large lorries and buses. The DVLA issue written guidelines for medical practitioners on the current 'Medical Standards of Fitness to Drive'. There is a section on respiratory and sleep disorders including OSAS causing excessive daytime/awake time sleepiness. Group 1 licence entitlement requires that if excessive sleepiness is present *driving must cease until satisfactory control of symptoms has been attained, confirmed by medical opinion.* Group 2 licence entitlement requires that if excessive sleepiness is present *driving must cease until satisfactory control of symptoms has been attained, with ongoing compliance with treatment, confirmed by consultant/ specialist opinion. Regular, normally annual, licensing review required.*

The guidelines include a section on neurological disorders which applies to narcolepsy and cataplexy. Group 1 licence entitlement requires an individual to *cease driving on diagnosis.* Driving will usually be permitted if symptoms are satisfactorily controlled when a licence will be granted for a period of 1, 2 or 3 years with regular medical review. Until the age of 70 a licence will be restored after at least seven years of satisfactory control. A patient is generally considered permanently unfit for a Group 2 licence, *but if a long period of control has been established licensing may be considered on an individual basis.*

Other sections of the guidelines include advice on cognitive impairment, blackouts and impaired consciousness which could be relevant to a sleepy patient. Other sleep disorders are not specifically mentioned.

Clinical approach: key points

Doctors in training should be assisted by a senior colleague in establishing the presence of symptoms of excessive sleepiness, the diagnosis of a sleep disorder, the appropriate therapy and advice regarding driving. Some patients describe few symptoms of sleepiness and it can be helpful to obtain information from a partner or relative.

History

- Symptoms of sleepiness, extent of sleepiness and examples of situations, involvement in MVAs or near misses, presence of cognitive impairment.
- Driving and type of licence held.
- Occupational history, e.g. driving, operating machinery, shift work.
- Medication causing sedation, alcohol consumption.
- Symptoms of sleep disorders and sleep pattern.

Examination

- Specific to detect enlarged tonsils, thyroid disease.
- General to detect respiratory, cardiology or neurological conditions.

Investigation

To establish a diagnosis

- Sleep investigation/study as evidence of the presence of OSAS, e.g. oximetry, multi-channel respiratory recording, polysomnography.
- Sleepiness score to estimate the presence of excessive sleepiness e.g. Epworth Sleepiness Score (ESS)

To obtain an objective measurement of sleepiness

- Maintenance of Wakefulness Test (MWT) or the behavioural version (MWTosler) thought to provide a measurement of the ability of the individual to stay awake.
- Multiple Sleep Latency Test (MSLT) thought to provide a measurement of ability of the individual to fall asleep.
- Simulation studies are sometimes performed but the relevance to driving on the real road is not clear.

Fitness to drive in the UK is not assessed by objective measurements of wakefulness/sleepiness, unlike some other countries. Debate continues about how these objective tests should be interpreted as an indication of fitness to drive.

Treatment

CPAP therapy is the treatment of choice for moderate to severe OSAS. Compliance with therapy can be estimated as most devices have a clock to measure running time. CPAP therapy improves steering simulator performance and reduces the risk of accidents in patients with OSAS to that of the normal population.

Patients with OSAS who drive for a living may require a facility for rapid set up with CPAP therapy.

Advice

This includes an explanation of the results of the investigations, the diagnosis and appropriate treatment.

- An explanation of the effect of the disorder on driving.
- Advice not to drive when the individual is sleepy or advice that driving must cease if excessive sleepiness is present. This may have implications on work which may have to cease prior to treatment.
- Explanation of therapy available.
- If possible, have a family member, partner or a friend present for information and to hear advice.
- Keep clear documentation.
- Recommend provision of written advice to the patient.

Notification to DVLA

In the UK it is the doctor's responsibility to advise the patient to notify the DVLA on diagnosis of a sleep disorder that may affect the ability to drive.

It is the responsibility of the patient who holds a licence to notify the DVLA by telephone or letter. The DVLA will then send forms both to the patient and doctor requesting information about diagnosis, treatment and satisfactory control of symptoms. The written consent of the patient is usually forwarded by the DVLA with the form. The doctor should ensure this is obtained before providing any information.

The DVLA considers the information provided and will then continue or revoke the driving licence. It is advisable to follow-up drivers to ensure adequate control of symptoms and compliance with therapy.

Insurance

The patient should be advised to notify the insurers of the diagnosis of a sleep disorder.

Difficult situations

If a symptomatic patient with a sleep disorder continues to drive against medical advice it is important to involve other people in discussions including general practitioners, nurses, family and friends.

Written information should be provided to the patient and general practitioner on the advice given. Copies of documentation should be kept. Every attempt should be made to resolve the issues whilst maintaining patient confidentiality. It may be useful to offer referral for a second opinion.

If a patient continues to drive against medical advice or fails to notify the DVLA, a senior doctor may have to consider notifying the DVLA by contacting a medical advisor. Verbal and written warnings of the intention to do so should be given to the patient where possible.

Further reading

American Academy of Sleep Medicine (2005). *The International Classification of Sleep Disorders* 2nd edn. Diagnostic and Coding Manual, Westchester: USA.

Driver and Vehicle Licensing Agency drivers medical group (2008) Guide to current medical standards of fitness to drive. www.dvla.gov.uk

George CF. Reduction of motor vehicle collisions following treatment of sleep apnea with nasal CPAP. *Thorax* 2001; **56**: 508–512.

George CF, Findley LJ, Hack MA. Across country viewpoints on sleepiness during driving. *Am J Resp Crit Care Med* 2002; **165**(6): 74 746–749.

National Institute of Clinical Excellence Technology Appraisal (2008). Sleep Apnoea- Continuous Positive Airway Pressure (CPAP) TA139. www.nice.org.uk/guidelines/TA/published

15.3 The overlap syndrome

Introductions

The overlap syndrome was first used to describe the coexistence of OSAS and COPD. Patients are prone to severe hypoxemia during sleep, especially rapid eye movement (REM) sleep, in addition to the hypoxaemic episodes from obstructive sleep apnoea. This is due to worsening of alveolar hypoventilation during sleep. The most marked falls in nocturnal arterial oxygen saturation occur in COPD patients who are hypoxic and hypercapnic when awake.

In recent years, the term has come to be used more widely and to include obesity-related hypoventilation. Obesity is not only associated with obstructive sleep apnoea but it is an increasingly common cause of hypoventilation. Daytime hypoxia and hypercapnia are increased in patients with a BMI >40.

Most authors now regard the overlap syndrome as any combination of two or more of these three conditions (Fig. 15.3.1). The syndrome is being diagnosed with increasing frequency, and as obesity levels continue to rise, it is set to become more prevalent in the future.

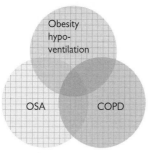

Fig. 15.3.1 The overlap syndrome.

Pathogenesis and implications for treatment

In pure obstructive sleep apnoea, the arterial oxygen saturation usually returns to baseline after each episode of hypoxaemia, and the arterial blood gas tensions when awake are usually normal. In contrast, in the overlap syndrome, the arterial oxygen saturation usually remains low between episodes of obstructive sleep apnoea, and these patients are usually hypoxaemic and hypercapnic when awake. Alveolar ventilation is reduced.

Ventilation falls normally during non-REM sleep and drops further during periods of REM sleep. In healthy individuals, the resulting falls in arterial oxygen tension cause little change in arterial oxygen saturation because they lie on the flat part of the oxyhaemoglobin dissociation curve. However, patients with severe COPD or obesity hypoventilation syndrome often have marked falls in arterial oxygen saturation during REM sleep. This is partly because they lie on a steeper part of the oxyhaemoglobin dissociation curve and partly because they hypoventilate more than healthy individuals, both when awake and during sleep.

When obstructive sleep apnoea coexists with severe COPD or obesity-related hypoventilation the level of ventilation tends to fall further because of the episodes of upper airway obstruction. The importance of this extra resistive load in contributing to alveolar hypoventilation is illustrated by the ability of CPAP alone to reverse hypercapnia and hypoxia in some patients with the overlap syndrome.

However, in other patients CPAP alone is insufficient to restore ventilation to adequate levels. In these patients, the other factors which contribute to non-apnoeic hypoventilation are presumably of more importance. These factors include decreased functional residual capacity, reduced ventilatory response to hypercapnia and hypoxia, decreased chest compliance in morbid obesity and generalized airway resistance in COPD.

The reduced ventilatory drive is of particular interest for there is evidence that it is not fixed. Some patients who do not respond well to CPAP at first can be established on CPAP after a period of non-invasive ventilation. The short-term ventilatory support improves arterial gas tensions and results in the ventilatory drive being re-set. After this, relatively normal oxygen and carbon dioxide levels can be maintained with CPAP alone.

Clinical aproach

General

The overlap syndrome should be suspected when COPD or morbid obesity is associated with sleep disruption and daytime sleepiness, especially if there is daytime hypoxia and hypercapnia. It should also be considered when patients already receiving CPAP treatment for OSAS have persistent symptoms of sleep disruption or carbon dioxide retention (especially if they are morbidly obese and/or have COPD).

History: key points

- Daytime sleepiness and/or poor sleep quality.
- Known COPD or significant smoking history.
- Morning headaches due to hypercapnia in a few patients.
- Inadequate or incomplete response to CPAP (in patients already on CPAP for OSA).

Examination: key points

- Morbid obesity – usually BMI >40 unless COPD also present.
- Physical signs of pulmonary hypertension and right ventricular failure.

Investigations

Overnight oximetry

- The baseline arterial oxygen saturation during sleep is usually lower and less stable than in pure obstructive sleep apnoea.
- In a typical study, gradual falls in arterial oxygen saturation caused by hypoventilation are combined with more rapid ('saw-tooth') fluctuations caused by obstructive sleep apnoea.
- However, note that, at low SaO_2, sharp falls in arterial oxygen saturation can also result from hypoventilation alone, because of the shape of the oxyhaemoglobin dissociation curve.

Arterial blood gas measurements

Daytime hypercapnia is common. Measure arterial blood gas tensions if the daytime oxygen saturation is low and/or symptoms of hypercapnia are present.

Transcutaneous CO_2

This is a useful adjunct if available. It can be used to help titrate the level of ventilation.

AUTHOR'S TIP

Polysomnography adds little in most cases. Assessment is usually based on skilled interpretation of the history and overnight oximetry, followed by trials of treatment.

Treatment

CPAP

- CPAP alone or with oxygen supplementation improves symptoms and daytime arterial gas tensions in many patients.
- However, others continue to have symptoms and significant desaturation during REM sleep, with ongoing hypercapnia despite the abolition of obstructive apnoeas and hypopnoeas with CPAP. These patients should be considered for non-invasive ventilation.

Non-invasive ventilation (NIV)

- NIV has been shown to be effective in treating OSA patients with hypercapnia.
- A short period of NIV can reset the central respiratory drive, enabling patients to continue with CPAP thereafter.

Supplemental oxygen

- Although oxygen therapy alone is safe in most patients with uncomplicated COPD, it can lead to dangerous hypercapnia in the overlap syndrome. However, oxygen therapy can be used in combination with NIV, and sometimes with CPAP, if hypoxaemia persists due to COPD.

Example case

A 50-year-old man with a 40 pack-year smoking history complained of tiredness, poor sleep quality, loud snoring and morning headaches. On clinical examination, he was morbidly obese with a BMI of 42kg/m^2 and had pedal oedema. The FEV_1 was 1.1 litres and the FVC 2.5 litres. The arterial oxygen saturation was 93% breathing air, PaO_2 6.5kPa, $PaCO_2$ 7.1kPa and pH 7.41

Overnight oximetry (Fig. 15.3.2a) showed a low baseline saturation during the night, gradual falls in arterial oxygen saturation due to hypoventilation and superimposed rapid falls in oxygen saturation due to obstructive sleep apnoea and hypoventilation.

After an unsuccessful trial of nasal CPAP, he was established on non-invasive ventilation. Overnight oxygenation improved markedly (Fig. 15.3.2b) and his symptoms resolved. He remains on long-term non-invasive ventilation.

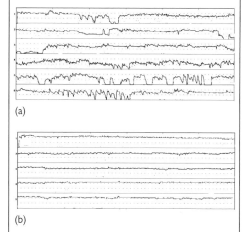

(a)

(b)

Fig. 15.3.2 Overnight arterial oxygen saturation (a) before treatment and (b) during treatment with non-invasive ventilation using an inspiratory pressure of 16 cmH$_2$O and an expiratory pressure of 6 cmH$_2$O without supplemental oxygen. Each line represents one hour and shows a continuous recording of the arterial oxygen saturation between 70 and 100%.

Further reading

Flenley DC. Disordered Breathing during sleep: discussion paper. *J Royal Soc Med* 1985; **78**: 1031–1033.

Mohsenin V. Sleep in Chronic obstructive Pulmonary Disease. *Sem Resp Crit Care Med* 2005; **26**(1): 109–116.

Laaban J, Chailleux E. Daytime Hypercapnia in Adult patients with Obstructive Sleep Apnoea Syndrome in France, before Initiating nocturnal nasal Continuous Positive Airway Pressure Therapy. *Chest* 2005; **127**(3): 710–715.

Piper AJ, Sullivan CE. Effects of Short-term NIPPV in the Treatment of Patients with Severe Obstructive Sleep apnoea and Hypercapnia. *Chest* 1994; **105**: 434–440.

Resta O, Foscino-Barbaro MP, Bonfitto P, *et al.* Prevalence and mechanisms of diurnal hypercapnia in a sample of morbidly obese subjects with obstructive sleep apnoea. *Resp Med* 2000; **94**: 240–246.

Resta O, Foschino-Barbaro MP, Brindicci C, *et al.* Hypercapnia in overlap syndrome: possible determinant factors. *Sleep Breath* 2002; **6**(1): 11–17.

15.4 Non-invasive ventilatory support in the acute setting

Overview
CPAP and non-invasive positive pressure ventilation (NIPPV or NIV) are the commonest forms of non-invasive ventilatory support. In the acute setting, CPAP is used as an adjunct in the management of pure hypoxic respiratory failure (type I), whereas NIV uses bi-level pressure ventilation to treat alveolar hypoventilation presenting as decompensated hypercapnic respiratory failure (type II). Despite their different indications, the two forms of ventilatory support share many practical aspects.

Indications in the acute setting
CPAP
Improves hypoxia in non-acidotic respiratory failure:
- Pneumonia and pneumonitis, as an interim measure before invasive ventilation or as ceiling of treatment.
- Acute cardiogenic pulmonary oedema.
- Severe obstructive sleep apnoea (OSA).

NIV
Treats hypercapnic respiratory failure with acidosis, including:
- Acute exacerbations of COPD.
- Decompensated chronic hypoventilation due to chest wall deformity, obesity hypoventilation (± OSA), neuromuscular disease.
- Rare conditions: congenital or acquired abnormalities of ventilatory control, metabolic disorders.
- Acute cardiogenic pulmonary oedema.

NIV will also improve oxygenation and may be better tolerated than CPAP, so can be used in type I respiratory failure.

Contra-indications
- Facial trauma or burns.
- Untreated pneumothorax.
- Vomiting or risk of aspiration.
- Fixed upper airway obstruction.

Caution is required in patients with decreased conscious level and unprotected airway, or excessive secretions.

Mechanisms of action
CPAP
- Recruits underventilated or collapsed lung units.
- Increases FiO_2 (due to mask efficiency).
- Splints the upper airway.
- Offloads inspiratory muscles to reduce work of breathing.

NIV
- Expiratory positive airway pressure (EPAP) overcomes elevated intrinsic positive end-expiratory pressure (PEEP), so delaying airway collapse in expiration.
- EPAP recruits underventilated or collapsed lung units.
- Inspiratory positive airway pressure (IPAP) assists inspiration and reduces the work of breathing against increased lung and chest wall compliance.
- The combined effect of EPAP and IPAP is to increase tidal volume and alveolar ventilation.

Clinical evaluation
A full clinical evaluation is required in all acute patients; the following are pointers that may help in the context of respiratory failure, and is not an exhaustive list.

History
Think about clues to disproportionate respiratory failure:
- Smoking history (undiagnosed COPD?).
- No smoking history (is this acute asthma, requiring urgent ITU referral rather than NIV?).
- Drug history (sedative or opiate overdose possible?).
- Somnolence and snoring (OSA or overlap syndromes).
- Morning headaches, fatigue (nocturnal hypoventilation).
- Old polio (physical disability not always obvious).
- Old TB (thoracoplasty or other collapse therapy?).
- Trauma or surgery affecting thoracic compliance, diaphragmatic movement or brainstem ventilatory control.

Examination
- Don't ignore the obvious: chest wall distortion or obesity may be longstanding but decompensate acutely.
- Signs of cor pulmonale suggest chronic hypoxia.
- Signs of pneumothorax or pleural effusion suggest alternative treatable causes.
- Reduced respiratory rate and conscious level are key indicators of CO_2 narcosis.

Investigation
Arterial blood gas measurements (ABGs) are essential to establish the pattern of respiratory failure. Simplified:
- PaO_2 <8.0kPa and normal/low $PaCO_2$ despite high FiO_2: type I respiratory failure, think about CPAP and ITU.
- High PaO_2 and high $PaCO_2$: FiO_2: too high in a hypoventilating patient, so give controlled FiO_2: and recheck.
- PaO_2 <8.0kPa and high CO_2 with pH <7.35 despite controlled FiO_2: suggests the need for NIV.

CXR is essential to exclude a pneumothorax and to investigate possible pneumonia or effusion. Look for CXR clues: hyperexpansion, old TB, elevated hemidiaphragm, scoliosis.

Investigation of persistent respiratory failure includes overnight oximetry (look for REM-related desaturation seen in hypoventilation, or saw-tooth desaturation of OSA), early morning ABGs or overnight capnography for CO_2 retention.

Commencing treatment
- Decide and document the ceiling of treatment in case NIV is unsuccessful: patients suitable for ITU, particularly those with type I failure, should be discussed early to anticipate the need for escalation and invasive ventilation.
- Patients unsuitable for escalation due to advanced disease, frailty or co-morbidity may still benefit from a trial period of CPAP or NIV.
- CPAP or NIV should be implemented by staff trained and familiar with the equipment and with mask fitting.
- A 'full-face mask' covering nose and mouth is most commonly used in the acute setting. Nasal masks or pillows are preferred by some patients but need more co-operation to avoid mouth breathing. Helmets are used less but may overcome intractable leakage problems.
- Allow the patient to hold the mask onto their face for familiarisation. The ease with which the mask can be removed should be demonstrated.

CPAP
Two types of equipment can deliver CPAP:
- Fixed pressure 'PEEP valve' on an airtight mask, with air/oxygen fed into the mask (flow rates of 40–60 l/min required).

This reliably delivers high FiO_2, and is the type usually used in emergency departments or ITU.

- An adjustable pressure-driven CPAP unit (or NIV unit with IPAP and EPAP settings equal). Most NIV units can deliver high FiO_2; CPAP units may require O_2 to be entrained and cannot guarantee $FiO_2 > 50\%$.

Initial pressure settings of 5 cmH_2O are suitable to familiarize the patient to the circuit. Increase the pressure over 30 minutes. Aim for 10–12.5 cmH_2O for pneumonia or pulmonary oedema; higher pressures may be required to treat severe OSA in obese patients.

NIV

- 'Spontaneous/timed' mode on a pressure-support ventilator is usually used, with breaths triggered by the patient's respiratory effort and a back-up rate of 8–12 breaths/minute if no effort is detected. The back-up rate must be below the patient's own respiratory rate; a patient with a very low rate is unlikely to be suitable for NIV.
- Start with IPAP/EPAP 10/4 cmH_2O aiming to titrate up over 30 minutes, e.g. to IPAP 16–18 and EPAP 5–6, according to the patient's response. The maximum practical IPAP is normally 20 cmH_2O.
- EPAP must overcome intrinsic PEEP (high in obstructive lung disease) or upper airway obstruction in OSA: up to 10 cmH_2O is sometimes needed.
- Use controlled oxygen at the lowest rate required to achieve target SaO_2; aim to improve oxygenation by optimal pressure support rather than high FiO_2. A target of 85–90% is often sufficient in COPD.
- Monitor respiratory rate, SaO_2 and conscious level as well as haemodynamics; observe patient comfort and synchonisation with the ventilator.
- Check ABGs after 1 hour, and again when a steady state is reached or if the patient's condition changes.
- Reduced conscious level due to CO_2 narcosis is a relative contraindication to NIV, but is acceptable if NIV is the ceiling of treatment. Doxapram has occasionally been used to improve respiratory drive to assist NIV.

Specific clinical presentations

COPD

NIV is of proven benefit in acute exacerbation of COPD with decompensated hypercapnic respiratory failure (pH <7.35). Poor response to NIV is often due to excessive FiO_2 with inadequate pressure support.

Pneumonia

CPAP can improve oxygenation in patients with pneumonia providing secretions can be controlled adequately. Hypercapnia and acidosis suggest co-existing COPD or a tiring patient and require an escalation in therapy.

Immunocompromised patients

Immunocompromised patients have an extremely poor prognosis when intubated for respiratory failure. Early NIV has been shown to reduce the need for intubation and to improve mortality in this group.

Obesity

Respiratory failure in obesity may be due to severe OSA, which responds to CPAP, or to obesity hypoventilation syndrome. The latter group hypoventilate despite treatment of upper airway obstruction, and so require NIV. These patients can present with acute-on-chronic respiratory failure: ask about the duration of symptoms of hypoventilation or cor pulmonale. They may require higher NIV pressures to overcome poor thoracic compliance, and may require a

prolonged period of NIV to treat the effects of long-term hypercapnia on central ventilatory control. Once stabilised, some can be converted to domiciliary CPAP for the longer term. Think about hypoventilation in obese patients labelled as having 'heart failure' despite well preserved cardiac function on echo: check ABGs. All obese patients with respiratory failure should be investigated with overnight oximetry. Weight loss is curative.

Neuromusculoskeletal disease

Respiratory failure in acute neuromuscular disease (e.g. Guillain–Barré syndrome, myasthenic crisis) should be managed in a high-dependency setting with immediate access to invasive ventilation; NIV may provide a holding measure. Patients with chronic neuromusculoskeletal disease (e.g. muscular dystrophy, post-polio syndrome, kyphoscoliosis) may decompensate and present acutely: NIV is often effective, and these patients are likely to require long-term domiciliary nocturnal NIV. Patients with chest wall deformity may require higher pressures.

Acute cardiogenic pulmonary oedema

CPAP and NIV are effective in cardiogenic pulmonary oedema and reduce the need for intubation. Their effects appear to be equivalent, and neither therapy increases the incidence of acute myocardial infarction. CPAP is usually cheaper and more rapidly available in the emergency department.

Other considerations

After the acute phase, breaks for food, drink and social interaction are usually feasible. Weaning is achieved by steadily increasing the length of breaks from ventilation. Patients requiring prolonged NIV may be more comfortable with a nasal mask, after stabilisation on a full-face mask. In severely unwell patients nutrition must be addressed early, by NG feeding if necessary. Thromboprophylaxis should be considered: most NIV patients will benefit.

Pitfalls and tips

- Skin breakdown can be disastrous. It may be due to poor or tight mask fitting with inadequate monitoring. Allow periods off ventilation; vary the mask type and position; protect the skin with a dressing.
- Think about the breathing circuit: we have seen exhalation ports blocked, removed or fouled with secretions.
- Humidification can aid tolerance of CPAP/NIV, but don't drown the patient: keep the reservoir below the level of the patient's head.
- Increase pressures cautiously in patients with severe emphysema or bullae: there is a risk of pneumothorax.
- Air swallowing is a problem. An NG tube can reduce subsequent gastric dilatation and prevent diaphragmatic splinting; rarely a flatus tube is necessary.

Further reading

British Thoracic Society Standards of Care Committee Non-invasive ventilation in acute respiratory failure. *Thorax.* 2002; **57**(3):192–211.

Perez de Llano LA, Golpe R, *et al.* Short-term and long-term effects of nasal intermittent positive pressure ventilation in patients with obesity-hypoventilation syndrome. *Chest* 2005; **128**(2): 587–594.

Peter JV, Moran JL, *et al.* Effect of non-invasive positive pressure ventilation (NIPPV) on mortality in patients with acute cardiogenic pulmonary oedema: a meta-analysis. *Lancet* 2006; **367**(9517): 1155–1163.

Ram FS, Picot J, Lightowler J, *et al.* Non-invasive positive pressure ventilation for treatment of respiratory failure due to exacerbations of chronic obstructive pulmonary disease. *Rev Cochrane Database Syst* 2004; **3**: CD004104.

15.5 Nocturnal hypoventilation

A reduction in overall ventilation is a natural accompaniment of sleep and in normal individuals arterial oxygen saturation falls by a few per cent and PCO_2 level rises by around 0.5kPa. These physiological changes are most marked during REM sleep.

Nocturnal hypoventilation becomes clinically significant in conditions where either the respiratory muscle pump is compromised or ventilatory drive is reduced (see Table 15.5.1), and may contribute to the development and progression of daytime (diurnal) respiratory failure in these groups.

Table 15.5.1

Reduced ventilatory pump: neuromuscular disease
Muscular dystrophies
Myopathies
Spinal muscular atrophy
High spinal cord injury
Motor neuron disease (amyotrophic lateral sclerosis)
High ventilatory load
COPD
Cystic fibrosis
Bronchiectasis
Morbid obesity
Scoliosis/chest wall disorder
Thoracoplasty

Reduced ventilatory drive
Congenital central hypoventilation syndromes
Acquired central hypoventilation syndromes
Sedative and analgesic drugs
Prader–Willi syndrome

Aetiology

A combination of factors of factors underlies the reduction in alveolar ventation. With the onset of sleep, ventilation falls due to a reduction in cortical ventilatory drive associated with wakefulness, upper airway resistance increases as tone in pharyngeal muscles falls and the ability to compensate for this increased resistance is diminished. Both hypercpanic and hypoxic ventilatory drive are also reduced. Particularly during REM sleep there is hypotonia of the intercostal and accessory muscles with a switch to a diaphragmatic pattern of breathing. REM sleep is therefore a challenging time for individuals with diaphragm weakness. In the supine position functional residual capacity will fall and ventlilation perfusion matching deteriorates especially in COPD patients. Nocturnal hypoxaemia alters pulmonary haemodynamics – COPD patients who desaturate at night have significantly higher pulmonary artery pressure and red cell mass than non-desaturators. Further adverse consequences include dysrhythmias, nocturnal ischaemia, sleep fragmentation and possible neurocognitive effects.

Predicting nocturnal hypoventilation

COPD

The extent on nocturnal desaturation in COPD patients is usually correlated with daytime SaO_2 and CO_2 levels.

It should not be forgotten that common conditions overlap. While there is no evidence that the prevalence of obstructive sleep apnoea (OSA) is increased in COPD, the coexistence of COPD and OSA is likely to produce nocturnal hypoxaemia disproportionate to daytime SaO_2 and will not be adequately addressed by long-term oxygen therapy (LTOT). Sleep studies in COPD patients are therefore indicated in COPD patients with witnessed apnoeas, crescendo decrescendo snoring, disproportionate hypoxaemia in relation to spirometry or daytime somnolence.

In LTOT recipients sleep studies are advisable in those with marked daytime hypercapnia or symptoms of CO_2 retention (e.g. morning headache, nocturnal confusion, frequent hypercapnic exacerbations), and also in those in whom features of right heart failure and polycythaemia persist while on LTOT (assuming compliance with LTOT has been confirmed).

Neuromuscular and chest wall patients

Routine evaluation of patients with neuromuscular disease and chest wall disorders includes assessment of symptoms and pulmonary function. Patients with isolated chest wall defects, e.g. idiopathic scoliosis and a vital capacity of >50% predicted are unlikely to develop ventilatory insufficiency long term, so respiratory clinic follow-up is unnecessary. However individuals with progressive conditions, e.g. Duchenne muscular dystrophy or motor neuron disease, should be seen regularly and a sleep study is indicated in those with symptoms of nocturnal hypoventilation, dyspnoea and FVC <60%. Special attention should be played to high-risk groups, e.g. motor neuron disease and a particular catch in congenital disorders is that profound hypoventilation can be seen in those with severe chest wall restriction, e.g. chest 'en cuirasse' or rigid spine syndrome, despite a relatively preserved vital capacity.

In a series of young patients with congenital myopathies, spinal muscular atrophy and muscular dystrophies, Ragette et al. found that a FVC capacity of <60% had a 91% sensitivity and 89% specificity for predicting the onset of sleep disordered breathing. Continuous hypoventilation was seen in REM and non-REM sleep once VC was less than 40% predicted and a VC of <25% predicted had a 92% sensitivity and 93% specificity for predicting daytime ventilatory failure. The authors also measured maximum inspiratory mouth pressures, but these were less accurate at predicting respiratory insufficiency and did not add to VC measurements. Cough peak flow measurement is useful to predict cough efficacy. In most neuromuscular conditons inspiratory and expiratory muscles are similarly affected. Discrepancies occur such as in isolated diaphragm paralysis due to phrenic nerve injury and in some spinal muscular atrophy patients in whom expiratory muscle weakness may outstrip inspiratory muscle weakness.

In motor neuron disease patients a sleep study is indicated if there is orthopnoea, rapid progression of symptoms, or VC <60%. There is no point in a sleep study if daytime PCO_2 is elevated. PCO_2 values will be inevitably higher at night and time is wasted as the appropriate action is to institute NIV if this is in accordance with the patient's wishes. Theoretically, multichannel studies to differentiate obstructive apnoeas and hypopnoeas from hypoventilation may be helpful, but in practice bi-level ventilators are commonly used and can be titrated to deal with all respiratory events regardless of aetiology.

Diagnosis of nocturnal hypoventilation

The characteristic features of nocturnal hypoventilation can often be detected from an oximetry trace. Whereas recurrent saw tooth dips are seen in OSA, in nocturnal hypovention several longer periods if desaturation are seen coinciding with the periodicity of REM sleep. (As a corollary, mild hypoventilation may therefore be missed if the patients sleep poorly and no REM sleep occur.)

Strictly speaking, alveolar hyopoventilation should be defined by a rise in PCO_2 and therefore endtidal of transcutaneous CO_2 monitoring is helpful. Intermittent arterial blood gas measurements or an arterial line overnight is not conducive to sleep.

Some centres rely on early morning blood gas measurements, but these may be misleading, depending on the relationship between the patient waking and measurement being made.

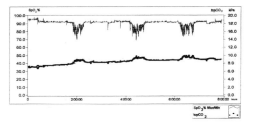

Fig. 15.5.1 Nocturnal hypoventilation: 3 cycles during REM sleep.

Transcutanous CO_2 ($TcCO_2$) monitoring has been criticised in the past, but a variety of machines are now in regular use and proving useful, providing the limitations of endtidal CO_2 are borne in mind. Transcutaneous measurements will always reveal a trend, not breath by breath results, and values are approx 0.5kPa above arterial values. Careful attentions should however be paid to calibrating the device with test gas mixtures, skin preparation and application of the CO_2 electrode. A printout of actual data (Fig. 15.5.1) should always be available rather than summary statistics so that artefacts can be detected and discarded from final analysis. In Europe polysomnography is rarely used to diagnose nocturnal hypoventilation or other respiratory sleep disorders or to titrate therapy, e.g. determine NIV settings. Occasionally it may be helpful when problem solving in difficult cases, or when treatment is not working optimally.

Treatment

Asymptomatic mild hypoventilation in a chest wall or neuromuscular patient does not require treatment, in a chest wall patient, yearly repeat sleep study would be reasonable although 6-monthly studies preferable in DMD. In Duchenne muscular dystrophy a randomised controlled trial showed no evidence that prophylactic non-invasive ventilation is indicated.

Around a decade ago, consensus conference recommendations were that NIV should be used once daytime PCO_2 exceeds 6kPa. However, the rate of progression of nocturnal hypoventilation may be difficult to predict and as a result many individuals may develop precipitous daytime ventilatory failure usually due to a chest infection. In one trial in which patients with neuromuscular and chest wall disease were randomised to NIV or control group at the onset of

nocturnal hypoventilation, 70% of the control group had developed daytime respiratory failure, recurrent chest infections or marked symptoms within a year and 90% experienced these problems with 2 years.

This would suggest that once nocturnal hypoventilation occurs, consideration should be given to initiating NIV in the next year. Progression can be more indolent in chest wall patients, and in these symptoms need to be marked or the trade off between nuisance value of NIV and symptom relief is not in the patients favour, and compliance likely to be poor.

COPD: LTOT is gold standard treatment in COPD patients who fulfil standard criteria. As indicated above a subgroup of patients may not tolerate LTOT due to hypercapnia, and in these and those with recurrent hypercapnic exacerbations domiciliary NIV may have a role. Tuggey et al. showed that NIV may be cost effective in the selective group of patients who are regularly admitted with acute exacerbations and tolerate NIV well. Randomised controlled trials are not conclusive on this point however, mostly as they have looked at mortality as an end point and have been underpowered.

NIV may also be helpful in other patients groups, e.g. in those with bronchiectasis or cystic fibrosis and marked symptoms of nocturnal hypoventilation or as a bridge to transplantation.

Central sleep apnoea

Central sleep apnoea in adults is defined by the presence of episodes of apnoea lasting for >10 seconds during which respiratory effort is absent. Central apnoeas may either occur as a result of a profound reduction in ventilatory drive, e.g. following brain stem stroke or as a result of heightened respiratory drive as in heart failure patients. In practice, the term embraces periodic breathing and Cheyne–Stokes respiration (Fig. 15.5.2) in which a crescendo decrescendo pattern of breathing is interspersed with central apnoeas. In the latter, pulmonary oedema stimulates lung receptors leading to hyperventilation. This drives down CO_2 such that an apnoea occurs, and the apnoea is terminated by an arousal associated with hyperpnoea which again reduces CO_2 precipitously and the cycle continues.

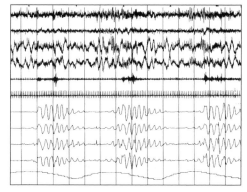

Fig. 15.5.2 Cheyne–Stokes ventilation.

The two types of central apnoea can easily be differentiated by measuring PCO_2 level. A further learning point is that in some patients with marked respiratory muscle dysfunction and obstructive apnoeas, inspiratory muscle weakness is insufficient to generate detectable effort (pseudocentral apnoea).

Sleep disordered breathing in chronic heart failure (CHF)

In severe CHF the prevalence of sleep disordered breathing (SDB) is at least 10 times greater than in the general population, and is associated with an increased risk of mortality. In mild to moderate CHF, it has recently been shown that the prevalence of SDB remains high at approximately 50% and about half of these patients have predominantly central sleep apnoea. While treatment of obstructive sleep apnoea in CHF with CPAP is clearly evidence-based, CPAP had not been shown to be beneficial in heart failure patients with central sleep apnoea. In these patients, presenting symptoms differ from OSA patients – sleepiness is not a major feature, and treatment remains controversial. Oxygen therapy may be helpful but recent work suggests that stabilising the respiratory pattern by a device that captures ventilation and smoothes the respiratory disturbance may be effective (Autoset CS, ResMed Inc.). This is being tested in a current European randomised controlled trial.

Key recommendations

- There should be a high suspicion of nocturnal hypoventilation in patients with conditions reducing ventilatory capacity and drive and disorders increasing ventilatory load – ask about symptoms of nocturnal hypoventilation, e.g. morning headaches, poor sleep quality, waking breathless, vivid dreams.
- Nocturnal hypoventilation can be diagnosed by overnight oximetry and PCO_2 measured continuously with transcutaneous or endtidal CO_2 probes.
- Central sleep apnoea is caused by either severely reduced ventilatory drive or in conditions that destabilise respiratory pattern as a result of enhanced ventilatory drive, e.g. heart failure, breathing at high altitude.

- Symptomatic nocturnal hypoventilation can be effectively treated with nocturnal NIV which improves survival and outcome in chest wall and neuromuscular disease and may help selected COPD patients with marked hypercapnia or recurrent hypercapnic exacerbations.

Further reading

American Thoracic Society Consensus Statement. Respiratory care of the patient with Duchenne muscular dystrophy. *American Journal of Respir Crit Care Med* 2004; **170**: 456–465.

Consensus Conference. Clinical Indications for Noninvasive Positive Pressure Ventilation in Chronic Respiratory Failure due to Restrictive Lung Disease, COPD, and nocturnal hypoventilation – a Consensus conference report. *Chest* 1999; **116**: 521–534.

Mellies U, Ragette R, Schwake C, et al. Long-term noninvasive ventilation in children and adolescents with neuromuscular disorders. *Eur Respir J* 2003; **22**: 631–636.

Ragette R, Mellies U, Schwake C, et al. Patterns and predictors of sleep disordered breathing in primary myopathies. *Thorax* 2002; **57**: 724–728.

Raphael J-C, Chevret S, Chastang C, et al. Randomised trial of preventive nasal ventilation in Duchenne muscular dystrophy. *Lancet* 1994; **343**: 1600–1604.

Takasaki Y, Orr D, Popkin J, et al. Effect of nasal continuous positive airway pressure on sleep apnea in congestive heart failure. *Am Rev Respir Dis* 1989; **140**: 1578–1584.

Teschler H, Dohring J, Wang YM, et al. Adaptive pressure support servo-ventilation: a novel treatment for Cheyne-Stokes respiration in heart failure and central sleep apnea. *Am J Resp Crit Care Med* 2001; **164**: 614–619.

Tuggey JM, Plant PK, Elliott MW. Domiciliary non-invasive ventilation for recurrent acidotic exacerbations of COPD: an economic analysis. *Thorax* 2003; **58**: 867–871.

Ward SA, Chatwin M, Heather S, et al. Randomised controlled trial of non-invasive ventilation (NIV) for nocturnal hypoventilation in neuromuscular and chest wall disease patients with daytime normocapnia. *Thorax* 2005; **60**: 1019–1024.

15.6 Cheyne–Stokes respiration associated with left ventricular failure

Cheyne–Stokes respiration (CSR) is characterised by the cyclical pattern of smooth crescendo decrescendo periods of hyperventilation with accompanying periods of central apnoea. It is variably called central sleep apnoea and periodic breathing. CSR is a respiratory complication of chronic left ventricular failure (LVF). CSR is important clinically because it can cause symptoms, worsens heart failure and is amenable to treatment.

Pathophysiology

CSR results from the following in heart failure:

- Increased ventilatory drive/hyperventilation.
- Low lung volumes and stores of oxygen.
- Reduced cardiac output.
- Haemodynamic alterations.

Hyperventilation is caused by a combination of stimulation of J receptors through increased left atrial pressure and pulmonary oedema, alongside changes in both central and peripheral chemosensitivity.

Hyperventilation lowers $PaCO_2$ levels and causes mild respiratory alkalosis (both common in patients with CSR).

At sleep onset, cortical input and respiratory drive reduce with an increase in apnoea threshold.

The $PaCO_2$ from awake hyperventilation falls below the apnoeic threshold (approx 35mmHg) initiating apnoea.

Low cardiac output prolongs circulation time and delays central perception of the apnoea induced blood gas changes.

The long apnoea duration, low lung volumes and oxygen stores contribute to hypoxaemia and hypercapnia.

Blood gas derangement may lead to cortical arousal and return of awake ventilatory drive.

A period of hyperventilation ensues to restore normal PaO_2 and $PaCO_2$ before sleep resumes and the cycle is repeated.

LVF-induced CSR also leads to stimulation of sympathetic activity, reduced renal blood flow, and sodium and water retention. Vasoconstriction, increased blood pressure and increased heart rate cause increased myocardial workload which further worsens LVF contributing to the poor prognosis seen in patients with CSR.

Depending on the different respiratory and cardiac components leading to CSR, it may settle with different sleep stages or spontaneously through the night. Any external arousals, obstructive events or deep sighs may trigger further episodes.

Symptoms and signs

- Poor quality of sleep.
- Frequent arousals.
- Choking episodes.
- Nocturnal dyspnoea, arrhythmias or angina.
- Daytime fatigue or sleepiness.

CSR and OSA have been correlated with more severe LV impairment, atrial fibrillation, ventricular dysrhythmias and earlier mortality in patients with cardiac disease.

> **AUTHOR'S TIPS**
> - CSR occurs in 50% of NYHA class III or IV heart failure or ejection fraction <45%.
> - CSR is more common in males, the elderly and patients with atrial fibrillation.

Investigations

Confirm LVF with Echo and brain natriuretic peptide.

Exclude type II respiratory failure with ABG sampling.

Overnight pulse oximetry

Approximately half of patients with NYHA class III and IV will have an apnoea hypoxia index (AHI) of between 0–10 per hour on multi channel sleep study. Oximetry is a simple screening tool looking for repetitive desaturations.

Compared to OSA, CSR tends to have a longer time period, lower amplitude desaturations through the apnoea and a slower rise in saturation at end apnoea (Fig. 15.6.1).

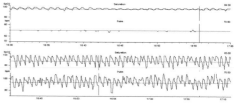

Fig. 15.6.1 Oximetry saturation and pulse rate for CSR, upper panel with reduced amplitude longer cycle length and slower end apnoea saturation rise versus OSA, lower panel.

Multichannel sleep studies

On full sleep study CSR is distinguished from OSA by the absence of respiratory effort. The gold standard to confirm this, invasive oesophageal pressure monitoring, is impractical for routine use. Several non-invasive surrogates for respiratory effort can be used combining abdominal and thoracic inductance bands, the nasal pressure trace, variations in pulse transit time (PTT, a marker of intrapleural pressure change) or dyssynchrony between abdominal and thoracic movements. In the examples in Fig. 15.6.2, CSR shows reduced nasal pressure accompanying reduced thoracic and abdominal effort and no swing in PTT.

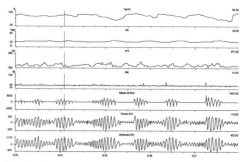

Fig. 15.6.2 Sleep study of CSR with desaturations (SpO_2), following decreased nasal airflow from reduced thoracic and abdominal effort. The PTT channel confirms no intrathoracic pressure swings of respiratory effort.

Treatment of heart failure

Medical management
CSR is related to heart failure severity and pulmonary capillary wedge pressure. Control of heart failure can reduce CSR and all patients should have their medical treatment optimised. Improve LV function and reduce circulatory time using diuretics, ACE inhibitors, β-blockers and digoxin. Shown to reduce CSR as well as mortality.

Cardiac re-synchronisation therapy (CRT)
Biventricular pacing can resynchronise myocardial contraction to increase left ventricular ejection fraction, cardiac output and exercise capacity. Increased cardiac output, reduced circulation time and uncoupling the cardiac and respiratory drive centres may all help stabilise CSR.

CRT can be considered in patients with the following:
- NYHA class III or IV.
- A prolonged QRS of greater than 150ms.
- Echo evidence of desynchronisation.

Treatment of CSR
The principles of treating CSR which remains after optimising LVF treatment are through pharmacological agents, oxygen or ventilation methods aiming to.
- Alter ventilatory drive.
- Prevent hypoxaemia.
- Reduce arousals.
- Control ventilation.

Opiates
Opiates decrease the sensitivity of peripheral chemoreceptors therefore lowering hypoxic ventilatory responses and may reduce arousal and afterload.

Theophylline
Use of short-term theophylline is associated with significant reduction in the AHI, but no reduction in the frequency of arousals or improvement in sleep structure or cardiac function. Detrimental effects however, include cardiac dysrhythmias as well as increased minute ventilation.

Acetazolamide
Acetazolamide causes a metabolic acidosis which leads to stimulation of central respiratory drive. It also increases the apnoeic threshold for pCO_2 thus reducing CSR. Effects seem to be long-lasting; however it is unlicensed. Metabolic acidosis and hyperventilation may be detrimental in LVF.

Oxygen
Low flow nasal oxygen (2–3L/min) administered at night has been shown in randomised control trials to reduce CSR, correct hypoxia, improve sleep quality and improve daytime cognitive function. CSR is probably reduced by increasing PaO_2 and lung oxygen stores and by suppressing peripheral chemoreceptor drive. Nocturnal oxygen has not yet been shown to improve left ventricular ejection fraction or exercise capacity.

Carbon dioxide
Inhaled carbon dioxide can eliminate CSR. By increasing the partial pressures of carbon dioxide ventilatory drive is maintained during sleep. Similar effects can be seen by increasing dead space ventilation via a facemask. Unfortunately CO_2 markedly increases sympathetic activation, may cause sleep fragmentation and is not recommended in the treatment of CSR.

CPAP
Nocturnal CPAP can reduce CSR in several ways. By increasing lung volumes and oxygen stores, decreasing lung water, reducing left ventricular transmural pressure and afterload to increase cardiac output, or by increasing dead space and CO_2 rebreathing.

It was hoped that CPAP would reduce mortality above it improvements in cardiac output and exercise capacity but this has not been confirmed by a recent large trial.

Those patients with cardiac failure with coexisting predominantly obstructive sleep apnoea do benefit from CPAP.

Bilevel positive airway pressure
There is no evidence that BiPAP is superior to CPAP in CSR. It may indeed lower pCO_2 levels leading to vocal cord opposition and arousal at night. BiPAP is reserved for those who do not tolerate CPAP.

Adaptive servo-ventilation (ASV)
ASV ventilators measure breathing frequency and tidal volume to calculate a minute volume averaged over the preceding 3 minutes. ASV aims to deliver only 90% of this recent minute volume to mimic the usual reduction in ventilation during sleep onset allowing pCO_2 levels to rise.

ASV delivers a stable end expiratory pressure (5 cmH$_2$O) but inspiratory pressure can vary between predefined levels (default 3–10 cmH$_2$0).

ASV predicts breath by breath variations in tidal volume from initial inspiratory effort and provides variable inspiratory pressure support to maintain target minute ventilation. During periods of apnoea ASV provides maximum pressure support at the preceding spontaneous respiratory rate.

ASV has a number of theoretical advantages to improve cardiac function. In practice it stabilises CSR over about 10–20 minutes, reducing AHI and arousals more than oxygen CPAP or BIPAP to improve sleep quality.

Small studies have shown improvement in daytime somnolence, quality of life, walking times and ejection fraction, with accompanying reduction in hospital admissions and improvement in survival time. This has not yet been proven in large trials and so although preliminary evidence suggests that ASV is superior to oxygen or CPAP, it is not yet recommended as first-line treatment.

AUTHOR'S TIP

For CSR causing sleep fragmentation despite optimising cardiac medications, nocturnal oxygen treatment may stabilise CSR simply prior to trials of CPAP, BiPAP or ASV.

Further reading
Bradley TD, Logan AG, Kimoff RJ, et al. Continuous positive airway pres-sure for central sleep apnoea and heart failure. N Eng J Med 2005; **353**(19): 2025–2033.

Cazeau S, Alonzo C, Jauvert G, et al. Cardiac resynchronization therapy. Europe 2004; **5**: S42-S48.

Hanly P, Zuberi N, Gray R. Pathogenesis of Cheyne-Stokes respiration in patients with congestive heart failure. Sleep 1994; **17**: 61.

Pevernagie D, Janssens JP, DeBacker W, et al. Ventilatory support and pharmacological treatment of patients with central apnoea or hypoventilation during sleep. European Respiratory Review, in press.

15.7 Other causes of sleepiness

Overview

There are a large number of other causes of sleepiness, the majority of which may be diagnosed with a careful history. True hypersomnolence must be differentiated from fatigue and tiredness, which are extremely common. The less common pathological causes of sleepiness will be rarely encountered by the respiratory physician; the parasomnias may be referred to a respiratory sleep clinic in the first instance, and a directed history will enable the appropriate investigation of the majority of disorders. Insomnia is not covered here.

History: key points

- Sleep hygiene/quality and duration of sleep – are enough hours being spent in bed, in an environment appropriate for sleep? Insufficient sleep is a very common cause of hypersomnolence.
- Associated sleep symptoms – including dreams and nightmares, and their timing (e.g. at sleep onset), sleep paralysis, cataplexy, hypnagogic hallucinations, leg movements or noises during sleep. A collateral history from the bed partner is paramount.
- Past medical history – including of neurological disease, anxiety/depression, previous neuro-surgery (especially pituitary surgery), cranial radiotherapy, and visual loss.
- Drug history – including prescribed drugs e.g. β-blockers, alcohol, caffeine and illicit drugs.
- Social history – current job and pattern of any shift work. Frequent long distance travel.
- Anything to suggest a neurological disease, e.g. Parkinson's disease, other movement disorder or muscle weakness.

Investigations: key points

- No further investigations may be needed in patients in whom there is a clear history of sleep disruption or inadequate sleep duration.
- Multiple sleep latency testing (MSLT) – this uses EEG to document the time to fall asleep in a dark and sound-isolated room, on five naps spaced throughout the day, and can be used to document objective sleepiness. The presence of sleep onset REM (SO-REM), may aid diagnosis of some parasomnias. An MSLT of <8 minutes is considered abnormal (normal is 10–15 minutes), though is not very specific. An abnormal MSLT alone is probably enough to diagnose narcolepsy confidently in those with a history of cataplexy and sleepiness.
- Patients with pathological hypersomnolence, in whom no cause is determined from the history, and without snoring or cataplexy, should have an MSLT. If the sleep latency is <10 minutes, further investigation may be warranted.
- Full polysomnography (including EEG, EOG and EMG, and measurement of respiratory signals and leg movements, usually via EMG) may be needed for confident diagnosis of less common disorders.

Causes of hypersomnolence

Shift work sleep disorder

Insufficient or disrupted sleep due to shift work is common, with variable shift patterns causing the most sleep disturbance. Individuals tend to become more intolerant of shift work (particularly night shifts) with increasing age.

Periodic leg movements in sleep (PLMS)

- This is the association between stereotyped, repetitive limb movements during REM sleep and daytime hypersomnolence or frequent nocturnal awakenings. Most commonly patients repeatedly flex and dorsiflex the ankle or great toe, every 20 to 40 seconds. Leg movements cause partial brain arousal, sleep fragmentation and thus daytime symptoms. There may be an association with Parkinson's disease.
- The night time syndrome can be associated with daytime restless legs syndrome (RLS), which is the sensation of continually needing to move the legs, in association with unpleasant parasthesia. The symptoms are relieved by movement. PLMS affects about 50% of individuals aged >65. Mild symptoms of PLMS may be present in up to 15%, but most will be asymptomatic. There may be a genetic basis for the disorder. RLS can be a feature of diabetic peripheral neuropathy, and is associated with lower leg venous insufficiency, hypothyroidism, spinal stenosis and excess caffeine intake.
- Dopaminergic lower spinal nerve dysfunction is postulated as a cause. Most commonly the disorder is idiopathic, but there is an association with iron deficiency anaemia, end stage renal disease (in up to 60%) and the use of tricyclic antidepressants and monoamine oxide inhibitors. All patients presenting with PLMS should have an FBC ± iron studies.
- Treatment – dopamine agonists tend to be more effective than benzodiazepines. Co-beneldopa has been shown to be effective (e.g. as Sinemet CR® 1 or 2 tablet nocte). Tachyphylaxis to L-dopa and an earlier onset of symptoms, or increased intensity of symptoms is recognised on L-dopa. Some recommend only intermittent L-dopa for these reasons. Clonazepam 0.5–2mg nocte may be better tolerated. Dopamine agonists, e.g. pramipexole 0.125–0.5mg nocte or pergolide 0.05–1mg nocte taken about 2 hours before the usual onset of symptoms may also help. Low potency opioids, e.g. tramadol and codeine, may be useful.

Parasomnias

These are disruptive sleep related disorders, which occur during arousal from REM sleep, or during partial arousal from non-REM sleep. They are characterised by physical phenomena which include autonomic involvement and/or skeletal muscle involvement. They can occur during specific sleep stages, or during the sleep-wake transition. The disorders are frequently bizarre, and patients are often labelled as having psychiatric disease. Parasomnias are more common in children than adults, and there may be a familial susceptibility. There are a number of related conditions; those most likely to be encountered are listed.

- REM behaviour disorder.
- Narcolepsy.
- Cataplexy.
- Sleep walking and sleep terrors.
- Sleep talking.
- Parasomnia overlap disorder.
- Nocturnal sleep-related eating disorder.
- Sleep paralysis.
- Sleep bruxism.

REM behaviour disorder

This typically occurs in men of late middle age, and involves the acting out of dreams which are often violent and action-packed. The nocturnal violent behaviour is usually out of keeping with the patient's awake personality. There may be a higher frequency in individuals who have seen active combat, and an association with the development of Parkinson's disease in later life. Clonazepam 0.5–1mg at night, along with maximising the safety of the sleep environment are the usual treatments.

Narcolepsy

This is a disorder of sleep–wake control, characterised by hypersomnolence, cataplexy, hypnagogic hallucinations and sleep paralysis. Hypnagogic hallucinations are vivid hallucinations occurring just before sleep onset, probably due to a mixture of REM sleep and wakefulness. Sleep paralysis is the complete inability to move for up to about 2 minutes after waking. Cataplexy is the sudden onset of loss of voluntary muscle tone, leading to partial or complete collapse, and may be triggered by emotion, such as laughter, joking or anger. Partial attacks are common, with, for example, just the head nodding, often with associated facial twitching. Paralysis typically lasts up to 2 minutes, with maintenance of consciousness. Cataplexy and sleep paralysis are probably due to inappropriate activation of the pathways usually causing muscle paralysis during REM sleep.

Narcolepsy has a prevalence of 25 to 50 per 100,000 (about 1/100th the prevalence of OSA), typically starting in the teens and early twenties. Only about one-third of patients will have all four classical symptoms. All affected individuals will have daytime hypersomnolence, often falling asleep with little warning, so called 'sleep-attacks', and in bizarre situations, such as eating. The sleepiness of narcolepsy often resolves after a brief nap, and individuals often feel refreshed in the morning, in comparison to other more common cause of hypersomnolence.

Pathophysiology

The disease is thought to be due to loss of neuropeptides orexin (hypocretin) A and B in the lateral hypothalamus. 90% of patients with narcolepsy have no detectable CSF orexin, due to reduced numbers of hypothalamic orexin-producing neurons.

The orexins have excitatory post-synaptic effects and are released during wakefulness, increasing the activity of many brain areas involved in the maintenance of wakefulness. Orexins inhibit REM sleep; it is the loss of orexin which promotes the disease specific REM sleep-related phenomena. Narcolepsy is usually sporadic; up to 90% have human leucocyte antigens HLA DR2 and DQ1. There is a strong association with the DQB1*0602 haplotype. Familial cataplexy is rare, thus environmental factors must also be important.

Diagnosis

This is usually made from the history, with a sleep study off stimulants and antidepressants, to avoid REM rebound. Polysomnography will show REM onset within 15–20 minutes of sleep onset (after 80 to 100 minutes is normal), with spontaneous awakenings and reduced sleep efficiency. MSLT may be useful.

Treatment

This includes pharmacological therapy for the daytime sleepiness and REM sleep intrusion phenomena, and frequent daytime naps. Psychosocial support is important.

Modafinil is a non-amphetamine based wakefulness promoting agent that probably increases dopaminergic signalling. 200–800mg OD, sometimes as a divided dose is effective. Modafinil is an enzyme inducer; side effects are uncommon, but include hypertension, dry mouth, nausea and diarrhoea. Mazidol, methyl-phenidate and selegiline are also used. Drugs increasing noradrenergic and serotinergic signalling suppress REM sleep and therefore reduce REM phenomena such as cataplexy: SSRIs, e.g. venlafaxine and fluoxetine, and tricyclic antidepressants may also be of use.

Neurological disease associated with hypersomnolence

Tumours and infarcts, particularly of the hypothalamus and upper brain stem, head injury and encephalitis may lead to hypersomnolence.

Parkinson's disease is associated with hypersomnolence due to sleep disturbance, often as a result of dopamine agonists. PMLS is common in Parkinson's disease, as are vivid dreams, nightmares and nocturnal tremor, all of which can cause sleep fragmentation. Other neurological diseases frequently associated with daytime hypersomnolence are listed:

- Myotonic dystrophy.
- Pituitary surgery.
- Cranial irradiation.

Multiple sclerosis – up to 80% suffer from severe fatigue, and sleep disruption is common, often due to pain or bladder spasms. There may be associated OSA.

Sleep disturbance related to blindness is due to disruption of the retino-hypothalamic pathways which cue circadian rhythm. Melatonin may be of use.

Rare causes of hypersomnolence

Delayed sleep phase syndrome

This most common in young adults and is characterised by late sleep onset with late awakening. Treatment is gradual phase advance (by 15–30 minutes each night), with bright light exposure on wakening.

Kleine Levine Syndrome

This rare syndrome is characterised by recurrent episodes of daytime sleepiness in association with bizarre eating patterns and hyper-sexuality.

- Magnesium toxicity.
- Idiopathic hypersomnolence.
- Idiopathic stupor.
- Post-infectious hypersomnolence.
- Post-traumatic hypersmonolence.
- Limbic encephalitis.

Idiopathic insomnia

This is a difficulty in maintaining normal sleep which stems from childhood. The aetiology is uncertain.

Further reading

Aldrich MS. *Sleep Medicine*. Oxford: Oxford University Press, 1999.
British Sleep Society `http://www.sleeping.org.uk/contents/homefrm.htm`
Douglas NJ. *Clinician's Guide to Sleep Medicine*, Arnold 2002.

Occupation and environment

Chapter contents

16.1 Drugs and toxins

Introduction

Respiratory disease may be caused by a wide range of drugs and toxins leading to diverse syndromes. Since 1950, knowledge has expanded in this area. It is important for all clinicians to consider, as it is potentially reversible and often forgotten. A few are quite common, most are not but reports are on the increase. Patients may present with protean symptoms, signs and radiological features to primary care and a variety of specialties including cardiology, oncology and rheumatology.

This chapter will outline the commonest presentation modes and some of the most commonly encountered drugs but is not exclusive: see the online databases.

Diagnosis

Diagnosis of drug-induced lung disease requires a number of criteria to be satisfied as shown in Table 16.1.1.

Table 16.1.1 Diagnostic criteria

Correct identification	Harder if occurs after drug stopped or multiple exposures
Timing consistent	Improvement on stopping Recurrence with re-challenge
Characteristic features	Clinical Imaging Broncho-alveolar lavage (BAL) Histology
Exclusion of common causes	Infection Oedema Underlying lung condition

Presentation modes

The commonest modes of presentation are shown in Table 16.1.2

Table 16.1.2 Modes of presentation

Interstitial lung disease	Pneumonitis Fibrosis Eosinophilia Organising pneumonia Acute respiratory distress syndrome (ARDS)
Pleural disease	Thickening Pleuritis Effusion Pneumothorax Pneumomediastinum
Airway disease	Direct injury Obliterative bronchiolitis Bronchospasm Bronchial hyper-reactivity (BHR)
Pulmonary vascular disease	Haemorrhage Infarction Thrombo-embolism Pulmonary hypertension
Infection	Pneumonia Aspiration Tuberculosis (TB)

Interstitial disease

The pathology can be variable but typically occurs after weeks or months, presenting commonly with dyspnoea, cough and fever. Common agents are shown in Table 16.1.3 below. Abnormal liver function tests or eosinophilia may be noted. Common causes of eosinophilia are also shown in Table 16.1.3.

Risk factors include multiple drugs at the same time. Bronchoscopy and BAL may reveal lymphocytosis but is helpful to exclude infection or cancer. Lung function is restrictive with impaired gas transfer as expected. High-resolution computed tomography (HRCT) is not specific, and increased uptake may be noted on Gallium scanning. Transbronchial biopsy (TBB) is not specific and a surgical lung biopsy may sometimes be needed. The drug must be stopped but steroids may be needed if there is extensive radiological change and impaired lung function.

Table 16.1.3 Common drugs causing interstitial lung disease and pulmonary eosinophilia

Interstitial lung disease	Eosinophilia
Bleomycin	Aspirin
Busulphan	Isoniazid
Chlorambucil	Penicillin
Cyclophosphamide	Sulphonamides
Methotrexate*	
Amiodarone*	
Nitrofurantoin*	
Sulphasalazine*	

*Denotes also causes eosinophilia.

Drug-induced lupus pleuritis

Lung involvement may occur in 50% of cases of drug-induced lupus, manifesting as pleuritis. Features discriminating it from spontaneous lupus are shown in Table 16.1.4.

Delayed metabolism (slow acetylation) is important in the pathogenesis of two of the commonest drugs. Treatment may include nonsteroidal anti-inflammatory drugs (NSAIDs) and anti-malarials for musculoskeletal symptoms. Corticosteroids have been used for serositis. The three commonest drugs are discussed here:

Procainamide

Drug-induced lupus often occurs in almost all after 2 years treatment but can occur in up to 33% after 1 year, especially in slow acetylators. Genetic factors have been implicated.

Hydralazine

Drug-induced lupus occurs in 5–10%, especially in those >200mg/day, cumulative dose >100g, female, slow acetylators and having a low C4 complement. Genetic factors have also been implicated.

Minocycline

Drug-induced lupus often occurs in young women on minocycline for acne. Fever and rashes are more common than with other drug-induced cases. Anti-histone Abs are often absent (<13%), although p-ANCA (anti-neutrophil cytoplasmic antibodies) may be positive in up to 85%.

Key points

- If both anti-histone Abs and p-ANCA are absent, this makes drug-induced lupus very unlikely.
- This diagnosis is often forgotten in patients investigated several times for pulmonary embolism (with negative findings) and ongoing unexplained pleuritis.
- If considering hydralazine-induced lupus, check ANCA as atypical p-ANCA (anti-elastase, not anti-MPO (myeloperoxidase)) is specific for hydralazine-induced vasculitis and may require immunosuppressant treatment.

Table 16.1.4 Discriminating features for drug-induced lupus

	Drug-induced lupus
Gender	No female predominance
Onset	Abrupt
Organs involved	Less for skin, renal and central nervous system
Auto-antibodies	95% anti-histone antibody (Ab) positive Double-stranded deoxyribonucleic acid (dsDNA) Ab rarely positive
Complement	Normal

Pleural eosinophilia

Pleural eosinophilia (>10%) can be due to air or blood in the pleural space, asbestos-related effusion, parasitic infections, but also drugs as listed in Table 16.1.5 below.

Table 16.1.5 Common drugs causing pleural eosinophilia.

Pleural eosinophilia
Nitrofurantoin*
Isotretinoin
Dantrolene
Valproate
Propylthiouracil
Bromocriptine*

*Denotes discussed later.

AUTHOR'S TIPS

- The presence of co-existing parenchymal infiltrates would support nitrofurantoin- or bromocriptine-induced lung toxicity amongst this select group of drugs.
- Concurrent peripheral blood eosinophilia would support nitrofurantoin, dantrolene or valproate-induced lung disease among this group.

Airway disease

β-blockers

β-blockers (including eye drops) and cholinergic drugs (e.g. pyridostigmine) cause bronchoconstriction via bronchial M2-receptor blockade and muscarinic M1 and M3 receptor activation.

However, a meta-analysis in reversible obstructive lung disease has confirmed no evidence of long-term decline in lung function with cardio-selective β-blockers (atenolol, metoprolol). A short-term decline of 8% in FEV_1 was seen, but this was not sustained and reversibility of bronchodilator increased to about 7%. In addition, respiratory symptoms were not increased lung term or quantities of inhaled β-agonists. Carvedilol has also shown to be well tolerated (in terms of FEV_1, FEF_{25-75} and VO_2 max) despite being a non-selective β-blocker, possibly because of mild broncho-dilation from its alpha (α)-blocking activity.

β-blockers have other (less well known) lung toxicities other than broncho-constriction including pulmonary infiltrates with eosinophilia, hypersensitivity pneumonitis, organising pneumonia, fibrosis, pleural thickening/effusion and drug-induced lupus.

NSAIDs cause bronchoconstriction in 5% of asthmatics by driving cysteinyl leukotriene production and inhibiting cyclo-oxygenase-1 (COX-1).

ACE inhibitors

Angiotensin converting enzyme (ACE) inhibitors (ACEI) cause dry nocturnal cough in 20% via bradykinin release, normally metabolised by ACE in the lungs. There is a poor dose response relationship and it usually occurs within 1 month but may take at least 3 months to subside after cessation of the drug. The main differentials are usually asthma and heart failure.

AUTHOR'S TIPS

- β-blockers can be cautiously trialled in mild–moderate reversible obstructive lung disease.
- Cardio-selective β-blockers are preferable (atenolol, metoprolol) or combined α- and β-blockers (carvedilol).
- Remember other lung toxicities of β-blockers, if broncho-constriction does account for the symptoms.
- Give it 3 months since stopping the ACEI, before referring or investigating for other causes of chronic cough.

Non-cardiogenic pulmonary oedema

ARDS has been associated with a variety of drugs. In overdose, it has been described with aspirin, cocaine (see later), opioids, phenothiazines and tricyclic antidepressants. At normal doses, nitrofurantoin (see later), protamine and certain radiographic contrast media have been implicated.

AUTHOR'S TIP

In ARDS of uncertain aetiology, consider drug-related causes especially if psychiatric issues are a possibility

Pulmonary arterial hypertension (PAH)

PAH has been described in relation to use of anorectic agents (fexflenuramine, dexflenfluramine) and stimulants including amphetamines and cocaine. In case control studies, odds ratios of 3–6 are reported with these agents. The mechanism is uncertain. The anorectics may block potassium channels leading to calcium influx increasing pulmonary vascular tone. Other studies have reported a higher prevalence of bone morphogenic protein receptor 2 (BMPR2) mutations in PAH due to anorectic agents.

AUTHOR'S TIP

In unexplained PAH, drugs must be considered

Individual drugs and toxins

Amiodarone

Amiodarone is one of the commonest drugs implicated (~5% of patients). Pneumotoxicity is more likely in males, with pre-existing lung disease, at daily doses ≥200mg

(5–15% chance at ≥400mg), > 2 months treatment, or cumulative doses >150g. The drug is directly cytotoxic but an immunological hypersensitivity also occurs. It has a long half-life (~45 days) and a high affinity for lung tissue. It presents insidiously most often as non-specific interstitial pneumonitis but can present as an organising pneumonia (25% of cases) or less often (but life threatening) ARDS and rarely as a solitary pulmonary mass. Foamy lipid macrophages are present in the airspaces and may be evident on BAL or biopsy but indicate exposure not injury. Lung function is as expected for interstitial lung disease. There are no predictors for who will develop lung toxicity.

Clinical features include dyspnoea, fever, malaise, weight loss with crackles and a high erythrocyte sedimentation rate (ESR), lactate dehydrogenase (LDH) and leucocytosis. Wheeze, pleuritic chest pain and a friction rub may occur. The CXR may show interstitial or alveolar shadowing but not pleural effusions.

An alternative drug should be used to control arrhythmias if possible or reduce dose with steroid cover (prednisolone 40–60mg od tapering over 2–6/12). If not, 80% will improve but up to 20% die with respiratory failure. If ARDS develops, mortality is 50%.

Key points
- Heart failure is the most important differential and should be suspected and treated if: pleural effusions, normal ESR, normal gallium scan, abnormal echocardiogram/pulmonary artery wedge pressure
- Consider an alternative anti-arrhythmic before starting amiodarone but if unavoidable, advise patient on potential lung effects, check baseline and serial lung function and aim for maximum 100mg OD maintenance dose
- BAL is helpful to exclude infection and also makes amiodarone-induced injury unlikely if there are no foamy macrophages
- Symptoms may progress despite stopping the drug due to accumulation in fatty tissue and long half-life

Methotrexate
Methotrexate pneumotoxicity is also very common, described in 2–8% of patients, even at doses < 20mg/week. Folic acid supplements do not prevent pneumotoxicity and the pathogenesis of lung toxicity remains unclear.

Pneumonitis (acute or subacute) develops over a 3–4 year period but most often after a few months treatment, it is often reversible (~1% mortality). (It has been reported after only day 12 and up to 18 years later). Systemic symptoms may occur before the respiratory symptoms. It may also present as eosinophilia, pleural effusions, organising pneumonia, ARDS or bronchitis with BHR. Table 16.1.6 summarises factors increasing the chances of lung toxicity.

Table 16.1.6 Factors increasing the risk of lung toxicity with methotrexate and bleomycin

Methotrexate	Bleomycin
Age > 60	Age
RA in lung	Cumulative dose
Previous DMARDs	Thoracic radiotherapy
Diabetes	Renal dysfunction
Low albumin	High FiO_2

BAL tends to show CD4+ lymphocytosis and/or eosinophilia. Granulomatous and eosinophilic inflammation is seen on biopsy. 10% of pneumonitis progresses to pulmonary fibrosis.

> ### AUTHOR'S TIPS
> - Exclude infection especially *Pneumocystis jiroveci* (PCP), cytomegalovirus, fungi, TB and non-tuberculous mycobacterium before steroid treatment.
> - Methotrexate lung toxicity is favoured over rheumatoid arthritis (RA) itself if biopsy shows granulomas rather than usual interstitial pneumonia (UIP) and if arthritis quiescent.

Bleomycin
Life-threatening fibrosing alveolitis can occur in up to 10% of patients. Bleomycin hydrolase is not active in the lung (or skin), which may explain toxicity in these tissues although the mechanism is unexplained.

Table 16.1.6 shows the factors associated with increased lung toxicity. Symptoms and signs are non-specific and may develop 1–6 months following treatment. A more acute hypersensitivity pneumonitis may occur more rapidly. The CXR features are variable, typically nodular but normal in 10%. Pleural effusions and adenopathy are rare. BAL is non-specific and sometimes lung biopsy may be needed. Histology resembles diffuse alveolar damage, although organising pneumonia or eosinophilia pneumonitis may be seen.

Steroids may help in pneumonitis with a 50–70% short-term improvement; the evidence is limited. Steroids should be considered in those with eosinophilic pneumonitis or organising pneumonia. Restarting bleomycin is only possible in those with hypersensitivity pneumonitis.

> ### AUTHOR'S TIPS
> - Use low inspired oxygen fractions when possible.
> - Consider steroids at 1mg/kg starting dose and taper to clinical response but later relapse may occur.
> - Pulmonary metastases are often the major differential on imaging.

Nitrofurantoin
Pneumotoxicity is rare (<1%) but can be severe, usually occurring in women (because of their greater likelihood of recurrent urinary infection). Acute reactions are more common, but sub acute and chronic forms are described. The mechanism of injury in the acute form is hypersensitivity leading to eosinophilia, inflammation and microvascular changes. In the more chronic form, an allergic/toxic response is thought to occur with septal thickening, fibrosis and organising pneumonia. It can be associated with ARDS.

Clinically, fever (>38°C), cough, rash and dyspnoea are the commonest symptoms of the acute from, typically 9 days after first exposure (much quicker with subsequent exposures). Eosinophilia, leucocytosis and elevated ESR can occur. The more chronic form develops after 1–6 months with more typical non-specific symptoms but not fever. CXR changes are usually present and BAL may show lymphocytosis, neutrophilia or eosinophilia. Pleural eosinophilia is also reported. The major differentials here are heart failure and infection.

Resolution occurs within 48 hours after stopping the drug in the acute form but takes weeks to 3 months in the less acute forms. The prognosis is very good if detected early, especially in the acute forms. Sometimes mild fibrosis persists.

> **AUTHOR'S TIPS**
> - There is no evidence to support steroids here.
> - If there is no rapid improvement in 72 hours following stopping the drug in the acute form, the diagnosis may well be wrong.

Tumour necrosis factor (TNF) blockers

TNF blockers include etanercept (soluble TNF receptor fusion protein), infliximab (dimeric anti-TNF antibody) and adalimumab (anti-TNF monoclonal antibody).

There are case reports of steroid responsive non-caseating granulomatous lung disease. In addition, there are reports of organising pneumonia developing in those with pre-existing lung disease.

More commonly, there is a well-recognised risk of reactivation of TB most reported with etanercept. The estimated incidence in a large database from 2000-2001 is 1.1% to 1.9%.

Drug-induced lupus is also described (see earlier) with up to nearly 90% developing positive anti-nuclear antibodies and 14% positive dsDNA antibodies with features of lupus syndrome, including pleuritis in 50%.

> **AUTHOR'S TIP**
> Consult the British Thoracic Society guidelines for advice on risk assessment regarding tuberculosis infection before starting TNF blockers: http://www.brit-thoracic.org.uk/c2/uploads/antitnf.pdf

Cyclophosphamide

This is less common but increased by the use of oxygen, radiation and other pneumotoxic drugs. Pneumonitis can occur early or late with fibrosis. Early pneumonitis occurs 1–6 months after onset, with symptoms akin to hypersensitivity pneumonia. Ground-glass change can be a feature. It often responds well to stopping the drug and steroids with complete recovery.

Late pneumonitis occurs after several months to years. It presents like UIP, does not respond to steroids and usually leads to respiratory failure in a chronic and progressive course. It can occur even 6 years after stopping the drug.

Histology is non-specific and may mimic UIP or ARDS. Lung biopsy can help in excluding extrinsic allergic alveolitis, infection or diffuse malignancy though. Genetic changes in metabolism may be important and there is no dose–response effect. Bloods, and lung function abnormalities are non-specific.

> **AUTHOR'S TIP**
> CT appearances in the late form of mid-upper region pleural thickening, lack of honeycombing and lack of basal predominance help distinguish it from UIP

Other DMARDs

Gold

After cumulative exposure >500mg, pneumonitis can occur which responds to stopping the drug and steroids. There are more rare reports of acute respiratory failure, obliterative bronchiolitis and pulmonary fibrosis.

Penicillamine

Bronchiolitis can develop between 3 and 14 months at doses between 375 and 1250mg. Presentation may be dry cough and dyspnoea with only hyperinflation on the CXR and progressive non-reversible airflow obstruction. Mosaicism and air trapping are evident on HRCT. Surgical lung biopsy may be needed. Prognosis is poor (50% mortality) and steroids, cyclophosphamide or azathioprine are often tried. Other less common lung toxicities include pulmonary haemorrhage, drug-induced lupus (see earlier) and pulmonary fibrosis.

Leflunomide

There are reports of accelerated interstitial disease and increases in lung nodules, but some of this may be due to previous exposure to methotrexate. The nodules stabilise when the drug is stopped.

> **AUTHOR'S TIP**
> Fever, other features of gold toxicity (proteinuria, liver dysfunction, rash, eosinophilia), and absence of clubbing with a lymphocytic BAL would favour pneumonitis due to gold rather than RA

Taxanes

Paclitaxel can lead to type 1 hypersensitivity reactions with urticaria, bronchospasm, dyspnoea, hypotension and rash in up to 30% of cases, although steroids and antihistamines can reduce this to 3%. A type 4 hypersensitivity reaction is also described with both and paclitaxel and docetaxel. Acute transient pneumonitis appears usually in the first 2 weeks after administration. With docetaxel, there are reports of severe and life-threatening pneumonitis despite high-dose steroids. The lung effects may be dose-related. As with bleomycin and other agents, concurrent radiotherapy can cause disproportionate toxicity. Sequential chest radiotherapy reduces the risk of pneumonitis. Lung toxicity has also been noted with gemcitabine and taxanes (without radiotherapy) in combination in lung and bladder cancer, developing over a few days with fever and dry cough but responding to high dose steroids.

> **AUTHOR'S TIP**
> In lung cancer patients on taxanes ± gemcitabine, lung toxicity must at least be considered as respiratory symptoms will not always be due to infection, the primary disease or co-morbid lung disease

Mitomycin

Table 16.1.7 summarises the variety of lung toxicities that have been associated with mitomycin. Pre-treatment with steroids can reduce this risk. Bronchospasm can occur in 5%, usually within a few hours and resolving by 24 hours, with/without broncho-dilators. Reticular CXR changes are described and usually resolve.

Table 16.1.7 Mitomycin lung toxicity

- Bronchospasm
- Acute pneumonitis
- Chronic pneumonitis
- Fibrosis
- Acute lung injury
- Pleural disease

Acute pneumonitis is characterised by acute dyspnoea that often partially resolves, although 60% can be left with impaired lung function not completely responding to steroids. CXR may show focal or diffuse interstitial opacities with physiologically reduced gas transfer and hypoxaemia. In one series, in those receiving thoracic radiotherapy and using oxygen therapy at an inspired oxygen fraction (FiO_2) > 0.5 incurred increased lung toxicity.

Chronic pneumonitis seems to be dose related (>30mg/m^2). Presentation is usually with insidious dyspnoea and dry cough with nodular appearances on imaging. Clinically and histologically, it resembles bleomycin pneumotoxicity. Lung function tests do not detect early disease and do not predict outcome. Steroids have been used with some success but early relapse after withdrawal does occur.

Acute lung injury with histological diffuse alveolar damage has been reported which sometimes responds to steroids. Haemolytic uraemic syndrome (with micro-angiopathic haemolytic anaemia, thrombocytopaenia, renal impairment, and acute lung injury in 50%) can occur. It appears to be dose-related and more common if preceding 5-fluorouracil or blood transfusions are given. The majority develop this syndrome 6–12 months after starting treatment. Lowering the dose (<30mg/m^2), increasing the dosing interval (>6 weeks) and reducing the FiO_2, steroids and plasmapharesis are often tried but mortality remains high.

Pleural exudates and fibrosis are described often with underlying parenchymal lung disease. There may be associated lymphocytes and eosinophils. There does not seem to be a dose effect.

> **AUTHOR'S TIP**
> Keep FiO_2 <0.3 to minimise acute pneumonitis and acute lung injury with sequential rather than concurrent radiotherapy if possible

Busulphan

Symptomatic injury occurs in 5%. No dose response effect occurs and the histology is variable. However, toxicity seems greater at cumulative doses >500mg.

Symptoms include dyspnoea, dry cough, weight loss and fever, typically 4 years after starting the drug but as early as 8 months sometimes. Basal reticular changes may occur on CXR. Lung function tests do not predict risk. BAL and lung biopsy are usually needed to exclude infection and cancer. Steroids have been tried with variable response but there is a relative lack of evidence.

> **AUTHOR'S TIP**
> Lung toxicity can occur as late as 10 years after exposure to the drug

Chlorambucil

Lung disease varies from mild pneumonitis to severe pulmonary fibrosis and toxicity is not dose dependent. Chronic interstitial pneumonitis is the commonest problem that may occur from five months to ten years after starting the drug and even several months after stopping the drug. Symptoms may include dry cough, fever, dyspnoea and weight loss. Haemoptysis and acute lung injury have been reported. Blood eosinophilia does not occur but BAL typically shows CD8+ lymphocytosis and eosinophilia. Imaging typically shows nodules and reticular changes. Lung function tests are as expected for interstitial lung disease.

Histology on TBB and surgical lung biopsy can vary enormously. Steroids are not effective in prevention but are used in those with acute respiratory failure or failing to improve after stopping the drug despite limited evidence. Prognosis is poor and 52% died in one series.

> **AUTHOR'S TIP**
> If pleural effusions and/or mediastinal lymphadenopathy, then an alternative cause should be sought

Ergoline drugs

Bromocriptine

Pleural effusion, thickening and parenchymal changes have been described. Toxicity occurs 1–4 years after starting the drug. Although pleural eosinophilia is reported, pleural lymphocytosis is more common.

Methysergide

Extensive pleural fibrosis can occur with/without effusions. Pleural fibrosis resolves in most cases where the drug is stopped. Increased serotonin is thought to increase fibroblast activity.

> **AUTHOR'S TIP**
> Effusions due to bromocriptine completely resolve on stopping it but thickening and infiltrates may persist

Radiation

Haemoptysis, airway disease (bronchitis, obstruction), pleural disease (effusion, pneumothorax), pulmonary vascular disease, and parenchymal lung disease (pneumonitis, pulmonary fibrosis) can occur. Pathogenesis may involve cytokines but also hypersensitivity.

Factors provoking greater lung toxicity are summarised in Table 16.1.8. Injury is detectable within hours histologically, but this is asymptomatic. Pneumonitis can occur histologically from 3 to 12 weeks, followed by fibrosis as early as 6 months if there is failure of resolution.

Pneumonitis occurs in 5–15% of patients with lung cancer, with CXR abnormalities in up to 66% although some of these may be related to the primary tumour. Clinical symptoms may include dry cough, dyspnoea, pleuritic chest pain, low grade fever and malaise. Signs may include crackles or a pleural rub.

Table 16.1.8 Summary of factors provoking greater radiation lung toxicity

Factors provoking greater radiation lung toxicity	
Lung architecture	'Serial': distal from proximal injury
Lung volume irradiated	>10%
Mean dose	20Gy to >35% of lung
Dose fraction	Single dose more toxic
Chemotherapy	Concurrent (sequential less toxic)
Other factors	Previous chest radiotherapy
	Smoking
	Low lung volumes
	Steroid withdrawal
	Female

The differential is wide and bloods show a non-specific increased CRP, ESR and LDH. Lung function tests are restrictive but the trend in DLCO may be the most useful predictive measurement.

Treatment requires prednisolone 60mg/day for 2 weeks then tapering over the next 12 weeks. Improvement does not usually occur beyond 18 months. There is no role for steroids in prophylaxis. Azathioprine or cyclosporin A can be used as steroid-sparing agents based on case reports. Initially promising results with amifostine and captopril have not been replicated. Pentoxifylline is a more promising future candidate.

> **AUTHOR'S TIPS**
> - Consider cardiac toxicity from radiotherapy (especially pericardial disease, valvular dysfunction, coronary artery disease, and cardiomyopathy) as an alternative cause of dyspnoea.
> - Skin erythema outside the port site does not predict the incidence of pneumonitis.
> - A straight-line effect on CXR not conforming to normal anatomy and the absence of lymphadenopathy are discriminating features.
> - A pleural effusion that is moderate or greater in size and/or increases in size following observation is unlikely to be due to radiotherapy.

Cocaine
Nearly 25% of cocaine users develop respiratory problems. 'Crack lung' can occur from 1–48 hours after smoking: fever, diffuse alveolar shadowing and eosinophilia with histology resembling ARDS. Cough, chest pain, dyspnoea and haemoptysis are common. Barotrauma can occur after the smoker performs a Valsalva manoeuvre (to improve drug delivery) leading to pneumothorax or pneumomediastinum. Chronic problems can also occur with ARDS, organising pneumonia, interstitial pneumonitis and fibrosis, pulmonary infarction or pulmonary artery hypertrophy and hypertension, and severe bullous emphysema. Pulmonary haemorrhage is also reported.

> **AUTHOR'S TIPS**
> - Consider cocaine toxicity in unexplained bullous emphysema or PAH.
> - If suspected crack lung, consider other adulterant lung toxicities e.g. talc lung.
> - Melanoptysis (carbon residue) and finger burns (from handling crack pipes) are suggestive.
> - Pulmonary embolic disease is a major differential.

Cannabis
Up to four times more tar content is inhaled because of different smoking technique, with no filter, greater inhalation depth and longer breath hold. In the short term, bronchodilation occurs that diminishes because of tachyphylaxis. Airflow obstruction can develop after 8 weeks.

Chronic lung toxicity includes a probable increased risk of lung cancer. The absolute excess risk is unknown and co-existing inhaled tobacco smoke may have a role. Bronchial epithelial metaplasia has been demonstrated in humans histologically.

Chronic cough, bronchitis, reduced exercise tolerance and reduced lung function occur. Smokers of 3–4 cannabis cigarettes daily have the same histological features as tobacco smokers of 20 cigarettes daily but this may reflect differences in smoking technique (discussed earlier). A probable increased risk of chronic obstructive pulmonary disease (often with co-existing large bullae) is though to occur.

Barotrauma including pneumomediastinum has been reported following Valsava manoeuvres and deep inhalation leading to alveolar rupture and dissection of air to the mediastinum. Aspergillus contamination of cannabis can lead to allergic bronchopulmonary aspergillosis (ABPA), or invasive aspergillosis following inhalation.

> **AUTHOR'S TIPS**
> - Unexplained large bullae with emphysema should prompt enquiry about cannabis (and cocaine).
> - Consider cannabis inhalation in ABPA and invasive aspergillosis.

> **AUTHOR'S TIPS**
> - A thorough drug and occupational history is mandatory.
> - A high index of suspicion is needed, check online: http://www.pneumotox.com/
> - Use online guidelines: http://www.brit-thoracic. org.uk/c2/uploads/antitnf.pdf
> - Stop the drug if possible.
> - Exclude infection and heart failure in particular.
> - If the patient fails to respond, reconsider the diagnosis.

Further reading
Albertson TE, Walby WF, Derlet RW. Stimulant-induced pulmonary toxicity. *Chest* 1995;**108**:1140–9.

Camus P, Fanton A, Bonniaud P, et al. Interstitial lung disease induced by drugs and radiation. *Respiration* 2004;**71**:301–326.

Camus P, Foucher P, Bonniaud P, et al. Drug-induced infiltrative lung disease. *ERJ* 2001;18:Suppl **32**:S93–100.

Costabel U, duBois RM, Egan JJ (eds). *Diffuse parenchymal lung disease.* Karger, 2007.

Foucher P, Biour M, Blayac JP, et al. Drugs that may injure the respiratory system. *ERJ* 1997;**10**:265–79.

Foucher P, Camus P, GEPPI (Groupe d'Etudes de la Pathologie Pulmonaire Iatrogene). The drug-induced lung diseases. Pneumotox online. http://www.pneumotox.com/

Gotway MB, Marder SR, Hanks DK, et al. Thoracic complications of illicit drug use: an organ system approach. *Radiographics* 2002;**22**: S119–35.

Haim DY, Lippmann ML, Goldberg SK, et al. The pulmonary complications of crack cocaine. A comprehensive review. *Chest* 1995;**107**:233–40.

Morelock SY, Sahn SA. Drugs and the pleura. *Chest* 1999; **116**:212–21.

Recommendations for assessing risk and for managing Mycobacterium tuberculosis infection and disease in patients due to start anti-TNF-α treatment. Joint Tuberculosis Committee of the British Thoracic Society. *Thorax* 2005; **60**: 800-805. http://www.brit-thoracic.org.uk/c2/ uploads/antitnf.pdf

Reed CR, Glauser FL. Drug-induced noncardiogenic pulmonary oedema. *Chest* 1991;**100**:1120–24.

Tashkin DP. Pulmonary complications of smoked substance abuse. *West J Med* 1990;**152**:525–30.

Whitcomb ME. Drug-induced lung disease. *Chest* 1973;**63**:418–22.

16.2 Pneumoconiosis

Pneumoconiosis is a term covering a group of dust-associated diseases of the lung. The main individual diseases are coal workers pneumoconiosis, silicosis and asbestosis.

Parkes suggests that pneumoconiosis may be defined as the non-neoplastic reaction of the lungs to inhaled mineral or organic dust and the resultant alteration in their structure but excluding asthma, bronchitis and emphysema.

This section will deal with pneumoconiosis caused by inorganic dusts only and will exclude asbestosis, which is dealt with elsewhere.

Epidemiology

With improved occupational hygiene and the decline of the coal mining industry pneumoconioses caused by inorganic dust exposure should become diseases of the past.

Fig. 16.2.1 shows the number of cases being compensated annually for pneumoconiosis other than asbestosis. Most cases occur in retired coal workers. A smaller number arise in quarry and foundry workers and in the potteries where silica was the main cause.

The recent increase in cases is probably due to more accurate recording and a publicity campaign in 2002. Death from pneumoconiosis is on a long-term downward trend.

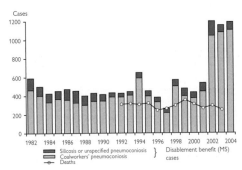

Fig. 16.2.1 Pneumoconiosis (other than asbestosis).

Diagnosis

The diagnosis of pneumoconiosis depends on three things:
- A high quality chest radiograph.
- A complete occupational history.
- Clinical examination.

The importance of a complete occupational history including every job since leaving school cannot be over emphasised, particularly as the relevant dust exposures are likely to have occurred many years ago.

Radiology

Pneumoconioses give rise to small round or irregular opacities on the CXR. In more severe cases of coal workers pneumoconiosis and silicosis large opacities can develop but these are not seen in asbestosis. Coal workers pneumoconiosis and silicosis give rise to predominantly round opacities situated in the middle and upper zones whereas asbestosis manifests with small irregular opacities at the lung bases.

The International Labour Office (ILO) Classification of Radiographs has been used to describe the profusion and type of radiographic opacity in pneumoconioses. The profusion of small opacities is categorised as follows:
- Category 1 indicates the presence of small opacities which are few in number.
- Category 2 indicates the presence of numerous small opacities but where the normal lung markings are still visible.
- Category 3 indicates very numerous small opacities which partially or totally obscure the normal lung markings.

The small opacities are usually rounded in coal workers pneumoconiosis and silicosis and are graded by size.
- 'p' describes opacities upto about 1.5mm.
- 'q' describes opacities between 1.5mm and 3mm.
- 'r' describes opacities between 3mm and 10mm.

Large opacities (see Fig. 16.2.2) are categorised as A, B or C as follows:
- Category A – an opacity with a greatest diameter between 1cm and 5cm or several opacities each greater than 1cm, the sum of whose greatest diameters does not exceed 5cm.
- Category B – one or more opacities larger than those in Category A whose combined area does not exceed the equivalent of the right upper zone.
- Category C – one or more opacities whose combined area exceeds the equivalent of the right upper zone.

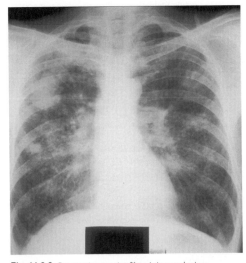

Fig. 16.2.2 Progressive massive fibrosis in a coal miner.

Small irregular opacities are designated 's', 't' and 'u'. Standard films are available to guide classification for epidemiological purposes.

Coal workers pneumoconiosis

This disease is caused by inhaling coal mine dust and its development is mainly dependent on the mass of respirable dust to which the miner has been exposed.

Pathology

Dust particles arriving in the alveoli are phagocytosed by macrophages and transported proximally to the respiratory bronchioles and the mucociliary escalator. When this system is overwhelmed dust laden macrophages accumulate near the centre of the secondary pulmonary lobule. Reticulin and later collagen are deposited in these macules giving rise to the discrete fibrotic lesions which constitute simple pneumoconiosis. In the case of coal workers pneumoconiosis collagen deposition is usually minimal.

Complicated pneumoconiosis or progressive massive fibrosis occurs when large opacities develop. These usually occur only in miners with well developed (category 2 or 3) simple pneumoconiosis. These lesions may cavitate.

Multiple well defined round opacities 0.5–5cm in diameter and distributed throughout the lung fields were observed by Caplan in miners with or who subsequently developed rheumatoid arthritis. The lesions tended to develop rapidly often against a background of minor simple pneumoconiosis and the lesions could cavitate. This pattern of disease is referred to as Caplan's syndrome.

Signs and symptoms

Simple coal workers pneumoconiosis does not give rise to any signs or symptoms. The early stages of complicated coal workers pneumoconiosis (Category A) is usually symptomless, but more advanced disease can lead to respiratory disability which may be severe.

Melanoptysis, the production of black sputum, can occur if an area of massive fibrosis cavitates. Coal dust can become incorporated into healing skin abrasions and thereby give rise to a form of tattooing. This is not particularly associated with pneumoconiosis but if observed should serve as a prompt for a full occupational history.

Lung function testing

Simple pneumoconiosis has little effect on lung function.

Complicated pneumoconiosis especially categories B and C lead to abnormalities of lung function which are poorly correlated with radiographic appearances. Decline may be found in FEV$_1$, and FVC often with an obstructive pattern. Total lung capacity and gas transfer are usually reduced.

Prognosis

Simple coal workers pneumoconiosis and Category A complicated pneumoconiosis do not shorten life.

Complicated coal workers pneumoconiosis of Categories B and C is associated with increased mortality mainly in association with airflow obstruction.

Differential diagnosis

Simple coal workers pneumoconiosis may be confused with:
- Sarcoidosis.
- Miliary tuberculosis.
- Extrinsic allergic alveolitis.

Complicated coal workers pneumoconiosis may be confused with:
- Lung cancer.
- Pulmonary metastases.
- Sarcoidosis.
- Tuberculosis.
- Wegener's granulomatosis.

Silicosis

Silicosis is probably the oldest pneumoconiosis to afflict man. Dusty trades have been associated with ill health since antiquity but silicosis should now be a disease of the past.

Silica exposure occurs in:
- Quarrying of slate, granite and sandstone.
- Hard rock mining.
- Tunnelling.
- Foundry work where silica was used in moulds and cores.
- Pottery and ceramic industries.

Occasional cases of silicosis are still reported often where workers have been exposed to silica by new industrial processes where the silica risk had not been appreciated.

Pathology

Silicosis is caused by inhaling crystalline silica dust. The prevalence and severity of disease is largely determined by the intensity of exposure.

Silica excites a more florid fibrotic reaction than coal mine dust. This leads to palpable nodules composed of concentric layers of fibrous tissue which may coalesce to produce massive fibrosis with associated distortion of lung architecture and scar emphysema.

Radiology

The nodules in silicosis tend to be denser and larger than those in coal workers pneumoconiosis and affect predominantly the upper lobes (see Fig. 16.2.3).

Eggshell calcification of hilar lymph nodes can occur.

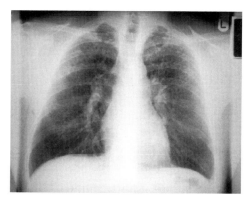

Fig. 16.2.3 Silicosis in a granite quarry worker.

Sings and symptoms

Early disease is usually symptomatic. Cough and breathlessness occur as the disease progresses and in severe cases respiratory failure may occur.

There are no signs that are specific to silicosis. Finger clubbing does not occur.

Lung function

Small reductions in vital capacity may occur in simple silicosis. As the disease advances there is a decrease in TLC, VC, RV, FRC and there may be evidence of airways obstruction.

Compilications

- Tuberculosis – silicosis predisposes to tuberculosis and in the past silicotuberculosis often lead to death.
- Environmental mycobacterial infection.
- Emphysema.
- Spontaneous pneumothorax.
- Cancer of the lung. Hard rock miners exposed to silica are often exposed to radon which is a known lung carcinogen but there is increasing concern that silica itself may be a lung carcinogen.

Prognosis

Uncomplicated silicosis does not usually shorten life but may do so if supervening tuberculosis is not diagnosed and treated promptly.

Complicated silicosis can lead to respiratory failure and thereby shorten life.

Differential diagnosis

- Sarcoidosis.
- Metastases.
- Lung cancer.
- Wegener's granulomatosis.

Acute silicosis (alveolar silico-lipoproteinosis)

Historically this disease was seen in sandblasters and was often rapidly fatal. Cases are still occasionally seen.

Exposure to very high concentrations of finely divided quartz can lead to a rapidly developing disease characterised by progressive breathlessness, malaise, fatigue and weight loss. Infection with tuberculosis or environmental mycobacteria commonly occurs.

The radiographic appearances vary from diffuse ground glass opacification to a mixture of coarse nodular opacities.

Mixed dust fibrosis

This disease occurs when the effects of silica are modified by accompanying non-fibrogenic dusts. It has been seen in haematite miners and in foundry workers. It gives rise to an irregular fibrotic upper lobe disease which radiographically resembles fibrocaseous tuberculosis. The lesions do not calcify nor is eggshell calcification seen.

Kaolinosis

Heavy exposure to kaolin (china clay) occurred in certain types of clay drying processes and could lead to a simple pneumoconiosis and very rarely to complicated pneumoconiosis. Simple pneumoconiosis cause by kaolin in the UK did not appear to cause symptoms or shorten life.

Talc

Talc has been used as a lubricant in the rubber industry and in roof felting.

Talc has a precise mineralogical definition but the term has been used loosely in industry. Commercial talc often contained impurities including significant amounts of quartz and asbestos minerals. It is unclear whether pure talc causes a pneumoconiosis but contaminated talc has given rise to pneumoconiosis with patterns similar to silicosis, asbestosis or combinations of the two diseases.

Further reading

International Labour Office (ILO) Guidelines for the use of the ILO International Classification of Radiographs of Pneumoconioses, Revised Edition 2000 (Occupational Safety and Health Series No22) International Labour Office: Geneva, 2002.

Parkes RW *Occupational Lung Disorders* 3rd edn. London: Butterworths, 1994.

16.3 Disability assessment

Respiratory disability is defined by the World Health Organization (WHO) as a reduction in exercise capacity secondary to impaired lung function. The social and occupational disadvantage resulting from disability is designated handicap. Assessment of respiratory disability requires information about lung function impairment and its effect on exercise performance. For clinical purposes exercise performance is usually assessed on the basis of the patient's account of symptoms. Various scales have been devised to standardise description of impairment of exercise tolerance in semi-quantitative terms. In the field of occupational lung disease disability assessment in quantitative terms is usually required for the purpose of financial compensation. The subject may therefore be motivated to exaggerate his disability. To deal with this problem attempts have been made to assess exercise capcity more objectively.

Assessment of symptoms

Various questionnaires and scales have been devised for the purpose of systematised semi-quantitative assessment of exercise tolerance impairment. A questionnaire devised by the Medical Research Council (MRC) has been modified a number of times. A currently used version is shown in Table 16.3.1.

Table 16.3.1 Medical Research Council Breathlessness Scale

Grade	Description
1	Breathless on strenuous exercise
2	Breathless hurrying on the level or up a slight hill
3	Breathless at a normal pace or has to stop after walking at own pace on the level
4	Has to stop after walking 100 yards or after a few minutes on the level
5	Too breathless to leave the home

The MRC scale is useful for clinical assessment of breathlessness and correlates with other measures of disability. Problems with using the MRC scale for more formal quantification of disability for the purpose of compensation for occupational lung disease is that it is based only upon subjective description of symptoms and the intervals are wide. A more detailed scale was devised by the authors of this chapter for assessing disability from COPD for the purposes of a compensation scheme for hundreds of thousands of UK coal miners. The scale is shown in Table 16.3.2.

This scale integrates information from a description of exercise performance with measures of static lung function. Where there is a discrepancy between the reported breathlessness and the lung function measurements more weight should be accorded to the objective evidence from the lung function tests. If reported breathlessness is greater than expected from the lung function measurements possible explanations include co-existing cardiac disease or other disorder such as anaemia contributing to breathlessness, or deliberate exaggeration.

Table 16.3.2 Coal Miners' Respiratory Disability Scale

Disability Score	Symptoms	Lung function impairment
0%	Not breathless on exercise	None
10%	Breathless on prolonged or heavy exertion	Mild
20%	Breathless on walking uphill or climbing stairs or on hurrying on level ground	Mild
40%	Breathless on walking 100 yards or climbing one flight of stairs at a normal pace	Moderate
50%	Breathless on walking 100 yards at a slow pace or climbing one flight of stairs at a slow pace	Moderate
60%	Breathlessness prevents walking 100 yards at a slow pace without stopping or climbing one flight of stairs without stopping	Severe
70%	Breathlessness prevents activity outside the home without assistance or supervision	Severe
80%	Breathlessness limits activities to within the home	Severe
90%	Able to walk only a few steps because of breathlessness	Severe
100%	Bed and chair bound, totally dependent on carers because of breathlessness	Severe

In the USA a different disability grading system is used which grades disability in four classes and then translates those into percentage 'impairment of total person' of up to 25%, up to 50% and up to 100% using American Medical Association criteria. This system has not been widely adopted in the UK.

Assessment of lung function

The coalminers' disability rating scale refers to impairment of lung function as mild, moderate or severe, as shown in Table 16.3.3.

Table 16.3.3 Rating of respiratory impairment

Grade	Criteria
None	FEV_1, FVC & DLCO $\geq$ 80% , FEV_1% $\geq$ 75%
Mild	FEV_1 or FVC or TLCO < 80% predicted or FEV_1/FVC < 70%
Moderate	FEV_1 or FVC or TLCO < 60% predicted or FEV_1/FVC < 60%
Severe	FEV_1 or TLCO < 40% predicted or FVC < 50% predicted or FEV_1/FVC < 50%

These grades are based on a slight modification of criteria formulated by the European Society for Clinical Respiratory

Physiology (SEPCR) and separately by the American Thoracic Society (ATS). They are arbitrary with no evidence base to confirm the validity of the boundaries between grades and hence they should be regarded as guidelines for assessment of disability rather than hard and fast rules. These grades are appropriate for persons with chronic stable lung function impairment.

Lung function test results are interpreted in relation to reference values, commonly but potentially misleadingly termed 'predicted values'. It is important to appreciate that these represent the mean values for persons of the same sex, age and height without known respiratory disease and are not actually 'predictive' of an individual's lung function. The 'normal range', statistically should be defined as the mean +/– 2 standard deviations (SD) to encompass 95% of the population. However, the concept of 'abnormally high' lung function is meaningless and so it is conventional to regard the upper 95th centile, defined by a value above the mean minus 1.64 SD as 'normal'. However, for convenience of calculation values $\geq$ 80% of the reference value are frequently taken as normal which gives a fair approximation. However the normal range is defined, a significant minority of healthy persons will have lung function 'below normal'. Conversely some patients with respiratory disease who have lost substantial lung function may have lung function which is still within the normal range. It is necessary to interpret the results in the context of clinical and radiological findings. For example FVC 85% of predicted is probably normal in a well man with normal exercise tolerance and a normal CXR whereas it is almost certainly abnormal in a man complaining of exertional breathlessness with interstitial shadowing on CXR.

Asthma

Since, by definition, asthma gives rise to respiratory function impairment which is variable over time it is necessary to take into account the pattern of impairment over a period in order to assess disability. A disability rating scheme for asthma has been devised by the ATS. A single set of 'normal' lung function test results does not necessarily imply that there is no disability due to asthma. Serial measurement of peak expiratory flow (PEF) three or more times daily is useful in assessing disability due to asthma. It is reasonable to take into account also treatment required to suppress symptoms and maintain lung function. For example, a person with normal PEF readings but who requires regular inhaled steroids and bronchodilator therapy may be regarded as mildly disabled whereas a person with the same PEF readings without any treatment would not be classed as disabled. A potential drawback of reliance on self-monitored peak flow readings is that an individual motivated to exaggerate his disability for the purposes of claiming compensation can easily fake low PEF readings unless an electronic recording peak flow meter which blinds the user to the results is available. A bronchial challenge with histamine or methacholine to measure bronchial hyper-reactivity can provide a more objective assessment of the activity of asthma. If a person complains of asthma symptoms but has normal resting lung function increased a finding of increased bronchial reactivity adds credibility to the clinical history. While normal bronchial reactivity does not exclude active asthma, it is rare to have disabling asthma with normal reactivity and normal lung function.

Exercise tests

Various types of exercise test have been devised to assist in assessment of disability. In healthy subjects exercise is limted mainly by the ability of the heart to deliver blood to muscles but in persons with respiratory impairment the ability of the lungs to deliver oxygen to the blood becomes the exercise limiting factor.

One of the simplest standardised exercise tests is the six minute walk. The subject is instructed to walk as far and as fast as he can along a measured route, such as a hospital corridor, in a period of 6 minutes. Additional information may be gained by assessing self-reported breathlessness and oxygen saturation before and at the end of exercise.

Another simple test is the shuttle walk in which the patient walks back and forth between two markers 10m apart at gradually increasing speed, paced by an audible signal until unable to keep up when the test is terminated. Inability to complete 25 shuttles suggested a maximal oxygen uptake (VO_{2max}) of < 10ml/kg/min.

Walking tests require motivation to cooperate which may be lacking in the context of assessment of disability for compensation. These simple exercise tests do not provide information as to the cause of reduced exercise capacity.

More information can be obtained from a progressive exercise test performed on a treadmill or cycle ergometer. A treadmill provides more familiar and relevant exercise for most patients with respiratory disease but a cycle is more logistically convenient in that the patient is stationary. Minute ventilation, oxygen consumption, heart rate, blood pressure and the electrocardiogram are monitored continuously. Results are compared with reference values. In a maximal exercise test the subject is asked to exercise until he cannot continue. Many patients cannot complete a maximal exercise test to the point at which their exercise capcity is limited by respiratory capacity because their ability to exercise is limited by non-respiratory factors such as arthritis, angina or simple fatigue. A sub-maximal test in which the subject exercises up to a pre-determined limit of oxygen consumption, commonly 45mmol min^{-1}, can be completed by more patients. From the measured ventilation at this oxygen uptake an equation can be used to estimate VO_{2max} with reasonable precision.

A disability rating scale based upon the results of maximal exercise testing has been devised by the SEPCR. Disability was assessed on a linear scale between zero, defined as a maximal oxygen uptake at or above the lower limit of the normal range, defined as (reference value – 1.64 residual SD) and 100% disability, defined as inability to achieve an oxygen uptake more than twice that at rest. Disability thus assessed correlates poorly with breathlessness and in practice disability is seldom assessed in this way in the UK. In the USA, however, the Social Security Administration requires some measure of exercise capacity in assessing disability for compensation purposes.

Lung function and disability

The relation between lung function impairment and consequent disability is highly variable. It depends upon the degree of exercise to which the individual was accustomed before respiratory impairment developed. There is a substantial reserve of respiratory function which is called upon only on strenuous physical exertion and people who do not engage in such exertion may lose 10–20% of their lung function without noticing breathlessness; they would not have any respiratory disability consequent upon the loss of lung function. The same lung function loss could cause significant disability to a person enjoying strenuous sports or in employment involving heavy manual labour.

Psychological factors also play an important part in determining disability. Mood affects the perception of breathlessness and attitude towards living with disability itself partly determines disability and contributes importantly to variation in reported breathlessness and in exercise performance associated with any given degree of lung function impairment. This phenomenon is separate from that of exaggeration of symptoms for the purpose of compensation which also may occur.

Co-existing impairments also affect the extent to which lung function impairment will cause disability. A person with sufficient lung function impairment to cause 30% disability if he were otherwise well may in fact have no respiratory disability if he also has a neurological disorder which renders him incapable of walking. Conversely, a person who was already breathless on minor exertion as a result of heart disease may suffer a significant increase in disablement from modest loss of lung function which would not have caused disability on its own if he had not had heart disease. Hence, while standardised scales relating lung function impairment to disability provide a useful framework it is important to take into account individual circumstances in assessing disability.

Further reading

American Medical Association. *Guidelines to the Evaluation of Permanent Impairment* 5th edn. Chicago 2001.

American Thoracic Society, Medical Section of the American Lung Association. Evaluation of impairment/disability secondary to respiratory disease. *Am Rev Respir Dis* 1986; **133**:1205–1209.

American Thoracic Society. Guidelines for the evaluation of impairment/disability in patients with asthma. *Am Rev Respir Dis* 1993; **147**: 956–1061.

Bestall JC, Paul EA, Garrod R, et al. Usefulness of the Medical Research Council (MRC) dyspnoea scale as a measure of disability in patients with chronic obstructive pulmonary disease. *Thorax* 1999; **54** 581–586.

Butland RJ, Pang J, Gross ER, et al. Two-, six-, and 12-minute walking tests in respiratory disease. *Br Med J (Clin Res Ed)* 1982; **284**: 1607–8.

Cotes JE. Rating respiratory disability: a report on behalf of a working group of the European Society for Clinical Respiratory Physiolo. Eur Respir J. 1990;**3**:1074–7.

Cotes JE, Chinn DJ, Reed JW, et al. Experience of a standardised method for assessing respiratory disability. *Eur Respir J* 1994; **7**: 875-880.

De Coster A. Respiratory impairment and disablement. *Bull Eur Physiopathol Respir* 1983; **19**: 1–3P.

Jones NL, Makrides L, Hitchcock C, et al. Normal standards for an incremental progressive cycle ergometer test. *Am Rev Respir Dis* 1985; **131**: 700–708.

King B, Cotes JE. Relation of lung function and exercise capacity to mood and attitudes to health. *Thorax* 1989; **44**: 402–409.

Revill SM, Morgan MD, Singh SJ, et al. The endurance shuttle walk: a new field test for the assessment of endurance capacity in chronic obstructive pulmonary disease. *Thorax* 1999; **54**: 213–222.

Weller JJ, el-Gamal FM, Parker L, et al. Indirect estimation of maximal oxygen uptake for study of working populations. *Br J Ind Med* 1988; **45**: 532–537.

World Health Organization. *International classification of impairments, disabilities and handicaps.* Geneva: WHO, 1980.

16.4 Occupational asthma

Occupational asthma is now the commonest occupational lung disease in westernised countries, it often affects people at the height of their working lives and may affect you. There are few diseases where it is so easy to do so much harm. Unsubstantiated diagnoses are as common as missed diagnoses. Advice to leave a job frequently leaves your patient unemployed and similar affected workers unprotected. There are now evidenced based guidelines and a BTS endorsed standard of care; they will form the backbone of this chapter.

Definition

The definition of occupational asthma is surprisingly difficult and a little controversial. Work-related asthma is asthma which deteriorates following work exposures and improves when away. If the worker has pre-existing asthma and the deterioration occurs with the first significant exposure the mechanism is likely to be irritant and the disease called work aggravated asthma. Examples would include asthmatics working in a cold store or in workplaces with significant sulphur dioxide exposure.

A single large exposure to an irritant can induce asthma for the first time, which may persist for months, or perhaps for ever, without sensitisation. This is usually called acute irritant induced (or toxic) asthma. After the acute exposure the worker should be able to work with low levels of the offending substance in the same way as a pre-existing asthmatic, so a job change is usually not needed. Chlorine exposure is the most commonly recognised cause.

Allergic occupational asthma is characterised by a latency period between first exposure to a respiratory sensitiser at work and the development of symptoms. Once sensitisation has occurred levels of exposure below those that were tolerated before cause deterioration. It can occur de novo or in those with pre-existing asthma, when a new sensitisation occurs, for instance a doctor with pre-existing asthma may develop latex sensitivity and be unable to tolerate the background latex exposures that are present in hospitals where latex gloves are used. Allergic occupational asthma is usually divided into high molecular weight (when specific IgE is usually found) and low molecular weight, (where an IgE mechanism is usually not evident).

How common is occupational asthma?

Occupational asthma accounts for about 15% of asthma in adults of working age, the great majority of which is allergic occupational asthma. The proportion of asthma attributable to work has been increasing over the last 30 years, newer estimates may be greater than this. If you think of the other causes of adult asthma this is not so surprising, as most asthma is allergic and occurs relatively soon after first exposure to the sensitising agent, which usually occurs in childhood. New exposures in adulthood are usually encountered at work. Other causes would include salicylates, drugs such as beta blockers, and acute airway insults from infection. The Health and Safety Executive (HSE) estimate that 1500–3000 people develop occupational asthma in the UK each year. This rises to 7000 cases a year if work-aggravated asthma is included. HSE estimates that the costs to society of new cases of occupational asthma are up to £1.1bn over 10 years.

What are the causes of occupational asthma?

Occupational asthma is nearly always due to something inhaled at work, occupational asthma tends to occur in clusters, it is often easier to start with the job, the most commonly identified include:

- paint sprayers and painters;
- bakers, pastry makers and food processors;
- nurses, dental workers and laboratory technicians;
- chemical, plastic and rubber workers;
- animal handlers and farm workers;
- welders and metal workers;
- timber and forestry workers;
- electrical and electronic production workers;
- textile workers;
- storage workers;
- waiters and cleaners.

In some of these the precise cause has been hard to pin down, the commonest identified agents include:

- isocyanates;
- flour and grain dust;
- colophony and fluxes;
- latex;
- animals;
- aldehydes;
- wood dust.

There are however more than 400 documented agents causing occupational asthma, finding the precise cause often needs specialist referral.

Diagnosis

> **AUTHOR'S TIPS**
>
> - Every worker with asthma or COPD should be asked whether their symptoms improve on days away from work or on holiday. Those who say yes to either should be investigated for occupational asthma.
> - You must decide whether you have the resources and knowledge to investigate and manage your patient yourself, or whether you would be advised to share care with a specialist in occupational lung diseases (as recommended in guidelines). You should start serial PEF measurements as soon as possible, whether you are going to manage the patient alone or are seeking help from a specialist.

The diagnosis of occupational asthma is compounded by pre-conceived beliefs of what is asthma. Occupational asthma is more commonly identified in the older smoking worker, who often have an initial label of COPD. Bronchodilator response, diurnal variation in PEF >20% and non-specific reactivity may all be within normal limits in workers with occupational asthma. Respiratory symptoms improving on days away from work or on holiday are the most sensitive screening questions, occupational asthma can be confirmed in a little over half of positive responders. A clinical history alone is insufficient to remove a worker from exposure. Workers denying respiratory symptoms may sometimes be identified from accelerated FEV_1 decline found during surveillance medicals.

The tests available are:

1 Specific IgE or skin prick tests.
2 Non-specific responsiveness at and away from work.
3 Serial measurements of PEF (or FEV_1).
4 Specific inhalation challenge tests.
5 Workplace challenge.

The production of specific IgE antibody may be detected by skin prick or serological tests. Testing is more helpful is defining the cause than the presence or absence of occupational asthma. The respective sensitivities and specificities of the ability of these tests to detect specific IgE vary between allergens but in any case are dependent on the specific content of the allergen extract and the setting of positive cut-offs. Blood testing for specific serum IgE may not be as sensitive as skin prick testing. The presence of specific IgE confirms sensitisation to an agent at work, but alone does not confirm the presence of occupational asthma. Testing is worthwhile for high molecular weight agents particularly enzymes (food and detergents), latex, rat and mouse urinary antigens, arthropods, flour, shellfish and fish. There is a high false-positive rate but few false-negatives. Some of those with positive tests may have occupational rhinitis, which may precede occupational asthma. Skin prick testing is useful for selected low molecular weight antigens including the ammonium hexachlorplatinate (platinum refiners), reactive dyes and acid anhydrides.

	Sensitivity	Specificity
Skin prick tests or specific IgE	Variable <100%	Often around 30%
3.2 × change in non-specific reactivity away from work	48%	64%
ΔPEF >44l/min pre/post shift	21%	77%
Serial PEF ≥4/day and ≥3 weeks	78%	92%
Serial PEF <4/day or <3 weeks	64%	83%
Specific challenge test	Unknown but <100%	Unknown but <100%

Sensitivity and specificity of diagnostic tests for occupational asthma

Non-specific reactivity as measured with methacholine or histamine is not sufficiently sensitive on its own to exclude occupational asthma (sensitivity 70-95% in different studies). The between visit variability in stable asthmatics has a 95% CI of around 3.2-fold. Changes greater than this after 2 weeks away from work have a sensitivity for the diagnosis of occupational asthma of <50%. Testing is useful but not sufficiently sensitive or specific on its own.

Serial measurements of PEF are the most appropriate first step in the physiological confirmation of occupational asthma and should be started at the earliest opportunity by the first clinician suspecting occupational asthma. The concept is simple but the precision is in the detail. Usual practice is to ask for approximately 2-hourly reading from waking to bedtime, with treatment kept constant on work and rest days, and times of starting and stopping work and waking and sleeping recorded each day. Suitable record forms and instructions can be downloaded from http://www.occupationalasthma.com/workers.aspx. The interpretation of the recordings is much easier if plotted as

daily maximum, mean and minimum with each 'day' starting with the first reading at work and finishing with the last reading before work on the next day, as shown in the Figs. 16.4.1 and 16.4.2. The computer plotter Oasys is a convenient tool for plotting and analysing serial PEF measurements and has the highest sensitivity and specificity of any diagnostic test for occupational asthma which has external validation. A positive record confirms occupational asthma but does not define the cause.

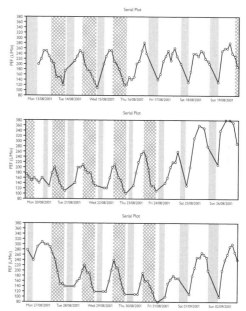

Fig. 16.4.1 A 40-year-old smoking nurse presented with increasing asthma and time off work. She had had quite bad asthma from the age of 6 which had remitted in her teens. She was better on days away from work, and better when working night shifts when she would use less latex gloves than on dayshifts. She was asked to keep 2-hourly measurements of peak flow from waking to sleeping, a sequential plot of the record is shown here figure. Shifts working at night are cross-hatched, periods sleeping are shaded. Her peak flow drops over night shifts and over night when away from work.

Asthmatics have a diurnal variation in peak flow which is usually lowest at the end of sleeping. As she works at night, the spontaneous diurnal variation might confound the record. Fig. 16.4.3 shows the same data plotted as the mean value from waking, separately for nightshifts and days away from work. The record shows similar waking values which increase after waking, but start to fall 8 hours after working on nightshifts. The bottom panel shows the time, the number of readings from which each datapoint is derived (blue days away from work, red work days, a minimum of 3 readings per datapoint required). The plot confirms that the night shift deterioration is not due to spontaneous diurnal variation.

AUTHOR'S TIP

If you suspect occupational asthma start a 2-hourly record of PEF using published guidelines

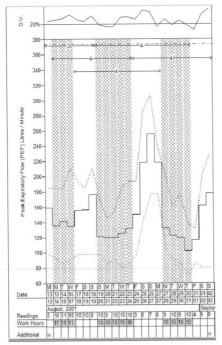

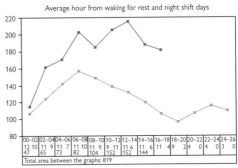

Average hour from waking for rest and night shift days

Total area between the graphs: 819

Hours from waking, number of readings and areas (night shifts) (rest)

Fig. 16.4.3

Fig. 16.4.2 Shows the same data as Fig. 16.4.1 plotted as the daily maximum, mean and minimum by the oasys plotter. The upper panel shows the daily diurnal variation in peak flow. The middle panel shows the predicted peak flow (the black dotted line at the top of the record), an assessment of the likelihood of each complex showing occupational asthma (4 definitely yes to 1 definitely no); below this the daily maximum (blue dotted), mean (black bars) and minimum (red dotted) peak flow. Nightshifts are cross-hatched, days away from work have a clear background. The bottom panel shows the date, the number of readings made per day and the number of hours worked. The deterioration on workdays in much more obvious on this plot.

Specific inhalation tests are the gold standard for diagnosing occupational asthma, and are standard practice in some countries with good resources for occupational lung disease (such as Finland, Belgium and Quebec). Occupational type bronchial provocation testing should not be attempted outside specialist centres. Control exposures with monitoring for 24 hours after exposure should always be done first. Exposures to specific occupational agents should start with exposures well below those at work and increase on subsequent days if no reactions have occurred. Measuring non-specific reactivity before and after exposure may help in the interpretation of borderline reactions. The resources for occupational type provocation testing are very limited in the UK. In practice a patient coming from a workplace with exposure to a well-identified antigen and a positive PEF record is sufficient for clinical purposes; examples would include a laboratory rat handler with a positive skin prick test to rat urinary antigen or a polyurethane moulder from a workplace with isocyanate exposure where others have previously developed occupational asthma. Specific challenge tests are underused in the UK by international standards and are particularly valuable when a worker is exposed to more than one possible cause, or the workplace has not had previous cases of occupational asthma.

Our nurse whose records are shown in Figs. 16.4.1–16.4.3 had specific challenge tests as her ward used powder-free latex gloves which her employer thought had removed the risk of latex allergy, also a domestic had developed occupational asthma on the ward from a cleaning agent (benzalkonium chloride) introduced to reduce the risks of cross infection. The results are shown in Fig. 16.4.4. The challenge clearly shows an immediate asthmatic reaction induced by donning and removing latex gloves, with no reaction following the use of nitrile gloves on another day. Her employer then knew what to remove from the work environment.

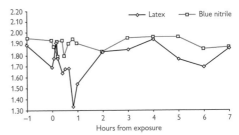

Fig. 16.4.4 Serial measurements of FEV$_1$ after donning blue nitrile gloves on a control day and latex gloves on the next day showing an immediate asthmatic reaction with an equivocal late fall in FEV$_1$ at 6 hours post exposure.

Workplace challenges can be done when laboratory challenges are impractical, for instance when the required heat is very high or the process too dangerous to reproduce in a hospital laboratory. There are no externally validated standards for assessing a response, they should not be attempted by non-experts. The principal is to establish a baseline for FEV$_1$ or PEF away from exposure, usually with hourly measurements over some days, then to accompany your patient to their workplace to be exposed to the putative agents while you monitor their response. You need to be able to cope with an acute asthmatic attack often in places without healthcare resources. Many employers are unhappy about allowing access for this kind of test, which is little more than a supervised longitudinal recording of PEF.

AUTHOR'S TIP
Never advise a patient with occupational asthma to leave their job unless you do not think they are fit to ever work again; advise their employer to remove them from exposure to the identified cause.

Management after a confirmed diagnosis

The aims of management are

- To remove the worker from the cause of their occupational asthma.
- To maintain their worthwhile employment.
- To advise about compensation.
- To prevent others from developing occupational asthma from the same workplace.
- To revise the risk assessment.
- (To preserve the viability of the workplace from which your patient came).

The next steps depend on the social, occupational and political system under which you work. In many countries all workers have access to an occupational health service, in the UK this is a minority. In theory the great majority of workers developing occupational asthma in the UK should have been under regular medical surveillance, following a risk assessment identifying exposure to a respiratory sensitiser. In practice many are not, for instance health-care workers in workplaces using latex gloves should be under surveillance (MS25), but few are. When surveillance is carried out, it is frequently contracted to companies whose contracts include only the questionnaires and lung function required for surveillance, rather than any responsibility for surveillance failures. In some countries (for instance, Germany) the treating physician has the responsibility for completing the notification and compensation assessments; in the UK the employer has the responsibility for notification (under the RIDDOR regulations) while the worker has the responsibility for seeking compensation which is decided by non-medical adjudicators. For all action is required in the workplace which is outside the brief of most treating physicians. Unless the worker has been referred from the workplace to you, you require your patients consent to communicate with the workplace, this is not always given.

AUTHOR'S TIPS

- Obtain the consent of your patient before communication with the employer or health and safety executive
- Once you have confirmed the diagnosis of occupational asthma you should inform your patient in writing of the diagnosis. In the UK the "date of knowledge" has legal significance as any common law claims should be made within three years of this date. The letter that I write is shown below.

Dear

I have told you today that in my opinion you have occupational asthma caused by .... You should no longer be exposed to this for the best outcome for your asthma. If you continue exposure you are likely to have worse asthma in the long term. You can claim for compensation from the Department of Works and Pensions using the forms I have given you. If you wish to make a common law claim you should do this within three years of knowing the diagnosis.

There is good evidence that early removal from exposure to the causative agent results in a greater chance of cure and less severe asthma in the remainder. Factors leading to a poor prognosis are the interval between the first work-related symptom and removal from exposure, the severity of asthma at the time of diagnosis and the interval between first exposure and first symptom (the shorter the better). I never advise the worker to leave their job, if you do your patient is likely to be unemployed, often for a long time (about one-third up to 6 years), and be poorer and less healthy because of poverty. No action is likely to happen in the workplace to prevent further cases as the workplace has no requirement to notify a diagnosis of occupational asthma in past employees (at least in the UK). My advice to the worker is to be removed from the causative agent; this requires the cooperation of the employer who will need to know of the diagnosis. It is then up to the employer to remove the cause or find suitable alternative employment. This is not always possible, in which case the worker will be dismissed or retired on medical grounds, allowing immediate social support and sometimes an enhanced pension. Once the employer is told of the diagnosis, in the UK it is his responsibility to notify the disease under the RIDDOR scheme, which usually results in a visit from the factory inspectorate.

Some workers are (rightly) concerned that communication with their employer will result in their dismissal. At least in the UK an employer has the right to dismiss a worker who is unable to do a particular job, which may be the situation in a worker with occupational asthma. In this case I reiterate the advice in the letter that continuing exposure to the cause is likely to lead to further loss of lung function and a worse prognosis in the long-term, and advise regular surveillance by myself or a clinician sharing care. Despite this general advice there are a minority of workers with occupational asthma who appear to tolerate further exposure without at least accelerated deterioration in FEV_1, however at present we have no method of identifying them at diagnosis.

Improvement can continue for at least 2 years after removal from exposure, and improvement in non-specific responsiveness sometimes for longer than this. Most agree than any assessment of residual disability should wait until removal from exposure for 2 years.

Prevention

Occupational asthma is more likely when exposure levels are higher and when the asthmagen is more potent. Some substances can cause occupational asthma in more than 50% of exposed workers, examples include castor beans in animal feed mills and platinum salts in platinum refiners. Catalytic car exhausts contain platinum, by substituting ammonium hexachlorplatinate with tetraamine platinum dichloride occupational asthma was prevented in those making the catalyst. In the health-care sector the substitution of use of 'powder-free' latex gloves has substantially reduced the incidence of latex allergy, which is further reduced by the substitution of latex with nitrile gloves allowing latex sensitive workers to work in a latex-free (at least in the air) environment. The removal of glutaraldehyde has prevented much asthma in endoscopy departments, however biocides themselves are a group of chemicals with sensitising properties, perhaps by their ability to denature protein. Biocides are responsible for at least some of the occupational asthma in cleaners and health care workers. Floors and surfaces are often sprayed with cleaning agents which contain potent biocides such as benzalkonium chloride and isothiozolinone.

Surveillance

Workers exposed to respiratory sensitising agents where there is a risk of occupational asthma should be under regular surveillance, usually with a sensitive (but non-specific) questionnaire and regular spirometry. This is the job of occupational health departments, but you may be asked to see surveillance failures. Investigation with serial measurements of peak flow is usually the first step in the confirmation or exclusion of occupational asthma.

Further reading

A comprehensive reference list on occupational asthma is available on www.occupationalasthma.com (under references). The evidence-based guidelines below are available in full on this website (Bohrf section). Help and forms for carrying out serial measurements of peak flow are in the workers section.

AsmaPro is an online occupational asthma database that can be searched by causative agent and job description. There is full and detailed information given on jobs, causative agents, substances, incidence, conditions, symptoms, methods of diagnosis, references and papers / abstracts.

http://www.remcomp.com/asmanet/asmapro/asma-work.htm

Occupational asthma hazard prediction program: an online program to predict the occupational asthma risk from any given chemical structure. This page contains links to the program and tools to help create the molfiles that the program uses.

http://www.medicine.manchester.ac.uk/coeh/research/asthma/

Burge PS, Pantin CFA, Newton DT, *et al*; and the Midlands Thoracic Society Research Group, Development of an expert system for the interpretation of serial peak expiratory flow measurements in the diagnosis of occupational asthma, *Occup Environ Med*. 1999; **56**: 758–764.

Haz-Map, A Relational Database of Hazardous Chemicals and Occupational Diseases EditHaz-Map® is an occupational toxicology database designed for physicians, physician assistants, occupational health nurses, and industrial hygienists to assist them in the recognition of diseases caused by toxic chemicals. Haz-Map links jobs to hazardous job tasks which are linked to occupational diseases and their symptoms.

http://hazmap.nlm.nih.gov

Medical aspects of occupational asthma, MS25, HSE Books London: 1998.

Nicholson PJ, Cullinan P, Newman Taylor AJ, *et al*. Evidence based guidelines for the prevention, identification, and management of occupational asthma, *Occup Environ Med*. 2005; **62**: 290–299.

16.5 The effects of high altitude on the lung

Introduction

More than 140 million people on this planet live at altitudes of above 2500m and many others travel to high altitude on expeditions and on holiday. It is estimated, for example, that more than 30,000 Britons travel to Nepal where they will experience altitudes of up to 5500m (Everest base camp). The lung takes the brunt of high altitude exposure. The lung is directly exposed to the external environment (just like the skin), but, unlike the skin, its function can become severely compromised by the environmental assault placed upon it. In this chapter I discuss the high altitude environment, discuss how this effects lung function (ventilation, gas exchange and the pulmonary circulation), describe the particular syndromes peculiar to high altitude (acute mountain sickness, high altitude pulmonary oedema and high altitude cerebral oedema), and consider how high altitude effects those with lung diseases wishing to travel to the higher regions of the planet or even to travel on a commercial aircraft.

The high altitude environment

The principle problem for humans travelling to high altitude is hypoxia. The fraction of oxygen in the air remains unchanged at 20.9% but, as we ascend, the atmospheric pressure falls and with it the partial pressure of oxygen. As a rule of thumb the atmospheric pressure is one-half of normal at 5500m, thus the partial pressure of oxygen is also one half of normal at that altitude. On the summit of Everest the atmospheric pressure is only one-third normal and, until recently, it was thought to be impossible that man could climb to that altitude without oxygen. In fact, Rheinhold Meissner and Peter Habeler did climb Everest without oxygen in 1978 and, since then, over 50 climbers have made it to the summit without the addition of bottled oxygen. These heroic physiological feats are rare however, and possible only for perfectly acclimatised supermen. The reason why some people can cope with this extraordinary altitude and other cannot remains unclear, but it is likely to be due to individual physiological susceptibility as a consequence of genetic adaptation. Not surprisingly, most people choose to live and work at lower altitudes, the highest place where people live continuously in North America is Leadville Colorado (3094m). The highest place in the world where people live and work continuously is Chacaltaya, Bolivia at 5300m, but only one population has lived for thousands of years at high altitude and that is the population living on the Tibetan plateau (approx. 3650m). The Tibetans have clearly adapted physiologically because the Tibetans, compared to lowlanders, maintain higher arterial oxygen saturation at rest and during exercise, and lose less aerobic performance with increasing altitude. This may be in part because they have larger lungs with better lung function and greater lung diffusion capacity than lowlanders. Furthermore, they only develop minimal hypoxic pulmonary hypertension and have higher levels of exhaled nitric oxide than lowlanders or Andeans.

The two other main environmental problems associated with high altitude are cold and dehydration (see Fig. 16.5.1). The fall in temperature is a feature of ascent; dehydration occurs partly because of the decreasing humidity of the air which falls to zero when the air temperature is below zero and also the decreased availability of water. For example, on the summit of Mount Everest temperatures can fall to minus 70°C. The only available water is melted ice and the insensible loss of water due to respiration can be huge because all the inspired gas must be warmed and humidified to body values. It is recommended that climbers drink at least 3 litres a day at altitudes above 4000m.

- **Cold**: T falls by 6.5° per 1000m

- **Hypobaric hypoxia**: PiO_2 falls by 13mmHg per 1000m

- **Dehydration**: humidity falls, insensible losses increase, water more difficult to obtain

---

Fig. 16.5.1 Environmental changes in temperature, humidity and inspired PO_2 at altitude.

AUTHOR'S TIPS
- Effects of altitude include hypoxia, dehydration and cold.
- Climbers can loose large amounts of fluid through insensible mechanisms such as respiration.

The effects of high altitude on the normal lung

Ventilation

Ventilation is controlled by the hypercapnic response (HCVR) and the hypoxic response (HVR). At sea level our breathing is controlled by our PCO_2 levels and PCO_2 is held at about 5kPa. The hypercapnic response is linear. In contrast the hypoxic ventilatory response is S shaped to PaO_2 (though linear to SaO_2) and no real increase in ventilation is seen until the inspired PO_2 falls below 12kPa (approx. 3000m). At altitude, there is competition between the two control mechanisms because, as hypoxia drives ventilation there is an increase in alveolar ventilation with fall in $PaCO_2$, and hence $PaCO_2$, which diminishes the hypercapnic response.

Hypoxic ventilatory response and mountain performance

Since gas exchange depends to a large extent on ventilation there have been many investigations into the hypoxic ventilatory response of successful versus unsuccessful climbers and successful high altitude people versus those that live at sea level. One of the greatest sociological experiments was the 1948 invasion of Tibet by lowland Chinese (Han people). Studies since that time have shown that the Han are much less able to cope with altitude than the native Tibetans. However, the Tibetans do not appear to have a brisker hypoxic ventilatory response. Likewise high altitude climbers do not necessarily have a better HVR than those who are less successful at altitude, in particular Peter Habeler has a normal HVR and so do many successful 8000m climbers. Ventilatory control is also important at night, during sleep. Naturally the oxygen saturations fall slightly during sleep due to suppressed ventilation and it is thought that loss of ventilatory control leads to the characteristic Cheyne–Stokes (periodic) type of breathing seen at altitude. (Fig. 16.5.2) It is likely that hypoxia during sleep is a significant cause of altitude illness and prevention of this by the use of the carbonic anhydrase inhibitor Acetazolamide may be a reason why people taking this drug are less susceptible to acute mountain sickness.

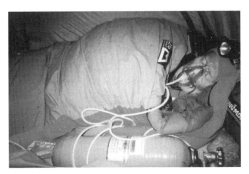

Fig. 16.5.2 Mountaineer sleeping on oxygen at camp 3 (7600m) on Mt Everest.

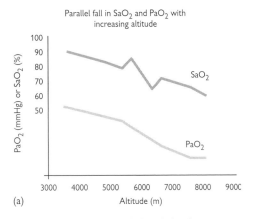

(a)

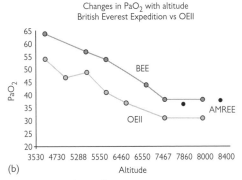

(b)

Figs. 16.5.4a and 16.5.4b: Comparison of British Everest Expedition (BEE) results with Operation Everest II (OEII).

Gas exchange

Once the oxygen is into the lung then it must be exchanged for CO_2 across the alveolar-capillary barrier. At sea level the gas exchange occurs one third the way along the capillary and the amount of gas exchanged depends entirely on the pulmonary flow rate (perfusion limitation). At altitude because of the lower PO_2 gradient across the alveolar-capillary membrane and also because of the higher flow rates due to higher cardiac output the exchange of gases may be incomplete by the end of the capillary and there is relative hypoxemia due to the high venous admixture. This is called diffusion limitation and is less severe in animals and man who have lived at high altitude for many generations. Interestingly, gas exchange appears to better on the mountain than in simulated high altitude chambers (see Fig. 16.5.3 (a and b) and Fig. 16.5.4). Experiments by both British and American teams have shown approximately a 1kPa (7.5mm Hg) difference in alveolar PO_2 between chamber and field values at various altitudes up to and including the South Col of Everest (8000m). The American project (Operation Everest II) was performed using a hypobaric chamber in contrast to the actual ascent of Everest by the British team. The reasons for the better performance on the mountain than in a hypoxic chamber are unknown.

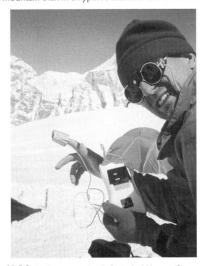

Fig. 16.5.3 Author measuring SaO_2 in the Western Cym.

Pulmonary circulation

Unlike the systemic circulation the pulmonary vasculature constricts to hypoxia (hypoxic pulmonary vasoconstriction; HPV) This reflex is present in all animals including man and birds so far studied. The purpose of HPV is two-fold: to keep the pulmonary circulation closed during gestation and also to promote matching of perfusion to ventilation when there is obstruction to ventilation such as inhaled foreign body or local lung disease. Unfortunately for normal people going to altitude this reflex is malign because there is global hypoxia and hence pulmonary vasoconstriction leading to pulmonary hypertension. The extent of hypoxic pulmonary vasoconstriction varies between individuals but, especially, between populations who are sea dwellers and populations who live at high altitude (e.g. Tibetans). It is highly likely that variation in the hypoxic pulmonary vasoconstrictive response to hypoxia is an important feature of long term acclimatisation to high altitude; for example the Yak, the Lhama and the Bar-headed Goose all have diminished hypoxic pulmonary vasoconstrictive responses yet function very well at altitude. (Fig. 16.5.5)

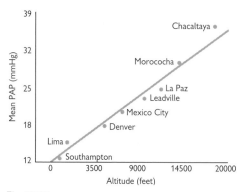

Fig. 16.5.5

AUTHOR'S TIPS

- At altitude ventilation is also controlled by hypoxia compared to control by $PaCO_2$ at sea level
- Cheyne–Stokes breathing occurs in sleep at altitude and can exacerbate hypoxia. This contributes to altitude related illness.
- Gas exchange at altitude can be diffusion limited.
- Hypoxic pulmonary vasoconstriction is a protective mechanism during gestation and in pulmonary disease in an attempt to maximise ventilation-perfusion matching. At altitude it can result in global vasoconstriction and elevated pulmonary vascular pressures.

Diseases specifically related to altitude

Acute mountain sickness

Acute mountain sickness is a syndrome comprising headache, dizziness, dyspnoea, drowsiness, poor appetite and is often associated with nausea and poor sleep related to the Cheyne–Stokes breathing as described above. Acute mountain sickness is a relatively benign condition providing there is appropriate treatment and no further ascent occurs until the symptoms subside. If these warning signs are ignored it can go on to develop into full blown high altitude cerebral oedema, with potentially fatal consequences. Severity of AMS is routinely assessed using the Lake Louise score. It can be prevented in many people by the use of the carbonic anhydrase inhibitor acetazolamide at a dose of 125–250mg BD. Acetazolamide is thought to work by acidifying the CSF and thus driving breathing.

High altitude cerebral oedema

This is a much more serious complication of hypoxia. Symptoms are headache, poor cerebral function, hallucinations, psychotic symptoms and ataxia. To the outside observer there is obvious poor decision making, the presence of ataxia and commonly there are retinal haemorrhages. The treatment is dexamethasone 8mg IV or IM then 4mg 6-hourly and descent.

High altitude pulmonary oedema

This enigmatic condition is due to the leak of high protein oedema fluid into the alveoli with consequent loss of gas exchange. This condition is difficult to distinguish from pneumonia, heart failure and other pulmonary conditions

(Fig. 16.5.6) and indeed was thought to be due to these conditions until 1960 when the first formal description was made of a skier in Aspen and Colorado who suffered a sudden onset of breathlessness which responded very quickly to decent. High altitude pulmonary oedema is always preceded by hypoxic pulmonary vasoconstriction with high pulmonary artery pressures and it is likely that the aetiology is related to this pulmonary hypertension. Other important factors may be alveolar capillary damage and loss of endothelial integrity. Symptoms are: breathlessness, orthopnoea, cough with haemoptysis, and chest discomfort. The principal sign is the presence of basal crackles. It is not surprising that the condition had previously been thought to be due to either chest infection or left heart failure. The treatment is oxygen, dexamethasone and the oral calcium-channel blocker nifedipine with emergency descent.

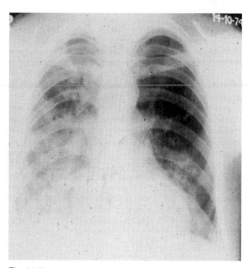

Fig. 16.5.6 CXR appearances of high altitude pulmonary oedema.

Treatment of altitude illness

Although there are bridging therapies that can be given to those who suffer the onset of altitude sickness, the most important treatment is descent. Indeed, just a few hundred metres can make a major difference to a person's condition. It can be difficult on the mountain but it is critical if the subject is going to survive.

Predicting those who are likely to get into trouble with altitude sickness

There have been a great many studies looking at the various causative factors for high altitude illness and some of these studies are summarised in Further reading. On current evidence it would appear that: the hypoxic ventilatory response, lung fluid clearance and the hypoxic pulmonary vasoconstrictor response are important elements that predispose the normal individual to development of high altitude pulmonary oedema. Of these the hypoxic pulmonary vasoconstrictor response is probably the most important and it is suppression of this by the calcium-channel blocker and/or dexamethasone that is the most successful treatment.

Going to altitude with lung disease

Asthma

There have been very few studies on asthma but there are potential benefits and draw-backs for the asthmatic going to altitude. The benefits include the relative absence of allergens – particularly the house dust mite – at altitude; so, for the atopic asthmatic, altitude can often improve symptoms and indeed was in the past used as a treatment for asthma. Opposing this benefit of altitude is the relative hypoxia (hypoxic broncho-constriction) and, more importantly, loss of humidity, leading to dehydration of the bronchial mucosa. Finally, there is the known effect of cold air on bronchial muscle tone. Overall asthmatics do well at altitude but must remember to take their inhalers and a course of steroids with them in their backpack in case of emergency.

COPD

These patients are at particular risk on travel to altitude for a number of reasons. Firstly, they have a diminished gas exchanging surface and therefore the problem of diffusion limitation is even greater. Secondly, they have fixed airflow obstruction and therefore the inability to raise ventilatory rates sufficiently to cope with the hypoxic environment. Thirdly, they are likely to already have alveolar hypoxia and pulmonary vasoconstriction and this is potentiated by the environmental hypoxia.

Pulmonary vascular disease

These patients are at particular risk at altitude and this was first shown in a case series of patients with pulmonary arterial atresia who developed high altitude pulmonary oedema when travelling to altitude. Because these patients already have pulmonary hypertension the addition of hypoxic pulmonary vasoconstriction to their condition can be fatal. With rare exceptions, patients with these groups of diseases are advised not to travel to high altitude.

Sleep disorders

As already stated earlier, normal people suffered from depressed ventilation during sleep with consequent alveolar hypoventilation and hypoxemia This is of course made worse at altitude so patients with sleep apnoea or hypopnoea are likely to do badly.

Air travel in patients with lung disease

It is not generally realised that the cabin altitude of commercial aircraft is between 1830–2430m. This is not a problem for normal people but for people with lung disease the consequences of hypoxia can be severe. There are various sea level formulae for calculating likely arterial oxygen saturation levels in a commercial aircraft and these are quoted in the BTS and other guidelines.

Further reading

Basnyat B, Gertsch JH, Johnson EW, et al. Efficacy of low-dose acetazolamide (125 mg BID) for the prophylaxis of acute mountain sickness: a prospective, double-blind, randomized, placebo-controlled trial. High Alt Med Biol. 2003; **4**(1):45–52.

Burgess KR, Johnson P, Edwards N, et al. Acute mountain sickness is associated with sleep desaturation at high altitude. Respirology 2004; **9**(4): 485–489.

Brutsaert TD. Genetic and environmental adaptation in high altitude natives. Conceptual, methodological, andstatistical concerns. Adv Exp Med Biol. 2001;**502**:133–151.

British Thoracic Society. Managing passengers with respiratory disease planning air travel: British Thoracic Society recommendations. Thorax. 2002;**57**(4):289–304.

Grant S, MacLeod N, Kay JW, et al. Sea level and acute responses to hypoxia: do they predict physiological responses and acute mountain sickness at altitude? Br J Sports Med. 2002;**36**(2): 141–146.

Hackett PH, Oelz O. The Lake Louise consensus on the definition and quantification of altitude illness. In: Sutton JR, Coates G, Houston CS (eds). Hypoxia and Mountain Medicine. Burlington, Vermont: Queen City Printers, 1992: pp. 327–30.

Imray CH, Myers SD, Pattinson KT, et al. Effect of exercise on cerebral perfusion in humans at high altitude. J Appl Physiol. 2005; **99**(2):699-706. Epub 26 May 2005.

Kriemler S, Kohler M, Zehnder M, et al. High Alt Med Biol. 2006;**7**(3):256–261.

Luks AM, Swenson ER. Travel to high altitude with pre-existing lung disease. Eur Respir J. 2007;**29**(4):770-792.

Maggiorini M. High altitude-induced pulmonary oedema. Cardiovasc Res 2006;**72**(1):41–50.

Peacock AJ, Jones PL. Gas exchange at extreme altitude: results from the British 40th Anniversary Everest Expedition. Eur Respir J 1997;10(7):1439–1444.

Pollard, AJ, Murdoch, DR. The High Altitude Medicine Handbook. New York: Radcliff Medical Press 1997.

Savourey G, Launay JC, Besnard Y, et al. Normo or hypobaric hypoxic tests: propositions for the determination of the individual susceptibility to altitude illnesses. Eur J Appl Physiol. 2007; **100**(2):193–205.

Seccombe LM, Kelly PT, Wong CK, et al. Effect of simulated commercial flight on oxygenation in patients with interstitial lung disease and chronic obstructive pulmonary disease. Thorax 2004;**59**(11):966-970.

Tsianos G, Eleftheriou KI, Hawe E, et al. Performance at altitude and angiotensin I-converting enzyme genotype. Eur J Appl Physiol. 2005;**93**(5-6):630–633.

Vachiery JL, McDonagh T, Moraine JJ, et al. Doppler assessment of hypoxic pulmonary vasoconstriction and susceptibility to high altitude pulmonary oedema. Thorax 1995;**50**(1):22–27.

Weiss J, Haefeli WE, Gasse C, et al. Lack of evidence for association of high altitude pulmonary edema and polymorphisms of the NO pathway. High Alt Med Biol. 2003;**4**(3):355–366.

West JB, Schoene R, Milledge JS. High Altitude Medicine & Physiology 4th edn. London: Hodder Arnold 2007.

Wu T, Kayser B. High altitude adaptation in Tibetans. High Alt Med Biol 2006:**7**(3); 193-208.

16.6 Diving

Diving involves immersion in fluid, usually water but sometimes other inhospitable media such as sewerage, or pressure exposure in a dry chamber.

- Water, a non-breathable fluid with a higher density, viscosity, thermal capacity and conductivity than air, exposes the diver to pressures in excess of one atmosphere (approximately 100kPa) as, for every increase in depth of seawater of 10 metres, ambient pressure rises by approximately 100kPa.
- This can compromise inspiratory or expiratory effort, depending on the diver's attitude in the water, and neutralises gravitational pooling of blood in veins of dependent limbs.
- Blood redistributes to the thorax, increases right heart filling and induces an immersion diuresis.
- Redistribution is potentiated by cold. Head-out immersion in water at 35°C (thermoneutral) reduces vital capacity by 5%, in 20°C by 10% and in 40°C by only 2%.

Alveolar gases at elevated pressure dissolve in greater quantity in blood. The circulation delivers the gases to other tissues into which they diffuse and dissolve. Oxygen is consumed by the tissues and CO_2 tension changes very little. Inert gases, however, accumulate until each tissue is saturated and no more can be dissolved at that pressure. The rate of saturation depends on a tissue's perfusion and its capacity for dissolved gas. The 'slowest' tissues, those with the lowest ratio of perfusion to capacity, take more than 24 hours to saturate. The fastest take minutes. On ascent, ambient pressure falls and, with it, the amount of gas that can remain dissolved. Some of the excess inert gas remains in solution in the venous blood as it returns to the lungs but, after most dives, at least some is liberated as free gas. Venous gas emboli are usually trapped in the alveolar capillaries until resorbed and the excess gas is exhaled. This lung 'filter' prevents gas emboli from reaching the systemic circulation but it can be circumvented by right-left shunts such as patent foramen ovale or pulmonary arteriovenous malformation. These potential pathways for 'undeserved' decompression illness can be identified using bubble-contrast echocardiography.

Carbon dioxide retention

Gas density increases in proportion to ambient pressure. Work of breathing, oxygen consumption, carbon dioxide production and physiological dead space increase. Maximal voluntary ventilation falls. Hypoxia is unlikely at raised ambient pressure but CO_2 removal may become critical when working hard at depth.

Some individuals become hypercapnic even when diving in favourable conditions. They often have a reduced ventilatory response to P_ICO_2 or a high end-breath-hold P_ACO_2 but these measurements are not sufficiently specific or sensitive for prediction of this response which is also found in a smaller proportion of non-divers.

CO_2 retainers can work hard underwater, enjoy good gas economy and avoid dyspnoea. They will, however, have little or no dyspnoeic warning of rising P_ICO_2 in the event of equipment malfunction. Also, hypercapnia sensitises to inert gas narcosis, cerebral O_2 toxicity, and decompression illness. Use of a less dense mixture, such as oxygen-in-helium, reduces retention but the precise mechanism of the phenomenon remains unclear. Inert gas narcosis does not cause respiratory depression. Elevated P_IO_2, however, has been shown to reduce the ventilatory response to exercise in some circumstances.

Pulmonary oxygen toxicity

P_IO_2 in excess of 50kPa causes a spreading tracheobronchitis typically starting at the carina. Early symptoms are retrosternal tickle, accentuated by inspiration, and occasional cough. These become progressively more intense and widespread until constant burning exacerbated by inspiration, uncontrollable cough and, eventually, dyspnoea at rest occur. Earliest symptoms appear within 6 hours at a P_IO_2 of 79–89kPa, 4 hours at 101kPa and 1 hour at 303kPa. Chest signs can be absent but fever, atelectasis, thick secretions, wheezes, crackles and bronchial breathing occur in advanced cases. Diffuse, bilateral opacities of varying extent are sometimes seen on CXR. Reduction in lung volumes and compliance, independent of any atelectatic effect of high fractional O_2, have been demonstrated, as has reduced DLCO. Lower P_IO_2 of greater duration is associated more with diffusion impairment while shorter exposure at high P_IO_2 preferentially affects lung mechanics. In general, alveolar-capillary permeability changes are thought to precede mechanical changes, such as drop in vital capacity. The latter are usually detectable before symptoms are reported.

Recovery after cessation of hyperoxia

- Advanced changes can be irreversible, but symptoms typically diminish rapidly in 2–4 hours with complete recovery in 1–3 days.
- An upper respiratory tract infection can cause symptom recurrence.
- Rates of onset and recovery tend to be symmetrical.
- Vital capacity improves rapidly in the first few hours usually returning to pre-exposure levels at around 30–35 hours, although some take several weeks.
- DLCO can correct almost completely in hours but a small residual impairment can persist for over a week.
- Large changes with rapid reversal are likely to be due to central nervous system oxygen toxicity, perhaps via a vagally mediated bronchoconstriction.

Decompression illness

Extravascular bubbles can occur in more severe decompression incidents, but excessive intravascular bubbles probably cause the majority of cases of decompression illness. Bubbles can embolise, damage vascular endothelium, induce 'foreign body' reactions or disrupt tissue, causing neurological, limb pain, cutaneous and cardiopulmonary manifestations.

> **AUTHOR'S TIP**
> 90% of cases present within 6 hours of returning to the surface.

If the venous bubbles overwhelm the capacity of the lungs to exchange gas, pulmonary capillary endothelial damage, dyspnoea, hypoxia, and pulmonary oedema can develop. Some bubbles might pass to the left heart before they have been resorbed, causing embolic complications. A very heavy bubble load can cause haemodynamic compromise. First aid for decompression illness is basic life support, oxygen and restoration of normovolaemia; definitive treatment is recompression.

Barotrauma and rupture

- Barotrauma is mechanical damage due to compression or expansion of gas. Although thoracic blood shift compensates for loss of gas volume and the lungs can tolerate compression far beyond residual volume, extreme exposures will cause damage leading to oedema and haemoptysis.
- If chest wall movement is unrestricted, lungs rupture when overpressurised by 9.3kPa, equivalent to ascent of barely 1m with closed glottis at total lung capacity or with a fully expanded, obstructed segment.
- If chest wall expansion is restricted 14.7kPa overpressure is required to cause rupture which is more likely to occur adjacent to less stiff areas of the chest wall.
- Gas can escape from the respiratory tract, including extrapulmonary sites, and present as pneumothorax, pneumomediastinum, subcutaneous emphysema, parenchymal emphysema or arterial gas embolism (AGE).
- AGE is a form of decompression illness which typically presents as diminution in level of consciousness or hemiplegia/paresis during ascent or within 10 minutes of reaching surface. First aid is basic life support, oxygen and restoration of normovolaemia; definitive treatment is recompression.
- Diving causes proportionately fewer cases of pneumothorax and more AGE than, for instance, intermittent positive-pressure ventilation or rapid decompression to altitude, perhaps because a diver's chest wall is less compliant and splints the lung peripheries.

Historical analyses of submarine escape training show that 33% of victims had pulmonary barotrauma (PBT) alone, 54% had neurological decompression alone and 13% had both. Only 5% of 'PBT alone' cases had significant pneumothorax.

- The true incidence of pneumomediastinum is not known as many are asymptomatic and only 50% are visible on a P-A CXR.
- Victims of PBT in submarine escape training are more likely to have a low FVC. The reason for this is not fully understood but reduced compliance and lack of support from the chest wall are two theories. No relationship has yet been demonstrated between PBT and FEV_1/FVC. It must be noted, however, that candidates with obstructive defects are screened out from submarine escape training.
- It is possible to rupture the respiratory tract with forceful exhalation against resistance or simply by maximal inhalation. This latter mechanism might be important in the rupture of lungs in divers who 'skip-breathe', deliberately holding themselves in prolonged inspiration in an attempt to reduce gas consumption.

Immersion pulmonary oedema

Symptoms of dyspnoea can develop while immersed in cold water despite minimal exertion, no aspiration of water, no evidence of cardiac dysfunction, no similar problems previously and unimpaired exercise tolerance on land. Cough, sometimes productive of blood and / or frothy sputum, and syncope are reported but no chest pain. Symptoms typically resolve within hours but third heart sounds, basal crackles and X-ray changes consistent with pulmonary oedema might be found earlier. A history of immersion pulmonary oedema is associated with a higher mean blood pressure and forearm vascular resistance, a greater increase in both when the head is cold challenged and an increased risk of developing hypertension. Immersion pulmonary oedema has occurred in warmer water especially during vigorous activity. Pulmonary capillary pressure is thought to be raised beyond plasma oncotic pressure by the combination of preload due to immersion with other factors such as increased cardiac output with, perhaps, overzealous rehydration, or greater afterload induced by the vascular reaction to cold. Pressures across the alveolar-capillary wall can be exaggerated further by breathing heavily or against an inspiratory resistance such as narrowed airways or a faulty demand valve. Treatment is rest and oxygen. The oedema usually resolves within hours although diuretics may be used in more severe cases. In one survey of divers some 1.1% of respondents reported symptoms suggestive of pulmonary oedema. Some have recurrent episodes and should be advised against diving.

Saltwater aspiration syndrome

Anyone active in or around water is at risk of near-drowning or drowning, the final common pathway in most diving fatalities. Smaller amounts of aspirated seawater can cause cough, sputum, retrosternal discomfort and haemoptysis during or within 2 hours of a dive. Extrapulmonary features develop such as fever, aches, malaise and even impaired consciousness. White cells can be elevated, PaO_2 is often low and $PaCO_2$ normal. Treatment is rest and oxygen. Warming often helps symptoms which usually resolve spontaneously within 6 to 24 hours.

Respiratory disorder and fitness to dive

In general a diver should have normal pulmonary function. Any deficiency which compromises gas flow or gas exchange could predispose to injury or an inability to cope with the respiratory demands of diving.

Contraindications to diving (BTS guidelines)
- Asthma precipitated by exercise, cold, or emotion.
- Active tuberculosis.
- Pulmonary cystic fibrosis.
- Lung bullae or cysts visible on chest x-rayfibrotic lung disease.
- Active sarcoidosis.
- COPD.
- Uninvestigated pneumothorax.

Specific questionable areas where diving permitted (BTS guidelines)
- Asymptomatic asthma with normal spirometry, negative exercise test, PEF no more than 10% below best values and requiring no more than regular inhaled anti-inflammatory agents.
- In cured tuberculosis or resolved sarcoidosis with normal chest radiography and pulmonary function testing.
- In spontaneous pneumothorax treated by bilateral surgical pleurectomy, or healed traumatic pneumothorax, if associated with normal lung function and thoracic CT.

Risk of recurrent spontaneous pneumothorax diminishes sharply if it does not recur in 2 years. Professor Denison permits diving without pleurectomy if there is no recurrence for 5 years and lungs are normal. In a review of 500 cases he noted that, if detailed lung function is normal, CT adds little to plain CXR findings and concludes that the radiation dose of CT cannot be justified routinely for assessment of fitness to dive.

Long-term pulmonary effects of diving

Findings vary. Some surveys show larger lung volumes, affecting vital capacity more than FEV_1, attributed to respiratory muscle training from dense gas and equipment resistance. Reduced expiratory flow rates at low lung volumes have been found, possibly reflecting small airway damage from bubble injury or chronic oxygen toxicity, but with no obvious clinical consequences. Vital capacity in some diver sub-populations may decline at an accelerated rate. DLCO falls during saturation dives, which last for many days but, once the dive is completed, it gradually returns to pre-dive values.

Further reading

British Thoracic Society guidelines on Respiratory Aspects of Fitness for Diving. *Thorax* 2003; **58**: 3–13.

Brubakk A, Neuman T (eds). *Bennett and Elliott's Physiology and Medicine of Diving* 5th edn. London: Saunders 2003.

Edmonds C, Lowry C, Pennefather J, et al. (eds). *Diving and Subaquatic Medicine* 4th edn. London: Arnold 2002.

Lundgren, CEG. Miller JN (eds). *The Lung at Depth*. New York: Dekker 1999.

Wilmshurst PT, Nuri M, Crowther A, et al. Cold-induced pulmonary oedema in scuba divers and swimmers and subsequent development of hypertension. *Lancet* 1989; **i**: 62–65.

16.7 Occupational chronic obstructive pulmonary disease

COPD is characterised by progressive fixed airflow obstruction. It is induced by inhaling noxious material, cigarette smoke, being the best recognised and discussed elsewhere. A recent definition emphasised that the disease is inflammatory and affects other systems as well as the lung.

The two COPD – chronic bronchitis and emphysema – have long been suspected to be induced by exposure to dust, organic material and fumes. The relationship between industrial exposure to dust and fumes and the development of obstructive airway pattern has often been an area of controversy. Some of the reasons for this are outlined in Table 16.7.1.

Table 16.7.1 Challenges in establishing relationship between occupation and COPD

- Concomitant cigarette smoking
- Inconsistency of pattern of work in one occupation
- Exposure to several materials in the same occupation
- Methods of diagnosis of chronic bronchitis and COPD in epidemiological analyses.
- Reliable comparative populations
- Estimation of exposure
- Individual susceptibility

A review of the literature on the relationship between chronic bronchitis and emphysema and occupational exposure was recently compiled by the Institute of Environmental Health a part of the Medical Research Council (MRC). Predictably, concomitant cigarette smoking was one of the most significant factors that have to be taken into account when regarding a material as independently responsible for causing chronic bronchitis and emphysema.

An independent relationship between an occupation and disease was regarded as present if there was doubling in the risk of chronic bronchitis and emphysema.

Table 16.7.2 outlines occupations associated with chronic bronchitis and emphysema independently from cigarette smoking.

Table 16.7.2 Occupations associated with more than double risk of incidence of chronic bronchitis and emphysema

- Underground coal exposure
- Agricultural and farm workers
- Cotton textile workers
- Flour mill and bakery workers
- Welders

Occupations associated with chronic bronchitis and COPD

Coal dust exposure

Due to political pressure, coal mining has been one occupation that attracted a significant amount of epidemiological and clinical research. There is an extensive body of literature that demonstrates a strong relationship between exposure to coal dust whilst working underground

(Figs. 16.7.1 and 16.7.2) and doubling the risk of chronic bronchitis and COPD even in the absence of any radiological changes of coal workers pneumonitis. The risk of COPD increases with the duration and intensity of exposure and in exposure at a young age. The relationship with emphysema in patients without pneumonitis is less clear.

The relationship between COPD and working on the surface of the mines or in open cast mines is less evident. A consensus has been that patients working on the surface handling loose coal are not associated with increased risk of chronic bronchitis.

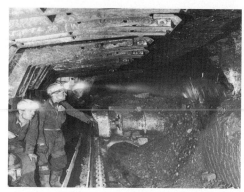

Fig. 16.7.1 Working in underground coal mines. The friable dust and the closed confined environment are responsible for inhalation of respirable coal dust.

Agricultural and farm workers

Farmers and agricultural workers are exposed to heterogeneous groups of components including parts of animal manure, gases that formed in silos and organic dusts.

Farm workers were found to be at increased risk of decline in lung function tests. The risk was more than doubled for those working with grains and in pig farms.

Cotton textile workers

The effect of cotton material on health is better recognised in the form of occupational asthma (byssinosis). Cotton fibres, bacteria and endotoxines are all implicated in the bronchospasm induced by exposure to cotton. Reduced peak expiratory flow rate, PEFR and FEV_1 in susceptible individuals is progressive. Airways disease becomes less reversible with continuous exposure The course of the disease and the symptoms resemble conventional COPD.

People working with cotton textiles for more than one year appear to have a more than double risk of accelerated decline in lung function tests in the short and long term. Cessation of exposure is associated with cessation in lung function decline.

Flour mills and bakery workers

Flour with its heterogeneous components is a well recognised sensitiser. As in cotton textile workers, repeated exposure especially in flour millers and bakers causes more than double risk of incidence of COPD especially in atopic individuals. Cessation of exposure is associated with cessation of decline in lung function and improvement of respiratory symptoms.

Welders

Welders are exposed to variety of particles, fumes and gases (Fig. 17.7.3). Welding has a known association with occupational asthma and with COPD. Considerable evidence exists of a relationship between welding and decline in lung function tests and the incidence of chronic bronchitis. The risk increases in current smokers.

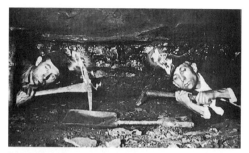

Fig. 16.7.2 Workers in underground coal mine.

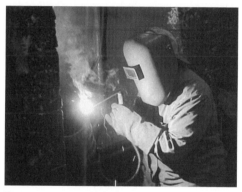

Fig. 16.7.3 A welder at work.

Management:

Cessation of exposure results in reduction of the decline in lung function in occupational COPD. In COPD associated with sensitisation, such as flour mill workers, bakers and cotton textile workers, lung function improvement was found after exposure was stopped.

As there is an additive effect of cigarette smoking, susceptible workers are urged to stop smoking. There is no evidence that screening for alpha-1 antitrypsin deficiency makes a significant difference, mainly due to rare occurrence of this condition.

Management of symptoms and COPD exacerbation in patients with occupational causes is similar to COPD cases induced by cigarette smoking.

Further reading

Chan-Yeung M, Enarson DA, Kennedy SM. The impact of grain dust on respiratory health. *Am Rev Respir Dis* 1992; **145**:476–467.

Enarson D, Chan Young M. Characterisation of health effects of wood dust exposure. *Am Rev Respir Dis Am J Ind Med* 1990; **17**: 33–38.

Glindmeyer HW, Lefante JJ, Jones RJ et al. Cotton dust and across shift change in FEV$_1$ as predictor of annual change in FEV$_1$. *Am J Respir Crit Care Med* 1994; **149**:584–590.

Kibelstis A, Morgan EJ, Roger R, et al. Prevalence of bronchitis and respiratory obstruction in American bituminous coal miners. *Am Rev Respir Dis* 1973; **168**: 886–893.

Rogan JM, Attfield MD, Jacobson M et al. Role of dust in the working environment in development of chronic bronchitis in British coal miners. *Br J Ind Med* 1973; **30**: 217–226.

Rudd R. Coal miner's respiratory disease litigation. *Thorax* 1998; **53**: 337–340.

Rushton L. Review of literature on chronic bronchitis and emphysema and occupational exposure. Publications of Institute for environment and health 2005.

Sferlazza SJ, Beckett WS. The respiratory health of welders. *Am Rev Respir Dis* 1991; **143**: 1134–1148.

16.8 Asbestos-related diseases (excluding mesothelioma)

Asbestos comprises of several naturally occurring fibrous mineral silicates. Due to its fantastic insulation qualities it was used extensively in the developed world until a 3–4 decades ago. Unfortunately, although the dangers of working with this material are well documented, it continues to be used regularly in the developing world.

Fibre types

The serpentine fibres of chrysotile (white asbestos) are curly and flexible; these fibres penetrate less readily to the periphery of the lung than the needle like amphiboles. The most important amphilboles are:

* crocidolite (blue asbestos);
* amosite (brown asbestos); and
* tremolite (a common contaminant of chrysotile).

Range of asbestos related disease

These include:

* Asbestos pleural plaques.
* Benign asbestos pleural effusion (BAPE).
* Diffuse pleural thickening.
* Asbestosis.
* Mesothelioma – pleura or peritoneum (covered in Chapter 14.7).

Pleural plaques

These can be calcified or non-calcified and affect the parietal pleura. They tend to occur in areas of maximum friction, i.e. the mid zones, diaphragms and pericardium. They tend to spare the costophrenic recess and apices.

Pleural plaques take approximately 12 years to appear on chest radiographs and 20 years to calcify. They are dose related and plain chest radiology tends to underestimate their number and extent. These lesions do not undergo malignant change.

They do not cause disability or pain and can occur after light exposure. Fig. 16.8.1 shows a chest radiograph with bilateral calcified pleural plaques

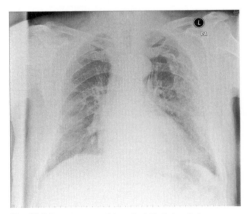

Fig. 16.8.1 CXR showing bilateral calcified pleural plaques.

BAPE

BAPE tend to occur earlier following asbestos exposure than mesothelioma does. The average latency is shorter than the development of pleural plaques. It is also an uncommon diagnosis beyond 25 years after first exposure. This contrasts with malignant mesothelioma with an exponentially rising incidence after initial exposure.

The pleural fluid is an exudate and may be blood stained but has no diagnostic characteristics. It is thought to be part of the inflammatory pathway that occurs before the development of diffuse pleural thickening.

> **KEY POINT**
> Benign asbestos pleural effusion is a diagnosis of exclusion

Diffuse pleural thickening

Diffuse pleural thickening of the pleura is less specific to asbestos exposure than pleural plaque development. Thickening and fibrosis of the visceral pleura occurs with fusion to the parietal pleura over a wide area.

Diffuse pleural thickening may result from exudative pleural effusions secondary to asbestos exposure, but other causes of pleural disease may also cause thickening (e.g. haemothorax, TB, chest surgery, drugs such as methysergide and parapneumonic effusions).

Diffuse pleural thickening on a chest radiograph presents as a smooth non-interrupted pleural density extending for at least 25% of the lateral chest wall, with or without blunting of the costophrenic angle. It has also been defined on CT scanning as a continuous sheet more than 5 cm wide, more than 8 cm in craniocaudal extent, and more than 3 mm thick. Diffuse pleural thickening may be difficult to differentiate from multiple pleural plaques, but the following may assist:

* plaques usually spare the costrophenic angles and lung apices;
* diffuse pleural thickening due to asbestos exposure rarely calcifies;
* diffuse pleural thickening is ill-defined and irregular from all angles, whereas plaques are well defined;
* plaques rarely extend over more than 4 rib interspaces unless multiple and confluent.

CT is more sensitive and specific for the detection of diffuse pleural thickening than chest radiography.

Symptoms include breathlessness and chest pain and lung function tests show a restrictive ventilatory defect with reduced total lung capacity.

A high resolution CT thorax is usually required as part of the initial work up (especially if pain is one of the symptoms) In cases of diffuse pleural thickening the pleura will be smooth, with no involvement of the mediastinal border. Whereas, in mesothelioma the pleural is likely to be irregularly thickened with mediastinal involvement (See Fig. 16.8.2a, a diffuse pleural thickening and 16.8.2b, mesothelioma). If there is diagnostic uncertainty a biopsy is recommended.

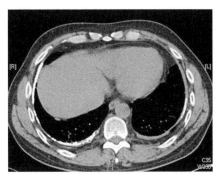

Fig. 16.8.2a Chest CT scan showing diffuse pleural thickening.

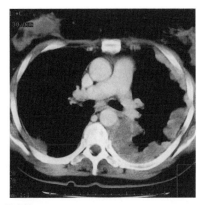

Fig. 16.8.2b Lobulated irregular pleural thickening in mesothelioma.

Not uncommonly patients with diffuse pleural thickening may have an area of folded lung. This is also known as Blesovsky syndrome or rounded atelectasis. It develops as contracting visceral pleura pulls and twists adjacent lung. This results is a subpleural opacity which often has a comet tail of vessels and bronchi converging toward the lesion (see Fig. 16.8.3).

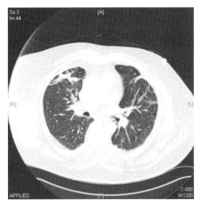

Fig. 16.8.3 Early folded lung in a patient with diffuse pleural thickening.

Patients with symptomatic diffuse pleural thickening may be eligible for compensation.

> **KEY POINT**
> Patients with pleural thickening involving the costophrenic angles are more likely to be symptomatic.

Asbestosis

Asbestosis is a diffuse interstitial fibrosis of the lung caused by asbestos dust.

It tends to be prominent in the lower lobes and subpleural areas. Radiographically, other than the presence of pleural plaques there a re no unique characteristics to differentiate it from usual interstitial fibrosis.

Asbestosis seldom develops less than 20 years after exposure and requires heavy asbestos exposure.

Pathogenesis

• Incomplete phagocytosis of asbestos fibres results in release of lysosomal enzymes, fibrogenic factors, cytokines and free radicals – all leading to fibrosis.
• Asbestos bodies are usually seen within areas of fibrosis.

Clinical features

• Presentation is usually with gradual exertional shortness of breath and a dry cough.
• Examination reveals late inspiratory fine crackles. Finger clubbing occurs in 40% of patients and is an adverse prognostic feature.
• Cyanosis and cor pulmonale may occur in advanced disease.

Investigations

HRCT is more sensitive than plain radiography and should be performed in all suspected cases. (See Fig. 16.8.4.)

• HRCT features include:
  • Parenchymal bands.
  • Basal ground glass opacities.
  • Subpleural curvilinear lines.
  • Interlobular septal thickening.
  • Fibrosis.
• Asbestos bodies may be found in sputum, BAL is more sensitive in detecting asbestos bodies.
• Histological confirmation of asbestosis is unnecessary unless there are atypical features. In these cases transbronchial biopsies are inadequate and a thoracoscopic or open lung biopsy will be needed.

Management

No drugs are of proven value. In advance cases palliative measures such as oxygen, diuretics, opioids should be used as appropriate.

Prognosis and complications

• Asbestosis usually progress slowly after removal from exposure and only 40% will progress over the following decade.
• There is an increased risk of lung cancer in patients with asbestosis.
• Due to the sensitivity of CT scanning some early cases are now being picked up in asymptomatic individuals. More research is required into the natural history of this subgroup.

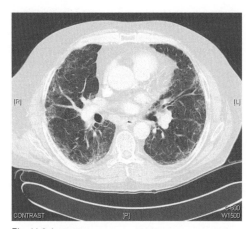

Fig. 16.8.4 HRCT showing interstitial fibrosis consistent with the diagnosis of asbestosis.

Further reading

ATS statement: Diagnosis and initial management of nonmalignant diseases related to asbestos. *Am J Respir Crit Care Med* 2004; **170**: 691.

Fletcher DE & JR Edge. 1970. The early radiological changes in pulmonary and pleural asbestosis. *Clin Radiol* 21:355-365

McLoud TC, BO Woods, CB Carrington, et al. 1978. Diffuse pleural thickening in an asbestos-exposed population. *Am J Roentgenol* 579-585

Lynch DA, G Gamsu& DR Aberle. 1989. Conventional and high resolution tomography in the diagnosis of asbestos-related diseases. Radiographic 9:523-551

Roggli VL, Oury TD, Sporn TA. *Pathology of Asbestos-associated Diseases* 2nd rev. edn. New York: Springer-Verlag 2004.

Lung transplantation/ITU

Chapter contents

17.1 Lung transplantation: considerations for referral and listing

Identifying potential lung transplant candidates

Lung transplantation offers a realistic therapeutic option to selected patients with end-stage respiratory disease who have failed to respond to maximal medical therapy. Potential lung transplant recipients need to demonstrate understanding of the risks and benefits of lung transplantation, appreciate the need for complicated mediation regimes and medication side-effects and be capable of and committed to following specific guidance from healthcare professionals within the transplant team. In the age of severe donor shortage it is essential that optimum use of this scarce resource occurs. This requires very careful assessment of potential candidates so that only patients in whom the benefit to risk ratio is favourable are taken on for lung transplantation.

General guidance

Indications and timing of referral

Patients with end-stage lung disease who have failed to respond to maximal medical treatment can be considered for lung transplantation.

Obviously many patients will have absolute or relative contra-indications and will not be suitable.

Those in whom survival chance is estimated to be 50% at 2–3 years should be considered to have disease of sufficient severity for referral.

Certain groups are at high risk of more rapidly progressive disease and are discussed below in disease specific guidance.

Absolute contra-indications to lung transplantation

- Smoking.
- Substance abuse (alcohol or illicit drugs).
- Severe dysfunction of other major organ.
- Unresolved extra-pulmonary infection.
- Chest wall or spinal deformity.
- Poor compliance with therapies or follow-up.
- Unstable psychiatric conditions.
- Absence of reliable social support system.
- Malignancy within last 5 years.

Adapted from International Guidelines for the selection of lung transplant candidates 2006 Update.

Smoking: current tobacco smoking is an absolute contra-indication to lung transplantation. Most centres will expect patients to demonstrate 3–6 months of complete abstinence before they would consider a patient's suitability for lung transplantation. It is important that patients are not simply still dependent on nicotine replacement products having given up smoking, but are free of nicotine addiction.

Malignancy: the risk of both lymphoproliferative and solid organ malignancy after lung transplantation is increased significantly due to the effect of powerful immunosuppressive drugs. Therefore patients with a history of recent malignancy would be at high risk of recurrence. Locally treated skin malignancy and certain very low grade tumours can be considered after definitive surgical treatment. In all other cases a 5-year disease free period after definitive treatment is required.

Unstable psychiatric conditions: compliance with a complex medication regimen, regular attendance at follow-up and early reporting of new symptoms are essential to producing good outcomes after lung transplantation. Patients who are unable to cope with these responsibilities are at high risk of a poor outcome after transplantation.

Relative contra-indications

- Age >65 years for single and >60 for bilateral lung.
- Poor rehabilitation potential.
- Colonisation with highly resistant micro-organisms.
- Obesity BMI >30.
- Poor nutritional status BMI <18.
- Severe symptomatic osteoporosis.
- Requirement for mechanical ventilation.
- Critical or unstable clinical condition.
- Other conditions causing significant end-organ damage.

Adapted from International Guidelines for the selection of lung transplant candidates 2006 Update.

Age

Increasing age above 55 years is an independent risk factor for a poor early and late outcome after lung transplantation.

Potential recipients over 55 years therefore require particular attention during assessment to exclude significant co-morbidities which will increase risk further.

The international guidelines recommend an upper age limit of 65 years for lung transplant. This acts as a guide and patients beyond this age limit can be successfully transplanted if they have no other co-morbidities and biologically are younger than their chronological age.

Weight and nutritional status

The physical stress associated with the transplant procedure causes most patients to lose 10% of their body weight in the post-operative period. This may be more if complications arise and there is a prolonged ITU stay.

If the patient is already underweight this is likely to be lost as muscle mass which will affect the ability to wean from ventilation and to rehabilitate. It is essential that patients therefore enter transplantation with sufficient nutritional reserve to cope with this stress.

Patients with cystic fibrosis (CF) are particularly at risk where pancreatic insufficiency, CF-related diabetes and advanced suppurative lung disease can cause a very poor nutritional status.

Patients with advanced COPD can also suffer from severe nutritional compromise due to the catabolic state and muscle dysfunction associated with the disease.

Careful attention to nutritional status is essential in these groups and in CF is achieved by aggressive enteral feeding (via NG tube or PEG), good glycaemic control and control of sepsis. Most centres would expect a minimum BMI of 18 in patients with CF or advanced Emphysema before listing for lung transplantation.

As important as being underweight are the risks associated with patients who are overweight or obese. As with all surgical interventions, obesity is associated with a higher complication rate.

After lung transplantation, poor mobility, poor wound healing and difficult weaning from ventilation can be experienced in those significantly overweight. This is seen as a correctable contra-indication to transplantation.

> **KEY FACT**
>
> BMI of 30 acts as an upper limit to consideration for listing for lung transplantation in most transplant centres.

Disease severity

Clearly, to be considered for lung transplantation patients will have advanced end-stage lung disease. However, potential transplant recipients also need to be fit enough to survive the physical stress of transplant surgery and to manage the rehabilitiation necessary as part of their recovery. There is thus a widow of opportunity for transplantation after which the severity of a patient's condition may make the chances of surviving the surgery and achieving recovery afterwards diminish rapidly (Fig. 17.1.1). In these cases, palliative care would be a more appropriate approach to management. Unfortunately, deterioration in a patient's condition beyond the window of opportunity may happen to those on the active lung transplant waiting list. This can necessitate removing them from the transplant waiting list and focusing on palliative approaches. This should be remembered when considering patients for initial referral. Many patients referred are already beyond the transplant window and the false hope that transplant referral can give may be detrimental to their remaining survival time.

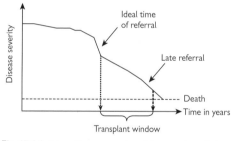

Fig. 17.1.1 Schematic representation of the transplant window and the timing of ideal referral for transplant assessment and when referral may be too late to successfully achieve transplantation.

Extra-pulmonary disease

Renal disease

- Calcineurin-inhibitors (ciclosporine and tacrolimus) form the cornerstone of immunosuppression regimens after lung transplantation.
- Both these agents have nephrotoxic potential.
- Most patients experience a deterioration in renal function after transplant and in some cases this can progress to renal failure requiring renal replacement therapy.

To minimise this possibility, patients being considered for lung transplantation should have well preserved renal function as demonstrated by an isotope glomerular filtration rate >60 ml/min. Acute renal failure in the early post-transplant failure can prolong intensive care unit stay and have an adverse effect on outcome.

Cardiac disease

The presence of known coronary disease or left ventricular dysfunction is a relative contra-indication for lung transplantation. However as with many relative contra-indications it needs to be assessed in its own right and also by examining its contribution to the individuals total risk.

Significant flow limiting or symptomatic coronary disease would increase risk of post-operative complications significantly and most centres would not accept such patients for lung transplant.

Patients with less severe disease may be suitable for pre-transplant coronary stenting or for consideration of bypass grafting at the time of transplant in these cases patients should be in otherwise excellent condition and have no other relative contraindications.

Mild left ventricular dysfunction can be treated with ACE inhibition and response followed by echocardiography.

Psychosocial aspects

Social support network

Undergoing lung transplantation places not only significant physical stress on an individual but also places many psychological and social strains on an individual. The complex nature of the follow-up arrangements, the travelling to and from the transplant centre and the complexity of the medication regimen means that transplant recipients need to be able to cope with these stresses as effetively as they can with physical stresses.

- Support from carers at the time of and in the post-transplant period is essentially to optimise the chances of a good outcome.
- Most transplant centres will insist that potential recipients have an identified primary carer or team of carers who will provide support in the post-transplant period.
- This individual(s) should also be involved in the pre-transplant assessment so they are fully informed as to what to expect in the post-transplant period.
- Social worker input is therefore an invaluable part of the assessment team.

Psychological status

The journey to successful lung transplantation involves many hurdles, each of which can cause significant stress to an individual and their family. The uncertainty in the assessment process, the waiting for a potential donor organ and the high risk of post-operative complications can place tremendous pressure on the individual and their carer(s).

- Potential recipients must therefore show that they are psychologically robust enough to get through this.
- A history of uncontrolled psychiatric illness, poor coping skills and extreme levels of anxiety may significantly impair the chance of achieving a good outcome from transplantation.
- Although these factors may be considered soft compared to other physical contraindications their importance should not be underestimated.

Disease-specific guidance

COPD and emphysema: worldwide this is the most common reason for referral and is the commonest indication for lung transplants performed. The value of the BODE score as guide to predicting prognosis in COPD has been adopted by the International Society of Heart and Lung Transplantation (ISHLT) in their disease specific guidance. However evidence that the BODE score is useful in guiding the decision to refer or list the younger COPD patient under consideration for lung transplant is lacking.

The international guidance suggests COPD patients with a BODE score of >5 should be considered for referral.

Those deemed unsuitable for lung volume reduction surgery may be considered for active listing when some or all of the following criteria are met:
● BODE >7.
● Repeated hospitalisations with acute hypercapnic respiratory failure.
● Pulmonary hypertension and cor pulmonale despite oxygen therapy.
● FEV_1 less than 20% predicted.
● Diffusing capacity less than 20% predicted.

The rate of progression of lung disease in COPD patients can be very slow and as a result lung transplantation may not offer a survival advantage to patients with this condition. In these cases lung transplantation can be performed predominantly for improvements in quality of life.

CF and bronchiectasis: patients with CF, of all the indications for lung transplantation, have a lot to gain in terms of an early survival advantage and the best long-term survival figures. However the multi-system nature of CF and chronic pulmonary sepsis with resistant organisms mean this group of patients require very careful assessment prior to acceptance for lung transplantation.

CF patients should be considered for referral when they have advanced lung disease as demonstrated by
● An FEV_1 of <30% predicted.
● A rapid loss of lung function (young female patients who appear to be at higher risk of rapidly progressive lung disease).
● An increasing frequency of exacerbations requiring admission or home intravenous antibiotics.
● Recurrent or refractory pneumothoraces or haemoptysis.

Assessment in potential CF recipients needs careful attention to the resistance patterns of organisms infecting their lungs, their nutritional status and the presence of liver disease. All of which can adversely affect outcomes after transplant.

> **KEY FACT**
>
> The ISHLT guidelines suggest a 10% or more fall in vital capacity or a 15% or more fall in diffusing capacity over 6 months indicate a need to list for transplant. This is probably more important than any absolute cut off for diffusing capacity or lung volumes.

Pulmonary fibrosis

Idiopathic pulmonary fibrosis is a common indication for referral for lung transplant assessment. Unfortunately many patients with this condition will lie outside the upper age limit for transplantation and will not be suitable for referral.
● Patients within the appropriate age group who have usual interstitial pneumonia (UIP) or fibrotic non-specific interstitial pneumonia (fibrotic NSIP) should be considered for referral early as they can progress very rapidly.
● Clinicians should not be falsely reassured by a diagnosis of NSIP as the mortality risk is as high as UIP in the first 2 years after diagnosis.
● Rate of progression of disease is an important indicator for need to list a patient for transplant.

Pulmonary arterial hypertension

The last 10 years has seen a dramatic increase in therapeutic options for patients with pulmonary arterial hypertension (PAH). As a result the prognosis for patients with PAH is better. Whether these therapies mean fewer PAH patients will ever be referred for lung transplant or will simply delay referrals by several years is too early to ascertain.

Patients who are WHO class III or IV who have progressive disease despite maximal medical therapies, including intravenous prostanoids, should be referred for assessment. When the following indicators are reached, patients should be considered for listing as these are markers of a poor prognosis.
● Six-minute walk distance falls well below 350m.
● Cardiac output <2 litres/min/m² or
● Right atrial pressure >15mmHg.

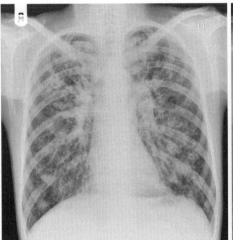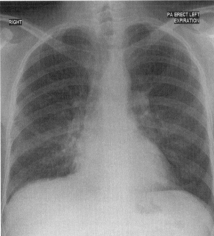

Fig. 17.1.2 Plain CXRs from a young male patient with CF before and after bilateral lung transplantation.

Others indications

There are a number of other rarer indications for lung transplant referral such as sarcoidosis, Langerhans cell histiocytosis (LCH) and lymphangioleimyomytosis (LAM). It is more difficult to provide disease specific guidance for these conditions due to their rarity. Disucssion with the transplant centre on a case-by-case basis is best to guide referral criteria in such cases.

Further reading

Orens J, Estenne M, Arcasoy S, et al. International guidelines for the selection of lung transplant candidates: 2006 update – a consensus report from the pulmonary scientific council of the international society of heart and lung transplantation. *J Heart Lung Transplant* 2006; **25**:745–755.

17.2 Complications after lung transplantation

The clinical course after lung transplantation varies markedly between individuals. This is due to development of common complications that range in severity from mild to potentially fatal and may impact on the recipient's quality of life. The common post-lung transplant complications can be categorised by their timing after transplant.

Early complications arise as a result of the surgical intervention and can affect the transplanted lungs themselves or other organ systems. Subsequent complications arise due to a loss of balance between alloimmune activity against the transplanted lungs and the level of immunosuppression used. Long-term complications arise due to the chronic toxic effects of immunosuppression and are due to chronic allograft dysfunction. Management of patients after lung transplantation can be complex but meticulous attention allows early detection and minimises the effect of such complications.

Survival after lung transplant

International registry shows survival figures of 50% at 5 years and 25% at 10 years. This compares poorly with other solid organ transplants such as liver, heart and kidney.

Improvements in lung transplant mortality in the first 3 months after transplantation have occurred over recent years largely due to improvements in surgical technique and postoperative critical care.

Morbidity and mortality after lung transplant can be considered in terms of time periods. Mortality within 30 days is mainly due to:

- Surgical complications (bleeding, anastomotic failure).
- Primary graft dysfunction (early acute lung injury or ARDS).
- Ventilator acquired lung injury or infection.
- Sepsis.

The leading cause of death at one year is infection as a consequence of common or opportunistic infections and immunosuppression. Infection is the leading cause of death after the first year reflecting increased susceptibility with impaired host defences, exposure of the allograft to the external environment and the development of chronic allograft dysfunction characterised by the development of the bronchiolitis obliterans syndrome (BOS).

> **KEY FACT**
>
> BOS is the leading cause of death in the long term and affects up to 70% of survivors by 5 years and accounts for 40–50% deaths at 3–5 years after lung transplant.

Surgical complications

Virtually all patients undergoing the procedure have reduced physical conditioning due to their significant underlying lung disease and are therefore at higher risk of post-operative complications.

Complications relating to the transplant surgery include haemorrhage, venous thrombosis, pulmonary arterial or venous stenosis, bronchial anastamotic dehiscence and intrathoracic sepsis. Vagus nerve injury may predispose to gastroparesis and gastroesophageal reflux disease. Phrenic nerve injury can occur and may be compromising if the diaphragmatic paralysis affects the side of single lung transplant. Anastomotic stenosis, due to ischaemia, affects only

3% patients in experienced centres but occur after several weeks and may require stenting to relieve the airflow obstruction.

Primary graft dysfunction

Primary graft dysfunction is a clinical diagnosis defined as significant impairment of oxygenation together with diffuse radiological infiltrates in the lung allograft within the first 72 hours after transplantation. It is analogous to acute lung injury and ARDS and requires exclusion of other causes such as hyperacute rejection, venous anastomotic obstruction, cardiogenic oedema and pneumonia.'

Primary graft dysfunction, previously called 'reperfusion oedema' or ischaemia-reperfusion-induced lung injury accounts for increased perioperative mortality, impaired lung function and worse longer-term survival.

Management of primary graft dysfunction is supportive with oxygen and ventilation strategies including permissive hypercapnia and prone positioning. Avoidance of fluid overload is important and approaches such as inhaled nitric oxide or prostaglandin infusions may be helpful to improve oxygenation. In severe cases extra-corporeal membrane oxygenation (ECMO) and surfactant therapy have been successfully used.

Infection

Infections, bacterial, viral and fungal can contribute substantially to both morbidity and mortality after lung transplant, the incidence is much higher than is seen after other solid organ transplants. The majority of infections occur within the thorax. The time after transplant is important when considering the possible cause.

Bacterial infections:

Usually presents as bronchopneumonia, commonest in the first few months after transplant. Responsible organisms include: *Pseudomonas aeruginosa* and other pseudomonas species, *Staphylococcus aureus*, coagulase-negative staphylococci, *Enterococcus* and *Haemophilus influenzae*. Infection with organisms such as Listeria, Nocardia and 'atypical' pneumonias are rare.

Patients with cystic fibrosis generally fare well with a rate of bacterial pulmonary infections comparable to those encountered in other patient populations. However, patients infected with the *Burkholderia cenocepacia* strain of the *Burkholderia cepacia* complex are at high risk of severe postoperative infections and septic death.

Subclinical colonisation with bacteria such as pseudomonas aeruginosa is seen in the later period after transplantation even in clinically stable allograft recipients. Clinically significant bacterial infection is a frequent complication of BOS with Gram-negative pathogens such as pseudomonas most frequently implicated.

Mycobacterial infection with *M. tuberculosis* or non-tuberculous mycobacteria is fortunately not frequent but is difficult to treat and effects long term outcomes. *M. tuberculosis* should be treated with the usual antituberculous drugs but blood levels of immunosuppressant drugs may be decreased due to cytochrome p450 activation. Non-tuberculous mycobacteria should only be treated if there is evidence of active disease. Infection with *M. abscessus* is a particular cause for concern.

Viral infections

Community respiratory viruses: infection with respiratory viruses (rhinovirus, respiratory syncytial virus, parainfluenza 1,2, and 3, influenza A and B) is common affecting up to 20% of recipients with significant associated morbidity. A possible link with the subsequent development of BOS has been suggested.

Cytomegalovirus (CMV) disease most frequently presents in the first 4 months after transplantation. Although the introduction of effective antiviral therapy, prophylaxis and viral surveillance has markedly reduced the frequency and severity of CMV infection, it remains a significant problem.

CMV predisposes to secondary bacterial and fungal infection and may be an independent risk factor for the development of BOS. Infection may be primary with seronegative recipients acquiring infection from a seropositive allograft, or secondary due to reactivation of endogenous virus acquired previously by the recipient.

Manifestations of CMV infection range from asymptomatic through to a mononucleosis like viraemia to severe invasive disease, most commonly affecting the lungs and sometimes disseminated to the central nervous system, gastrointestinal tract and retina.

CMV pneumonitis, the commonest form of invasive disease may be difficult to diagnose. The use of lung biopsy or bronchoalveolar lavage to demonstrate specific viral cytopathic changes has a low sensitivity. A significantly rising viral titre on PCR may be diagnostic.

Treatment is with an appropriate anti-viral such as oral valganciclovir with foscarnet being an alternative in cases of ganciclovir resistance. Some centres also add anti-CMV immunoglobulin to the treatment of severe and relapsing disease.

Relapse—rates following treatment are high, up to 60% for primary and 20% for secondary infection. Routine antiviral prophylaxis to prevent CMV has been shown to reduce the incidence and severity of CMV infection.

Epstein–Barr Virus (EBV) is common within the general population with more than 90% of adults over the age of 35 seropositive for the virus. Reactivation of the virus occurs in a significant number of patients post transplant and EBV is the major risk factor for the development of post-transplant lymphoproliferative disease (PTLD).

Fungal infection

Routine trimethoprim-sulfamethoxazole prophylaxis has reduced *Pneumocystis carinii* infection rates from 70% to virtually zero.

Other fungi causing infections in lung transplant recipients include *Cryptococcus, Candida* species and *Aspergillus*.

Aspergillus is a ubiquitous environmental fungus that is common in lung transplant recipients, affecting 30–50%. Despite this only 3% develop invasive disease that presents as pneumonia occasionally complicated by systemic dissemination with mortality rates as high as 60%. Treatment is with intravenous or nebulised amphotericin or oral voriconazole and surgical resection of affected areas in refractory cases.

Renal disease

Chronic kidney disease (CKD) is common after transplant, eventually affecting up to 90% of patients. Deterioration in

renal function begins in the first 6 months post transplant and 4–10% progress to end-stage renal failure requiring renal replacement therapy.

The renal toxicity of the calcineurin inhibitor immunosuppressants is the most important cause of renal dysfunction after lung transplant. These drugs cause a dose dependent acute renal injury due to intense afferent arteriolar vasoconstriction that may be reversible. However chronic use produces irreversible injury associated with structural remodelling of the glomeruli.

Complications of CKD include hypertension, anaemia and cardiovascular disease, patients with CKD post lung transplant have a 4–5-fold increase in mortality. Strategies aimed at minimising renal failure include introducing an alternative immunosuppressive agent such as rapamycin to allow a reduction in calcineurin inhibitor dose, aggressive control of blood pressure and therapy for hyperlipidaemia.

Patients with end-stage renal failure should ideally be listed for a renal transplant as it carries a significantly lower risk of death than long term dialysis.

Osteoporosis

Osteoporosis defined as a bone mineral density more than 2.5 standard deviations below the age related mean confers an increased risk of fracture.

An increased rate of non-traumatic fractures has been reported in lung transplant recipients, studies indicate over 70% of transplant recipients having osteoporosis with BMI and cumulative steroid dose being the main predictors.

Osteoporosis related fractures are painful, debilitating and may impair lung function as a result of thoracic restriction secondary to vertebral compression fractures. For this reason many centres consider patients with significant osteoporosis to be unsuitable for lung transplantation.

Treatment of osteoporosis in post-transplant patients includes calcium and vitamin D supplementation and oral bisphosphonates.

Neoplastic complications

Immunosuppression impairs T-lymphocyte mediated tumour surveillance, predisposing patients to malignancy. Tumours tend to be more aggressive than is seen in the general population.

The commonest tumour is PTLD. Other tumours include Kaposi's sarcoma and cancers involving the skin, lung, prostate, colon, head and neck and kidneys.

PTLD is a non Hodgkin's lymphoma predominantly of B cell type whose proliferation is driven by EBV. The risk of PTLD is highest in EBV seronegative recipients who receive an EBV positive graft.

Most PTLD occurs in the first year after transplant and involves the allograft with pulmonary nodules and possible mediastinal lymphadenopathy. Disease presenting later tends to be more disseminated and carries a worse prognosis with an overall mortality of 40–50%.

Diagnosis of PTLD is best achieved by tissue biopsy. Patients are staged by CT scanning. The main treatment is a significant reduction in immunosuppression to restore some host immunity to EBV. If this fails, other options include surgical resection of localised disease and chemotherapy/radiotherapy in refractory cases. Chemotherapy is poorly tolerated, infectious complications are frequently seen as a result of the additional immunosuppression.

Gastrointestinal complications

Gastrointestinal problems, mainly due to immunosuppressive drug toxicity, are common (incidence of up to 50%) in lung transplant recipients, the majority are self-limiting and respond to conservative management.

Complications include: peptic ulcer disease, gastritis, gastroparesis, pseudomembranous colitis, and CMV infection. Bowel perforation in an immunosuppressed patient carries a particularly high mortality of up to 75%.

KEY FACT

Gastroesophageal reflux disease appears to be a particular problem after lung transplant and has been linked to the development of BOS.

Neurological complications

Most non-infectious neurological complications are due to calcineurin inhibitor side effects. Manifestations are usually mild and include tremor, headaches and paraesthesia.

Drug-induced leukoencephalopathy is a more serious problem, manifesting as a wide range of possible symptoms including confusion, coma, seizures, cortical blindness and quadriplegia. Occipital lobe involvement is common with CT scans showing non-enhancing areas of reduced attenuation in the cerebral white matter. The cause of the injury is not clear and may relate to either a direct toxic effect of the drug or possible vasospasm and consequent ischaemic injury. Dose reduction or withdrawal of the offending drug is usually results in a substantial improvement.

Acute rejection

Acute rejection of the transplanted lung affects up to 40% of patients in the first 30 days after transplant and its incidence markedly declines after 6 months.

Acute rejection presents with non specific symptoms such as fever, cough, breathlessness and malaise and may be associated with infiltrates or pleural effusions on the CXR. Rejection may be clinically silent, particularly later on and as many as 20% of cases are picked up unexpectedly during surveillance transbronchial biopsy.

Bronchoscopy and transbronchial biopsy is required for diagnosis. Histologically it is characterised by perivascular and interstitial mononuclear cell infiltrates that may extend into the alveolar septae and affect the airway depending on severity. Acute rejection is graded according to an ISHLT formulation from A0 (no evidence of rejection) to A4 (severe acute rejection).

Early acute rejection is treated with pulsed IV methylprednisolone followed by an augmented dose of oral corticosteroids tapered over the course of a month. Most patients respond rapidly with improvements seen as early as 24 hours after treatment is commenced. Acute rejection occurring after the first month can be adequately treated with augmented oral corticosteroids

The frequency and severity of acute rejection episodes are recognised as predisposing to BOS, the principal cause of late mortality.

The bronchiolitis obliterans syndrome (BOS)

Diagnosis and clinical features of BOS
Obliterative bronchiolitis (OB) is the pathological manifestation of chronic allograft dysfunction in the transplanted lung with affected individuals showing obliteration of the

Table 17.2.1 International Society of Heart and Lung Transplantation scoring criteria

Grade	Histology
A0 (no rejection)	No significant abnormality
A1 (Minimal)	Infrequent perivascular mononuclear cell infiltrates around venules
A2 (Mild)	More frequent infiltrates, more than a few cells thick, involving veins and arteries
A3 (Moderate)	More exuberant mononuclear cell infiltrates from the perivascular space into the alveolar interstitium.
A4 (Severe)	Infiltrates extend into the alveolar space with pneumocytes damage: there may be necrosis of vessels and lung parenchyma.

small and medium sized airways airways with connective tissue.

OB is a histological diagnosis obtained from lung biopsy but patchy distribution of disease results in a low diagnostic sensitivity (15–28%). This lead to the use of a clinical correlate, the 'bronchiolitis obliterans syndrome' (BOS) based on the development of airflow limitation with decline in FEV_1 and reduced FEF25–75, from a stable post transplant baseline value. Staging of the disease (BOS level 0–3) depends on the magnitude of the decrease in FEV_1. The loss of function was considered to be irreversible (present >3 weeks) and requires exclusion of other conditions that can alter allograft function such as infection or acute rejection.

BOS is variable in its clinical presentation and natural history. Initial symptoms are often non specific or absent. As the disease progresses patients develop exertional dyspnoea, cough, and wheezing and can suffer frequent respiratory tract infections.

Table 17.2.2. BOS Scoring System (Estenne, 2002)

BOS 0	FEV_1 >90% of baseline and FEF25–75% >75% of baseline
BOS 0 p ('potential' BOS)	FEV_1 81–90% of baseline and/or FEF25–75% <75% of baseline
BOS 1	FEV_1 66–80% of baseline
BOS 2	FEV_1 51–65% of baseline
BOS 3	FEV_1 <50% of baseline

The median time from transplantation to initial diagnosis is 16–20 months, yet the range is very wide. The disease is progressive with a poor long-term survival rate of 30–40% at 5 years.

Progression of BOS tends to follow one of three patterns:
- Sudden onset of symptoms with a rapid decline in lung function.
- Insidious onset and slow progression over time.
- Initial rapid decline followed by a period of stable lung function.
- BOS impacts on quality of life; patients have less energy, more depressive symptoms and impaired functional capacity compared to those who are BOS-free. Worse outcomes are seen with acute onset, female gender, single lung transplant and pretransplant diagnosis of idiopathic pulmonary fibrosis.

Treatment of BOS

Most treatments for BOS are disappointing and the disease remains the major barrier to long-term survival after transplant. Most therapies seem to work by an anti-inflammatory rather than antifibrotic effect and therefore early detection and prevention of BOS should be emphasised.

Augmentation of immunosuppression with antilymphocyte antibodies, cyclophosphamide, methotrexate and total lymphoid irradiation has shown only modest success. These therapies may slow progression but offer little chance to reverse disease.

Altering immunosuppressive therapy from ciclosporine to tacrolimus may have some benefit but there is concern that this effect may not be specific.

The macrolide antibiotic azithromycin seems to partially reverse airflow obstruction seen in some patients with established BOS. Currently placebo controlled randomised trial are not available but are awaited.

Gastroesophageal reflux disease has been implicated in the aetiology of BOS and intervention with early gastric fundoplication may offer some protection.

Retransplantation is a controversial issue. Outcomes compare favourably with primary lung transplant in highly selected individuals and rates of BOS recurrence are not increased. Most centres will consider patients on a case by case basis but the lack of suitable donor organs has resulted in this procedure only being performed in exceptional cases.

Further reading

Alexander BD, Tapson VF. Infectious complications of lung transplantation. *Transpl Infect Dis* 2001; **3**: 128–137.

Boehler A, Estenne M. Post transplant bronchiolitis obliterans. *Eur Resp Monograph* 2003; **26**: 158–178.

Kotloff RM, Ahya VN. Medical complications of lung transplantation. *Eur Resp J* 2004; **23**: 334–342.

Perrot M, Mingyao M, Waddell TK, et al. Ischaemia-reperfusion-induced lung injury. *Am J Resp Crit Care Med* 2003; **167**: 490–511.

Studer SM, Levy RD, McNeil K, et al. Lung transplant outcomes: a review of survival, graft function, physiology, health related quality of life and cost effectiveness. *Eur Resp J* 2004; **24**: 674–685.

van der Bij W, Speich R. Infectious complications after lung transplantation. *Eur Resp Monograph* 2003; **26**: 193–207.

17.3 The care of lung transplant candidate or recipient

Clinical updates

Once a patient has been accepted as a suitable lung transplant candidate and is placed on an active waiting list it is essential that they remain in the best possible condition. It is important that lung transplant candidates remain under the care of their referring respiratory physician while on the transplant waiting list and are regularly reviewed at least every 3 months, and in many cases monthly would be more appropriate. Copies of clinic letters should be sent to the transplant team and any change in the patient's condition should be communicated to the transplant centre immediately.

Use of antibiotics

Although many patients with COPD or pulmonary fibrosis may become accustomed to regular use of antibiotics before referral for lung transplantation, once on the waiting list antibiotic use should be kept to a minimum. Over zealous use of antibiotics is associated with the emergence of more resistant bacterial species such as *Pseudomonas* spp. This can also produce fungal contamination which may be problematic after transplantation due to the powerful immunosuppression used. It is recommended therefore that antibiotics are reserved for microbiologically proven and clinically relevant infections only.

Patients with cystic fibrosis however, will have complex anti-microbial regimens and will likely need ongoing courses of antibiotics while waiting for lung transplant. Use of powerful combinations of antibiotics for atypical mycobacteria or resistant fungi or mould infections must be discussed with the transplant centre. Many of these treatments may need to be reserved for the post-transplant period where they would have much more chance of penetrating lung tissue if there is any recurrence of these infections.

Ventilation

Some patients awaiting lung transplantation will deteriorate either acutely due to an exacerbation of their disease or slowly due to progressive respiratory failure. The question as to whether individuals with end-stage lung disease should be intubated and ventilated is made more complicated when the patient is actively waiting for a lung transplant.

> **KEY POINT**
>
> Currently in the UK, no lung transplantations are performed on patients who are mechanically ventilated. This is because the outcomes from this group are very poor compared to non-ventilated patients.

In essence therefore, intubation and ventilation should be avoided in virtually all patients on the lung transplant waiting list as it is likely to be a futile intervention which will render the individual non-transplantable.

If the cause of an acute deterioration is felt to be highly reversible then it maybe justifiable to intubate and ventilate the patient. They would however need to demonstrate survivability and a capability to rehabilitate from the episode before they would become active on the transplant waiting list again.

Non-invasive ventilatory support (NIV) however is to be encouraged in patients with progressive hypercapnic respiratory failure on the transplant waiting list as it allows the patient to maintain their level of fitness for possible transplant.

Palliative care

The widening gap between the demand for lung transplantation and the shortage of donor organs accounts for a waiting list mortality of approximately 30–40%. As a result it is not infrequent for patients to die while waiting for a suitable donor lung. It is important to identify when a lung transplant candidate has moved beyond the transplant window and has become too sick to survive the transplant surgery.

There should be no reluctance to commence palliative care in such individuals as being on the transplant waiting list should not exclude giving appropriate palliative care to patients with end-stage disease. The decision to switch to a purely palliative approach and remove a patient from the lung transplant waiting list can be traumatic for both patient and their next of kin. Such decisions should be made in conjunction with the transplant centre.

The lung transplant recipient

Sudden changes in clinical condition

The first 6 months and especially the first 3 months after lung transplantation represents the time of highest risk for the development of acute rejection of the transplanted lungs. This is also a key period when a number of transplant-associated infections are common. The symptoms, signs and investigation findings shown in Table 17.3.1 can be caused by both acute rejection and infection. Clearly rejection and infection will require very different interventions and so the presence these indicators warrant immediate further investigation and discussion with the transplant centre.

Table 17.3.1 Changes in condition

Symptoms	Investigations
New or worsening cough	Fall in FEV_1 of greater than 15%
Breathlessness	New pleural effusion
Persisting fever	New pulmonary infiltrate
General malaise	

The high risk of acute rejection during this period means an urgent transbronchial lung biopsy is indicated. This is best carried out at the transplant centre where specialist transplant histopathologists are available to interpret the potentially difficult histological appearances. At the same time detailed microbiological evaluation of bronchoalveolar lavage (BAL) can be performed. If a patient is too unwell to be transferred to the transplant centre then a management plan should be agreed with the transplant team and there should be daily communication about progress. It is important to note that the risk of acute rejection is most marked in the first month following transplantation and the risk reduces each month until after 6 months, after which it is quite rare for patients to have an episode of acute rejection.

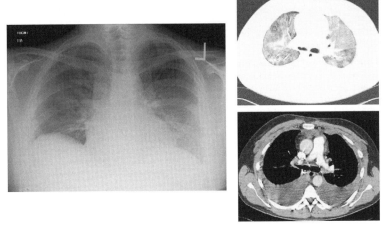

Fig. 17.3.1 Patient presenting 2 months flowing bilateral lung transplant with severe acute rejection. Plain CXR shows diffuse alveolitic shadowing in both lung fields and small lung volumes. CT chest images demonstrate the extent of the alveolitis and also the presence of large bilateral pleural effusions not seen on the plain CXR.

Immunosuppression

The immunosuppression regimen used by an individual recipient will have been tailored to their specific needs by the transplant centre. In general this will comprise a triple drug approach with a calcineurin inhibitor either ciclosporin or tacrolimus, corticosteroids and a cell cycle inhibitor such as azathioprine or mycophenolate mofetil. Other agents such as methotrexate or sirolimus may be used in addition. The transplant centre will assume responsibility for appropriate dosing of immunosuppression and for any changes in the immunosuppression regimen. In order to do this it is necessary to monitor the serum level of immunosuppressive drugs as well as liver and renal function. These will be checked every time the patient attends the transplant clinic but it will be necessary to check these bloods at least every 6 weeks. It is essential that the immunosuppression is not stopped or changed without prior consultation with the transplant team.

The danger of drug interactions

There are many interactions between immunosuppressive drugs and other medications in common use. Extreme care should be exercised whenever a new medication is prescribed to ensure that it will not decrease or significantly increase serum levels of immunosuppression and either expose the patient to the risk of rejection or to drug toxicity. The *British National Formulary* provides a comprehensive list of important interactions. For example, the macrolide antibiotics clairthromycin or erythromycin must not be given without a significant reduction in the dose of ciclosporin or tacrolimus and preferably they should be avoided altogether. This is because these drugs will increase significantly the area under the serum concentration curve for these drugs and may lead to marked renal dysfunction and in severe cases haemolytic uraemic syndrome.

The vomiting lung transplant recipient

If a lung transplant recipient presents with prolonged vomiting they may not be able to take or be absorbing sufficient immunosuppression. Every effort should be made to identify the cause and to control the vomiting with appropriate anti-emetics. Missing one or two doses of immunosuppressive medication is unlikely to cause any problems and it is important to exclude toxic levels of ciclosporin or tacrolimus as causes for the vomiting. If this is excluded and if control of the vomiting is unsuccessful then immunosuppression can be given intravenously and an appropriate regime should be discussed with the transplant centre. Dehydration in the presence of only moderately elevated serum concentrations of the calcineurin inhibitors can precipitate renal failure and care must be made to avoid dehydration in the vomiting lung transplant patient. In such circumstances daily measurements of serum drug levels may be necessary to aid prescribing.

Seizures

A new lung transplant recipient who experiences a seizure shortly after discharge from the transplant centre may have developed leuco-encephalopathy as a result of their immunosuppressive drugs. Warning signs of this complication include prior visual disturbance, hypertension and a low serum magnesium level.

Patients who have seizures usually do so within the first week or two following commencement of immunosuppression though rarely it may occur in the first month, which might include after discharge from the transplant centre. Initial management should be as for any other patient with a seizure and the transplant centre should be informed as soon as possible.

MRI scanning of the brain is the most useful investigation in determining the presence of leuco-encephalopathy. CT scanning of the brain will not diagnose this condition but may be useful in excluding other intra-cranial pathology. If a CT scan is performed as an initial investigation then it should be done with intravenous contrast.

If boluses of diazepam are unable to control the seizures or there is a need to give anti-convulsant therapy then sodium valproate is the anticonvulsant of choice because it will not interact with the patient's immunosuppression.

If there is difficulty in controlling seizures then phenytoin can be given but this will interact and dose changes in immunosuppression will be required. The calcineurin inhibitors (ciclosporin or tacrolimus) should be stopped until seizure activity is controlled.

Infections in the lung transplant recipient

Although lung recipients are at increased risk of opportunistic infections, it is much more frequent for them to present with common viral or bacterial infections than an opportunistic pathogen. These infections may, however, be more severe than in an immunocompetent patient. It is important to note that lung transplant recipients are rarely neutropenic and therefore it is unnecessary to commence high dose broad spectrum antibiotics immediately on presentation with a fever or other clinical signs of infection. However a recipient presenting very unwell with signs suggestive of sepsis should receive appropriate broad spectrum antibiotics as per any acutely unwell patient.

Appropriate sampling:
- blood cultures;
- urine cultures;
- sputum cultures or BAL culture.

In many cases identification of causative organisms can be made on culture allowing more targeted antibiotic therapy is commenced.

Lung recipients will receive prophylaxis against specific opportunistic infections, such as pneumocystis and herpes virus infection. Prophylaxis against pneumocystis should be continued lifelong with the standard regimen of co-trimoxazole 480mg daily or an alternative if necessary. pneumocystis infection is vanishingly rare in patients on prophylaxis.

This therapy therefore should not be stopped without consultation with the transplant centre. Herpes virus prophylaxis is provided by oral acyclovir which can be stopped after 3–6 months when levels of immunosuppression are lowered.

Cytomegalovirus (CMV) infection is an important cause of disease in lung transplant recipients. CMV may present with generalised malaise and flu-like symptoms or with specific gastrointestinal symptoms or respiratory symptoms. When there is a mismatch between the donor and recipients CMV status the risk of CMV disease is much higher. In these cases prophylactic treatment against CMV is given for the first 3 months with an anti-viral agent such as oral valganciclovir when the risk of developing CMV disease is at its highest. Other patients will be under surveillance for a rise in CMV activity using a PCR-based assay of viral load measured on a weekly basis. In these patients viral load will increase before symptoms develop allowing pre-emptive treatment with valganciclovir before a full blown CMV syndrome develops. If CMV disease is suspected then early discussion with the transplant centre should occur.

Some recipients may also be receiving nebulised anti-infective agents such as anti-pseudomonal antibiotics and/or anti-fungal therapy on the basis of organisms they were culturing pre-transplant or guided by positive cultures from pre-discharge bronchoalveolar lavages. These should be continued until reassessed by the transplant centre and may be required lifelong.

Blood pressure and renal function

Hypertension and renal dysfunction are very common in lung transplant recipients. This is due to side effects of their immunosuppressive therapy and as the two complications are interrelated it is important that careful attention is paid to both. Blood pressure should be controlled within standard guideline limits in an attempt to preserve good renal function and reduce other cardiovascular risks. The calcineurin inhibitors have potent nephrotoxic side-effects due to their vasoconstrictive actions on renal arterioles. Excellent blood pressure control, diabetes control and reducing levels of immunsuppression can help improve or stabilise renal function for many years. However in some patients renal dysfunction will progress despite these measures and may require renal replacement therapy and consideration for renal transplant.

The balance between the level of immunosuppression and its evidence on renal function will depend on the rejection history of the recipient and recent allograft biopsies. In recipients with stable lung function and a low risk of rejection ciclosporin or tacrolimus levels can be reduced significantly to protect renal function. Any change to a patients immunosuppression regime must be made in consultation with the transplant centre.

Increased cancer risk

Lung transplant recipients have an increased risk of cancer as a result of their immunosuppression. Skin cancers are particularly common and recipients are advised to avoid excessive periods in the sun or to use very high factor sun protection. Recipients should be advised to be vigilant for new skin lesions and report them immediately. The risk of solid organ cancers is also increased.

Any patient presenting with tonsil enlargement, peripheral lymph nodes, recurrent abdominal pain suggestive of intussuception, bowel obstruction, perforation or the presence of pulmonary nodules on CXR may have developed post transplant lymphoproliferative disease (PTLD). Rarely, a patient with PTLD may present with perforation or bowel obstruction and will require emergency surgery. In such cases biopsies of any lymph nodes and abnormal tissue should be taken for frozen section as well as placed in formalin so that appropriate molecular typing can be undertaken.

PTLD is usually an Epstein–Barr virus-driven B-cell proliferative process that responds in a majority of cases to a reduction in immunosuppression. Such patients should not therefore be fast-tracked into local lymphoma services to receive chemotherapy. It is very important that the transplant team is informed immediately should a recipient present in this way so that a management plan can be formulated. Ideally Patients presenting in an emergency situation with nodules or lymph nodes including tonsillar enlargement should be referred back to the transplant centre for investigation and subsequent management.

Lung transplant recipient needing routine surgery

Lung transplant recipients may require routine surgery and advice may be sought from local respiratory physicians by surgeons or anaesthetists.

KEY POINT

A lung transplant recipient with stable and adequate lung function has no excessive risk associated with routine surgery. There is no need to give prophylactic antibiotics to lung recipients specifically unless they would normally be used for that procedure anyway.

Special attention should be given to maintain good hydration, monitor renal function and serum levels of immunosuppressive drugs. Immunosuppression can be omitted the morning of surgery and restarted when the recipient is safely passing urine again usually within 24 hours. If a patient will be unable to take oral medication for some time a treatment regimen should be agreed with the transplant centre in advance.

17.4 Acute respiratory distress syndrome

ARDS is the most extreme manifestation of acute lung injury (ALI). This condition can develop as the result of a wide range of both direct and indirect insults.

Prevention is the best strategy in that the outcome is usually dependent on prompt identification and management of the precipitating cause which is a key role for the respiratory team.

Definition of ALI/ARDS

Radiology: new, bilateral, diffuse pulmonary infiltrates on CXR consistent with pulmonary oedema.

Oxygenation: PaO_2:FiO_2 ratio of <40kPa (acute lung injury); PaO_2: FiO_2 ratio of <26kPa (acute respiratory distress syndrome).

No clinical evidence that heart failure, fluid overload, or chronic lung disease are responsible for the infiltrates; or pulmonary artery occlusion pressure of <18mmHg.

The advantages of this definition are that it is simple to apply in the clinical setting, it recognises that the spectrum of lung injury severity and also attempts to exclude cardiogenic pulmonary oedema and chronic lung disease. It has limitations

- No account of the amount of PEEP applied, which may profoundly affect oxygenation or lung compliance the cause of ARDS or consideration of different pathophysiology according to the site of the original injury.
- Presence of multiorgan dysfunction and the radiographic findings are not specific.

> **AUTHOR'S TIP**
>
> The definition does not demand the automatic mesurement of PAOP. It can be elevated over 18 mmHg in ARDS patients particularly if volume overloaded or with high intrathoracic pressures.

Epidemiology

Using the 1994 consensus definition the reported incidence has varied from 13.5 per 100,000 to 75 per 100,000. Ongoing prospective studies using the 1994 consensus definition will clarify this issue.

The number of patients at risk of ARDS is unknown. The proportion of those which develop ARDS varies with the aetiology from 2% following cardiopulmonary bypass to 35% following aspiration. In the critically ill an incidence of 16–18 % is reported.

Risk factors

- Direct injury: pneumonia, aspiration, pulmonary contusion, fat emboli, near-drowning, inhalational injury.
- Indirect injury: sepsis, trauma, cardiopulmonary by pass, drug overdose, acute pancreatitis, massive blood transfusion.

> **AUTHOR'S TIP**
>
> Sepsis is the factor most associated with development of ARDS (40% of cases) and the presence of multiple predisposing factors substantially increases the risk.

Pathophysiology

ARDS is characterised by evidence of alveolar inflammation and injury leading to breakdown of the alveolar-capillary membrane and resultant pulmonary capillary permeability. It involves through exudative, inflammatory, and fibroproliferative processes which are not sequential.

Presentation

- <50% of patients with acute lung injury present either with acute lung injury or full-blown ARDS, which may have prognostic seem to develop ARDS within three days of admission to an intensive care unit.
- Most patients present clinically with dyspnoea, which may be masked by symptoms of the precipitating condition.

Differential diagnosis

- Cardiogenic pulmonary oedema: excluded by using echocardiography.
- Acute interstitial pneumonia: rapidly progressing form of lung injury. BAL characteristics shows both eosinophils and neutrophils.

> **AUTHOR'S TIP**
>
> Prognostic factors predicting death at the time of diagnosis include chronic liver disease, nonpulmonary organ dysfunctions, sepsis and age. Oxygenation (P_aO_2/F_iO_2) is not a prognostic factor at onset of ARDS but 24–48 hours later predicts outcome.

- Diffuse alveolar haemorrhage: seen at bronchoscopy (post-intubation). Diagnostic haemosiderin laden macrophages appear after 48 hours.
- Idiopathic acute eosinophilic pneumonia: raised eosinophils (typically 40%) are seen in the BAL fluid and usually in the blood.
- Lymphangitis carcinomatosis: bronchoscopy with BAL (and biopsy) aids diagnosis.

Investigation

These will depend on the mode and severity of presentation. The respiratory team will be involved both with patients at risk of developing ARDS (e.g. those with pneumonia) also with management and investigation of patients on ITU with the condition.

- Radiology: CXR and CT to exclude other diagnoses.
- Physiology: blood gases will establish severity of respiratory failure.
- Bronchoscopy and BAL, will be useful both diagnostically (especially in the immunocompromised) and therapeutically to remove mucus plugs.

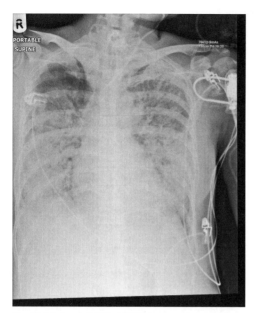

Fig. 17.4.1 A typical CXR of ARDS showing widespread diffuse alveolar shadowing.

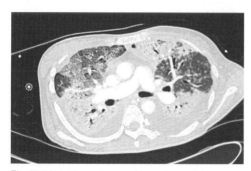

Fig. 17.4.2 A CT scan showing widespread ground glass showing with areas of consolidation and some areas of more normal appearance.

Treatment
Treatment is essentially supportive ventilation with aggressive management of the precipitating condition. Nutritional support and tight glycaemic control are essential Complications include the exacerbation of lung injury, multiple organ system failure, nosocomial pneumonia, deep vein thrombosis, and gastrointestinal bleeding must be minimised.

- *Mechanical ventilation* is discussed in detail in Chapter 17.6. Low tidal volumes have been shown to be protective but can result in reduced carbon dioxide clearance. Permissive hypercapnia is acceptable as long as oxygenation is not compromised and the pH is maintained above 7.2. The use of positive end expiratory pressure (PEEP) and prone ventilation are other techniques which may be helpful.
- *Corticosteroids:* these drugs remain controversial and no clear cut advantage has been shown by Cochrane review.
- *Inhaled nitric oxide:* an improvement in oxygenation occurs in 60% of patients but the effect is transient (48 hours) and does not improve mortality.
- *Nebulised prostacyclin:* this is another vasodilator with similar physiological effects to nitric oxide. When nebulised, it has an equivalent effect on pulmonary vasodilation and oxygenation but is easier to administer, and requires no special monitoring.

Outcome
- Most studies until recently have reported a mortality rate of 40–60%.
- Death occurs mainly due to sepsis or multiorgan dysfunction and not respiratory failure.
- The therapeutic success of low tidal volume ventilation in the ARDS Network Trial indicates some deaths are directly related to lung injury.
- Some data suggest mortality is falling. Possible reasons for this include improved treatment of sepsis, better ventilation strategies and improved supportive care.
- Pulmonary function in most survivors returns to normal or near-normal levels by 6 months.
- Mild restriction, reduced, bronchial hyper-reactivity and air trapping can persist.

AUTHOR'S TIP

ARDS survivors may have a persistent extrapulmonary functional disability 12 months after discharge mainly due to muscle wasting and weakness with minimal lung function changes.

Further reading

Bernard GR, Artigas A, Brigham KL, et al. The American-European consensus conference on ARDS. Definitions, mechanisms, relevant outcomes, and clinical trial coordination. *Am J Respir Crit Care Med* 1994; **149**: 818–824.

Gattinoni L, Caironi P, Cressoni M, et al. Lung recruitment in patients with the acute respiratory distress syndrome. *N Engl J Med* 2006; **354**: 1775–1786.

Peter JV, John P, Graham PL, et al. Corticosteroids in the prevention and treatment of acute respiratory distress syndrome (ARDS) in adults: meta-analysis. *BMJ* 2008; **336**: 1006–1009.

Useful Website: NHLBI Acute Respiratory Distress Syndrome network for trial details and results. www.ardsnet.org

17.5 Severe acute respiratory syndrome

Epidemiology

- SARS was first recognized in Guangdong Province, China in November 2002 and spread to 26 countries over the subsequent 9 months.
- 8098 infected people and 774 deaths were reported to the World Health Organization before the outbreak was declared over in July 2003.
- Four isolated cases of SARS with no associated transmission were identified in China in December 2003 and January 2004. Two isolated cases and a cluster of 11 cases (one death) were identified in South-East Asia related to breaches in biosafety practices in laboratories culturing SARS-CoV.
- Whether or not a large-scale re-emergence of SARS will occur is debatable.

Aetiology

- SARS Coronavirus (SARS-CoV) was identified in 2003.
- SARS-CoV likely evolved from animal SARS-like CoV (found most frequently in Himalayan civet cats and bats in China).
- SARS-CoV, like other coronaviruses, is an enveloped non-segmented, single-stranded, positive sense, RNA virus.

Incubation period

- Based on the 2003 outbreak, the typical incubation period for SARS is 2 to 10 days (mean of 4 to 6 days). A small proportion of cases may have incubation periods as short as 1 day and as long as 14 days.
- SARS is not communicable prior to symptom onset but transmission may occur soon after. Risk of transmission increases as symptoms progress, peaking during the second week of illness corresponding to peak viral load. Most countries considered patients to be potentially infectious and kept them in isolation precautions until 10 days after resolution of fever and signs of clinical improvement. There was no evidence of transmission from anyone treated in this manner, and it is possible that isolation for a shorter period of time may be sufficient.

Modes of transmission

- SARS-CoV has been found in respiratory specimens, stool, and to a lesser extent, blood, urine, and conjunctival secretions antemortem. At autopsy, SARS-CoV has been found in lung, gastrointestinal and lymphopoetic tissue and to a lesser extent heart and kidney tissues.
- Transmission primarily occurs by nasal mucosa or conjunctiva exposure to respiratory droplets either directly from an infected person or indirectly through inoculation with contaminated hands. It is possible that airborne transmission or transmission via contaminated fomites may also with SARS, but infrequently, if at all.
- Faecal-oral or faecal-droplet transmission has also been postulated but plays only a minor role if any.
- Given that SARS-CoV has been found in multiple organs and body substances, transmission through blood and organ transplantation is possible but there is no evidence of such transmission to date.
- No evidence of vertical transmission.
- In the 2003 outbreak, transmission was mostly limited to households, hospitals/immediate pre-hospital care.

Clinical course

Clinical presentation

- Clinical presentation ranges from asymptomatic disease to mild respiratory symptoms to the severe acute respiratory syndrome after which the virus was named.
- Typical SARS presents with fever, chills, malaise, headache, and myalgia; non-productive cough, dyspnoea, and sometimes watery diarrhoea seen 3 to 5 days later.
- If infants and children acquire the infection (rare), they follow a milder course frequently with rhinorrhea.

Routine laboratory investigations

- Normal total white blood cell count, lymphopenia, increased lactate dehydrogenase and creatinine kinase levels are typical.
- Laboratory abnormalities progress and peak at/just after the second week of disease.

Chest radiography

- 75% of patients have uni- or bilateral infiltrates on CXR at the time of presentation.
- If CXR clear, ground glass opacities often detectable on HRCT or will progress to develop CXR infiltrates.
- Typically see air-space opacities with ill-defined margins in a predominant peripheral location progressing from unilateral focal involvement to unilateral or bilateral multifocal involvement.
- CXR opacities peak between 8 and 10 days after illness onset and then improve.
- Progressive radiographic deterioration may occur associated with a more protracted clinical course.
- Cavitation, lymphadenopathy, and pleural effusions are not typically seen. Pneumothoraces have been found in critically ill patients receiving mechanical ventilation.

Prognosis

- 20% of patients develop worsening respiratory distress requiring intensive care.
- Approximately 10% of patients die from progressive respiratory distress or complications of their hospital admission, typically during the third or fourth week of symptomatic illness.
- Increased risk of death with age (50% mortality if >60 years), co-morbidity, elevated lactate dehydrogenase, elevated CRP, and elevated neutrophil counts.

Complications

- In women infected during pregnancy who survive, high incidences of spontaneous miscarriage, preterm delivery, and intrauterine growth restriction have been seen.
- At 3 months post symptom onset, most survivors have normal lung function but muscle weakness fatigue may account for residual disability.

Pathogenesis

- SARS-CoV most likely enters the human body via the respiratory tract mucosa, leading to viraemia and then replication in the lung and gastrointestinal tract.
- Viral replication is maximal during the second week of symptoms, correlating with worsening of symptoms and increased efficiency of transmission to others.
- Paradoxically, despite a fall in SARS-CoV viral load and a rise in SARS-specific antibodies during the third week of illness, clinical deterioration may occur in some. Immune dysregulation may play a role in these situations.

Diagnosis

The diagnosis of SARS relies on the combination of:
- identifying epidemiologic and clinical features consistent with SARS;
- ruling out infections other than SARS;
- laboratory confirmation of SARS-CoV infection.

SARS-CoV laboratory tests

- Available tests include reverse-transcription PCR (RT-PCR), enzyme immunoassays (EIAs), and viral culture for the detection of SARS-CoV. Serological tests including immunofluorescent assays, EIAs, immunoblots, and neutralization assays for the detection of IgM and IgG directed against SARS-CoV.
- RT-PCR is the mainstay of laboratory diagnosis at the time of patient presentation. Highest percent RT-PCR positivity seen in upper and lower respiratory samples (such as nasopharyngeal swabs/aspirates and sputum), stool samples, and serum or plasma.
- During the first 5 days of symptoms RT-PCR yield from serum or plasma ~80%, whereas the yield from respiratory and stool specimens is considerably lower. Days 10–14, yield from respiratory and stool specimens increases to 80 to 90%.
- Serologic tests are useful for the retrospective diagnosis of SARS in the weeks following illness. Seroconversion (IgM and IgG) usually 1 to 4 weeks after symptom onset, occasionally later at weeks 7 and 8.

Laboratory confirmation of SARS-CoV infection

Laboratory confirmation of SARS-CoV infection is based on one or more of the following diagnostic criteria:

(a) Detection of SARS-CoV by a validated RT-PCR method from:
- Two or more clinical specimens from different sources *or*
- Two or more clinical specimens collected from the same source at different time periods *or*
- Two different RT-PCR assays or repeat RT-PCR using a new RNA extract from the original clinical sample on each occasion of testing

(b) Detection of SARS-CoV antibodies in any of the following ways using a validated test:
- Negative SARS-CoV antibody test result on acute phase serum and positive SARS-CoV antibody test results on convalescent phase serum tested in parallel *or*
- A fourfold or greater rise in antibody titre between acute and convalescent phase sera tested in parallel

(c) Isolation in cell culture of SARS-COV from a clinical specimen in a reference laboratory, with confirmation using a validated method such as RT-PCR.

AUTHOR'S TIPS
- A single test result is insufficient for the definitive diagnosis of SARS-CoV infection because both false-negative and false-positive results are known to occur.
- Testing for SARS-CoV in the 2003 outbreak period needs to be done with caution given the potential for false-positives and the associated major public health and economic implications.

Treatment

- During the 2003 outbreak, ribavirin, steroids, type 1 interferons, convalescent plasma, and lopinavir/ritonavir were used in varying doses and combinations to treat patients with SARS.
- All of these agents have varying reports of associated anecdotal clinical improvement and some have been supported by studies using in-vitro assays and animal models. Some, such as ribavirin, were associated with significant toxicity. No definitive conclusions regarding the efficacy of any of these treatments can be made.
- Currently, of all of the agents studied that are already approved for clinical use, type 1 interferons, steroids, and lopinavir/ritonavir appear to be the most promising.

Prevention

- One of the keys to prevention is the early identification of cases of SARS through surveillance i.e. screening of patients who have compatible clinical features in the context of potential SARS–CoV exposure followed by appropriate laboratory testing. Epidemiologic risks to consider include: 1) exposure to settings where SARS activity is suspected or documented; and/or 2) being a laboratory worker in a laboratory that contains live SARS-CoV.
- Droplet, contact, and respiratory precautions should be used when caring for patients with SARS in order to prevent transmission to health care providers (gown, gloves, eye protection, in addition to an N95 respirator and private negative pressure room)
- Attempts should be made to: minimize the time spent by healthcare workers and visitors in the room and specifically minimize the time spent in close contact with the patient; keep to the side of the patient out of direct droplet range; assign the most experienced personnel to perform procedures on the patient; and avoid transporting SARS patients where possible.
- Public health authorities should immediately be notified of any suspected or confirmed case of SARS in order to search for and isolate symptomatic contacts and quarantine asymptomatic contacts for the 10 day incubation period following exposure.
- Many candidate SARS vaccines have been proposed but none are currently available for clinical use.

Further reading

Kamps BS, Hoffman C (eds.). SARS Reference. www.sarsreference.com/index.htm. Accessed April 2008.

Poutanen SM, Low DE. SARS. In Torres A, Ewig S, Mandell L, *et al.* (eds.) *Respiratory Infections*, pp. 515–34. Hodder Arnold: London.

World Health Organization. Severe acute respiratory syndrome. www.who.int/csr/sars/en/. Accessed April 2008.

17.6 The ventilated patient

Intensive care units (ICUs) were first developed in the 1950s to provide acute respiratory support for the victims of polio epidemics in Europe and North America. Ventilatory management remains a core competency for the intensivist today and continues to present significant challenges. This chapter outlines the principles underpinning the care of the intubated, ventilated patient.

Epidemiology

A recent, large international study found that 33% of patients admitted to an ICU required mechanical ventilation for at least 12 hours:

- Indications for ventilation included acute respiratory failure (ARF) (69%), coma (16%), and respiratory failure on a background of chronic lung (13%) or neuro-muscular (2%) diseases.
- Duration of ventilation was for a median of 5 days, but 1% of patients required support for more than 28 days.
- Overall mortality was 31% (ICU) and 39% (hospital). ICU mortality was associated with age, severity of illness, prior functional impairment, severe hypoxaemia, difficult ventilation, and specific clinical conditions (coma, sepsis, ARDS). Those who developed ARDS, coagulopathy or metabolic acidosis while ventilated, or who developed a second organ failure, were at greatest risk (mortality 60–70%). Ventilated patients usually die from multiple organ failure rather than from hypoxaemia.
- A study of over 20,000 medical ICU patients in the USA found that units treating over 400 ventilated patients per year had a lower hospital mortality (25.5%) compared with those treating less than 150 ventilated patients per year (34.2%).
- Patients with an acute exacerbation of COPD who received mechanical ventilation suffered mortality of 22% (ICU) and 28% (hospital), which is lower than for ventilated patients in general. The duration of ventilatory support (median 6 days), and ICU (8 days) and hospital (17 days) length of stay were similar to those for ventilated patients as a whole. These results probably indicate that more patients with COPD should be offered mechanical ventilation, but a difficult decision remains to be made for each individual patient.
- In patients with ARDS, ICU mortality was 52–63%, in accordance with other cohort studies. Mortality in clinical trials is lower (e.g. 31–40%), possibly due to trial selection criteria.

Indications for invasive ventilation

Acute hypoxic (type I) respiratory failure

Common causes include community-acquired or nosocomial pneumonia, cardiogenic pulmonary oedema, ARDS, atelectasis after major abdominal or thoracic surgery, severe asthma and COPD. There is no absolute value for arterial oxygen tension (PaO_2), or for the ratio of PaO_2 to fractional inspired oxygenation concentration (FiO_2) which triggers the need for invasive ventilation. That decision also depends upon the underlying pathology, the likelihood of success using non-invasive ventilation (NIV), and the mental and physical condition of the patient. For example, a patient with cardiogenic pulmonary oedema will often recover rapidly from severe hypoxaemic respiratory failure using only continuous positive airways pressure (CPAP) or NIV and standard drug therapies, but if the patient is exhausted and cerebrally obtunded they will need intubation and conventional ventilatory support. If in doubt, it is usually safer to intubate a patient with severe hypoxaemia, (e.g. with a PaO_2 <8kPa, receiving an FiO_2 of 0.6 or above). This permits greater control of the patient's physiology and avoids the risk of respiratory arrest.

Hypercapnic (type II) respiratory failure

The most common cause of type II respiratory failure in the ICU is exhaustion due to increased work of breathing. This usually occurs in patients who have already developed type I respiratory failure, or in those with severe metabolic acidosis (e.g. septic shock) who attempt to compensate through hyperventilation. In such cases, a rising arterial carbon dioxide tension ($PaCO_2$) may be a sign of impending respiratory arrest, even if the level remains within normal limits, and invasive ventilation should be considered immediately. Other causes of type II failure include acute on chronic respiratory failure, acute neuromuscular diseases (Guillain–Barré syndrome, myasthenia gravis, botulism), chest wall or diaphragmatic trauma, drug overdose, post-operative pain, opiate analgesia, intracranial pathology, and partial airway obstruction. Once again, the decision to intubate depends on assessment of the patient as a whole, including the severity of respiratory acidosis, the ability of the patient to protect their airway, and the reversibility of the pathology, as well as physiological parameters such as $PaCO_2$ and FVC.

Reduction of oxygen demand

Invasive ventilation is indicated in the initial resuscitation of some patients (e.g. those with severe sepsis) in order to reduce tissue oxygen requirements, even in the absence of respiratory failure or other absolute indications for ventilation.

Post-operative management

Ventilation for 4–12 hours is routine after certain types of surgery, including cardiothoracic surgery requiring cardiopulmonary bypass, and major head and neck surgery.

Decreased conscious level

Intubation and ventilation may be indicated in order to:

- Maintain a patent airway. In patients with a traumatic brain injury, hypoxaemia related to airway obstruction is a major cause of secondary brain injury.
- Protect the lungs from aspiration of gastric contents.
- Control $PaCO_2$ between 4.5–5.0kPa as part of an algorithm to control raised intra-cranial pressure (ICP).
- Enable deep sedation in patients with status epilepticus or severe traumatic brain injury, in order to reduce cerebral oxygen demand.

A Glasgow Coma Score (GCS) of 7 is sometimes used as a threshold for intubation. However, other factors may favour intubation when the GCS is higher.

The role of NIV and facemask CPAP

NIV and facemask CPAP have an established role in patients with an exacerbation of COPD, acute on chronic respiratory failure from chest wall deformities and neuromuscular disease, cardiogenic pulmonary oedema, thoracic trauma, respiratory failure after thoracic surgery, and respiratory failure in the setting of immunosuppression. There are many reports of the successful use of NIV and CPAP in other conditions. For some patients these techniques may represent an appropriate ceiling to support when invasive ventilation is not considered to be in a patient's best interests.

However, when NIV or CPAP fail and intubation beomes necessary, prognosis may be worse than if intubation had been performed at the outset. In ARDS, an attempt at NIV before intubation was associated with an increase in ICU mortality from 31% to 48%. In patients who were weaned from invasive ventilation but in whom respiratory failure recurred, NIV did not reduce the rate of re-intubation, and was associated with a mortality increase from 14% to 25%. NIV should therefore be used with caution in the majority of patients admitted to the ICU. Beyond its recognised indications it should be used only when the underlying condition is likely to improve rapidly. Patients should be monitored closely. Those who fail to improve rapidly should be considered for early intubation before they become exhausted.

Ethical considerations

The decision to commence or withhold invasive mechanical ventilation is frequently difficult. In the UK, the decision should be made in accordance with the guidance of the General Medical Council on withholding and withdrawing treatment. In summary, competent adults have the right to refuse treatment, even if this results in harm to themselves or death, but do not have a right to demand treatment which the doctor thinks is not clinically indicated. The aim should be to achieve consensus between the patient, their close family and friends and the healthcare team. A second opinion should be sought where there is disagreement.

There is no ethical or legal distinction between withholding and withdrawing treatment. When there is uncertainty about the patient's best interests, as in many emergency situations, treatment should be started until a clearer assessment of best interests can be made.

Airway management

Rapid sequence intubation (RSI)

The intubation of a critically ill patient is a time of particular risk, with high rates of complications including severe hypoxaemia (26%), difficult intubation (12%), oesophageal intubation (5%), aspiration of gastric contents (2%), haemodynamic collapse (25%), arrhythmias (10%), and cardiac arrest (2%). Although intubation is traditionally an area of expertise of the anaesthetist, it is increasingly seen as a core skill for all physicians working in the critical care setting. Specific considerations are:

- The patient may need to be intubated on a ward distant from the ICU or theatre complex with limited equipment or assistance. Essential equipment, drugs, and a trained assistant should be immediately available to go to a ward to manage this situation. If possible, the patient should be attached to a monitor and transferred to a more suitable location before intubation.
- Critically ill patients desaturate quickly during apnoea at the time of intubation. It is therefore vital to pre-oxygenate fully before induction. This requires at least 3 minutes of normal tidal breathing while inhaling 100% oxygen (but as few as 5 vital capacity breaths). To maximise the functional residual capacity (FRC), i.e. the oxygen reservoir in the lungs, the patient should be kept head-up and positive pressure applied via the anaesthetic breathing system to recruit collapsed airways.
- ICU patients have an increased risk of difficult intubation. Even if a pre-intubation assessment of the airway is normal, difficulties may arise (e.g. due to laryngeal oedema),

especially if the patient has only recently been extubated or is hypoproteinemic. It is essential that RSI is performed by those who are familiar with a difficult airway algorithm, and who know how to use the difficult airway equipment. A maximum of four attempts should be made at intubation before handing over to a more experienced colleague. The emphasis should be on maintaining oxygenation rather than on achieving intubation. Other means of oxygenation including bag-and-mask ventilation, insertion of a laryngeal mask airway, or cricothyroid puncture should be considered without delay.

- Patients are at increased risk of regurgitation and aspiration until the endotracheal tube is in place with the cuff inflated. They should therefore be anaesthetised and intubated in the head-up position. Cricoid pressure helps to prevent regurgitation, but may make intubation more difficult, and may have to be relaxed to allow the endotracheal tube to pass through the larynx.
- A critically ill patient is at risk of cardiovascular collapse due to the negative inotropic and vasodilatory effects of anaesthetic drugs, and due to positive pressure ventilation which increases the intra-thoracic pressure and reduces cardiac preload. To minimise these risks, ensure reliable IV access for fluid loading. Invasive arterial blood pressure monitoring is desirable before induction if time allows. Reduced and incremental doses of the IV anaesthetic agent should be used, with a short-acting vasopressor agent such as metaraminol immediately available. The choice of induction agent is less important than the dose that is given. However, many ICU doctors avoid etomidate despite its cardiovascular stability, as even a single dose may cause adrenal suppression.
- The paralysing agent suxamethonium should be used with caution. It provides optimum conditions for intubation, but may cause an exaggerated release of potassium from muscle cells in patients with burns or neuromuscular diseases, including those with prolonged immobility or ICU neuro-myopathy. Cardiac arrests from hyperkalaemia have occurred in ICU patients as a result.
- Given the significant risk of oesophageal intubation, capnography should always be used to confirm the position of the ETT in the trachea. Listening for breath sounds with a stethoscope may be misleading.

Management of the endotracheal tube (ETT)

The most common artificial airway when invasive ventilation begins is a cuffed oral ETT. Nasotracheal tubes are preferred in paediatric ICUs, but in adults are only generally employed after major head and neck surgery when surgical access to the oral cavity has been required. A small number of patients already have a tracheostomy in situ (2%).

- The ETT should be secured firmly, but without obstructing venous drainage from the head (especially if there is raised ICP). Accidental extubation occurs in 3–5% of ventilated patients. If this occurs, the priority is to maintain oxygenation and ventilation via a bag-and-mask until equipment and drugs are prepared for re-intubation, but this may only be necessary in 41%.
- An air leak around the cuff of the ETT may indicate cuff rupture, but more commonly the tube has migrated above the vocal cords. Further cuff inflation stops the leak temporarily but also pushes the ETT further up into the pharynx, so the leak soon recurs. The correct response is to check the position of the ETT immediately, and if necessary push it back down the trachea to prevent accidental extubation.

- Modern ETTs typically have a high-volume/low-pressure cuff to spread the pressure over the tracheal mucosa and minimise the risk of pressure necrosis and subsequent tracheal stenosis. Cuff pressures should be measured regularly and should not exceed 30cmH$_2$O.
- Pharyngeal secretions pool above the ETT cuff and can pass into the lower airway. Such micro-aspiration occurs in 89% of intubated critically ill patients, and is thought to be the main route of access for organisms causing ventilator-associated pneumonia (VAP). To minimise the problem a subglottic drainage tube (an integral part of the ETT) just above the cuff should be aspirated either periodically or continuously. Subglottic drainage reduces the incidence of VAP by 50%, the duration of ventilation by 2 days, and the length of stay in ITU by 3 days. However, these tubes are not widely used, partly because of concern about an increased risk of mucosal injury.
- Suction via the ETT lumen is performed routinely, both to reduce micro-aspiration and to maintain tube patency. Closed suction systems have not been found to reduce the incidence of VAP, mortality or ICU length of stay compared with open suction.
- Artificial humidification is necessary to prevent drying of the airways and thickening of secretions. This is normally achieved with a heat and moisture exchanger (HME), which also functions as the breathing system filter. However, HMEs can increase work of breathing, particularly when saturated with water vapour. The alternative, water-bath humidifiers, may increase the risk of VAP.

Tracheostomy

Until the mid-1980s, tracheostomy was almost exclusively performed as an open, surgical procedure. Since that time several percutaneous techniques have been described which can be performed at the bedside in the ICU. The most popular is that described by Ciaglia, using a seldinger guidewire and either serial dilators or a single tapered dilator.

- The most common indication for tracheostomy in the ICU is to aid weaning from respiratory support in patients who need ventilation for more than a few days. Other indications include upper airway obstruction and impaired bulbar function. A mini-tracheostomy may help in the management of secretions in self-ventilating patients with an inadequate cough.
- The major benefit is improved comfort (compared to an oral ETT), allowing sedation to be stopped. Airway resistance and anatomical dead space are reduced, and easier mouth care may reduce the risk of VAP.
- Risks of tracheostomy include hypoxaemia, bleeding, infection, and damage to the trachea or oesophagus. Severe hypoxia may be due to loss of airway control at the time of tracheostomy formation, or dislodgement or obstruction of the tube at a later time. To reduce the risk of blockage, a tracheostomy tube may have an inner lining tube which can be removed and cleaned. Bleeding may occur at the time of the procedure or due to erosion through an adjacent vessel days or weeks later. Infection is usually not severe but mediastinitis, especially in the presence of a median sternotomy wound, may be catastrophic. The risk of infection is less with percutaneous tracheostomy than with open tracheostomy, probably due to the difference in the amount of tissue trauma.
- Contra-indications to tracheostomy include soft tissue infection of the neck, and significant thrombocytopenia or coagulopathy. Patients with abnormal neck anatomy such as a goitre or a pulsatile vessel above the sternal notch should have an open surgical tracheostomy rather than a percutaneous procedure. Percutaneous tracheostomy may be performed in morbidly obese patients, but the risk of complications is much higher, and many ICU doctors routinely refer these patients for surgical tracheostomy.
- The optimal timing for tracheostomy is unknown. As an aid to weaning, a tracheostomy is of no benefit until a patient has recovered from the acute phase of their illness and is ready to wean from ventilatory support. However, one study found a reduction in mortality from 61.7% to 31.7% when tracheostomy was performed within 48 hours of intubation rather than 14–16 days after intubation. The Tracman study is currently recruiting patients to compare tracheostomy performed at day 1–4 versus day 10 after ICU admission.

Ventilator terminology

- Intermittent positive pressure ventilation (IPPV) is a general term for all forms of positive pressure ventilation. However, it is also sometimes used to indicate controlled mechanical ventilation (CMV).
- Ventilator cycling refers to the signal which tells the ventilator to switch from inspiration to expiration. Time cycling occurs after a set inspiratory time. Pressure, volume or flow cycling occurs after the target pressure, volume or flow has been reached. The method of cycling depends on the mode of ventilation used.
- CMV delivers a set tidal volume and respiratory rate, and is time-cycled. The tidal volume is usually delivered in the first part of the inspiratory phase, and is followed by the inspiratory plateau before expiration begins. Peak inspiratory pressure depends on the interaction of tidal volume, inspiratory flow rate, airway resistance, and lung compliance. Plateau pressure is an indicator of the pressure transmitted to the alveoli, and is an important determinant of ventilator-induced lung injury (VILI). CMV does not allow spontaneous breaths, and is appropriate for patients who have no respiratory effort. If the patient coughs or tries to take a breath, high airway pressures and work of breathing may be generated.
- Pressure controlled ventilation (PCV) delivers a set airway pressure and respiratory rate, and is time-cycled. Tidal volume depends upon the inspiratory pressure, inspiratory time, airway resistance and lung compliance. PCV does not permit spontaneous respiration. The risk of high airway pressure is avoided, but tidal volumes and minute ventilation are variable.
- Assist-control ventilation (ACV) delivers a set tidal volume. Each breath is triggered by the patient's inspiratory effort (assist). If the patient does not trigger the ventilator, the set tidal volume is delivered at a set back-up respiratory rate (control). ACV is the mode of ventilation employed in the ARDS Network studies.
- Synchronised intermittent mandatory ventilation (SIMV) enables a set number of ventilator breaths (either volume controlled or pressure controlled) to be synchronised with the patient's spontaneous respiratory efforts. Patients can also breathe between these mandatory breaths, with pressure support added to the extra breaths. Patient-ventilator dyssynchrony may still occur, with increased work of breathing.
- Biphasic positive airway pressure (BIPAP) alternates between two levels of airway pressure, providing tidal ventilation but permitting spontaneous breaths throughout the ventilator cycle. Spontaneous breaths can be

augmented by pressure support. Like SIMV, BIPAP can provide complete or partial ventilatory support, but the ability to take a spontaneous breath at any time renders it better tolerated than SIMV.

- Pressure support ventilation (PSV). The patient triggers each breath. The ventilator delivers a set level of inspiratory pressure, and cycles to expiration when the inspiratory flow rate drops below a certain level. Tidal volume depends upon the interaction between inspiratory pressure, inspiratory time, airway resistance and lung compliance. PSV is used for weaning patients from respiratory support, once they have recovered from the acute phase of critical illness. A mandatory mode of ventilation acts as a back up, activated by apnoea.

- Triggering is the mechanism by which the ventilator recognises a patient's attempt to take a spontaneous breath. The ventilator measures either a small negative deflection in airway pressure, or a change in the rate of air flow within the breathing system. Modern ICU ventilators measure changes in both pressure and flow. Flow can be measured earlier, and provides a more sensitive trigger which reduces work of breathing.

- Positive end-expiratory pressure (PEEP) occurs when airway pressure remains above atmospheric pressure at the end of expiration. It may be set externally by the ventilator, or may be intrinsic (PEEPi) when there is increased resistance to expiratory flow in the airways, as in asthma or COPD. PEEP is used therapeutically to recruit collapsed areas of lung, increase FRC, and improve ventilation-perfusion matching, leading to better arterial oxygenation. There is less cyclical opening and closing of small airways with each breath, reducing shear forces and lung injury ('open lung ventilation'). Tidal ventilation occurs on the steeper part of the pressure-volume curve, with improved lung compliance and reduced work of breathing. Excessive PEEP may cause barotrauma, increase pulmonary vascular resistance and paradoxically worsen shunt by diverting blood flow away from over-distended lung units. 'Best PEEP' is defined by the minimum level which achieves an acceptable PaO_2. Different levels of PEEP did not affect mortality in ARDS patients receiving carefully controlled tidal volumes and inspiratory pressures.

- Continuous positive airway pressure (CPAP) is delivered by a ventilator or by specific CPAP equipment. It gives no support for tidal ventilation but, like PEEP, it improves lung compliance and oxygenation. It is useful to reduce work of breathing and maintain FRC during the final stages of weaning from ventilation.

- Prone ventilation may be used in patients with refractory hypoxia, and improves oxygenation in about 60% of patients with ARDS. However, it may cause haemodynamic instability and airway compromise, and has not been shown to reduce mortality or duration of ventilation.

- High frequency oscillatory ventilation (HFOV) typically delivers 180–360 breaths per minute, the tidal volume being smaller than the anatomical dead space. The mechanism of gas exchange is not completely understood, but both oxygenation and CO_2 removal may be improved. Randomised trials in adults with ARDS have revealed no significant benefits over conventional ventilation for either mortality or duration of ventilation. HFOV may be used as a rescue therapy in patients with ARDS or a broncho-pleural fistula when conventional ventilation is failing.

- Extra-corporeal membrane oxygenation (ECMO) achieves gas exchange via an extra-corporeal circuit similar to that used for cardio-pulmonary bypass during surgery. It is used as a rescue therapy in patients with severe, refractory hypoxia. There is currently no good evidence of benefit in adults, but the results of the CESAR trial in patients with severe ARDS are awaited.

Ventilator settings

It is important to understand the various modes of ventilation, but current evidence suggests that other ventilator settings such as tidal volume and airway pressure have more influence on outcome:

- FiO_2 should start at 0.6–1.0, and be titrated according to PaO_2 (aiming for 8–10kPa) and SpO_2 (aiming for at least 90–95%). Until the patient has been stabilised, the over-riding concern is to avoid hypoxaemia. In patients with severe chronic respiratory failure or severe ARDS, a lower PaO_2 or SpO_2 may be accepted, as long as tissue oxygenation appears to be adequate, as assessed by end-organ function, central venous oxygen saturation, lactate and base deficit. The duration and severity of an SpO_2 less than 90% is correlated with cognitive impairment in survivors of severe ARDS. The effect of oxygen therapy on the hypoxic respiratory drive is irrelevant in the mechanically ventilated patient in the acute setting. However, it may become important during weaning. Hyperoxia is beneficial in the treatment of carbon monoxide poisoning but should be avoided in other circumstances. Oxygen toxicity occurs after 12–36 hours at an FiO_2 above 0.5, and is characterised by lung inflammation and atelectasis, the clinical importance of which is not clear.

- Respiratory rate is typically 12–16 breaths per minute, adjusted with the tidal volume in order to achieve an acceptable CO_2 clearance and arterial pH. In severe asthma or COPD a slower rate (8–10 breaths per minute) may be necessary. This allows sufficient time for inspiration without excessive peak airway pressures, and for full expiration without dynamic hyperinflation.

- Tidal volume used to be set routinely at 10–12ml/kg. However, there is evidence that in patients with ARDS these tidal volumes contribute to ventilator-induced lung injury and increase mortality. A target of 6ml/kg in patients with ARDS is appropriate, based on body weight predicted from height and sex. In other ICU patients the evidence is less clear, but it is prudent to limit tidal volume in all patients where possible.

- Inspiratory pressure should be set to achieve the desired tidal volume and minute ventilation, while keeping the plateau pressure below 30cmH$_2$O. Once again the evidence for this comes from trials in patients with ARDS, and its applicability to other populations is uncertain.

- Inspiratory: expiratory ratio is normally 1:2. A ratio approaching 1:1 or inverse ratio ventilation (2:1) increases mean airway pressure, recruits alveoli, allows more even distribution of ventilation and improves V/Q matching. It is used as part of a strategy to manage severe hypoxaemia. Ensure that there is enough time for full expiration, by observing the expiratory flow waveform return to zero between breaths. Prolonged expiration with a ratio of 1:3 or 1:4 may be necessary in COPD or asthma.

- PEEP may be set at 5 cmH$_2$O in ventilated patients with relatively normal lungs requiring an FiO_2 of up to 0.4, in order to prevent atelectasis. In patients requiring a higher FiO_2, PEEP may be increased up to 10–15cmH$_2$O on a sliding scale as the FiO_2 also increases towards 1.0. The ARDS Network trials used a sliding scale of PEEP up to a maximum of $24cmH_2O$. However, such high PEEP is rarely used in practice. An alternative method of setting PEEP is to look at the pressure-volume curve and adjust PEEP so that tidal ventilation takes place on the steep part of the curve. In patients with expiratory air flow limitation the external PEEP should be set just below intrinsic levels (PEEPi) in order to reduce the work of breathing required to trigger a pressure supported breath.

- Lung-protective ventilation is the ventilator strategy used in ARDS to minimise VILI. It includes limitation of tidal volume (6ml/kg) and plateau pressure ($30cmH_2O$), and use of PEEP for open lung ventilation.
- Permissive hypercapnia may be necessary in ARDS or in other patients who are difficult to ventilate such as those with severe asthma or persistent pleural air leaks. The $PaCO_2$ is allowed to rise to 8–10kPa in order to limit tidal volume and airway pressure. However, arterial pH should be maintained above 7.2–7.25 by limiting the rise in $PaCO_2$.

Monitoring the ventilated patient

- Routine monitoring includes continuous pulse oximetry, ECG and invasive arterial pressure measurement.
- Arterial blood gas (ABG) analysis should be performed 15–30 minutes after adjusting the ventilator, and 1–4 hourly depending on the severity of illness and the need for other measurements such as blood glucose.
- Important ventilator measurements include inspiratory and expiratory tidal volume, airway pressures, inspiratory and expiratory flow rate, respiratory rate and FiO_2. Observation of the expiratory flow curve is a useful way to ensure that intrinsic PEEP is minimised and that breaths are not being 'stacked' leading to hyperinflation.
- End-tidal CO_2 ($ETCO_2$) may correlate poorly with the $PaCO_2$ in ICU patients due to V/Q mismatch and shunt, and is not routinely monitored. However, it is essential for confirmation of tracheal placement of the ETT at the time of intubation. It may also be used continuously in patients with raised intracranial pressure, for whom tight control of the $PaCO_2$ is necessary.
- Alarms on the ventilator and monitor should be set to provide adequate warning of deterioration, and to minimise false alarms caused by minor changes. Alarms should not simply be disabled in order to reduce noise.
- Plain CXR should be performed when clinically indicated, rather than as part of the daily routine for every ICU patient. Routine CXR is not associated with an improvement in ICU or hospital length-of-stay or in-hospital mortality. Targeted CXR is a useful investigation in the ICU, but almost all films are taken in recumbent patients and may not reveal clinically significant pleural effusions or pneumothoraces. When the lungs are very stiff, even a small pneumothorax may be under tension and may cause haemodynamic instability. Ultrasound scanning or CT should be considered when the CXR is equivocal.
- Extra-vascular lung water (EVLW) is a variable derived from the thermodilution curve of some cardiac output monitors. It provides an estimate of lung oedema, and may help to guide fluid balance management in conjunction

with other haemodynamic data, clinical examination and the CXR. However, there are no studies to show that measuring the EVLW by single thermodilution reduces either mortality or duration of ventilation.
- Clinical examination is limited by the patient's recumbent position and their inability to perform the usual manoeuvres required for full assessment. However, within these limits, thorough clinical examination is essential in order to put the monitored data in context and to pick up problems which would not otherwise be apparent. Inadequate clinical examination may lead to missed or delayed diagnoses which a critically ill patient will tolerate poorly.

Weaning from invasive ventilation

Weaning is the process of withdrawing ventilatory support until the patient breathes unaided. In 80% of patients this is achieved quickly and easily once the original reason for ventilation has resolved, but in 20% of patients it may take prolonged efforts over several days or weeks.

- Patients should be screened every day for readiness to wean, looking for: resolution of the problem which required ventilation; haemodynamic stability; adequate gas exchange; absence of serious acid-base or electrolyte abnormalities, and an alert cooperative patient. Many physiological parameters have been studied in attempts to predict readiness to wean, but none have been found to be consistently accurate.
- Having fulfilled the screening criteria, a patient should undergo a spontaneous breathing trial (SBT) for 30–120 minutes, using a low level of PSV, CPAP or a T-piece. Success is indicated by comfortable breathing at a rate <35/min, adequate gas exchange, and cardiovascular stability at the end of the trial.
- If a patient fails the SBT, they are returned to supported ventilation. Weaning may then progress by repeated breathing trials, or by incremental reduction of PSV over the following days. The level of support may be varied during the day in order to exercise the respiratory muscles. In patients with COPD or cardiogenic pulmonary oedema, weaning may be expedited by extubation directly onto NIV.
- After short-term ventilation with rapid weaning, the artificial airway is usually removed immediately. The risk of reintubation within 48 hours is about 13%. After prolonged weaning, removal of a tracheostomy is usually delayed for 24 hours in case respiratory failure recurs. After successful weaning, an artificial airway may still be needed in some patients to prevent airway obstruction, to enable suctioning or prevent aspiration.
- Weaning protocols have been shown to reduce the duration of ventilation and ICU length of stay in some studies, but other studies have found no difference. Protocols may be less important in intensivist managed ICUs which have high levels of physician staffing and structured ward rounds.

General care of the ventilated patient

General care of the ventilated patient includes adequate sedation and analgesia, preventive measures against deep vein thrombosis and gastric stress ulceration, nutrition, meticulous infection control and one-to-one nursing care. Raising the head of the bed by 45° above horizontal has been shown to significantly reduce the incidence of VAP.

Further reading

Drakulovic MB, Torres A, Bauer TT *et al*. Supine body position as a risk factor for nosocomial pneumonia in mechanically ventilated patients: a randomised trial. *Lancet* 1999; **354**: 1851–1858.

Esteban A, Anzueto A, Frutos F, *et al*. Characteristics and outcomes in adult patients receiving mechanical ventilation. *JAMA* 2002; **287**: 345–355.

Esteban A, Alia A, Tobin MJ, *et al*: Effect of spontaneous breathing trial duration on outcome of attempts to discontinue mechanical ventilation. *Am J Respir Crit Care Med* 1999; **159**: 512–518.

Esteban A, Frutos-Vivar F, Ferguson N, *et al*. Noninvasive positive pressure ventilation for respiratory failure after extubation. *N Engl J Med* 2004; **350**: 2452–2460.

Ferrer M, Esquinas A, Arancibia F, *et al*. Non-invasive ventilation during persistent weaning failure: a randomised controlled trial. *Am J Respir Crit Care Med* 2003; **168**: 70–76.

Guerin C, Gaillard S, Lemasson S, *et al*. Effects of systematic prone positioning in hypoxemic acute respiratory failure, a randomised controlled trial. *JAMA* 2004; **292**: 2379–2387.

Henderson JJ, Popat MT, Latto IP, Pearce AC. Difficult airway society guidelines for management of the unanticipated difficult intubation. *Anaesthesia* 2004; **59**: 675–694.

Kahn JM, Goss CH, Heagerty PJ *et al*. Hospital volume and the outcomes of mechanical ventilation. *N Engl J Med* 2006; **355**: 41–50.

Kripoval M, Shlobin OA, Schwartzstein RM. Utility of daily routine portable chest radiographs in mechanically ventilated patients in the medical ICU. *Chest* 2003; **123**: 1607–1614.

Krishnan JA, Moore D, Robeson C *et al*. A prospective controlled trial of a protocol-based strategy to discontinue mechanical ventilation. *Am J Respir Crit Care Med* 2004, **169**: 673–8.

Meade M, Guyatt G, Cook D, *et al*. Predicting successful weaning from mechanical ventilation. *Chest* 2001; **120**: S400–404.

Rivers E, Nguyen B, Havstad S, *et al*. Early goal-directed therapy in the treatment of severe sepsis and septic shock. *N Engl J Med* 2001; **345**: 1368–1377.

The ARDS Network. Ventilation with lower tidal volumes as compared with traditional tidal volumes for acute lung injury and the acute respiratory distress syndrome. *N Engl J Med* 2000; **342**: 1301–1308.

The ARDS Network. Higher versus lower positive end-expiratory pressures in patients with the acute respiratory distress syndrome. *N Engl J Med* 2004; **351**: 327–36.

Withholding and withdrawing life-prolonging treatments: Good practice in decision-making. General Medical Council, London 2002.

Orphan lung diseases/BOLD

Chapter contents

18.1 Pulmonary alveolar proteinosis

Pulmonary alveolar proteinosis (PAP) is extremely rare (prevalence around 0.2 per million) but nevertheless important because when optimally managed it should generally have a good prognosis, but ignored or poorly managed may well lead to preventable death. There have been important developments in the understanding of the pathogenesis and following this, the treatment of PAP in the last decade. This is all the more remarkable considering the rarity of PAP and the fact that it was only first described as a clinical entity in 1958. Indeed, unravelling the mystery of this enigmatic syndrome may shed important light on the pathophysiology and cell biology of more common diseases.

Epidemiology

There are 3 distinct forms of PAP which share practically identical clinical features but have very different triggers or aetiology. These forms are

- Congenital (extremely rare and least amenable to treatment – almost universally fatal in early infancy). Unlikely to present to many clinicians because of rarity and absence of therapeutic options.
- Secondary (PAP in association with or caused by a range of **severe** clinical entities such as haematological malignancy, lung cancer, infection, massive exposure to inhaled irritants such as petrol fumes or silica dust). The outcome is generally dependant entirely on the management of the precipitating condition, for example, control of the leukaemia may lead to remission of the secondary PAP.
- Primary (previously referred to as idiopathic, now increasingly referred to as auto-immune). This is the most common form at around 0.2 per million and the form that requires specific management.

It is primary PAP that is best studied and understood and accounts for more than 90% of cases of PAP. Most reported series show an average age at onset in the late 30s but all ages can be affected with a 5 to 1 male predominance. There is no apparent ethnic propensity other than PAP being more common in Japan where first presentation is typically at an older (late 50s) stage.

Clinical presentation

In most cases there is an insidious progressive decline in exercise tolerance and increasing dyspnoea. Some patients have a non-productive cough and some report various types of chest pain (neither pleuritic nor anginal in nature) while some patients present with combinations of the above. In some cases there is an apparently acute onset with features of respiratory infection, fever and even sweats. It is possible that this may be the true onset of acute PAP but more likely that an infection (PAP patients prone to opportunistic and conventional infection) exacerbates the insidious decline. There may be central cyanosis which worsens on activity and measured pulse oximetry may show SpO_2 in the low 90s falling to the 80s on exercise or stress. Finger clubbing is rare but reported. A very small minority of PAP patients present with relatively rapid onset respiratory failure. Since the earliest published reports of PAP there has been an apparent 'rule of thirds':

- One-third of patients have very mild disease which has only a small impact on their health, may not progress and may even get spontaneously better
- One-third of patients have moderate to severe disease which has a significant impact and may progress and require a series of treatment options (see later)

- One-third of patients suffer very severe symptoms and extreme limitation of function, progress despite treatment and die of chronic hypoxaemia, cor pulmonale or superseding infection.

While the 'rule of thirds' is undoubtedly an oversimplification, it nevertheless stands as a guide to prognosis.

Aetiology and pathophysiology

The key appears to be the function of the alveolar macrophage (AM) which has a central role in both surfactant turnover and in pulmonary host defence, both of which are disordered in PAP. The AM migrates to the pulmonary interstitium and then matures to full functional capacity under the influence of granulocyte monocyte colony stimulating factor (GMCSF). In the absence of proper function of the AM there is a progressive build up of effete surfactant lipoproteins within the alveolar space together with other debris such as foamy and immature AMs. This reduces lung volumes, prevents effective gas exchange across the alveolar-capillary membrane and causes the typical hypxaemia. In the congenital form of PAP there is a fundamental (and fatal) failure of GMCSF receptor sensitivity but in the cases of primary PAP there is an IgG autoantibody to circulating GMCSF so that GMCSF expression is neutralised. This is similar to a mouse model where genetically modified (gene knock-out) homozygotes incapable of expressing GMCSF develop a pulmonary syndrome identical to PAP. It is not possible to explain all cases of secondary PAP along similar lines but is intriguing that the vast majority of cases of secondary PAP are secondary to a haematological malignancy, implying that there may be some as yet unexplained acquired defect of GMCSF sensitivity.

Diagnosis (and differential diagnosis)

The diagnosis is in two parts, one to confirm the clinical features of PAP and two, to look for evidence for provocative processes associated with secondary PAP. The typical gradual onset of exercise intolerance and dyspnoea in the absence of features of heart disease or serious pulmonary disease is suggestive. The plain chest radiograph typically reveals diffuse bilateral airspace shadowing and the absence of features of cardiac disease or lymphadenopathy is important.

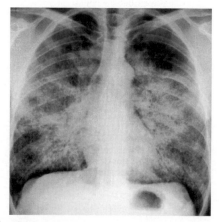

Fig. 18.1.1 CXR of PAP.

Pulmonary function studies often confirm a restrictive lung defect with reduced lung volumes and impaired gas transfer. Routine blood tests are generally normal apart from elevated lactate dehydrogenase (LDH). In fact the elevated LDH is a fairly consistent feature and may even be a useful proxy for adequacy of control of the PAP. Unfortunately many clinical biochemistry laboratories now omit LDH from the standard panel of 'liver function tests' and LDH is obsolete as a 'cardiac enzyme' so it needs to be specifically requested as a marker of PAP. The typical sequence of events is that the patient presents, initial investigations are inconclusive for anything, a course of antibiotics is consumed with no improvement and the chest radiograph which is still abnormal leads on to referral to pulmonary specialist, then high resolution CT scan of the thorax, fibre-optic bronchoscopy (FOB) and diagnostic broncho-alveolar lavage (BAL) which is ideal because this sequence will unequivocally seal the diagnosis in the majority of cases.

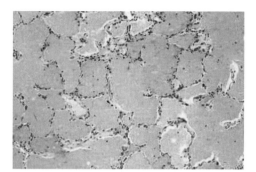

Fig. 18.1.3 Pathology PAS stain of alveoli filled with lipo-protein. (see Plate 15.)

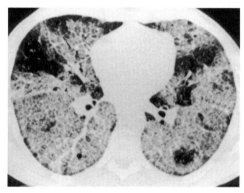

Fig. 18.1.2 Chest CT of PAP.

The CT is almost pathognemonic because the features of 'crazy paving', geographic distribution of airspace shadowing and ground glass opacities and the absence of other features (mediastinal lymphadenopathy, pulmonary fibrosis, cardiac anomalies etc.) are specific for PAP. The extent of PAP features on the CT may be a useful guide to the likely progression or response to therapy. The FOB should reveal normal airways but the BAL is very striking. The saline goes in clear but comes back laden with lipoproteins and macrophages and looks like a milky, yellowish, opalescent colloid which is unique to PAP. Light microscopy of the BAL reveals typical features of periodic acid–Schiff (PAS) staining material with cholesterol clefts and abundant macrophages. The BAL should be sent for microbiological analysis because there is a well-reported tendency to opportunistic infection in PAP, typically with pneumocystis, nocardia and mycobacterium (including atypical mycombacteria). Only rarely should it be necessary to resort to open lung biopsy to confirm the diagnosis of PAP if the other elements are typical. The next question is to differentiate between forms of PAP. Features suggestive of any of the serious conditions associated with secondary PAP should be carefully excluded. The presence of high titres of the anti-GMCSF antibody and the absence of any suggestion of a secondary aetiology confirms primary PAP. This distinction is important in terms of planning and assessing subsequent therapy.

The differential diagnosis includes a text book full of potential causes of dyspnoea, restrictive pulmonary defect and diffuse pulmonary infiltrates but the strikingly individual features of PAP, despite its extreme rarity usually makes the elimination of alternatives relatively easy.

Treatment

Treatment options include:

- Observation.
- Lung lavage:
  - Segmental therapeutic lavage during FOB.
  - Whole lung lavage.
- GMCSF-related:
  - Exogenous GMCSF by injection.
  - Exogenous GMCSF by aerosol inhalation.
- Immunotherapy:
  - Anti-B lymphocyte – using rituximab.
  - Plasmapheresis.

In patients who are stable, with only mild physiological impairment compatible with their personal needs and daily activities, it is reasonable to observe for a while because some patients in this group enjoy spontaneous remission. Where symptoms are more significant and interfere with normal life and work, treatment should be offered. Repeated segmental therapeutic lavage via FOB has been used and can be effective but most patients prefer the greater potency of whole lung lavage (WLL) under general anaesthesia. This is a specialist procedure and should be confined to a small number of dedicated units worldwide. The safety and efficacy depends on the absolute perfect placement of a double-lumen endobronchial tube to separate left and right lungs so that one lung can be adequately ventilated with 100% oxygen (because of the exacerbation of the resting hypoxaemia by single-lung ventilation) while the other is filled and indeed 'ventilated' with saline until all the lipoproteinaceous material is lavaged out and subsequent effluent is clear. This may take 40 or more litres and more than 3 hours. Some of the saline remains in the lung despite attempts at complete drainage so it is essential the patient is kept asleep and ventilated for several hours after the procedure during which time all residual saline is absorbed and the full benefits of the 'washed-out' lung start to manifest. In some cases both lungs are lavaged in sequence. In most cases the WLL has to be repeated several times before satisfactory and prolonged remission is achieved. There are well documented data showing improvement in pulmonary function, resting SpO_2, exercise tolerance and imaging after WLL. Symptoms such as dyspnoea and even cough and chest pain can be relieved by a successful programme of WLL. Most importantly the patient feels better. Though invasive, the procedure is inherently safe provided it is undertaken appropriately and the airway management is secure.

Alternative treatments

A minority of patients either fail to respond to WLL or they re-accumulate alveolar material so quickly that the WLL has to be repeated at excessively short intervals (e.g. less than 1 month). Then alternative options should be considered. The option with by far the most experience so far is the use of exogenous GMCSF. It may seem odd trying to treat an auto-immune disorder with the target of the auto-immunity but John Seymour in Melbourne treated several PAP patients with daily sub-cutaneous GMCSF injections successfully *before* the existence of the anti-GMCSF antibody was appreciated. Around half of that series of patients obtained remission and the non-responders suffered no obvious harm. Many more patients have subsequently demonstrated a similar response rate and absence of serious side effects. The drug is very expensive however, and there have been great difficulties with reliable supply because of pharmaceutical issues. An alternative approach, to save money and to deliver the drug to its actual site of action is to use the aerosol inhalation route and there have been very promising results from this approach (11 out of 12 patients in Mayo Clinic study).

There have been anecdotal reports of use of plasmapheresis to remove the causative antibody or to switch off its production using the selective agent rituximab but much less experience than for WLL and GMCSF.

The ideal management of PAP:
* Confirm the diagnosis of PAP.
* Look for and rule out differential diagnoses or conditions which cause secondary PAP or aggravate primary PAP.
* Confirm the presence of the anti-GMCSF antibody (requires assay at specialist centre).
* Treat – WLL first then move on to aerosol inhaled GMCSF in patients who do not remit after 6 episodes of WLL.

* Consider rituximab or other options if the above does not produce remission.
* Keep all patients under review until long established remission is obtained.

Other things to consider:
* The psychological impact of prolonged chronic dyspnoea and repeated hospital episodes.
* The ever present risk of infection of lung and other sites with conventional and unconventional opportunistic organisms.
* The principles of rare disease management – the need for concentration of effort and increase in knowledge.

Further reading

Beccaria M, Luisetti M, Rodi G, et al. Long-term durable benefit after whole lung lavage in pulmonary alveolar proteinosis. *Eur Respir J* 2004; **23**: 526–531.

Characteristic pulmonary pathology. *Proc. Natl. Acad Sci* 1994; **91**:5592–5596.

Kitamura T, Tanaka N, Watanabe J, et al. Idiopathic pulmonary alveolar proteinosis as an autoimmune disease with neutralizing antibody against granulocyte-macrophage colony stimulating factor. *J Exp Med* 1999; **190**:875–880.

Ramirez RJ, Schult RB, Dutton RE. Pulmonary alveolar proteinosis: a new technique and rationale for treatment. *Arch Intern Med* 1963; **112**:419–431.

Rosen SH, Castleman B, Liebow AA. Pulmonary Alveolar Proteinosis. *N Engl J Med* 1958; **258**:1123–1142.

Seymour JF, Dunn AR, Vincent JM, et al. Efficacy of granulocyte-macrophage colony-stimulating factor in acquired alveolar proteinosis. *N Engl J Med* 1996; **335**: 1924–1925.

Seymour JF, Presneill JJ. Pulmonary alveolar proteinosis: progress in the first 44 years. *Am J Respir Crit Care Med* 2002; **166**: 215–235.

Stanley E, Lieschke GJ, Grail D, et al. Granulocyte/macrophage colony-stimulating factor-deficient mice show no major perturbation of hematopoiesis but develop a characteristic paulmonary pathology. *Proc Natl Acad Sci USA* 1994; **91**: 5592–5596.

Trapnell BC, Whitsett JA, Nakata K. Pulmonary alveolar proteinosis. *N Eng J Med* 2003; **349**: 2527–2539.

Wylam ME, Ten R, Prakash UBS, et al. Aerosol granulocyte-macrophage colony-stimulating factor for pulmonary alveolar proteinosis. *Eur Respir J* 2006; **27**: 585–593.

18.2 Churg–Strauss syndrome

- Churg–Strauss syndrome is a multi-system disorder that typically occurs in severe asthmatics. It is characterised pathologically by granulomata and necrotising eosinophilic vasculitis.
- Estimated annual incidence is 2.4–6.8 per million. Mean age of onset is 48 years. Males and females are equally affected.
- Aetiology is poorly understood; key factors in the development of Churg–Strauss syndrome appear to be atopy and asthma, anti-MPO (myeloperoxidase) autoantibodies and the toxic effects on tissues of activated eosinophils.
- Leukotriene antagonists have been linked to over 160 cases of Churg–Strauss syndrome. It is postulated that this is due to a tapering of corticosteroid dosage in patients with hitherto unsuspected Churg–Strauss syndrome rather than direct drug toxicity.

Disease classification

Individuals with Churg–Strauss syndrome may manifest a spectrum of abnormalities that frequently make the diagnosis a challenging one to confirm. A number of classification schemes have been developed in an attempt to systematize the diagnosis of this condition. The American College of Rheumatology classification criteria (Table 18.2.1) are the most applicable in the clinical setting.

Table 18.2.1 American college of rheumatology classification scheme for Churg–Strauss syndrome

Diagnosis of Churg–Strauss syndrome is likely when at least four criteria are present (sensitivity 85%, specificity 99.7%)
(1) Asthma
(2) Blood eosinophilia >10%
(3) Neuropathy (mononeuropathy or polyneuropathy)
(4) Pulmonary infiltrates
(5) Paranasal sinus abnormality
(6) Extravascular eosinophil infiltration on biopsy

History

Classically, Churg–Strauss syndrome occurs in phases, beginning with asthma, then eosinophilia and ultimately multi-system necrotising vasculitis. Onset of systemic disease is typically heralded by fever, weight loss, fatigue and malaise. Other symptoms reflect the specific pattern of organ involvement.

- Pulmonary: almost all patients have pre-existing asthma and this tends to worsen over the course of the disease. Occasionally there is paradoxical improvement in asthma with the onset of vasculitis. Pulmonary vasculitis, pleuritis and effusions may also lead to symptoms.
- Upper airway: three-quarters of patients have allergic rhinitis. Other disease manifestations include; recurrent sinusitis, nasal polyps, purulent or bloody nasal discharge and, more rarely, septal perforation.
- Neurological: mononeuritis multiplex occurs in up to 65% of cases. The lower limbs are more commonly affected than the upper limbs. Rarer manifestations occur include; ischaemic optic neuropathy, cerebral haemorrhage, psychosis and seizures.

- Cardiac: this occurs in 40% of patients and is associated with significant mortality. May present as: eosinophilic endomyocarditis, coronary vasculitis, valvular dysfunction, or pericarditis. Cardiac failure is the commonest presentation.
- Gastrointestinal: abdominal pain, diarrhoea, and or bleeding occurs in up to 60% of patients. Histological changes can occur throughout the GI tract but are most common in the small intestine and colon. Bowel perforation is the most serious pcomplication.
- Renal glomerulonephritis is common, renal failure however, is rare
- Cutaneous may include: erythema, pustules, vesicles, ulcers, skin nodules or palpable purpura.

Examination

Examination findings are dictated by pattern of organ involvement. The focus of examination in the patient with suspected Churg–Strauss syndrome should be: (1) confirming the diagnosis; (2) identifying sites for biopsy and (3) characterising the extent of organ involvement.

Investigation

As with examination, investigations should be aimed at confirming diagnosis and assessing the pattern and extent of organ involvement.

Laboratory

- FBC characteristically shows a marked eosinophilia (>1500 cells/μL). This may fluctuate and is often masked by corticosteroids.
- ANCA (anti-neutrophil cytoplasmic antibodies) is positive in a peri-nuclear pattern in half of patients with Churg–Strauss syndrome. This should be confirmed by demonstration of anti-MPO antibodies.
- Inflammatory markers (ESR, CRP) will be raised in active disease and provide a useful measure of response to therapy.

Radiology

The most common finding on chest imaging is transient, multi-focal, non-segmental consolidation (Fig. 18.2.1). Other features include; ground glass change, interlobular septal thickening, nodules (which may become miliary), adenopathy and pleural effusions.

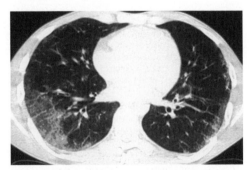

Fig. 18.2.1 HRCT of Churg–Strauss syndrome showing patchy peripheral consolidation, ground glass attenuation and interlobular septal thickening.

Histology

The classical histological lesion of Churg–Strauss is a necrotising small vessel vasculitis with associated granulomata and eosinophilic tissue invasion. It is unusual to find all features present within a single biopsy.

Other

Will depend on organ involvement but should include; urine dipstick, 24-hour urine collection for protein estimation, ECG and echocardiogram.

Differential diagnosis

The range of possible differential diagnoses is wide and is dictated by the predominant phase of the disease.

- Allergic phase: poorly controlled asthma, allergic bronchopulmonary aspergillosis (ABPA), or acute extrinsic allergic alveolitis.
- Eosinophilic phase: eosinophilic pneumonia (acute or chronic), drug induced eosinophilia, helminth infection, Loeffler's syndrome, or ABPA.
- Vasculitic phase: Wegener's granulomatosis, microscopic polyangiitis or polyarteritis nodosa.

AUTHOR'S TIP

The vasculitides are generally considered to be separate diseases. However, in clinical practice there is considerable overlap between these conditions, often to the extent that it is not possible to make a precise diagnosis.

Management

Disease stratification

Five factors predict poor prognosis disease. These are: proteinuria >1g/day, serum creatinine >140 μmoles/l, cardiomyopathy, GI involvement and central nervous system involvement. The presence of one or more of these features should prompt treatment for bad prognosis disease.

Good prognosis disease

Initial management revolves around high dose corticosteroids. Consider oral prednisolone 1mg/kg/day. In severe cases initial treatment with pulsed intravenous methylprednisolone (15mg/kg every 24 hours for 3 days) enables more rapid establishment of disease control

Corticosteroids can be gradually tapered once an improvement in clinical and inflammatory marker parameters is seen. No hard and fast rules are available to guide long term steroid dosage. A proportion of patients with Churg–Strauss syndrome remain on lifelong, low dose corticosteroids.

Bad prognosis disease

Cyclophosphamide in combination with corticosteroids should be used in disease with bad prognostic features. Cyclophosphamide is best tolerated when given intravenously. The typical dosing regimen for IV cyclophosphamide is 600mg/m² every 2 weeks for 4 weeks then monthly for 6 to 12 months.

Maintenance therapy

Once stopped, cyclophosphamide should be replaced with a less toxic immunosuppressant. There is little evidence to guide choice. amcmmAlternatives include; azathioprine, methotrexate, ciclosporin or mycophenolate mofetil.

Once long-term remission is established, immunosuppressant therapy and corticosteroids should be cautiously weaned over a prolonged period.

Treatment failure/disease relapse

For patients with good prognosis disease who fail to respond to corticosteroids or who relapse following initial response, second-line therapy should be with intravenous cyclophosphamide (as for bad prognosis disease).

Patients relapsing after initial successful treatment for bad prognosis disease should undergo re-induction therapy with corticosteroids and cyclophosphamide.

Intravenous immunoglobulins (2mg/kg over two days every month) and/or monthly plasma exchange are accepted therapy for cases refractory to corticosteroids and cyclophosphamide.

Because of the rarity of Churg–Strauss syndrome few treatments have been subject to rigorous evaluation. The biological therapies, rituximab, interferon α and omalizumab have been reported, in small numbers of patients, to be effective in treating Churg–Strauss syndrome and should be considered in cases refractory to conventional therapy.

Prognosis

Generally prognosis in Churg–Strauss syndrome is good. overall remission rates are 81–92 %. Approximately a quarter of patients in remission relapse. Half do so within the first year and the remainder after a mean period of 5 years. Five year survival exceeds 90%. Ten-year survival in a French cohort of patients was 79%.

Complications

Patients with Churg–Strauss syndrome may deteriorate due to: (1) infection; (2) drug toxicity; (3) disease relapse; or (4) new unrelated pathology. Infection can be particularly difficult to discriminate from disease relapse. Relapses often present with a recrudescence of symptoms present at original diagnosis. However, in a proportion of patients, previously uninvolved organs may become affected resulting in new symptoms and signs.

Follow up and disease monitoring

Churg–Strauss syndrome can relapse after many years remission. Furthermore, asthma often remains a significant problem even when systemic vasculitis is controlled. Patients should therefore remain under long term follow-up.

No serological marker exists to discriminate between quiescent and active Churg–Strauss syndrome. Assessment at follow up should consist of clinical history and examination with judicious use of ancillary investigations such as inflammatory markers, FBC (for eosinophilia) and serum ANCA.

Further reading

Bosch X, Guilabert A, Espinosa G et al. Treatment of antineutrophil cytoplasmic antibody associated vasculitis: a systematic review. *JAMA* 2007; **298**: 655–669.

Guillevin L, Lhote F, Gayraud M et al. Prognostic factors in Polyarteritis nodosa and Churg–Strauss syndrome: a prospective study in 342 patients. *Medicine (Baltimore)* 1996; **75**: 17–28.

Keogh KA, Specks U. Churg–Strauss syndrome: clinical presentation, ANCA, and leukotriene antagonists. *Am J Med* 2003; **115**: 284–290.

Masi AT, Hunder GG, Lie JT, et al. American College of Rheumatology 1990 criteria for classification of Churg–Strauss syndrome, allergic granulomatosis and angiitis. *Arthritis Rheum* 1990; **33**: 1094–1100.

Noth I, Strek ME, Leff AR. Churg–Strauss syndrome. *Lancet* 2003; **361**: 587–594.

18.3 Ciliary dyskinesia

Mucociliary clearance is a first-line defence mechanism which protects epithelial surfaces against inhaled particulate matter, including infectious agents. These are trapped in the mucus layer which is cleared by ciliary beating. Primary ciliary dyskinesia (PCD), also known as Kartagener's syndrome (triad of situs inversus, bronchiectasis and sinusitis) and immotile cilia syndrome, is a rare disorder of impaired ciliary activity. Cilia are found on the cell surface in the upper respiratory tract and bronchial tree, fallopian tubes, ductus epididymis and brain ventricles. In the lung they move mucus continually toward the pharynx. Abnormal cilia do not beat in the normal fashion resulting in reduced mucociliary clearance and susceptibility to infection which causes structural lung damage (bronchiectasis).

Cilia are made up of microtubules with outer and inner dynein arms containing ATPase which provides energy for movement at about 14 beats per second (Fig. 18.3.1). Many gene defects have been identified causing cilia abnormalities, the most common being the absence of the outer dynein arms (Fig. 18.3.2). Other defects include absence of the inner dynein arms, absence of radial spokes, absence of central microtubules, abnormal length of cilia, supernumerary microtubules, abnormal basal bodies, total absence of cilia, and anatomically normal but functionally abnormal cilia.

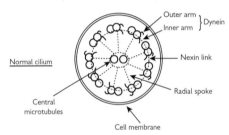

Fig. 18.3.1 Diagram of cilia ultrastructure.

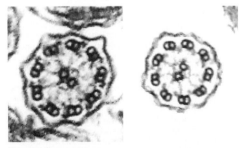

Fig. 18.3.2 (a) Cilia in cross section with normal ultrastructure showing the nine microtubular doublets that form a circle surrounding two central microtubules. (b) A cross section of a cilia with an outer dynein arm defect.

Ciliary dysfunction may also be acquired by pathologies associated with increased airway inflammation such as viral and bacterial infection, allergy and cigarette smoking. Mucociliary clearance is also impaired by abnormal airway surface fluid production (e.g. cystic fibrosis) and abnormal mucus (e.g. watery mucus following viral infection, viscous mucous with bacterial infection).

Epidemiology

PCD inheritance is predominantly autosomal recessive but other inheritance patterns are possible and extensive loci of mutations are suspected. There is equal prevalence in men and women and it affects between one in 15,000 to 60,000 individuals.

Clinical approach

There is considerable variation in the clinical presentation but the most common features are persistent cough (which in the absence of mucociliary clearance is relied on to expel mucus) and recurrent upper and lower respiratory infections.

History: key points

- Neonates may present with respiratory distress and/or pneumonia.
- Chronic cough and daily sputum production.
- Recurrent lower respiratory tract infections are common.
- Patients may report intermittent haemoptysis.
- Wheeze occurs in 20% of cases and individuals may have been previously diagnosed as 'asthmatic'.
- Chronic rhinosinusitis and nasal polyposis are frequently reported.
- Hearing problems with a history of otitis media and grommets in childhood
- Fatigue and headaches may be caused by chronic sinusitis and bronchiectasis; however, hydrocephalus has also been associated with PCD.
- Male infertility may occur due to immotile spermatozoa and women may have subfertility including ectopic pregnancy.
- Other congenital abnormalities occasionally associated with PCD include transposition of the great vessels, cardiac abnormalities, pyloric stenosis and epispadias.

Examination: key points

- Situs inversus occurs in about 50% but only 20–25% of persons with situs inversus have chronic bronchitis and sinusitis.
- Coarse inspiratory and expiratory crackles may be present on auscultation.
- Airflow obstruction with wheeze.
- Conductive hearing loss from chronic otitis media.
- Voice may be nasal in tone due to absence of frontal sinuses.

> **AUTHOR'S TIP**
> PCD is an important differential diagnosis of neonatal respiratory distress, bronchiectasis when the history begins in childhood, atypical asthma in childhood, unusually severe upper airways disease, situs inversus, and male infertility.

Investigations

A diagnosis of PCD is usually made by the identification of immotile, dysmotile or missing cilia.

Saccharin test

A 0.5mm particle of saccharin is placed on the inferior turbinate of the nose and the time taken for it to be tasted in the mouth is measured. The patient is sat quietly with head bent forward and instructed not to sniff or blow their nose. A normal result is less than 30 minutes. This technique is less reliable than other tests and should only be used in patients older than 10 years.

Nasal and exhaled nitric oxide
Nitric oxide (NO) is produced by both the upper and lower respiratory tract. In PCD nasal and exhaled NO are low. Nasal NO <100 ppb indicates need for cilia biopsy. Nasal polyps (obstruction) also causes low nasal NO.

Nasal brush or scrape biopsy
Biopsies from the inferior turbinate of the nose are examined by light microscopy and equipment to determine ciliary beat frequency and pattern. Electron microscopy is used to assess ciliary morphology and orientation. It is important not to confuse primary and secondary abnormalities and tests should be repeated after treatment of infections if there is any uncertainty.

Spermatozoa assessment
Spermatozoa may be examined for motility and ultrastructure however some patients have immotile cilia but normally motile spermatozoa.

Chest radiography
Chest radiograph may be normal or may show peribronchial thickening, hyperinflation, atelectasis and bronchiectasis. Dextrocardia is present in up to 50% of cases.

HRCT
Bronchiectasis predominantly affects the middle and lower lobes.

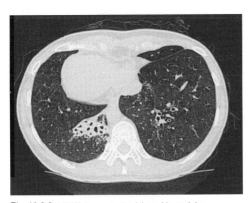

Fig. 18.3.3 HRCT demonstrating bilateral lower lobe bronchiectasis with an area of collapse on the right and dextrocardia.

Pulmonary function tests
Spirometry may show mild to moderate airway obstruction with variable responsiveness to bronchodilators. Gas trapping occurs, and gas transfer values corrected for alveolar volume are usually normal.

Microbiology
Routine culture of sputum should be completed. *Haemophilus influenzae* is common and *Pseudomonas aeruginosa* when bronchiectasis is more severe.

Management
Early diagnosis is important because early treatment may delay the development of bronchiectasis as well as avoid unnecessary otorhinolaryngological procedures. Patients should be managed by multidisciplinary teams in units with a special interest in PCD with paediatric and adult chest

physicians, otolaryngologists, audiologists, physiotherapists, counselling services and fertility clinics.

Respiratory
Daily physiotherapy is essential to prevent exacerbations and progression of disease. Techniques include postural or autogenic drainage, active cycle of breathing technique, flutter devices and exercise programmes. Compliance can be very challenging in paediatric and adolescent patients.

Early and effective antimicrobial treatment of exacerbations is essential to minimise progressive lung damage. Antibiotic courses need to be longer and of higher dose than in people without bronchiectasis (usually 10–14 days minimum). Antibiotics may be oral, intravenous or nebulised and regular sputum surveillance will guide empiric treatment. Antibiotic prophylaxis may be considered in more severe cases.

Variable airflow obstruction should be treated with bronchodilators and inhaled steroids. Routine pneumococcal vaccination and annual influenza vaccinations should be administered. Education on smoking cessation should be provided.

ENT
A multidisciplinary approach should be used to manage upper airways disease with surgical intervention in selected patients for middle ear disease, sinusitis and nasal polyposis. Hearing should be monitored.

Fertility
Infertility is not inevitable however patients with PCD will need access to fertility services.

> **AUTHOR'S TIP**
> Mucus clearance by physical exercise, physiotherapy and flutter devices reduces the rate of infective episodes. Early and effective treatment of exacerbations is essential to minimise progressive lung damage.

Prognosis
The prognosis for PCD is generally good. However a subset of patients exhibit a more rapid decline with considerable morbidity and mortality, and the cause is usually more serious infections causing bronchiectasis, and then chronic infection and more frequent exacerbations.

Further reading
Afzelius B, Stenram U. Prevalence and genetics of immotile-cilia syndrome and left handedness. *Int J Dev Biol* 2006; **50**: 2132.

Bush A, Cole P, Hariri M, et al. Primary ciliary dyskinesia: diagnosis and standards of care. *Eur Resp J* 1998; **12**: 982–988.

Corbelli R, Bringof-Isler B, Amacher A, et al. Nasal nitric oxide measurements to screen children for primary ciliary dyskinesia. *Chest* 2004; **126**: 1054–1059.

Greenstone M, Stanley P, MacWilliam L, et al. Mucociliary function and ciliary ultrastructure in patients presenting with rhinitis at Brompton Hospital Nose Clinic. *Eur J Respir Dis Suppl* 1983; **128**: 457–459.

Jain K, Padley S, Goldstraw E, et al. Primary ciliary dyskinesia in the paediatric population: range and severity of radiological findings in a cohort of patients receiving tertiary care. *Clin Rad* 2007; **62**: 986–993.

Kennedy M, Noone P, Leigh M, et al. High Resolution CT of patients with primary ciliary dyskinesia. *Am J Roentgenol* 2007; **188**: 1232–1238.

Noone P, Leigh M, Sannuti A, et al. Primary ciliary dyskinesia: diagnostic and phenotypic features. *Am J Respir Crit Care Med* 2004; **169**: 459–467.

Wilson R. Secondary ciliary dysfunction. *Clin Sci (Lond)* 1988; **75**: 113–120.

18.4 Pulmonary Langerhans' cell histiocytosis

Pulmonary Langerhans' cell histiocytosis (PLCH) is a rare interstitial lung disease (ILD), characterised by the presence of granulomas containing large numbers of Langerhans' cells (LC) that invade and destroy distal bronchioles.

The clinical spectrum of Langerhans' cell histiocytosis (LCH) is large, ranging from an acute disseminated form, which has a very poor prognosis and occurs in children, to a more benign form of the disease where lesions are localised in single tissues. LCH can be classified according to the level of the infiltration to organs. It may affect a single organ, i.e. the lung, bone, lymph nodes, or multiple organs.

Epidemiology

PLCH affects 2–5 per 1,000,000 individuals per year and accounts for fewer than 5% of ILDs diagnosed by surgical lung biopsy.

Numerous studies have shown that over 90% of patients have a history of heavy smoking, and adding to this, the bronchiolar distribution of the pathologic lesion supports the possibility that an inhaled antigen is involved in the pathogenesis of the disease.

Although no precise epidemiological data are available, it has a peak incidence in young white adults between 20–40 years old. The relative frequency of disease in males in comparison to females is unclear, as evidence is mainly from case series rather than inclusive trials. Early studies suggested a male predominance. However, more recently an equal incidence or slight predominance in women has been found. This may be due to the increased prevalence of female smokers over recent years.

Clinical presentation

The presentation of PLCH varies:

- 66% patients present with persistent respiratory symptoms, commonly dyspnoea and a non-productive cough.
- 25% of patients are asymptomatic and the disease is revealed on a routine chest radiograph.
- 10% patients present with spontaneous pneumothorax.

Constitutional symptoms (33%), haemoptysis (<5%) and rarely chest pain may occur.

Physical examination is commonly normal.

The affect of PLCH on pulmonary function depends on the stage of disease and the abnormalities present. Restrictive, obstructive and mixed patterns have been observed. Approximately 50% patients show an obstructive pattern, particularly patients with cystic lesions from long standing disease. As most ILDs show a restrictive pattern, the presence of obstructive abnormalities helps in the diagnosis of PLCH. However, obstructive changes may also be a result of co-existing COPD. The most commonly described abnormality in pulmonary function is a reduction in carbon monoxide transfer factor (70–100% patients). However, it is difficult to determine the effect of the disease from that of cigarette smoking.

PLCH is isolated to the lungs in more than 85% of patients.

Extra-pulmonary manifestations (<15%) include:

- Bone pain (20% of patients) due to lesions often in the skull, ribs and pelvis.
- Polyuria and polydipsia from pituitary involvement producing diabetes insipidus.
- Abdominal discomfort due to infiltration of liver and spleen.
- Skin rashes and adenopathy.

Investigation and diagnosis

Radiography

Abnormalities seen depend on disease stage as the lesions are thought to evolve from nodules to cavitary nodules into thick walled cysts, thin walled cysts and finally fibrosis.

A normal chest radiograph seen in <10% patients.

Typical chest radiograph findings:

- Disease is found in upper and middle lung fields, bilateral, diffuse, with sparing of the costophrenic angles. Lung volumes appear normal or increased, unlike the reduced volumes seen in other ILDs (with exception of lymphangioleiomyomatosis (LAM)).
- Recent onset – poorly demarcated micronodular lesions (<5mm).
- Medium term– reticulonodular shadows with underlying cystic lesions.
- Long standing – cystic cavities (few nodules). Appearance is indistinguishable from advanced emphysema and LAM.

HRCT

This allows the nature and distribution of parenchymal abnormalities to be excellently determined, and is capable of showing disease in patients whose chest radiographs are normal. HRCT frequently shows that reticular abnormalities on chest radiograph are actually shadows produced by multiple cysts (Fig.18.4.1).

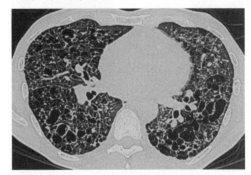

Fig. 18.4.1 HRCT showing multiple cysts in a patient with advanced LCH.

Typically abnormalities are seen interspersed in normal parenchyma, and lesions are equally distributed between central and peripheral portions of the lung with partial sparing of the bases.

NB sparing of lung bases and an irregular shape of cysts help distinguish PLCH from LAM.

In cases where ground-glass attenuation and/or adenopathy are seen, biopsy may be needed to establish diagnosis.

Biopsy

Biopsy has largely been replaced by HRCT due to the high sensitivity of imaging. Brochoalveolar lavage, transbronchial biopsy, or surgical lung biopsy may be performed to provide morphological evidence for diagnosis. Samples show an increased number of LC, which can be detected under light microscope, positive for CD1 antigen or S-100 staining. If the proportion of CD1a-stained cells is greater than 5%, PLCH is very likely. However, this is not particularly helpful as an increased CD1a level is also found in heavy smokers and other ILDs. Under electron microscopy, characteristic intracytoplasmic Birbeck granules may be seen. VATS biopsy is mainly used to exclude alternative diagnostic possibilities (Fig.18.4.2).

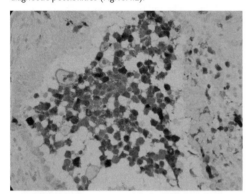

Fig. 18.4.2 Lung biopsy with Langerhans cells labelled with labelled for S-100 protein. (See Plate 16.)

Differential diagnosis

The ability to establish a diagnosis of PLCH depends on the clinical and radiological findings.

The diagnosis is simple in young smokers presenting with nodular and cystic lesions.

If a patient has systemic symptoms and prominent cavitary nodules the following diseases must be considered: mycobacterial infection, sarcoidosis, silicosis, Wegener's disease, cavitary metastatic lesions, alveolar cell carcinoma, septic emboli, or excavated pneumocystis.

LAM must be distinguished from PLCH in women with purely cystic lesions.

Treatment and prognosis

There are no reliable guidelines regarding treatment and prognosis due to the large variation in outcome seen across patients. Generally, PLCH patients' life expectancy is shorter than that of the general population.

Poor prognostic factors include: a very young or very old age at onset of disease, ongoing systemic symptoms, recurrent pneumothoraces and extrapulmonary features (excluding bone involvement).

It is uncommon for the disease to progress to advanced pulmonary fibrosis and death. Approximately 10–20%

patients will deteriorate with progressive respiratory insufficiency and cor pulmonale. 30–40% will regress to a lesser extent to be left with persisting thin walled cysts. 50% patients will undergo partial or complete resolution of radiographic abnormalities. Long-term follow-up of all patients is necessary, as even after years of remission, new nodules may form, causing lung function to again deteriorate.

Patients' outcome is likely to improve with the cessation of smoking, therefore this should strongly be encouraged.

Corticosteroids are thought to help accelerate resolution of the disease, particularly in symptomatic patients with systemic symptoms, but precise benefits remain unclear.

Chemotherapeutic agents such as vinblastine and cyclophosphamide are used to treat diffuse LCH in children. However limited data is available on their efficacy in PLCH.

Lung transplant has been successful in patients with advanced disease causing severe respiratory impairment, or severe pulmonary arterial hypertension. Interestingly, PLCH has later recurred in the transplanted lung in several cases. Although this complication reduces the transplanted lung's function, the effect on overall survival has not been established.

AUTHOR'S TIPS

- Lack of exposure to smoking and age >60 make diagnosis unlikely.
- Typical cases show impaired diffusing capacity and upper-lobe predominance.
- Smoking cessation is vital to treatment
- 50% patients undergo resolution. Death from disease is rare.

Further reading

Caminati A, Harari S. Smoking-related interstitial pneumonias and pulmonary Langerhans cell histiocytosis. *Proc Am Thorac Soc* 2006; **3**: 299–306.

Kim CK, Park BP. Pulmonary Langerhans' cell histiocytosis presented with recurrent pneumothorax. *Interact CardioVasc Thorac Surg* 2006; **5**: 512–513.

Tazi A, Soler P, Hance AJ. Adult pulmonary Langerhans' cell histiocytosis. *Thorax* 2000; **55**: 405–416.

Vassallo R, Ryu JH, Colby TV, *et al.* Medical progress: pulmonary Langerhans'-cell histiocytosis. *N Engl J Med* 2003; **342**(26): 1969–1978.

Vassallo R, Ryu JH, Schroeder DR, *et al.* Clinical outcomes of Pulmonary Langerhans'-cell histiocytosis in adults. *N Engl J Med* 2002; **346**(7): 484–490.

Vassallo R, Jensen EA, Colby TV, *et al.* The Overlap Between Respiratory Bronchiolitis and Desquamative Interstitial Pneumonia in Pulmonary Langerhans Cell Histiocytosis. *Chest* 2003; **124**(4): 1199–1205.

18.5 Lymphangioleiomyomatosis

Lymphangioleiomyomatosis (LAM) is a rare cystic lung disease which almost exclusively affects women. The disease is associated with angiomyolipomas, benign tumours generally occurring in the kidneys and abnormalities of the axial lymphatics.

Epidemiology
LAM affects 1–2 per million of the general population (sporadic-LAM) but is common in tuberous sclerosis complex (TSC-LAM) where lung cysts are present in up to 40% of adult women.

Presentation and clinical features
Most patients present between 20 and 50 years of age with dyspnoea or pneumothorax. Cough and wheezing are common in LAM and can lead to misdiagnosis of more common conditions. Diagnosis may follow CT scanning performed for other purposes. Less often haemorrhage from renal angiomyolipoma or symptomatic abdominal or pelvic lymphatic masses are the first symptom. LAM is exacerbated by, and may present during, pregnancy.

Missed presentations of LAM
- 'Emphysema' in younger women.
- 'Asthma' unresponsive to therapy.
- Pneumothorax during pregnancy.
- Respiratory symptoms in TSC.

Cysts develop in the lungs causing dyspnoea in most patients. Pneumothorax occurs in two thirds of patients and is frequently recurrent. Occlusion of the axial lymphatics results in lymphadenopathy, cystic abdominal and pelvic masses (lymphangioleiomyomas), chylous pleural effusions and ascites. Abdominal discomfort, bloating, or pressure symptoms occur in up to 20%.

Half of patients have one or more angiomyolipomas, benign tumours of smooth muscle, fat, and blood vessels. Angiomyolipomas occur mainly in the kidneys and can bleed when large. A small number of patients have meningiomas.

Investigation and diagnosis
Plain radiographs may be normal in early disease or show interstitial markings with preserved lung volumes. HRCT scanning shows lung cysts with thin walls evenly distributed within normal lung parenchyma (Fig. 18.5.1). The cysts become more numerous as the disease progresses. 80% of patients have abnormalities on abdominal imaging: 50% with renal angiomyolipomas and a significant number with lymphadenopathy, lymphangioleiomyomas, or chylous ascites. Abdominal CT is recommended to identify these complications, to explain abdominal symptoms and to screen for angiomyolipoma which has a characteristic appearance due to its fat content (Fig. 18.5.2).

Lung function tests may be normal in early disease but airflow obstruction with impaired gas transfer is commonly seen. Pleural complications and their treatment may lead to restrictive changes. Pathological samples show abnormal smooth muscle type cells (LAM cells) proliferating in the lung to form nodules which protrude into small airways and line the walls of cysts (Fig. 18.5.3). Biopsy of extra-thoracic lymphatics shows tissue infiltrated LAM cells.

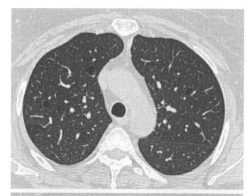

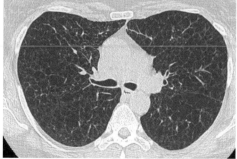

Fig. 18.5.1 HRCT of patients with LAM. Upper panel is asymptomatic disease with minimal cysts (arrowed) and normal parenchyma. Lower panel shows extensive disease.

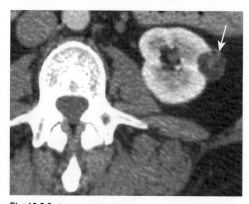

Fig. 18.5.2 Angiomyolipoma in the left kidney. Characteristic mixed attenuation tumour (arrow) of low density suggesting presence of fat.

Although morphology is characteristic, immunostaining for the melanoma-related protein GP100 with the antibody HMB45 is a helpful marker especially in early disease. LAM cells are also smooth muscle actin and often oestrogen and progesterone-receptor positive.

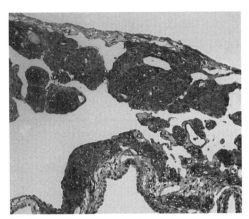

Fig. 18.5.3 Lung biopsy showing LAM nodules stained with α-smooth muscle actin.

Diagnostic criteria for LAM have not been formally agreed, however a suggested scheme is:

Definite LAM
• characteristic HRCT.

Plus one or more of:
• Lung or extra-pulmonary biopsy.
• Angiomyolipoma.
• Chylous collection.
• Tuberous sclerosis.

Probable LAM (consider biopsy)
• Characteristic HRCT plus compatible clinical history only.

Differential diagnosis

Emphysema may mimic LAM and vice-versa. A cystic lung appearance on CT can be seen in LCH, metastatic endometrial sarcoma, Birt–Hogg–Dubé syndrome, light chain deposition disease and lymphocytic interstitial pneumonia.

It is important to consider TSC in LAM patients. The diagnosis can be overlooked, particularly as 2/3 of TSC patients have no family history of TSC and many have no learning difficulties and only minor skin involvement.

Clinical course

Many patients develop progressive airflow obstruction although rates are variable, on average, FEV$_1$ falls by 120 ml/year. Pneumothorax and chylous effusions may occur and can be recurrent. Respiratory failure may develop and overall survival is between 70–95% at 10 years. Some patients with sporadic LAM and many with TSC-LAM do not have progressive disease. At present there are no prognostic markers with which to predict the clinical course.

Management

General measures: patients should avoid exogenous oestrogen including the combined oral contraceptive and HRT.

Pregnancy is associated with an increased risk of pneumothorax and premature birth: patients should be warned of this. Those with airflow obstruction should be given a trial of bronchodilators. Smoking cessation and pulmonary rehabilitation are likely to be of benefit.

Patients should be warned of the symptoms of pneumothorax which is recurrent in 2/3 and early liaison with thoracic surgeons is suggested. Chylous effusions may also require surgical treatment if symptomatic.

Anti-oestrogen therapies have been used, most commonly progesterone but also the GnRH agonists, tamoxifen and oophorectomy. Although no prospective studies support their use.

Clinical trials of newer agents including the mTOR inhibitor rapamycin are currently underway and participation in clinical trials is a potential option for patients.

Angiomyolipomas can bleed, resulting in severe haemorrhage requiring nephrectomy. Bleeding is associated with larger size, rapid growth and aneurysmal blood vessels. If present, angiomyolipoma should be screened regularly to detect growth. Those >4cm should be examined twice yearly and if symptomatic or enlarging rapidly; evaluated for possible embolisation or nephron sparing surgery. Angiomyolipomas may need specialist management especially in TSC-LAM patients who almost always have angiomyolipomas which are often large and multiple.

Lung transplantation has been used for severe disease. Referral criteria have not been formalised although NYHA functional class III or IV, severe impairment in lung function and exercise capacity (VO$_2$ max <50%) with hypoxemia at rest are often used. Previous pleural surgery is associated with increased peri-operative bleeding but has no effect on overall survival. Although LAM may occasionally recur in the graft this does not affect the outcome and survival data is at least as good as other indications for transplant.

LAM in tuberous sclerosis complex

LAM is common in women with TSC with 40% having cystic lung disease if examined by CT. Although less than 5% have symptoms some have severe disease and develop respiratory failure. These patients should be managed in the standard way including transplant evaluation where appropriate. Asymptomatic patients identified by screening should probably avoid oestrogen and receive advice regarding pneumothorax and pregnancy.

TSC-LAM patients are likely to have other problems including epilepsy, angiomyolipoma, and skin lesions requiring specialist or multidisciplinary assessment, possibly though a TSC clinic.

Further reading

Johnson SR. Lymphangioleiomyomatosis. *Eur Respir J* 2006; **27**: 1056–1065.

Juvet SC, McCormack FX, Kwiatkowski DJ, *et al.* Molecular pathogenesis of lymphangioleiomyomatosis: lessons learned from orphans. *Am J Respir Cell Mol Biol* 2007; **36**: 398–408.

NHLBI LAM Registry Group. The NHLBI lymphangioleiomyomatosis registry: characteristics of 230 patients at enrollment. *Am J Respir Crit Care Med* 2006; **173**: 105–111.

18.6 Primary tracheal tumours

Definition
Primary tracheal tumours arise within the trachea itself and should be distinguished from other adjacent or distant tumours that have simply extended or metastasised to the trachea.

Tracheal tumours can be either malignant (90%) or benign (10%).

Epidemiology
Possibly as result of heightened local immunosurveillance, primary tracheal tumours are rare and constitute less than 0.2% of all respiratory tract malignancies.

It is estimated that there are just 2.6 new cases per million population per year.

Pathology
More than 30 different tumours have been described, originating within the surface epithelium, salivary glands or mesenchymal structures of the trachea.

Squamous cell carcinoma (SCC) accounts for 50% of cases and is most commonly found in male smokers in their sixth and seventh decades. The tumour grows rapidly and has metastasised in one-third of patients by the time of presentation.

Adenoid cystic carcinoma (ACC) is the second most common tumour (20%), has no male/female predominance, is not associated with smoking and most often presents in the fourth and fifth decades. ACCs are slow growing and metastasise less commonly than SCCs.

Clinical presentation
Upper airways obstruction
- Patients present with dyspnoea, inspiratory stridor or expiratory wheeze and are often initially misdiagnosed as having asthma or COPD.
- Tumours are typically advanced at presentation as symptoms only occur once the tracheal lumen is compromised by 50–75%.

Mucosal irritation and ulceration
SCCs can present with cough or haemoptysis and as a result may be diagnosed earlier.

Direct invasion of adjacent structures
- Involvement of the right recurrent laryngeal nerve may lead to a right vocal cord palsy and hoarseness.
- Dysphagia and superior vena caval obstruction (SVCO) can also result from local tumour spread.

Investigations
Pulmonary function tests
- PEFR is characteristically disproportionately lower than FEV_1 in upper airways obstruction. This can be quantified by an Empey index > 10, where:

- Empey index = FEV_1 (mls)/PEFR (L/min).
- Flow-volume loops demonstrate flattening of both inspiratory and expiratory phases. This is because of the fixed nature of the upper airway obstruction typically associated with tracheal tumours.

Radiology
- CXR is often falsely reassuring but can reveal narrowing, distortion or deviation of the trachea, mediastinal widening or evidence of metastatic spread.
- CT with multiplanar reconstruction provides an excellent non-invasive tool for assessing tumour stage and operability.
- MRI offers no clear advantages over CT at present.

Bronchoscopy
- Bronchoscopy is essential for both obtaining a tissue diagnosis and for adequately assessing tumour stage.
- Flexible bronchoscopy can be safely performed in the majority of individuals. However biopsies should be avoided in patients with severe airway compromise as consequent haemorrhage and oedema may convert critical narrowing to complete upper airway obstruction.
- Rigid bronchoscopy allows biopsies to be performed whilst maintaining upper airway stability and ventilation and is thus the investigation of choice in patients with severe airway compromise.

Acute management
Patients occasionally present with acute respiratory distress at their initial presentation. It is essential that airway

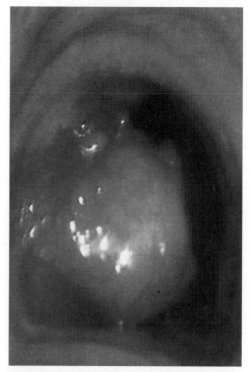

Fig. 18.6.2 Tracheal tumour visible at flexible bronchoscopy. (See Plate 17.)

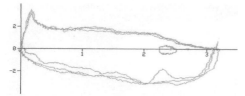

Fig. 18.6.1 Flow volume loop demonstrating flattening of both inspiratory and expiratory limbs.

control is optimised early, using the minimum number of interventions.

- Nebulised racemic adrenaline may help acutely reduce local airway inflammation and oedema.
- Intravenous dexamethasone can similarly provide more sustained anti-inflammatory effects.
- Inhaled Heliox, a oxyhelium mixture in which relatively dense nitrogen is replaced by lower density helium, helps temporarily reduce the work of breathing.
- CT should ideally be performed, although many patients will be unable to tolerate this.
- Flexible bronchoscopy should be avoided in life-threatening upper airway obstruction.
- Rigid bronchoscopy under general anaesthesia, however, can both obtain tissue for diagnosis and help alleviate upper airway obstruction through a variety of endoscopic resection techniques (see Endoscopic interventions).
- Radiotherapy and endobronchial stenting are contraindicated until the tumour has been fully characterised and staged, as both interventions can preclude later curative surgical resection.

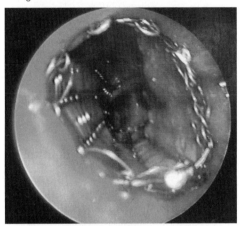

Fig. 18.6.3 View seen at bronchoscopy following endoscopic resection and stenting. (See Plate 18.)

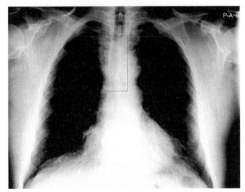

Fig. 18.6.4 CXR showing presence of a tracheal stent.

Long-term management

A histological diagnosis must be obtained in all patients, as benign and malignant tumours cannot be distinguished radiologically. Subsequent treatment options include:

Surgery (i.e. complete resection with tracheal reconstruction)

All patients must be adequately staged and considered for surgery at an experienced centre. Although up to 70% of patients have resectable disease, many are denied this potentially curative treatment option through a lack of awareness.

Contraindications to surgery include:

- Extensive local lymphatic spread.
- Mediastinal invasion of unresectable organs.
- Distant metastases.
- Involvement of >50% of the trachea.
- Prior radiotherapy >60Gy to the mediastinum.

External beam radiotherapy

As both SCC and ACC are radiosensitive, external beam radiotherapy can be utilised as either:

- Adjuvant therapy following surgery, to ensure clear resection margins.
- Palliative therapy, in conjunction with endoscopic debridement, in patients with inoperable disease.

Although no clear RCT evidence exists it is commonly believed that radiotherapy is inferior to surgery in achieving complete disease clearance.

Endoscopic interventions

The following endoscopic techniques can alleviate upper airway obstruction and thus provide long term palliative relief. All are possible via rigid bronchoscopy, whilst some can also be delivered via flexible bronchoscopy.

- Endoscopic debridement using biopsy forceps.
- Diathermy or electrocautery/radiofrequency ablation.
- Cryotherapy.
- Laser photoresection.
- Brachytherapy, particularly as second line therapy.
- Endoscopic stenting is typically reserved for extrinsic compression of the trachea, but also has a role in the palliative management of intraluminal obstruction.

Prognosis

Given its rarity there is relatively little published data on survival in patients with primary tracheal tumours. It is well recognised, however, that patients with ACC have a more favourable outcome than those with SCC. A large UK based postal survey examining patients receiving a variety of treatment modalities suggested five-year survival rates of 80% and 25% for ACC and SCC respectively.

> **AUTHOR'S TIPS**
>
> - Always consider upper airway obstruction in patients with 'late onset asthma' or 'COPD' who fail to respond to bronchodilator therapy.
> - Ensure all patients with primary tracheal tumours are fully staged and actively considered for curative surgery before embarking on palliative therapy.

Further reading

Gelder CM, Hetzel MR. Primary tracheal tumours: a national survey. *Thorax* 1993; **48**(7):688–692.

Henning A, Gaissert MD. Primary tracheal tumours. *Chest Surg Clin N Am* 2003; **13**: 247–256.

Macchiarini P. Primary tracheal tumours. *Lancet Oncology* 2006; **7**:83–91.

18.7 Pulmonary arteriovenous malformations

Pulmonary arteriovenous malformations (PAVMs) are thin-walled abnormal vessels which replace normal capillaries between the pulmonary arterial and venous circulations (Fig. 18.7.1) providing a right-to-left (R-L) shunt.

Epidemiology

Association with HHT

More than 90% of macroscopic PAVMs are associated with hereditary haemorrhagic telangiectasia. HHT affects 1 in 5000–8000 and is inherited as an autosomal dominant trait, caused by mutations in one of at least 5 different genes. HHT is usually diagnosed clinically, with 3 of 4 separate criteria (nosebleeds; telangiectasia; visceral involvement and/or family history) required for a definite diagnosis of HHT. Most HHT patients are unaware of their diagnosis but

- commonly experience nosebleeds (>90%) and/or have a family history of recurrent nosebleeds;
- display mucocutaneous telangiectasia (Fig. 18.7.2) which may not be prominent until over 40ys;
- commonly have silent visceral AVMs including PAVMs (50%), hepatic AVMs (30%), and cerebral AVMs (10%);
- rarely, have additional genotype-specific features (pulmonary hypertension; juvenile polyposis).

Other PAVMs

Macroscopic PAVMs occasionally occur sporadically (when they are usually single) or secondary to surgically generated cavopulmonary shunts.

Microscopic PAVMs merge into the spectrum of functional right-to-left shunting associated most commonly with the hepatopulmonary syndrome.

Natural history

Most PAVMs appear to develop at puberty, though some are present in childhood. Affected individuals are at risk of four main complications:

- hypoxaemia (due to R-L shunt);
- paradoxical emboli (due to R-L shunt): by aged 65ys, a third of PAVM patients will have suffered a stroke or brain abscess;
- haemorrhage: this affects fewer than 10%, but can be life-threatening, especially during pregnancy;
- Migraine.

Respiratory symptoms and PAVM severity do not appear to influence the risk of later stroke/abscess or pregnancy complications.

Clinical approach

The aims of management are to

- reduce the risk of PAVM complications;
- establish whether HHT is present in the family.

Establishing a diagnosis of HHT will facilitate PAVM screening of relatives, and appropriate management of HHT for all affected individuals. This should be performed without introducing unnecessary alarm life expectancy in HHT patients over the age of 60ys is normal.

History key points

- PAVM: dyspnoea, haemoptysis; stroke, brain abscess, TIAs, migraine.
- HHT: nosebleeds; GI bleeds; liver disease; epilepsy.
- FH: Pedigree to establish presence of these.
- Potential future pregnancies (for women).

Examination – key points

- General: cyanosis, clubbing (for R-L shunt).
- HHT telangiectasia (lips; oral cavity, fingers; nose).
- Dental hygiene (risk of brain abscess).
- CVS: BP (especially if nose bleeds), JVP, heart sounds and peripheral oedema (concern re pulmonary hypertension).

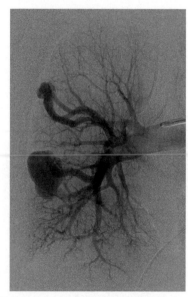

Fig. 18.7.1

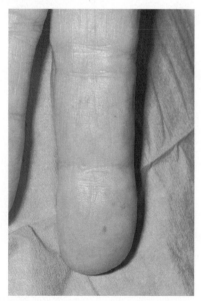

Fig. 18.7.2

- RS: Bruits (PAVM).
- Abdo: liver bruit (hepatic AVM).
- CNS: focal neurology indicative of earlier CVA.

Investigations

- Radiology to confirm PAVM structure (CXR, dedicated CT scan) and amenability to embolisation.
- Assessment of hypoxaemia: recommend comparison of erect and supine SaO_2 after 10 mins in each posture to detect orthodeoxia.
- Measurement of R-L shunt: perfusion scan or 100% O_2 rebreathe shunt study (beware air bubbles in blood gas syringe leading to false positive).
- Haematological investigations for polycythaemia, anaemia.
- Consider echocardiogram if clinical evidence of pulmonary hypertension.
- Consider cerebral MRI if neurological symptoms (?less stable cerebral AVM), or if more than one family member has had a cerebral haemorrhage (? HHT-independent familial Berry aneurysms).
- Consider hepatic AVM screening particularly if evidence of pulmonary hypertension or cardiac failure.

Differential diagnosis

- Microscopic shunt consider HPS/liver disease.
- Single PAVM and no FH: consider sporadic.

Management

Dental hygiene

Advise to optimise dental hygiene and use antibiotic prophylaxis for dental and surgical procedures (reapproved post NICE).

Embolisation treatment

Patients with PAVMs large enough for embolisation should be offered embolisation by an experienced interventional radiologist to reduce stroke/abscess risk, and improve oxygenation if hypoxaemic. These considerations do not apply to individuals with severe pulmonary arterial hypertension.

Pregnancy advice

Inform obstetric team that while most PAVM/HHT pregnancies proceed normally, pregnancy should be considered high risk. Inform patient that any haemoptysis or sudden severe dyspnoea may be a medical emergency and should precipitate admission.

Other HHT considerations

Manage nasal and gastrointestinal bleeding, and other visceral involvement symptomatically by appropriate specialists.

Educate patients (and medical practitioners) that screening for cerebral or hepatic involvement is the subject of intense debate and is currently not offered in the UK except in circumstances listed earlier.

When patients ask about their children:

- Each child of an HHT-affected parent has a 50% chance of inheriting HHT: add 'possible HHT' to medical records. Consider for all PAVM patients' children unless clear alternative cause of PAVMs.
- The overwhelming majority of HHT-affected children are completely healthy.
- Aim to screen for PAVMs post puberty. Early PAVM development is usually symptomatic resulting in breathlessness or dizziness that prompts investigation, diagnosis and treatment.

HHT genes

- *Endoglin* (HHT type I) most common cause of PAVMs: also associated with higher risk of cerebral AVMs.
- *ACVRL-1/ALK-1* (HHT type 2) most common genotype for HHT patients with pulmonary hypertension.
- *Smad4* (JP-HT) causes combined HHT–juvenile polyposis syndrome: If *Smad4* mutation detected, consult gastroenterologists for management as juvenile polyposis (inherited GI cancer) family.
- *HHT3, HHT4 and further genes*: mutation screening not yet available.

Due to late onset penetrance, no child of an HHT-affected relative should be told they do not have HHT without a molecular diagnosis, but if no gene mutation is found in the family, this does not mean that HHT is not present (maximum test sensitivity ≈80%).

Patient FAQs

Can I fly? Yes consider DVT prophylaxis

Are there any self-help groups? Yes:

- UK Telangiectasia Self help group: http://www.telangiectasia.co.uk, email info@ telangiectasia.co.uk
- HHT Foundation International: http://www.hht.org– highly informative website, advice sometimes more applicable to North American healthcare, particularly with regard to cerebral AVM screening.

Further reading

Buscarini E, Plauchu H, Garcia Tsao G, et al. Liver involvement in hereditary hemorrhagic telangiectasia: consensus recommendations. *Liver Int* 2006; **26**: 1040–1046.

Cottin V, Plauchu H, Bayle JY, et al. Pulmonary arteriovenous malformations in patients with hereditary hemorrhagic telangiectasia. *Am J Resp Crit Care Med* 2004; **169**:994–1000.

Govani PS, Shovlin CL. Hereditary haemorrhagic telangiectasia. *Eur J Hum Genet* 2009 (accepted subject to revisons).

Kjeldsen AD, Vase P, Green A. Hereditary hemorrhagic telangiectasia (HHT): a population-based study of prevalence and mortality in Danish HHT patients. *J Intern Med* 1999; **245**: 31–39.

Pierucci P, Murphy J, Henderson KJ, et al. Screening for pulmonary arteriovenous malformations: twenty-seven-year experience. *Chest* 2008; **133**: 653–61.

Post MC, van Gent MWF, Snijder RJ, et al. Pulmonary arteriovenous malformations and migrane: a new vision. *Respiration* 2008; **76**:228-33.

Shovlin CL, Guttmacher AE, Buscarini E, et al. Diagnostic criteria for hereditary hemorrhagic telangiectasia (Rendu-Osler-Weber syndrome). *Am J Med Genet* 2000; **91**: 66–67.

Shovlin CL, Jackson JE, Bamford KB, et al. Primary determinants of ischaemic stroke and cerebral abscess are unrelated to severity of pulmonary arteriovenous malformations in HHT. *Thorax* 2008; **63**: 259–266.

Shovlin CL, Sodhi V, McCarthy A, et al. Estimates of maternal risks of pregnancy for women with hereditary haemorrhagic telangiectasia (HHT, Osler-Weber-Rendu syndrome): suggested approach for obstetric services. *BJOG* 2008; **115**:1108–1115.

Shovlin CL, Tighe HC, Zukotynski/Chan Chow, et al. Embolization of PAVMs: no consistent effect on pulmonary artery pressure. *ERJ* 2008, in press.

van Gent MWF, Post MC, Luermans JG, et al. Screenng for pulmonary arteriovenous malformations: using transthoracic contrast echocardiography: a prospective study. *Eur Respire J* 2008; **33**: 85–91.

Zukotynski K,Chan RP, Chow CM, et al. Contact echocardiography grading predicts pulmonary arteriovenous malformations on CT. *Chest* 2007; **132**: 18–23.

18.8 Pulmonary amyloidosis

Definition

Amyloidosis encompasses a heterogeneous collection of diseases, characterised by local or systemic over-expression of amyloidogenic precursor proteins. These proteins undergo abnormal conformational changes, resulting in local or systemic deposition of an insoluble fibrillar form that subsequently causes organ dysfunction. Pulmonary involvement occurs in up to 50% of amyloidosis cases, although it often does not contribute significantly to overall disease burden.

Classification and pathophysiology

The various forms of amyloidosis can be classified by their precursor proteins:

- AL amyloidosis results from production of monoclonal immunoglobulin light chains (typically κ or λ chains).
- AA amyloidosis occurs following production of acute phase serum amyloid A in response to chronic inflammatory conditions.
- ATTR amyloidosis is an autosomal dominant condition that leads to production of mutant transthyretin (TTR) protein.
- $A\beta_2M$ amyloidosis is due to accumulation of β_2 microglobulin in patients receiving dialysis.

Despite this wide variation in precursor proteins, the resulting insoluble protein deposit in amyloidosis is structurally alike in all forms of the disease, comprising β-pleated sheets complexed with serum amyloid P (SAP) and glycosaminoglycans (GAG). This configuration can resist proteolysis and is thus extremely stable, to the detriment of the organ affected.

Whilst all forms of amyloidosis can lead to systemic disease, AL amyloidosis is unique in that it can be associated with either local ('organ-limited') or systemic disease.

- Local AL disease results from localised clonal expansion of B cells or plasma cells. The light chains secreted by these cells do not circulate outside of their target organ, but instead produce local amyloid deposits.
- Systemic AL disease develops following the release of monoclonal light chains into the circulation by bone marrow-derived plasma cells. The cause of plasma cell expansion can range from a low grade plasma cell dyscrasia (i.e. primary systemic amyloidosis) to an overt malignancy (i.e. amyloidosis associated with myeloma).

Clinical manifestations

Although pulmonary involvement can occur with AA and ATTR disease, this is usually an incidental finding and is rarely of any clinical significance.

Conversely, AL amyloidosis can present in a number of ways, some of which can overlap

- Laryngeal amyloidosis (local AL) presents with hoarseness, stridor or dyspnoea as a result of nodular or diffuse infiltrative changes within the larynx.
- Tracheobronchial amyloidosis (TBA) (local AL) appears as discrete nodules that can macroscopically mimic tumour (28%), as submucosal infiltrative plaques (44%) or as cirumferential wall thickening (28%). All forms cause upper airway obstructive symptoms (cough, haemoptysis, dyspnoea, and recurrent infections) and are not infrequently initially misdiagnosed as asthma.

- Nodular pulmonary amyloidosis (local AL) presents with solitary or multiple discrete parenchymal nodules which range from 0.4–15cm and are typically located peripherally or subpleurally within both lower lobes. In most cases they are asymptomatic, but must be distinguished from lung cancer, particularly if any of the nodules demonstrate dyssynchronous growth.
- Diffuse alveolar-septal amyloidosis (systemic AL) occurs whenever amyloid is diffusely deposited within the interstitium and can vary in severity depending upon the degree to which gas exchange is affected. The burden of lung disease, however, tends to parallel cardiac involvement and as a result overall morbidity and mortality is typically governed more by cardiac than pulmonary disease.
- Hilar and mediastinal adenopathy (local and systemic AL) can occur with and without pulmonary involvement.
- Pleural effusions (systemic AL) usually result from parietal pleural involvement producing an exudative lymphocytic (and occasionally chylous) effusion. Transudative pleural effusions can also occur in association with cardiac disease and nephrotic syndrome.
- Other reported manifestations include:
  - Respiratory failure secondary to diaphragmatic involvement.
  - Haemoptysis, AV fistula formation and precapillary pulmonary hypertension as a result of pulmonary arteriolar involvement.

History

The diagnosis of amyloidosis will rarely be made at initial presentation. However, do consider the diagnosis in patients who present with:

- Upper airway obstructive symptoms.
- Haemoptysis.
- Incidental pulmonary nodules.
- Dyspnoea and parenchymal infiltrates.
- Respiratory symptoms in the presence of an underlying paraproteinaemia.

Examination

Patients may exhibit:

- Macroglossia (systemic AL).
- Inspiratory stridor (TBA).
- Fine inspiratory crepitations and hypoxia (diffuse alveolar septal amyloidosis).

Investigations

Initial investigations

- PFTs may demonstrate upper airways obstruction (i.e. low PEFR, abnormal flow volume loops) in TBA, or restrictive lung disease (i.e. reduced transfer factor and vital capacity) in diffuse alveolar septal disease.
- CXR may reveal pulmonary nodules, diffuse parenchymal infiltrates or pleural effusions.

Diagnostic investigations

- Biopsy material can be obtained as appropriate at:
  - laryngoscopy or bronchoscopy, although note that amyloid lesions can bleed readily;
  - thoracoscopy; and
  - thoracotomy.

- A biopsy demonstrating both congo red staining and green birefringence under polarised light confirms the diagnosis.
- Further histological analysis should be performed to identify the precursor protein subtype as distinguishing AA and ATTR from AL disease can alter subsequent management (Fig. 18.8.1).

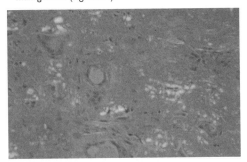

Fig. 18.8.1 Histological example demonstrating the presence of apple-green birefringence.

Staging investigations

- HRCT and/or MRI may demonstrate pulmonary nodules, honeycombing, heterogeneous ground glass opacification or generalised lymphadenopathy.
- Serum electrophoresis, urinary Bence Jones protein and bone marrow aspirate can identify an underlying paraproteinaemia in systemic AL.
- An elevated serum ALP and hepatomegaly on ultrasound suggest liver involvement.
- Echocardiography ±myocardial biopsy can identify restrictive and dilated cardiomyopathy.
- 24-hour urinary protein collection is required to exclude or confirm nephrotic syndrome.
- Radiolabelled SAP scanning can help quantify and monitor overall disease burden, although this test is not widely available.
- Beware FDG-PET which can give false-positive results in pulmonary nodular amyloidosis.

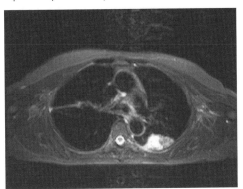

Fig. 18.8.2 MRI thorax demonstrating both TBA disease affecting the carina and nodular parenchymal disease involving the left lower lobe.

Management

- In many cases, particularly AA disease, ATTR disease and pulmonary nodular disease, pulmonary involvement is an incidental finding and needs no specific treatment.
- In localised laryngeal or proximal tracheobronchial amyloidosis repeated local interventions may be required for symptom control, including endoscopic resection, YAG laser therapy, stenting and tracheostomy. In more diffuse and/or severe disease, management takes on a more supportive role and includes prompt treatment of infections and emergency treatment of haemoptysis (e. g. with tranexamic acid and therapeutic bronchoscopy).
- In systemic AL disease chemotherapy can be given to target B cell clonal disease and thus limit the supply of precursor proteins. Both low dose melphalan and prednisolone and high dose melphalan with autologous stem cell rescue have been used in this role and should be considered when detectable levels of paraprotein are present.
- A centrally funded tertiary referral service for amyloidosis is currently provided in the UK by the National Amyloidosis Centre at the Royal Free Hospital, London.
- Patients and clinicians may obtain further information at www.ucl.ac.uk/medicine/amyloidosis/nac/index. html

Prognosis

Systemic AL disease has an unfavourable outcome with median survival estimated at just 13 months. Prognosis of local AL disease can vary, ranging from several months for those with diffuse TBA disease to unlimited for those with parenchymal nodular disease.

AUTHOR'S TIPS

- Amyloidosis is one of many conditions that can mimic lung cancer always aim to obtain a tissue diagnosis.
- Once amyloidosis is diagnosed it is essential that systemic AL be distinguished from local AL disease, given the change this can make to management.

Further reading

Aylwin AC, Gishen P, Copley SJ. Imaging appearance of thoracic amyloidosis. *J Thorac Imaging* 2005;**20**(1):41–46.

Berk JL, O'Regan A, Skinner M. Pulmonary and tracheobronchial amyloidosis. *Semin Respir Crit Care Med* 2002;**23**(2):155–515.

Cordier JF (2005). Pulmonary amyloidosis in hematological disorders. *Semin Respir Crit Care Med* 2005;**26**(5):502–513

Index
Index

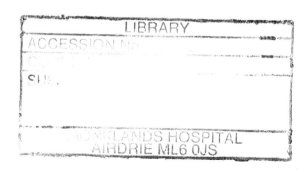